Essential
Clinica

Handbook

Seventh Edition

Editors:
Justin Hall
Katrina Piggott
Miliana Vojvodic
Kirill Zaslavsky

TMSP
TORONTO MEDICAL STUDENT PUBLICATIONS

Thieme

Toronto Medical Student Publications
Toronto, Ontario, Canada

Thieme
New York • Stuttgart

Editors:
Justin Hall
Katrina Piggott
Miliana Vojvodic
Kirill Zaslavsky

Cover Design: Nigel Tan, A Different Lens Photography (www.adifferentlensphotography.com)

Thieme Publishers (www.thieme.com) is the exclusive worldwide distributor of
Essentials of Clinical Examination Handbook, Seventh Edition.

In the Americas:
Thieme Publishers New York
333 Seventh Avenue
New York, NY 10001
United States of America
Email: customerservice@thieme.com
Tel: +1 800-782-3488 (Toll-free in US only)
Tel: +1-212-760-0888
Fax: +1-212-947-0108

In Europe, Asia, Africa, and Australia:
Thieme Publishers Stuttgart
P.O. Box 30 11 20
70469 Stuttgart, Germany
Email: customerservice@thieme.de
Tel: +49 711-8931-421
Fax: +49 711-8931-410

In India, Bangladesh, Pakistan, Nepal, Sri Lanka, and Bhutan:
Thieme Medical and Scientific Publishers Private Limited
A-12, Second Floor
Sector 2
NOIDA-201301
Uttar Pradesh, India
Email: customerservice@thieme.in
Tel: +91 120 427 4461 to 4464
Fax: +91 120 427 4465

Sixth Edition copyright © 2010 Editors: Matthew Lincoln, Christopher Tran, Gordon McSheffrey, Denise Wong
Fifth Edition copyright © 2005 Editors: Woganee Filate, Dawn Ng, Rico Leung, Mark Sinyor
Fourth Edition copyright © 2002 Editors: Sonial Butalia, Catherine Lam, Hin Hin Ko, Jensen Tan
Third Edition copyright © 2000 Editors: Tyler Rouse, Cory Torgerson, Gilbert Tang, Hariette Van Spall
Second Edition copyright © 1999 Editors: Ashis Chawla, Rizwan Somani
First Edition copyright © 1997 Editors: Shane Burch, Derek Plausinis

Library and Archives Canada Cataloguing in Publication Information is available from the publisher.

ISBN 978-1-60406-911-2
eISBN 978-1-60406-912-9

Printed in the United States
5 4 3 2 1

Table of Contents

Preface and Acknowledgements

First published in 1997, the *Essentials of Clinical Examination Handbook* was created by medical students to fill a need for a concise, portable, and affordable guide to clinical examinations. The *Handbook* is used as a study resource and reference by medical students and trainees of allied health programs around the world.

The *Handbook* emphasizes the knowledge that is most relevant to clinicians-in-training, and is designed to be a concise, on-the-job reference for history-taking and physical examinations. Our users describe it as their go-to resource on the wards for up-to-date, succinct, and easy-to-understand information.

The *Seventh Edition* of the *Essentials of Clinical Examination Handbook* has been revised to reflect new advances in clinical examination and to improve usability for students. The *Handbook* has a more rigorous and comprehensive focus on evidence-based medicine. It also includes citations to sources of information used in preparing the edition to allow for easy access for further study and an improved index for quick access to information on the wards. We have also worked diligently to describe the nuances of physical examination with greater clarity. This includes numerous high-quality charts, graphs, tables, algorithms, and illustrations of examination techniques and findings.

The new edition is entirely written, illustrated, and edited by over 90 students and 60 faculty members at the University of Toronto. The University of Toronto's Faculty of Medicine has a long tradition of excellence and innovation in research and medical education dating back to its founding as a medical school in 1843. Much of our success stems from our well-established affiliation with nine academic Toronto hospitals and their world-class clinicians and educators.

The *Essentials of Clinical Examination Handbook* is also proud to be a part of the strong tradition of enabling social welfare and community service by undergraduate medical students at the University of Toronto. All revenue supports student charities and community health initiatives in Toronto and Mississauga, Ontario, Canada.

We would like to express our utmost appreciation to all who made the publication of this edition a reality – the chapter editors, illustrators, photographer, layout editors, copy editors, and faculty advisors. Their dedication, passion, and hard work have been invaluable. We would also like to acknowledge members of the University of Toronto Medical Society, as well as the Fitzgerald Academy, for their help in the production of this text. We extend our gratitude to our predecessors, who have provided a strong foundation for the current edition. Finally, we thank our new international distributor, Thieme, for helping us bring the *Handbook* to a worldwide audience. We hope you enjoy using the *Handbook* as much as we enjoyed working on it.

Sincerely,

Essentials of Clinical Examination Handbook Editors In Chief
Justin Hall, Katrina Piggott, Miliana Vojvodic, and Kirill Zaslavsky

Contributors

Editors in Chief

Justin Hall
Katrina Piggott
Miliana Vojvodic
Kirill Zaslavsky

Chief Layout Editor

Jenny Hong

Art Directors

Amanda Hird
Olivia Yonsoo Shim

Chapter Editors

Sena Aflaki
Marko Balan
Harleen Bedi
Miranda Boggild
Michal Bohdanowicz
Kimberly Cai
William K. Chan
Justin Chow
Neil Dinesh Dattani
Joel Davies
Christopher Davis
Holly Delaney
Ayan K. Dey
Bailey Dyck
James England
Mostafa Fatehi
Lior Flor
Jonathan Fuller
Mary Ellen Gedye
Sharleen Gill
Anandita Gokhale
Cassandra Greenberg
Tara He
Thanh-Cat Ho
Mackenzie Howatt
Jane Hsieh
Yayi Huang
Maria Jogova
Eric Kaplovitch
Vahagn Karapetyan
Jieun Kim
Minji Kim
Aneta Krakowski
Anna Krylova
Esther Lau
Ashley Leckie
Jessica Leen
Evan Lilly
Ryan Lo
Tenneille T. Loo
Waed Mallah
Tom McLaughlin
Howard Meng
Kaspar Ng
Sabrina Nurmohamed
Ashna Patel
Sheron Perera
Khaled Ramadan
Bhupinder Sahota
Ashwin Sankar
Suparna Sharma
Theodore W. Small
Alia Sunderji
Chris Tang
Jennifer M. Tran
Emily Trenker
Shivangi Trivedi
Giorgia Tropini
David Tsui
Yuliya Velykoredko
Yao Wang
Brad Wiggers
Fanyu Yang
Alex Zhao

Faculty Editors

Anne Agur PhD, MSc, BSc(OT)
Nupura Bakshi MD, FRCS(C)
Meyer Balter MD, FRCP(C)
Marisa Battistella BSc Phm, Pharm D, ACPR
Alan Berger MD, FRCS(C)
Michael Bernstein MD, FRCP(C)
John Bohnen MD, FACS, FRCS(C)
Tina Borschel MD, MSc
Adrian Brown MD, FRCS(C)
Nadia Bugada MD, CCFP
David Chan MD, FRCP(C)
Chi-Ming Chow MD, CM, MSc, FACC, FASE, FRCP(C)
Jeremy Edwards MD, FRCP(C)
Kenneth Eng MD, FRCS(C)
Jaime Escallon MD, FACS, FRCS(C)
Scott Fung MD, FRCP(C)
Jeannette Goguen MD, FRCP(C)
Wayne L. Gold MD, FRCP(C)

Contributors

Faculty Editors (continued)

David Hall MD, FRCP(C)
Raed Hawa MD, MSc, DABSM, FRCP(C)
Ruth Heisey MD, CCFP, FCFP
Sender Herschorn BSc, MDCM, FRCS(C)
Kevin M. Higgins MD, FRCS(C)
Darryl Irwin MD, FRCP(C)
Sheila Jacobson MBBCh, FRCP(C)
Nasir Jaffer MD, FRCP(C)
Raymond Jang MD, FRCP(C)
Michael Jewett MD, FRCS(C)
David Juurlink BPhm, MD, PhD, FRCP(C)
Gabor Kandel MD, FRCP(C)
Yoo-Joung Ko MD, MSc, FRCP(C)
Paul Kuzyk MD, MASc, FRCS(C)
Prateek Lala MD, MSc
Liesly Lee MD, FRCP(C)
Nick Lo MD, FRCP(C)
Jodi Lofchy MD, FRCP(C)
Yvette Miller-Monthrope MD, FRCP(C)
Tony Moloney MD, MB, HDip, FRCS(C)
Andrew Morris MD, SM, FRCP(C)
George Oreopoulos MD, MSc, FRCS(C)
Daniel M. Panisko MD, MPH, FRCP(C)
Sev Perelman MD, MSc, CCFP(EM)
Richard Pittini MD, MEd, FACOG, FRCS(C)
Susan M. Poutanen MD, MPH, FRCP(C)
Atul Prabhu MD, FRCA
Mark J. Rapoport MD, FRCP(C)
James Shaw MD, FRCP(C)
Martin Schreiber MD, MEd, FRCS(C)
Shawna Silver MD, FAAP, PEng, FRCP(C)
Samir Sinha MD, DPhil, FRCP(C)
Donna Steele MD, MA, FRCS(C)
Khalid Syed MD, FRCS(C)
Lisa Thurgur MD, MSc, MCFP
Richard Tsang MD, FRCP(C)
Ross Upshur MD, MSc, FRCP(C)
Allan D. Vescan MD, FRCS(C)
Daniel Weisbrod MD, FRCS(C)
Rory Windrim MD, FRCS(C)
Camilla Wong MD, FRCP(C)
Cindy Woodland PhD
Jeff Zaltzman MD, FCFP(C)

Artists

Ahmed Aly
Zaria Chowdhury
Jan Cyril Fundano
Justin Hall
Caitlin Monney
Prerna Patel
Joy Qu
Miguel Luis Reyes
Olivia Yonsoo Shim
Bonnie Tang
Miliana Vojvodic
Minyan Wang
Anosha Zanjani

Layout Editors

Josephine Hai
Maggie Siu
William Tu

Copy Editors

Toni Burbidge
Pinky Gaidhu
Rubeeta Gill
Eric Grayson
Ritesh Gupta
Jordan Hutson
Alexander Leung
Hiten Naik
Azra Premji
Carl Shen
Erin Spicer
Ann Young
Monica Yu
Jeremy Zung

Technology Consultant

Matthew Turnock

Photographer

Nigel Tan
www.adifferentlensphotography.com

Common Abbreviations

ACE	Angiotensin converting enzyme
ACTH	Adrenocorticotropic hormone
ALP	Alkaline phosphatase
ALT	Alanine transaminase
AP	Anterior-Posterior
aPTT	Activated partial thromboplastin time
ASA	Acetylsalicylic acid
AST	Aspartate aminotransferase
β-hCG	β-human chorionic gonadotropin
BMI	Body mass index
BP	Blood pressure
BPM	Beats per minute
BUN	Blood urea nitrogen
C&S	Culture and sensitivity
CAD	Coronary artery disease
CBC	Complete blood count
CC	Chief complaint
CHF	Congestive heart failure
CN	Cranial nerve
CNS	Central nervous system
COPD	Chronic obstructive pulmonary disease
Cr	Creatinine
CRP	C-reactive protein
CSF	Cerebrospinal fluid
CT	Computerized tomography
CVS	Cardiovascular system
CXR	Chest X-ray
DDx	Differential diagnosis
DHEAS	Dehydroepiandrosterone
DIP	Distal interphalangeal
DM	Diabetes mellitus
DOB	Date of birth
DRE	Digital rectal exam
DVT	Deep vein thrombosis
ECG	Electrocardiogram
EEG	Electroencephalography
ESR	Erythrocyte sedimentation rate
FHx	Family history
FI	Functional inquiry
FNAB	Fine needle aspiration biopsy
FSH	Follicle-stimulating hormone
GCS	Glasgow coma scale
GERD	Gastroesophageal reflux disease
GI	Gastrointestinal
GU	Genitourinary
Hb	Hemoglobin
HIV	Human immunodeficiency virus
HPI	History of present illness
HPV	Human papilloma virus
HR	Heart rate
HSV	Herpes simplex virus
HTN	Hypertension
Hx	History

Common Abbreviations

IBD	Inflammatory bowel disease
ICU	Intensive care unit
ID	Identifying data
INR	International normalized ratio
IV	Intravenous
JVP	Jugular venous pressure
LFT	Liver function test
LOC	Level of consciousness
LR	Likelihood ratio
MAOI	Monoamine oxidase inhibitor
MI	Myocardial infarct
MMSE	Mini mental status exam
MRI	Magnetic resonance imaging
MS	Multiple sclerosis
MSK	Musculoskeletal
N/V	Nausea, vomiting
NSAID	Non-steroidal anti-inflammatory drug
OPQRST	Onset, palliating/provoking factors, quality, radiation, severity, temporal (progression)
OTC	Over-the-counter
PA	Posterior-Anterior
PE	Pulmonary embolism
PIP	Proximal interphalangeal
PMHx	Past medical history
PRN	*Pro Re Nata*, as needed
PSA	Prostate specific antigen
PT	Prothrombin time
PTH	Parathyroid hormone
PTT	Partial thromboplastin time
RBC	Red blood cells
ROM	Range of motion
ROS	Review of systems
RR	Respiratory rate
SHx	Social history
SLE	Systemic lupus erythematosus
SSRI	Selective serotonin reuptake inhibitors
STI	Sexually transmitted infections
TB	Tuberculosis
TCA	Tricyclic antidepressant
TIA	Transient ischemic attack
TSH	Thyroid stimulating hormone
U/S	Ultrasound
URTI	Upper respiratory tract infection
UTI	Urinary tract infection
WBC	White blood cells

The General History and Physical Exam

Editors:
Justin Chow
Tara He

Faculty Reviewers:
Nadia Bugada, MD, CCFP
Daniel M. Panisko, MD, MPH, FRCP(C)

TABLE OF CONTENTS

1. PREPARATION FOR THE INTERVIEW

- Introduce yourself and explain your role
- If a third party is present, explain his/her role in the interview (e.g. evaluator, tutor, colleague)
- Explain to the patient that the contents of the interview will be kept confidential. Recognize, however, that certain cases (e.g. child abuse, gunshot wounds, certain infectious diseases) may require mandatory reporting depending on government policies
- **Posture and Positioning:** sit at the same or at a lower level than the patient, in a position that permits but does not force eye contact. It is preferable to be on the patient's right side, at a comfortable distance that facilitates conversation but does not invade the patient's personal space
- Maintain eye contact and show interest
- Ask the patient how he/she would like to be addressed
- If the patient is accompanied by someone, suggest that he/she wait outside while you conduct the interview and physical exam

EBM: Perspective on Greetings in Medical Encounters

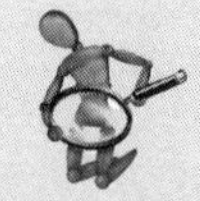

Physicians are encouraged to shake hands with patients but should remain sensitive to nonverbal cues that might indicate whether patients are open to this behavior or not. As a general rule for the initial interview, physicians should use both first and last names when introducing themselves and addressing patients.

Makoul G, Lick A, Green M. 2007. *Arch Intern Med* 167(11):1172-1176.

GENERAL H&P

2. GENERAL HISTORY

The general history is organized into the following sections:

- Identifying data (ID)
- Chief complaint (CC)
- History of the present illness (HPI)
- Past medical history (PMHx)
- Family history (FHx)
- Medications (MEDS) and Allergies (ALL)
- Social history (SHx)
- Review of systems or functional inquiry (ROS/FI)

Identifying Data

- Record date of interview
- Patient's name, age, gender, relationship status, dependents, occupation, ethnicity, and living status
- If applicable, document translators and family members present during the interview

Chief Complaint

- Brief statement of why the patient is seeking medical attention using the descriptors and words that the patient provides
- Include duration of symptoms

History of Present Illness

- A comprehensive and chronological account of the presenting chief complaint
- Symptom characterization:
  - **O** = Onset and duration
  - **P** = Provoking and alleviating factors
  - **Q** = Quality of pain (e.g. sharp, dull, throbbing)
  - **R** = Does the pain radiate?
  - **S** = Severity of pain ("on a scale from 1 to 10, 10 being the most severe")
  - **T** = Timing and progression ("Is the pain constant or intermittent? Worse in the morning or at nighttime?")
  - **U** = "How does it affect 'U' in your daily life?"
  - **V** = Déjà vu ("Has this happened before?")
  - **W** = "What do you think it is?"
- Explore relevant risk factors, relevant past medical and family history, and associated symptoms
- Include pertinent positive and negative symptoms in the HPI
- Explore the patient's thoughts/feelings of presenting problem

Past Medical History

- Inquire about childhood illnesses, past medical illnesses, injuries, operations, gynecological and obstetrical history for women, immunizations, and screening procedures (e.g. Pap smear, mammogram, colonoscopy)
- Record dates

Family History

- Inquire about all serious illnesses within immediate family (first-degree relatives); if relevant, include grandparents, aunts, and uncles
- Pay attention to illnesses/disorders that are familial or genetically transmitted
- Construct a genogram (also called a family tree or pedigree); record ages of family members, illnesses, and causes of death if applicable

- e.g. Mrs. Jill Hill, the consultant, and Mr. Jack Hill are consanguineous in that their mothers are sisters. They have a healthy son and a healthy daughter who is 16 weeks pregnant. Jack has a healthy older sister and an older brother who died of an autosomal recessive (AR) disease. Jill has a healthy younger brother. Jill's uncle (mother's youngest brother) had a son who passed away of the same AR disease and two other healthy boys (see **Figure 1**)

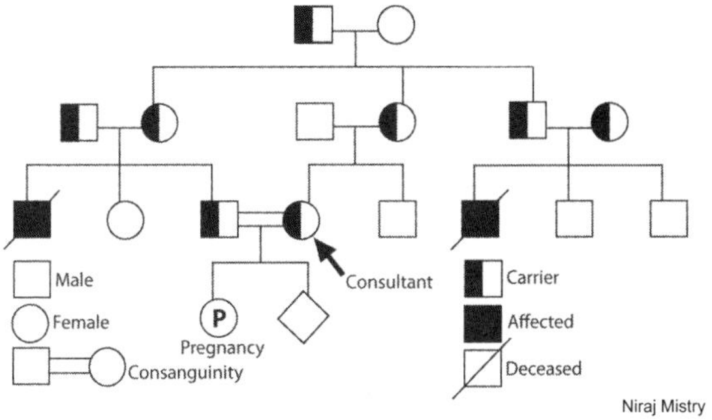

Figure 1. Family Tree

Medications

- Record prescription drugs (name, dosage, frequency, and route of administration), over-the-counter medications, all nutritional supplements and herbal remedies

Allergies

- Record all environmental, ingestible, and drug-related allergies
- Include the response (rash, anaphylaxis) and timing (immediate or delayed)

Social History

- Living arrangements
  - Type of home (e.g. apartment, basement, house), location, occupants, privacy
- Education (highest level obtained)
- Occupation (current and past)
  - **WHACS**[1]: **W**hat do you do? **H**ow do you do it? **A**re you concerned about any of your exposures or experiences? **C**oworkers or others exposed? **S**atisfied with your job?
- Hobbies and leisure activities (e.g. sports, reading, traveling)
- Marital/relationship status, social support, finances, and living conditions; primary caregiver if applicable
- Sexual history ("Do you have sex with men, women, or both?") (see **Review of Systems/Functional Inquiry** and **Difficult Interviews**)
- Spirituality ("Do you have any religious beliefs concerning your health or medical treatment?")
- Smoking ("Have you ever smoked?" to determine pack years)
  - 1 pack year = (1 pack or 20 cigarettes a day) x (1 year)
- Alcohol (type, how much, how often)
  - Use **CAGE**[2] to assess alcoholism: Have you ever felt the need to **C**ut down on your drinking? Have people **A**nnoyed you by criticizing your drinking? Have you ever felt bad or **G**uilty about your drinking? Have you ever had a drink first thing in the morning to steady your nerves or to get rid of a hangover – an **E**ye opener?
- Recreational drugs (type, how much, how often)
- Diet and stress

Review of Systems/Functional Inquiry

- A head-to-toe review of the patient's current state of health ("at this time is there anything new?" or "has anything changed recently?")
- Primarily yes/no questions; positive answers should be explored in greater detail and be moved to HPI/PMHx if appropriate
- **General:** weight gain/loss, loss of appetite, fever, chills, fatigue, night sweats
- **Dermatological (DERM):** rashes, lumps, sores, skin discoloration, pruritus, changes to nails or hair
- **Head:** headaches, dizziness, light-headedness
- **Eyes:** visual changes, visual field deficits, dry eyes, excessive tearing, red eyes, pain
- **Ears:** tinnitus, vertigo, hearing loss, earaches, discharges
- **Nose:** epistaxis, nasal stuffiness, sinus pain
- **Mouth and Throat:** dental disease, dry mouth, hoarseness, throat pain, difficulty swallowing
- **Neck:** swollen glands, lumps, goiter
- **Breasts:** lumps, pain, nipple discharge, skin changes
- **Respiratory (RESP):** cough, dyspnea, sputum (color, quantity), hemoptysis, wheezing, chest pain
- **Cardiovascular (CV):** chest pain, murmurs, dyspnea, orthopnea, paroxysmal nocturnal dyspnea, edema, palpitations, syncope, intermittent claudication, leg cramps, change in color of fingers and toes with cold exposure, varicose veins
- **Gastrointestinal (GI):** dysphagia, heartburn, abdominal pain, nausea, vomiting and/or hematemesis, diarrhea, constipation, hemorrhoids, food intolerance, hyperflatulence, changes in frequency of bowel movements or stool appearance (e.g. color, size, melena, hematochezia)
- **Urinary (GU):** dysuria, frequency, urgency, polyuria, nocturia, hematuria, and in males: hesitancy, dribbling or decrease in caliber of urinary stream
- **Sexual:** sexual orientation, interest and function, number of partners, birth control methods, history of sexually transmitted diseases
    - **Female:** age of menarche, regularity, frequency and duration of periods, amount of bleeding, bleeding between periods or after intercourse, last period, dysmenorrhea, age of menopause, vaginal discharge, sores or lesions, pregnancies (number, type of delivery, complications), abortions
    - **Male:** penile discharge, genital sores, testicular pain or masses
- **Endocrine:** polydipsia, polyuria, skin or hair changes, heat or cold intolerance, change in glove/shoe size
- **Musculoskeletal (MSK):** joint pain, swelling, redness, arthritis, myalgias, stiffness (note onset and timing)
- **Neuropsychiatric (PSYCH):** weakness, seizures, problems with gait, paresthesia, memory loss, depression
- **Hematologic:** anemia, easy bruising or bleeding, blood transfusions

EBM: Accuracy of the History and Physical Exam

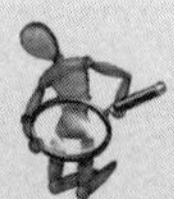

One study that surveyed hospitalists and senior residents found that in correctly diagnosed cases, history alone was identified as the most useful tool 20% of the time, whereas the physical examination alone was most useful less than 1% of the time. A combination of both history and physical examination was identified as most useful in 39% of correctly diagnosed cases. Together, these account for 60% of all correct diagnoses.

Paley L, et al. 2011. *Arch Intern Med* 171(15):1394-1396.

3. INTERVIEW SKILLS

- Progress from open-ended questions ("Can you describe the pain?") to directed questions ("Is the pain sharp, dull, or burning?", "Does the pain radiate to your left arm?")
- Encourage the patient to continue ("uh-huh", "yes") and do not interrupt the patient
- Redirect the patient when necessary ("it seems this is important to you and maybe we can discuss it further, but right now I would like to focus on…")
- Ask the patient to define vague terms (suddenly, a little, tired, dizzy, hurts, sick, weak)
- Summarize to refocus the interview or to transition into a new topic
- Ask one question at a time
- Avoid leading questions ("You don't smoke, right?")
- Avoid jargon

At the end of the interview, summarize and ask the patient if there is anything else they wish to add to ensure all has been covered

EBM: Verbal and Nonverbal Behaviors Associated with Positive Health Outcomes

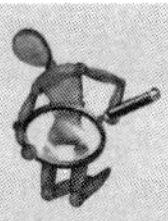

Verbal behaviors associated with positive health outcomes include empathy; support/encouragement for patient's questions; high proportion of objective statements in the concluding part of the visit; positive reinforcement; addressing problems of daily living, social relations, feelings and emotions; increased time on health education, sharing medical data with the patient; discussion of treatment effects; friendliness; courtesy; summarization, talking at the patient's level, and clarifying statements; humor; and increased encounter length.

Nonverbal behaviors associated with positive health outcome include forward leaning, head nodding, uncrossed arms and legs, arm symmetry, and less mutual eye contact.

Beck RS, Daughtridge R, Sloane PD. 2002. *JABFP* 15(1):25-38.

Emotion Handling Skills: NURSE[3]

- **N**: **N**ame the emotion
- **U**: Show **U**nderstanding
- **R**: Handle the issue with **R**espect
- **S**: Show **S**upport
- **E**: Ask the patient to **E**laborate on the emotion

Understanding the Patient's Perspective: FIFE[1]

- **F**: **F**eelings and **F**ears ("What concerns you the most?")
- **I**: **I**deas ("What do you think is going on?")
- **F**: **F**unction ("How has your illness affected you day-to-day?")
- **E**: **E**xpectations ("How do you expect this treatment to help?" "What do you think will happen with your illness?")

Breaking Bad News: SPIKES[4]

- **S**: **S**etting up the interview
  - Deliver the news while sitting
  - Ensure privacy
  - Involve significant others (if appropriate)
  - Inform the patient about time constraints or interruptions
- **P**: **P**erception of the patient
  - Use open-ended questions to assess the patient's understanding of his/her situation
- **I**: **I**nvitation to disclose information
  - Ask the patient what he/she would like to know

- **K**: **K**nowledge Giving
  - Warn the patient ("Unfortunately I have some bad news…")
  - Deliver information in small chunks using non-technical words
  - Avoid being too blunt; be careful and considerate in your choice of words and phrasing
- **E**: **E**mpathizing with the Patient's Emotions
  - Allow the patient to express his/her emotions, identify the reason behind his/her emotions, and validate his/her emotions
- **S**: **S**trategize and Summarize
  - Ask the patient to summarize his/her understanding of what was discussed
  - Elicit treatment goals and discuss suitable treatment plans

4. DIFFICULT INTERVIEWS

Sexual History

- It is especially important to take a sexual history if the patient presents with:
  - Urethral and/or vaginal discharge
  - Painful urination
  - Genital rash and/or ulcers
  - Abdominal pain
  - Pain during or after intercourse
  - Anorectal symptoms
  - Suspected sexually transmitted infection(s)
- Preface the interview by explaining why the sexual history is necessary, and ask the patient for permission
- Ask about the last date of intercourse, number of partners (in the last 6 months and lifetime partners), pregnancy risk, condom use, whether they have sex with men, women, or both, contact with sex workers, and sexual practices
- Sexual abuse history may be relevant

Cross-Cultural History Taking

- To improve communication it is important to be familiar with diverse cultures and beliefs
- Avoid using stereotypes
- If language is a barrier, use an interpreter who is not a relative of the patient
- Introduce the interpreter to the patient and ask the interpreter to translate in the patient's own words
- Maintain eye contact with and direct questions toward the patient
- Keep your sentences short and simple
- Ensure the patient's understanding of the content of the interview

Spousal/Partner Abuse

- Types of Abuse
  - Physical: pushing, choking
  - Sexual: forced sexual contact, pregnancy, abortion
  - Emotional: name-calling
  - Psychological: social isolation, controlling behavior
  - Financial control
- Common Signs of Spousal Abuse[5]
  - Unexplained traumatic injuries inconsistent with history taken
  - Head or neck injuries: facial lacerations, fractures, burns, perforated eardrums, fractured teeth, retinal detachment, orbital blow-out fracture, retinal hemorrhages, skull fractures, subdural and epidural hematomas, multiple bruises at different stages of healing

- o Chest, abdominal, pelvic or back pain
- o Multiple visits for nonspecific and often stress-related complaints
- o Headaches, insomnia, anxiety, depression
- o Suicidal ideation, suicide attempts
- o Chronic pain syndromes
- o Substance abuse
- o Eating disorders
- o Pregnancy complications (miscarriage, stillbirth, abruptio placentae, premature labor) or injuries during pregnancy
- o Recovery from illness/injury inappropriately delayed
- o Nonadherence with medications, treatment or follow-up appointments
- o Partner appears overly supportive
- o Cancelled appointments, especially if cancellation call was made by partner

- Approach to History and Physical Exam
  - o Interview the patient alone (document if this is impossible)
  - o Ensure confidentiality
  - o Ask direct and specific questions:
    - » "What happens when your partner loses his/her temper?"
    - » "Do you feel safe at home?"
    - » "Does your partner ever hit or abuse your children?" (inform the patient that suspected child abuse must be reported to Children's Aid Society)
  - o Remind the patient he/she is not to blame
  - o Assess his/her risk
    - » Has the severity/frequency of assaults increased?
    - » Have threats of homicide or suicide been made? Have these threats increased?
    - » Have threats to any children been made?
    - » Does your partner have access to a firearm?
    - » Do you know where to call for help in an emergency?
  - o If the patient is not in immediate risk, do not tell him/her what to do; help the patient explore each option and be supportive
  - o If the patient is in immediate risk, help him/her develop a safety plan that includes emergency numbers, key documents, a packed suitcase and money
    - » Encourage the patient to stay with family, friends or at a shelter
  - o Provide information on available community resources
  - o Document the patient's history, physical exam, and medical treatment in detail as well as your suspicions
  - o If patient consents, take measurements or photographs of physical injuries
  - o Arrange to follow-up
  - o Do not be frustrated if abuse is denied or help is declined; remain empathic and nonjudgmental

EBM: Prevalence of Intimate Partner Violence

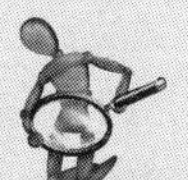

A group family practice clinic in inner city Toronto surveyed their female patients and found the overall prevalence of intimate partner violence in current or recent relationships to be 14.6%. Emotional abuse was reported by 10.4%, threat of violence by 8.3%, and physical or sexual violence by 7.6% of respondents.

Ahmad F, et al. 2007. *Can Fam Physician* 53(3):460-468.

5. PREPARATION FOR THE PHYSICAL EXAM

- Prepare the patient by explaining what you are about to do before proceeding
- Ensure patient comfort, and proper draping, positioning and lighting
- By convention, examine patients from the right side
- Avoid showing extreme reactions during the examination

Principles of Infection Control

- Hand Hygiene
  - If hands are not heavily soiled, use alcohol-based hand cleanser before and after seeing each patient; if hands are soiled (i.e. with dirt, blood, etc.) use soap and warm water for 15 s
- Barriers
  - Body substances include blood, oral secretions, sputum, emesis, urine, feces, wound drainage, and any additional moist body substances (excluding tears or sweat)
  - Assume that all patients are potentially infected with pathogens and all body substances are potential sources of transmission
  - Use barriers (gloves, gown, mask, eyewear) when appropriate (e.g. gloves when in contact with any bodily substances, masks when dealing with respiratory infections)
- Minimize Needlestick Injury
  - Never recap needles; immediately dispose of any sharps in designated containers

Note: additional precautions may apply when working with specific airborne pathogens and antibiotic-resistant organisms

6. GENERAL INSPECTION

General Appearance

- Apparent state of health: any signs of distress (cardiac, respiratory, pain, anxiety, depression)? Any lines or tubes present (e.g. Foley catheter, IV line)? Quickly scan the room (e.g. bedside items, number of pillows for orthopnea, etc.)
- Physical appearance: dress, grooming, personal hygiene, level of consciousness, skin (color and obvious lesions), diagnostic facies, appears stated age (see **Table 1** and **Table 2**)
- Body structure: height, habitus, sexual development, fat distribution, symmetry, body posture and position, bony abnormalities (see **Figure 2**)
- Mobility: gait (normally, shoulder-width base, with smooth, even strides), range of motion, involuntary movements (see **Geriatric Exam** and **Neurological Exam**, p.69 and 171 respectively)
- Behavior: facial expression, mood, affect, speech (articulation, fluency, hoarseness)
- Any odors of the breath or body

Head

- Look for diagnostic facies, color abnormalities, swelling, scalp lesions, and abnormal hair distribution (alopecia, hirsutism)

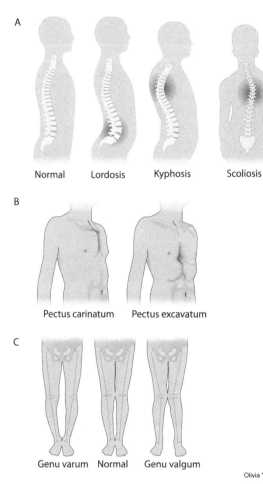

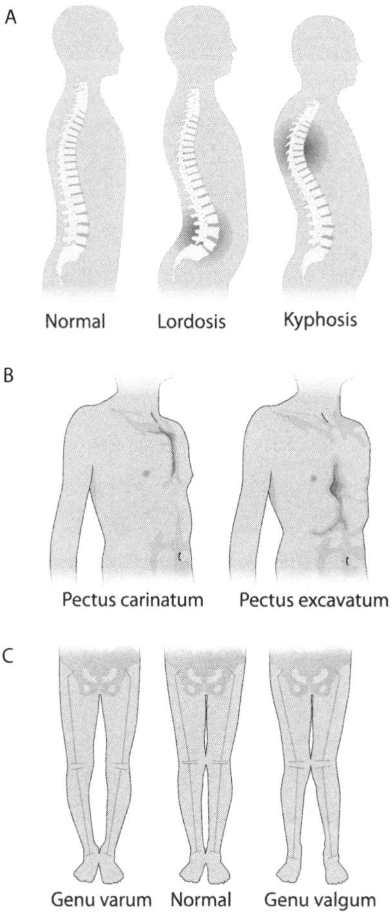

Olivia Yonsoo Shim

Figure 2. Common Bony Abnormalities

Table 1. Color Abnormalities and Possible Causes

Color Abnormality	Where to Look	Possible Causes
Blue	Tongue and mouth	Central cyanosis (pulmonary and/or cardiac disease)
	Lips, hands, and feet	Peripheral cyanosis
Blue-gray	General appearance	Hemochromatosis
Pale	Conjunctiva and oral mucosa	Anemia
Red	Can be generalized to whole body or localized to a specific part	Polycythemia, infections or drug reactions
Yellow	Sclera (jaundice)	Cholestasis, hepatic failure, hemolysis

Table 2. Common Diagnostic Facies and Possible Causes

Signs and Symptoms	Possible Causes
Thick dry skin, loss of hair on head and lateral eyebrows	Hypothyroidism
Lid retraction, exophthalmos, sweating	Hyperthyroidism
Moon facies, acne, hirsutism, thinning of skin, and erythema	Cushing's syndrome
Large protruding jaw, wide spacing of teeth, protruding tongue, thick skin, prominent supraorbital ridges	Acromegaly
Periorbital edema (puffy eyes)	Nephrotic syndrome or thyroid disorder
Sunken eyes, temporal wasting	Malignancy, AIDS, advanced peritonitis
Dry sunken eyes, dry mucous membranes, reduced skin turgor	Dehydration
Malar flush with facial telangiectasias	Alcoholism
Expressionless face, depressed affect, infrequent blinking	Parkinson's disease
Flat occiput and forehead, down-slanting palpebral fissures, low nasal bridge, large tongue	Down syndrome

Hands and Nails

- Inspect the hand for abnormal color or morphology (see **Table 3**)
- Inspect shape, size, color, and consistency of nails
- See **Essentials of Dermatology**, **Table 3**, p.397

Table 3. Hand Abnormalities and Possible Causes

Signs and Symptoms	Possible Causes
Enlarged	Acromegaly
Bouchard's (PIP) and Heberden's (DIP) nodes	Arthritis
Tremor or Muscle Wasting	Neurological disease
Asterixis (Flapping Tremor)	Metabolic encephalopathy
Blue	Peripheral cyanosis
Pigmented	Jaundice
Pallor of Palmar Creases	Anemia

7. VITAL SIGNS

Temperature

- Body temperature is influenced by age, the diurnal cycle, the menstrual cycle, and exercise (see **Table 4**)

Table 4. Normal Body Temperatures for Adult Men and Women

Location	Mean Temperature (°C)	Temperature Range (°C)
Oral	36.4	33.2-38.2
Rectal	36.9	34.4-37.8
Tympanic	36.5	35.4-37.8
Axillary	36.3	35.5-37.0

Sund-Levander M, Forsberg C, Wahren LK. 2002. *Scand J Caring Sci* 16(2):122-128.

Pulse Measurement

- Use the radial or carotid artery to determine:
  - Rhythm: regular, regularly irregular, irregularly irregular
  - Rate:
    - Regular rhythm: count for 30 s
    - Regularly irregular: count for 1 min
    - Irregularly irregular: count for 1 min using apex beat
  - Magnitude: normal, diminished, or increased
  - Symmetry: left vs. right
- Before palpating the carotid artery, auscultate for carotid bruits
- Never palpate both carotid arteries at the same time
- Normal adult pulse rate is 50-100 bpm[6]
  - **Bradycardia:** an abnormally slow heart rate (<60 bpm)
  - **Tachycardia:** an abnormally fast heart rate (>100 bpm)

Respiratory Assessment

- Look for signs of respiratory distress (the use of accessory muscles, intercostal indrawing, pursed lip breathing, tripod positioning, heaving or audible wheezing)
- RR most reliably measured when patient is distracted from his/her own conscious breathing (e.g. pretending to take their pulse)
- Count for 30 s if breathing is normal and for 1 min if you suspect abnormality
- Normal adult RR is 16-25 breaths/min[7]
  - **Bradypnea:** an abnormal decrease in RR (<16 breaths/min)
  - **Tachypnea:** an abnormal increase in RR (>25 breaths/min)
  - **Apnea:** absence of breathing, either periodic or sustained (i.e. cardiac arrest, CNS lesion)

Blood Pressure Measurement

- Terminology
  - Systolic blood pressure (SBP): maximum arterial pressure during left ventricular contraction (see **Table 5**)
  - Diastolic blood pressure (DBP): resting arterial pressure between ventricular contractions (see **Table 5**)
  - Pulse pressure = SBP – DBP
  - Korotkoff sounds: arterial sounds heard during blood pressure measurement by auscultation
  - Auscultatory gap: transient loss of Korotkoff sounds during measurement of SBP

- Preparation (see **Figure 3**)
  - Patient should be relaxed, sitting with his/her back supported and feet flat on the floor
  - Wrap cuff around upper arm, 2-3 cm above antecubital fossa, with brachial marker over brachial artery
  - Ask the following questions:
    - "In the last 30 min, have you smoked, had caffeine, or exercised?"
    - "Is there any reason that you should not have your blood pressure taken on either of your arms?"

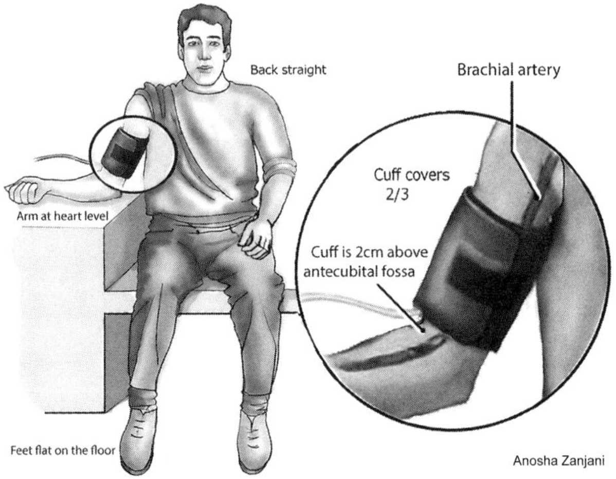

Figure 3. Blood Pressure Measurement Setup

- Systolic Pressure by Palpation
  - Usually performed to avoid missing the auscultatory gap which could result in underestimating SBP
  - Palpate radial artery on arm
  - Inflate blood pressure cuff until radial pulse disappears
  - Slowly deflate approximately 2 mmHg/s
  - SBP is estimated when radial pulse can be felt again
- Systolic and Diastolic Pressure by Auscultation (see **Figure 4**)
  - Note in which arm BP is being measured
  - Support upper arm at heart level
  - Place stethoscope over brachial artery
  - Inflate cuff to 20-30 mmHg above estimated SBP
  - Slowly deflate approximately 2 mmHg/s
  - SBP is read at the first Korotkoff sound
  - DBP is read when the Korotkoff sounds disappear
  - Repeat using other arm to assess symmetry
- Orthostatic Hypotension Measurement
  - Measure BP with the patient supine, then standing
  - Positive test: ≥20 mmHg fall in SBP or ≥10 mmHg fall in DBP upon standing[8]
  - Patients may also experience symptoms of cerebral hypoperfusion upon standing: dizziness, weakness, lightheadedness, visual blurring, darkening of visual fields, syncope (due to abrupt peripheral vasodilation without compensatory increase in cardiac output)

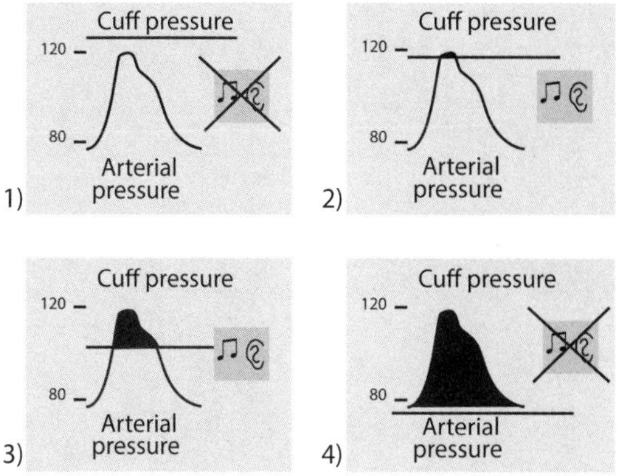

Prerna Patel

Figure 4. Korotkoff Sounds During BP Measurement

1. When cuff pressure is above SBP, blood flow is stopped; no Korotkoff sounds are heard.
2. When cuff pressure falls below SBP, turbulent blood flow causes Korotkoff sounds; a clear tapping sound is initially heard. This marks the SBP.
3. As cuff pressure continues to fall, the quality of the Korotkoff sounds changes.
4. When cuff pressure falls below DBP, laminar blood flow is restored and Korotkoff sounds disappear. This marks the DBP.

Table 5. Blood Pressure Levels for Adults

Classification*	Systolic Pressure (mmHg)	Diastolic Pressure (mmHg)
Normal	<120	<80
Prehypertension	120-139	80-89
Stage 1 Hypertension	140-159	90-99
Stage 2 Hypertension	>160	>100

*If the patient's SBP and DBP categories are not the same, classify them according to the more severe category

Chobanian AV, et al. 2003. *JAMA* 289(19):2560-2572.

Factors Influencing Blood Pressure

- Age (gradually rises throughout childhood until adulthood)
- Sex (generally lower in females until menopause, after which point females have higher blood pressure)
- Diurnal rhythm (lower in morning and higher in afternoon)
- Weight (higher in obese individuals)
- Exercise (lower in physically active individuals)
- Stress
- Ethnicity

EBM: Benefits of Home Blood Pressure Monitoring

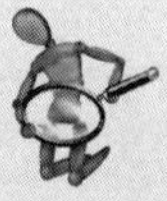

Blood pressure measurements taken at home have stronger associations with cardiovascular prognosis than readings taken at a medical center. Home measurements are also associated with positive outcomes such as improving blood pressure control and medication adherence, and may help identify white coat or masked hypertension.

Canadian Hypertension Education Program. 2008. *Can J Cardio* 24(6):447-452.

Body Mass Index (BMI)

- BMI is an internationally designated measure of nutritional status used in adults and is based on height and weight (see **Table 6**)
  - Disadvantage: does not account for differences in body composition (%fat/muscle/fluid)
- BMI = weight (kg)/height^2 (m^2) = weight (lbs)/height^2 (inches^2) x 703

Table 6. BMI Classifications for Adults (Male and Female)

Classification	Body Mass Index (kg/m^2)
Underweight	<18.5
Healthy Weight	18.5-24.9
Overweight	25.0-29.9
Obese (Class I)	30.0-34.9
Obese (Class II)	35.0-39.9
Obese (Class III)	≥40.0

Katzmarzyk PT, Mason C. 2006. *CMAJ* 172(2):156-157.

Waist Circumference (WC) Measurement

- Measure WC when the patient is standing, with abdominal muscles relaxed at the end of normal expiration (see **Table 7**)
- Position the measuring tape in a horizontal plane, level with the top of the iliac crest
- The circumference should be measured to the nearest 0.5 cm

Table 7. Ethnic-Specific Values for Waist Circumference

Ethnicity/Country	Waist Circumference (as a measure of central obesity), cm	
	Male	Female
European*	≤94	≤80
Asian (East Asian, Chinese, South Asian)†	≤85	≤80
African American, Hispanic or Middle Eastern†	Use European-based cutoffs	
Aboriginal, African, Pacific Islanders, or South American†	Unable to recommend	

*Lau DC, et al. 2007. *CMAJ* 176(8):S1-13.
†Lear SA, et al. 2010. *European Journal of Clinical Nutrition* 64(1):42-61.

EBM: Identifying Cardiovascular Risk

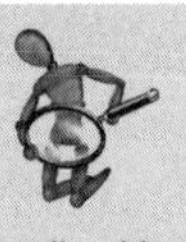

Although the predictive value of BMI vs. WC is hotly debated in the literature, both are useful clinical tools in identifying cardiovascular risk. One study found that WC was an independent predictor of CVD incidence in overweight females (BMI 25-30), but did not substantially add to prediction of risk over BMI in men (regardless of BMI category), or women in other BMI categories.

Freiberg MS, et al. 2008. *Obesity* 16(2):463-469.

8. OVERVIEW OF THE PHYSICAL EXAM

Four Principles of the Physical Exam for Each Body System

- **I**nspection
- **P**alpation
- **P**ercussion
- **A**uscultation

The following is a guideline for a general screening exam:

- **General Appearance:** note patient's apparent state of health, any tubes or IV lines present?
- **Vitals:** temperature, pulse, respiration, blood pressure
- **Skin, Hair, Nails:**
  - Skin: color, integrity, texture, temperature, hydration, excessive perspiration, unusual odors, presence of lesions
  - Hair: texture, distribution
  - Nail: morphology, texture, color, condition
- **Lymph Nodes:** occipital, posterior and preauricular, tonsillar, submandibular, submental, cervical (superficial, deep, posterior), supra- and infra-clavicular, epitrochlear, axillary, inguinal nodes; note size, shape, mobility, tenderness (see **Head and Neck Exam** and **Lymphatic System and Lymph Node Exam**, p.114 and p.125)
- **Head:** bruising, masses; check fontanelles in infants/young children
- **Eyes:** pupils (equal, round, pupillary light and accommodation reflexes), extraocular movements, visual fields and acuity, ptosis, fundoscopy (red reflex, optic disc, retinal vessels), scleral icterus (see **Ophthalmological Exam**, p.235)
- **Ears:** external ear, otoscopic findings in canals (cerumen, discharge, foreign body) and tympanic membranes (integrity, color, landmarks, and mobility), tenderness. Hearing: Weber and Rinne tests (see **Head and Neck Exam**, p.101)
- **Nose, Mouth and Throat:** nasal discharge, sense of smell, mucous membrane color and moisture, oral lesions, dentition, pharynx, tonsils, tongue, palate, uvula (see **Head and Neck Exam**, p.106, 108)
- **Neck:** tracheal position, thyroid enlargement/nodules, lymphadenopathy, masses, carotid or thyroid bruits (see **Head and Neck Exam**, p.114)
- **Respiratory:** inspection, palpation, percussion, and auscultation (IPPA) – chest configuration, clubbing, central and peripheral cyanosis, chest expansion, tactile fremitus, percussion, diaphragmatic excursion, auscultation for adventitious sounds, egophony, whispered pectoriloquy (see **Respiratory Exam**, p.351)
- **Heart:** JVP at 30° incline, hepatojugular reflux; regular rate and rhythm (RRR), apex beat, first and second heart sounds (S1, S2), gallops (S3, S4), murmurs (graded 1-6) and thrills, pulses (graded 0-4), (see **Cardiovascular Exam**, p.52)
- **Peripheral Vascular:** Carotid, temporal, renal, femoral, abdominal aortic bruits; temperature, capillary refill, edema, pulses, pallor on elevation and rubor on dependency (see **Peripheral Vascular Exam**, p.297)
- **Breast:** dimpling, tenderness, lumps, nipple discharge, axillary masses (see **Breast Exam**, p.39)
- **Abdomen:** IAPP – contour (e.g. flat, obese, distended), scars, dilated veins, visible peristalsis, ascites, ecchymoses, bowel sounds, bruits, tenderness, guarding, masses, liver and spleen size, costovertebral angle tenderness (see **Abdominal Exam**, p.20)

GENERAL H&P

- **Urological:** inguinal masses or hernias, scrotal swelling, anal sphincter tone, rectal masses, prostate gland (nodules, tenderness, size), discharge, lesions, varicoceles (see **Urological Exam**, p.366)
- **Gynecological:** external genitalia, vaginal mucosa, cervical discharge and color, ovaries, uterine size and shape, masses (including adnexal), lesions (see **Gynecological Exam**, p.82)
- **MSK:** inspection, palpation, ROM, tenderness, heat, erythema, crepitus, edema, muscle atrophy, deformities, symmetry, joint swelling, joint stability (see **Musculoskeletal Exam**, p.134)
- **Neuropsychiatric:** LOC, cranial nerves, mental status, speech, mood and affect
  - Sensory: 1° sensory modalities (pain, temperature, fine touch, vibration, proprioception), 2° sensory modalities (stereognosis, graphesthesia, 2-pt discrimination)
  - Motor: tone, power (0-5), reflexes (0-4+), gait and coordination tests (see **Neurological Exam** and **Psychiatric Exam**, p.174 and p.322)

REFERENCES

1. Schuman SH, Simpson WM. 1999. WHACS your patients. *J Occup Environ Med* 41(10):829.
2. Paley L, Zornitzki T, Cohen J, Friedman J, Kozak N, Schattner A. 2011. Utility of clinical examination in the diagnosis of emergency department patients admitted to the department of medicine of an academic hospital. *Arch Intern Med* 171(15):1394-1396.
3. Pollak KI, Arnold RM, Jeffreys AS, Alexander SC, Olsen MK, Abernethy AP, et al. 2007. Oncologist communication about emotion during visits with patients with advanced cancer. *J Clin Oncol* 25(36):5748-5752.
4. Baile WF, Buckman R, Lenzi R, Glober G, Beale EA, Kudelka AP. 2000. SPIKES-A six-step protocol for delivering bad news: Application to the patient with cancer. *Oncologist* 5(4):302-311.
5. Statistics Canada. *Family Violence in Canada: A Statistical Profile 2004.* Ottawa: Canadian Centre for Justice Statistics; 2004.
6. McGee S. *Evidence-based Physical Diagnosis: Expert Consult.* Philadelphia: Elsevier Saunders; 2012.
7. Hooker EA, O'Brien DJ, Danzl DF, Barefoot JA, Brown JE. 1989. Respiratory rates in emergency department patients. *J Emerg Med* 7(2):129-132.
8. Lanier JB, Mote MB, Clay EC. 2011. Evaluation and management of orthostatic hypotension. *Am Fam Physician* 84(5):527-536.
9. Bickley LS. *Bates' Pocket Guide to Physical Examination and History Taking.* Philadelphia: Lippincott Williams & Wilkins; 2009.
10. Bickley LS, Szilagyi PG, Bates B. *Bates' Guide to Physical Examination and History Taking,* 10th ed. Philadelphia: Lippincott Williams & Wilkins; 2009.
11. Seidel HM, Ball JW, Dains JE, Flynn JA, Solomon BS, Stewart RW. *Mosby's Guide to Physical Examination.* Missouri: Mosby, Inc; 2010.

The Abdominal Exam

Editors:
Christopher Davis
Jessica Leen

Faculty Reviewers:
Michael Bernstein, MD, FRCP(C)
Scott Fung, MD, FRCP(C)
Gabor Kandel, MD, FRCP(C)

TABLE OF CONTENTS

1. ESSENTIAL ANATOMY

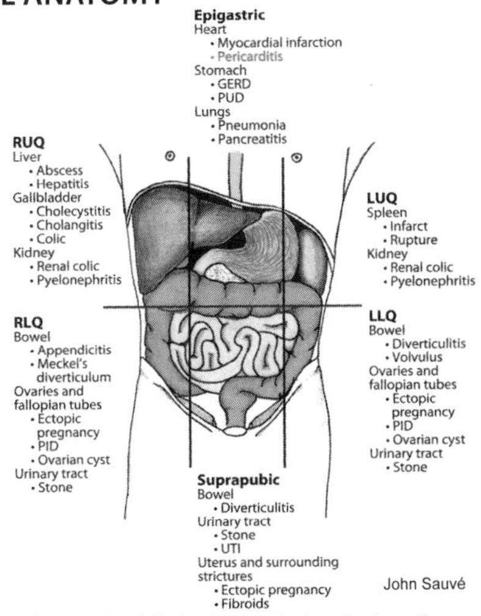

Figure 1. Differential Diagnosis of Abdominal Pathology by Location

2. COMMON CHIEF COMPLAINTS

- Abdominal pain
- Fever
- Jaundice (yellowing skin)
- Dysphagia (difficulty swallowing)
- Odynophagia (painful swallowing)
- Vomiting
- Hematemesis (vomiting blood)
- Nausea
- Gas/bloating
- Abdominal distension
- Reflux (heartburn)
- Mass
- Diarrhea
- Constipation
- Irregular bowel habits (alternating constipation and diarrhea)
- Melena or hematochezia (blood in stool)
- Weight loss
- Hepatic encephalopathy (confusion/poor sleep)

3. FOCUSED HISTORY

Pain

- **OPQRSTUVW** (see **General History and Physical Exam**, p.2)
- Location and aggravating/alleviating factors are especially important

> **Clinical Pearl: Abnormal Etiology of Abdominal Pain**
> Diseases of the heart and lungs, such as coronary artery disease and pneumonia, can present with upper abdominal pain, especially in pediatric and geriatric populations.

Table 1. Area of Pain May Suggest Its Cause

Location of Pain	Possible Pathology
RUQ	Cholecystitis, hepatitis, pancreatitis, hepatic abscess, choledocolithiasis, cholangitis, tumor (e.g. colon, kidney, liver)
Epigastric	PUD (complicated or perforated), pancreatitis, thoracic causes (pericarditis, aortic aneurysm, MI), gallstones
LUQ	Splenic infarct, ruptured spleen, pancreatitis, abscess, gastric ulcer, gastric cancer
Flank	Pyelonephritis, nephrolithiasis, retrocecal appendicitis, retroperitoneal bleeding, sarcoma, abscess
Lower Abdomen	Aortic aneurysm, appendicitis, diverticulitis, colorectal cancer, PID, bowel perforation, sigmoid volvulus
Variably Located	Gastroenteritis, GI obstruction, IBD, mesenteric colitis, visceral angina
Diffuse, Steady or Sharp	Peritonitis

IBD = inflammatory bowel disease, MI = myocardial infarction, PID = pelvic inflammatory disease, PUD = peptic ulcer disease, R/LUQ = right/left upper quadrant

Table 2. Character of Pain Suggests Its Cause

Character	Possible Pathology
Abrupt, Excruciating	MI, perforated ulcer, ruptured aneurysm, renal colic, biliary colic
Rapid Onset, Steady and Severe	Acute pancreatitis, strangulated bowel, ectopic pregnancy, mesenteric ischemia (may present with pain disproportionate to signs)
Gradual, Steady	Acute cholecystitis, acute cholangitis, acute hepatitis, appendicitis
Colicky	Small bowel obstruction, IBD

IBD = inflammatory bowel disease, MI = myocardial infarction

Bowel Habits

- Chronic or acute change in bowel patterns: establish baseline bowel habits
- Change in number of stools per day
- Constipation, diarrhea, tenesmus (straining, passing little or no feces, sense that all stool has not been passed)
- Character of stools: solid/loose, floating, malodorous, presence of blood (mixed with stool/on the surface/separate), mucus (true mucus in irritable bowel syndrome vs pus in inflammatory bowel disease), color (red, black, or pale; other colors have no diagnostic significance)
- If bowel obstruction suspected: absence of flatus suggests obstruction is complete
- Association with:
  - Weight loss
  - Other constitutional symptoms
  - Pain (aggravating or alleviating)
  - Meals
  - Risk factors for food poisoning
  - Travel history

Gastrointestinal Bleeding

- Hematemesis: vomiting blood from gut (bright red or "coffee-grounds")
- Melena: black, tarry, malodorous stools

> **Clinical Pearl: Melena vs. Hematochezia**
> Color of stool in GI bleeding depends on (1) location of bleeding (higher in the GI tract, more likely melena rather than hematochezia); (2) rate of bleeding (slower, more likely melena rather than hematochezia); (3) transit time (slower, more likely melena rather than hematochezia).

- Hematochezia: blood in stools (bright red/maroon)

Jaundice and Scleral Icterus

- Best seen in full spectrum natural light (artificial lighting may impair detection of cyanosis, pallor, and jaundice)
- Pale stools and dark urine point toward hepatobiliary disease, away from hemolysis, and can be an indicator of hepatobiliary disease before jaundice develops
- Inquire about associated symptoms, duration, fever, medications, herbals, alcohol, and industrial chemical exposure
- Pruritus (indicates the cholestasis is chronic)

Medications

- If epigastric pain, ask about NSAIDs, steroids, ulcer medications (antacids, proton pump inhibitor (PPI), H2-receptor antagonists), laxatives, herbal products, OTCs, etc.
- If altered bowel habits, ask about narcotics as well as pro-motility agents

Family History

- Colorectal cancer or colonic polyps (especially if diagnosed <50 yr)
- Ovarian/endometrial cancer
- Gallstones
- IBD: ulcerative colitis (UC) or Crohn's disease (CD)
- Celiac disease or other autoimmune diseases
- Functional bowel disease
- Diverticulosis
- Family history of similar symptoms
- Genetic conditions (including hereditary nonpolyposis colorectal cancer [HNPCC], familial adenomatous polyposis [FAP])
- Liver disease including hepatitis B and hepatocellular carcinoma

Past Medical History

- Past abdominal/GI/GU pathology
- Past abdominal/GI/GU surgery

Social History

- Sexual practices (e.g. anal intercourse)
- Dietary history including triggers
- Menstrual patterns as a clue to onset of a chronic disease
- Alcohol intake: CAGE questionnaire* (see **Psychiatric Exam**, p.320)
  *to be used for screening only and not for diagnosis
- Smoking history

> **Clinical Pearl: Jaundice**
> In a patient with jaundice, long-standing history of decreased libido and abnormal menstruation suggests chronic liver disease or cirrhosis.

4. FOCUSED PHYSICAL EXAM

Prepare the Patient

- Adequate lighting, warm room, comfortable environment
- Adjust bed to flat position
- Patient lying supine, arms at his/her side
- Appropriate draping
- Stand on the patient's right side
- If abdominal wall is tense, it can be relaxed by maximally flexing knees (heels close to buttocks), by placing a pillow under patient's head and/or knees or by placing the patient's hand onto your palpating hand (this may also help with "ticklish" patients, and children)

Vital Signs

- BP, HR, RR, and temperature

Inspection

- Most commonly missed: nail and skin changes, subtle lower limb edema, elevated neck veins, stigmata of liver disease

- State of the patient
  - Completely still: suggests peritonitis
  - Writhing: suggests colic
  - Curled up in fetal position: suggests visceral pain
  - One hip flexed: suggests splinting
  - Sitting up and leaning forward: suggests retroperitoneal irritation
- **Skin**
  - Skin color
    - Jaundice, pallor, cyanosis, erythema
    - Ecchymoses of the abdomen and flanks (Grey-Turner's sign, Cullen's sign, see **Table 3**)
  - Skin abnormalities
  - Striae (recent = pink, blue; purple = Cushing's; silver = old, obese, postpartum)
  - Scars (surgical and hypertrophic/keloid)
  - Spider angiomas
  - Gynecomastia in men
- **Hands and Nails**
  - Thenar wasting
  - Palmar erythema
  - Dupuytren's contracture
  - Clubbing
  - Leukonychia (white spots, streaks on nails)
- **Abdomen:** look at the abdomen from the foot of the bed
  - Contour
    - Normal: note symmetry
    - Scaphoid: normal, malnourished
    - Protuberant: **6 F**'s (Fat, Fluid, Feces, Flatus, Fetus, Fetal growth)
    - Distended lower half: suggests pregnancy, leiomyoma (fibroid), ovarian tumor
    - Distended upper half: suggests gastric dilatation, enlarged lobe of liver
    - Bulging flanks: suggests ascites but need to differentiate from obesity
  - Umbilicus
    - Everted: increased abdominal pressure: suggests fluid, mass
    - Umbilical hernia
    - Bluish (Cullen's sign, see **Table 3**)
    - Nodular: suggests metastatic cancer
  - Hernias (see **Urological Exam**, p.373)
  - Superficial veins
    - Visible in thin patients and in vena cava obstruction
    - Caput medusae (surrounding umbilicus)
    - Cephalad drainage pattern in IVC obstruction, caudad drainage in SVC obstruction, normal flow pattern (cephalad above umbilicus and caudad below umbilicus) in portal hypertension without caval obstruction
- **JVP** (see **Cardiovascular Exam**, p.52)

> **Clinical Pearl: Liver Disease and JVP**
> In ascites, elevated JVP may be the only clinical clue to a cardiac cause of liver disease (tricuspid insufficiency, pericarditis), whereas in other causes of cirrhosis, JVP is low. Also be alert to a pulsatile liver.

- **Stigmata of Chronic Liver Disease** (due to hyperestrogenism)
  - Spider angioma
  - Gynecomastia
  - Testicular atrophy
  - Frontal balding

ABDOMINAL

Auscultation

- Bowel sounds (least useful portion of the physical exam)
- Listening to one quadrant is sufficient
- Listen for 2 min before concluding absent
- Vascular bruits
  - Aortic (midline)
  - Renal arteries (above umbilicus off midline)
  - Bifurcation of the common iliac arteries (below umbilicus off midline)
- Liver
  - Bruit: suggests hepatocellular carcinoma, alcoholic hepatitis
  - Venous hum: suggests portal hypertension
- Other
  - If vomiting, assess for succussion splash: gently shake patient from side-to-side while auscultating in the epigastrium for the "whoosh" noise indicating gastric outlet obstruction

Percussion

- Percuss all 4 quadrants (usually tympanic; note any dullness)

Liver

- Lower border: start below umbilicus (tympanic) and percuss upward in right mid-clavicular line (MCL) or mid-sternal line (MSL) until liver dullness
- Upper border: start from lung resonance in MCL or MSL and percuss downward to liver dullness
- Measure the span
  - Normal: M: 8-12 cm, F: 6-10cm MCL
  - Falsely increased span (lung dullness, e.g. right pleural effusion)
  - Falsely decreased span (gas in the right upper quadrant, e.g. gas in the colon)

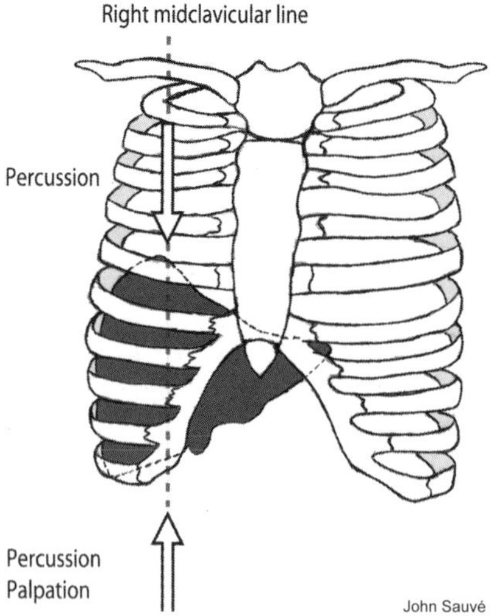

Figure 2. Liver Percussion and Palpation

Spleen

- **Traube's Space**
  - Have the patient lie supine and breathe normally
  - Percuss in the area bounded by the sixth rib superiorly, left anterior axillary line laterally, and the left costal margin inferiorly (Traube's space)
  - Normal or small spleen sounds resonant or tympanic
  - Enlarged spleen sounds dull[1]
- **Castell's Sign**
  - Have the patient lie supine and breathe in and out deeply in a continuous manner
  - While patient is breathing continuously, percuss the lowest intercostal space in the left anterior axillary line
  - Have the patient take a full inspiration, percuss in the same area and compare the percussion notes
  - Normal or small spleen sounds tympanic on inspiration
  - Enlarged spleen sounds dull on inspiration[2]

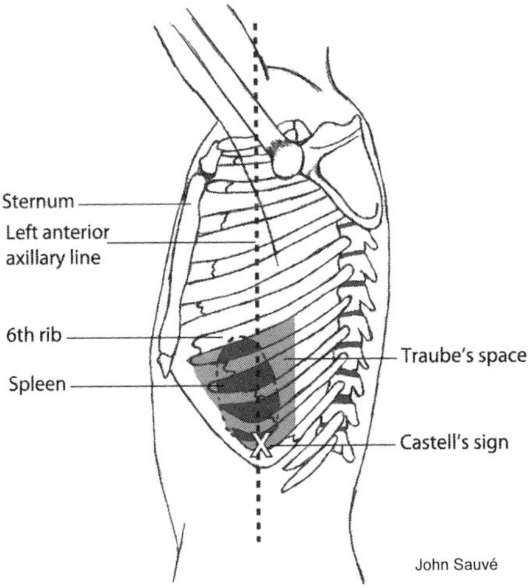

Figure 3. Spleen Percussion

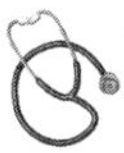

Clinical Pearl: Percussing the Spleen Postprandially
Since food in the stomach causes dullness in the left upper quadrant, interpret dullness cautiously if patient has eaten within the past four hours.

EBM: Splenomegaly

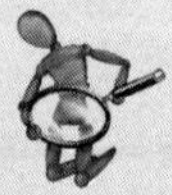

Percussion is more sensitive but less specific than palpation as a diagnostic test for splenomegaly. Percussion (Castell's sign) should therefore be done first, followed by palpation. If both percussion and palpation are positive, the diagnosis of splenomegaly can be ruled in, provided there is a pretest probability of at least 10%.

Grover SA, Barkun AN, Sackett DL. 1993. *JAMA* 270(18):2218-2221.

Ascites

- **Shifting Dullness**
  - Determine the border of tympany and dullness by percussion in supine position, beginning at the umbilicus and moving laterally (mark this spot with a pen). Repeat percussion in the same direction with the patient rolled to that same side
  - In the presence of ascites, the tympany-dullness margin will move 'upward' (toward the umbilicus) as the ascitic fluid pools in the dependent side of the peritoneal cavity
  - In the absence of ascites, the margin does not move
- **Fluid Wave**
  - Ask the patient to place the ulnar side of his/her hand in the midline of the abdomen (this prevents a false positive due to the patient's fat and flatus)
  - Tap on lateral side of abdomen and assess the transmission of a wave to contralateral side using the other hand – if the fluid thrill can be palpated by this hand, the abdominal distension is likely due to ascites
    - ***Note:*** the tap must be below the level of tympany

Palpation

- Warm hands
- Ask the patient to locate the area of maximum tenderness; examine this area last

Light Palpation

- Detects abdominal tenderness, areas of muscle spasm/rigidity
  - Lightly palpate entire abdomen using palmar surface of either hand
  - Lift hand entirely from the skin when moving from area to area
  - In the case of a ticklish patient try placing the patient's hand on top of your hand while palpating
  - If areas of tenderness are identified, further palpation can be used to delineate the area
- If hernia suspected, examine inguinal hernial rings and male genitalia
- Palpate costovertebral angle tenderness:
  - Place one hand flat on the costovertebral angle to assess for tenderness
  - If pain not elicited, attempt fist palpation (using the ulnar surface of your open hand, strike the costovertebral angle and assess for pain)
  - For assessment of retroperitoneal abscess, retrocecal appendicitis, and pyelonephritis
- Elicit cough tenderness (examine this last)
  - Coughing often elicits localized pain in an inflamed area
- Shake tenderness: shake the bed
  - Sudden movements can be used to elicit peritoneal signs

Deep Palpation

- Detects presence of masses, inflamed gallbladder, appendiceal abscess, etc.
- Using both hands, rest one hand on the abdomen and apply gentle but steady pressure with the other over top
- Ask patient to breathe through his/her mouth

> **Clinical Pearl: The Equivocal Patient**
> To differentiate between involuntary or malingering pain try to distract patient by pretending to auscultate by pushing in the stethoscope.
> ***Note:*** Do not do this routinely, only when pain is questionable!

Palpation of Liver, Spleen, and Kidney

- Determines presence of organ enlargement and/or tenderness
- Ask patient to breathe deeply through his/her mouth
- Palpate during inspiration; move hand during expiration
- Palpate for the liver beginning along the MCL at the right lower quadrant (RLQ) moving superiorly
- Palpate for the spleen beginning at the RLQ moving toward left upper quadrant (LUQ)
- May feel the liver or spleen edges touch the fingertips

Palpation of Liver Edge

- **Method 1**
  - Place the right hand on the abdomen with fingertips positioned superiorly parallel to the rectus abdominus muscle and push inwards and upward toward patient's head during each inspiration until the liver edge is felt
  - The hand inches forward/upward during expiration
  - To check for tenderness, the examiner's left hand is placed on the liver while the ulnar side of the right fist strikes the left hand
- **Method 2** (useful method if a patient is obese)
  - Stand near the head of the patient with examiner facing patient's feet
  - Place both hands below the right costal margin to "hook" over the liver edge
  - The examiner pushes inward and toward the patient's head during inspiration
- When describing your examination of the liver, always include:
  - Length of liver below costal margin
  - Total liver span
  - Texture of liver edge (i.e. smooth or nodular)
  - Consistency of liver edge (i.e. firm or soft)
  - Tenderness of liver edge
  - Presence of bruits
- ***Note:*** the edge of an enlarged liver may be missed by starting palpation too high on the abdomen

EBM: Hepatomegaly

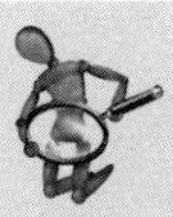

Combined results of 3 studies:

Palpability	Hepatomegaly		LR	95%CI
	Yes	No		
Yes	231	301	LR+ 2.5	2.2-2.8
No	112	818	LR- 0.45	0.38-0.52

A palpable liver is not necessarily enlarged, but increases the likelihood of hepatomegaly. A nonpalpable liver edge does not rule out hepatomegaly, but reduces its likelihood.

Naylor CD. 1994. *JAMA* 271(23):1859-1865.

Palpation of Spleen

- Stand on the right side of the supine patient
- Place left hand behind the patient's left rib cage and right hand in the right lower quadrant (area of the appendix) angled toward the left anterior axillary line
- Use the right hand to push inwards and upwards toward patient's head during each inspiration
- Incrementally move the right hand diagonally upward to the left costal margin palpating for the spleen

- When the right hand reaches the left costal margin, gently dig deep under the left costal margin while the patient inspires deeply, searching for an enlarged spleen (i.e. palpate for the tip of the spleen coming forward against fingertips)

Palpation of Kidney

- The kidney is not usually palpable in an adult except in polycystic kidney disease
- Stand on the patient's right side
- Palpate deeply with the right hand below the right costal margin
- Left hand is placed on the patient's back between the right costal margin and the right iliac crest and is used to lift upward
- For the left kidney, stand on the left side of the patient and repeat the maneuvers switching hands
- To check for tenderness, ask patient to sit up; strike the two costovertebral angles with the ulnar side of your fist (lightly)
  - Proceed in a downward vertical direction

Table 3. Specific Signs and Their Possible Interpretation

Sign/Special Test	Description	Possible Pathology
Rovsing's Sign	RLQ pain on LLQ palpation	Appendicitis
McBurney's Sign	Tenderness at McBurney's point (1/3 along line extending from the ASIS to the umbilicus)	Appendicitis
Rebound Tenderness	Pain on quick withdrawal of palpation Check for peritonitis before assessing rebound tenderness by asking patient to cough or by lightly jarring the bed; if this reproduces the abdominal pain, there is no need to maximize the pain by demonstrating rebound tenderness	Peritonitis
Murphy's Sign	Arrest of deep inspiration on RUQ palpation (hand contact with gallbladder elicits pain)	Cholecystitis
Courvoisier's Sign	Painless, palpable distended gallbladder	Pancreatic cancer
Cullen's Sign	Blue discoloration of periumbilical area caused by retroperitoneal hemorrhage tracking around to anterior abdominal wall	Acute hemorrhagic pancreatitis Ectopic pregnancy
Grey-Turner's Sign	Blue discoloration of the flank area caused by retroperitoneal hemorrhage	Acute hemorrhagic pancreatitis Ruptured abdominal aortic aneurysm Strangulated bowel
Kehr's Sign	Severe left shoulder pain exacerbated by elevating foot of bed (referred pain; diaphragmatic involvement)	Splenic rupture

Table 3. Specific Signs and Their Possible Interpretation (continued)

Sign/Special Test	Description	Possible Pathology
Psoas Test	Pain on flexion of the hip against resistance	Appendicitis Other causes of inflammation in region of psoas muscle (e.g. retroperitoneal abscess)
Obturator Test	Pain when thigh is flexed to a right angle (with the hip and knee at 90º), gently rotate the hip, first internally then externally	Pelvic appendicitis diverticulitis PID Other causes of inflammation in region of obturator internus muscle
Positive Carnett's Sign	Abdominal pain/tenderness exacerbated when patient lifts feet above the bed without bending knees	Source of pain is abdominal wall (strain/sprain/abdominal wall hernia) because stretching of abdominal wall worsens any lesion within wall (positive Carnett's sign)
Negative Carnett's Sign	Abdominal pain/tenderness alleviated when patient lifts feet above the bed without bending knees	Source of pain is inside abdominal cavity because stabilizing abdominal wall protects the organs within the abdominal cavity (negative Carnett's sign)

ASIS = anterior superior iliac spine, PID = pelvic inflammatory disease, R/LLQ = right/left lower quadrant, RUQ = right upper quadrant

EBM: Appendicitis

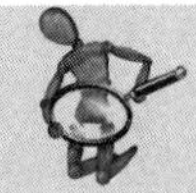

Sign	Sensitivity (%)	Specificity (%)	LR+
RLQ Pain	81	53	8.0
Rigidity	27	83	3.76
Pain Migration	64	82	3.18
Psoas Sign	16	95	2.38

Wagner JM, et al. 1996. *JAMA* 276(19):1589-1594.

Clinical Pearl: The Epigastrium
The most common cause of an epigastric mass is an enlarged liver.

Abdominal Aortic Aneurysm

- See **Peripheral Vascular Exam**, p.307

Digital Rectal Exam

- Male (see **Urological Exam,** p.368)
- Female (see **Gynecological Exam,** p.85)

5. COMMON INVESTIGATIONS

Table 4. Common GI Investigations

Test	Description	Indication for Test
Stool C&S and/or Microscopy	Detection of microbes in stool	To rule out infection (ask specifically for *Clostridium difficile* toxin assay if patient has been on antibiotics or recent hospitalization)
FOBT	Detects small volumes of blood in the stool	Colon cancer screening
Colonoscopy*	Provides best direct view of colon mucosa and opportunities for biopsy	Used to rule out or establish diagnosis of multiple mucosal conditions (e.g. colorectal cancer, IBD)
CT Colonography	CT examination of colon after introduction of air into anorectum	To detect diverticula, fistulae, look for extrinsic compression of the colon If colonic mucosal visualization is indicated but colonoscopy too risky or contraindicated
MRCP	MRI evaluation of the bile duct, gallbladder, and pancreatic duct	To diagnose biliary obstruction as a cause of jaundice or elevated liver enzymes
ERCP*	Endoscopic procedure to examine the common bile duct and pancreatic duct	Suspect bile duct obstruction requiring intervention such as sphincterotomy, stent, biopsy
Upper Endoscopy (OGD)	Provides a direct view of the esophagus, stomach, and duodenum	Look for esophageal varices, esophagitis, peptic ulcer, small bowel biopsy to rule out intestinal disease, such as celiac disease, etc.
Schilling Test*	Measurement of urinary radioactive labeled vitamin B12 following oral ingestion	Evaluate vitamin B12 absorption to test for pernicious anemia, ileal disease, bacterial small bowel overgrowth, pancreatic insufficiency
C-14 Urea Breath Test C-13 Non-Radioactive	Detection of the enzyme urease, produced by *Helicobacter pylori*. If gastric urease present, then orally administered C-14 urea will be hydrolyzed into ammonia and $^{14}CO_2$. The $^{14}CO_2$ can be detected in the expired breath. Analogous test possible with non-radioactive $^{13}CO_2$, but is more expensive	*Helicobacter pylori* infection of stomach

*Gold standard in indicated pathology
FOBT = fecal occult blood test, ERCP = endoscopic retrograde cholangiopancreatography, MRCP = magnetic resonance cholangiopancreatography, OGD = oesophago-gastro-duodenoscopy

6. COMMON DISORDERS

Disorders marked with (✓) are discussed in **Common Clinical Scenarios**

✓ Alcoholic liver disease
✓ Appendicitis
✓ Celiac disease
✓ Cirrhosis: including complications (ascites, encephalopathy, variceal bleeding, spontaneous bacterial peritonitis, liver cancer)
✓ Colorectal cancer
✓ Diarrhea
✓ Gallstones
✓ GI bleeding
✓ Pancreatitis
✓ Inflammatory bowel disease
✓ Irritable bowel syndrome
✓ Peptic ulcer disease

- Diverticulitis
- Hemochromatosis
- Hepatitis: alcoholic, viral, drug-related/toxic
- Non-alcoholic fatty liver disease (NAFLD)
- GERD
- Other GI malignancies (esophageal cancer, gastric carcinoma, pancreatic cancer, and hepatocellular carcinoma)
- Vascular disease of the bowel

7. COMMON CLINICAL SCENARIOS

7.1 Acute Diarrhea

History

- Associated signs and symptoms include vomiting, fever, arthritis, skin rash, anorexia, and weight loss
- Onset (abrupt onset suggests infection) and duration (longer duration suggests initial phase of a chronic illness)
- Urgency to defecate suggests rectal involvement
- Frequency of movements (Does it wake you at night?) indicates severity of diarrhea and rectal involvement
- Quantity of each bowel movement:
  - The small bowel tends to be the source if the bowel movements are large and relatively infrequent
  - The colorectum is more likely the source of disease if the feces are small in volume, passed frequently, and are mixed with blood, mucus or pus
- Quality:
  - Bloody (bright red) suggests large bowel problem, black suggests upper GI problem, watery suggests small bowel problem; mucus, foul smelling, floating in toilet, difficult to flush all suggest steatorrhea
- Abdominal pain: cramping before defecation has no diagnostic significance but abdominal pain between movements suggests involvement of bowel serosa

Risk Factors

- Antibiotic history (*Clostridium difficile*)
- Food history, especially potential for undercooked poultry or eggs (*Campylobacter*, *Salmonella*), beef products (*E. coli* O157:H7), seafood (*Vibrio parahaemolyticus*, cholera, viral agents), food poisoning due to *S. aureus* or *Clostridium perfringens*, fresh fruits such as raspberries (*Cyclospora*)
- Contact with infected person (all bacterial and viral agents), exposure to healthcare, chronic care, child care facilities

- Travel history/camping/well water
- Immunosuppression
- Laxative use
- Anal intercourse
- Malignancy

ABDOMINAL

Physical Exam

- Assessment of intravascular volume by BP/HR with postural changes, JVP evaluation, capillary refill, skin turgor (not useful in adults)
- Hydration status is essential especially in infants, children, and the elderly, all of whom can potentially die from diarrhea by dehydration
- Is patient in distress? (toxic?)
- GI: peritonitis (guarding), masses, tenderness, sigmoidoscopy or proctoscopy with appropriate swabs and cultures if rectal urgency not yet diagnosed and/or question of anorectal problems associated with anal intercourse
- MSK: myalgias and arthritis

7.2 Acute Pancreatitis

- Upper abdominal pain, usually with fever, vomiting
- Characterized by elevated serum lipase or amylase, often with increase in liver enzymes/serum glucose, dilated loop of bowel may be visualized radiologically
- First step: rule out syndromes other than pancreatitis, such as bowel perforation, infarction, obstruction, since pancreatitis itself not amenable to specific therapy
- This may require CT scan if diagnosis unclear
- Ultrasound allows to look for gallstones and/or dilated bile ducts suggesting obstructing stone as a cause of the pancreatitis. May require endoscopic retrograde cholangiopancreatography (ERCP) if gallstone pancreatitis suspected
- Delayed CT with contrast (at 72 h) rules out complications and determines severity by estimating proportion of necrosis of pancreatic gland (inflamed gland does not take up the contrast)

7.3 Alcoholic Liver Disease

- **Spectrum:** alcoholic fatty liver, alcoholic hepatitis, and cirrhosis
- **Fatty Liver:** characteristically asymptomatic, but hepatomegaly may be present
- **Alcoholic Hepatitis:** variable symptoms and signs but characteristically presents as dull RUQ discomfort, N/V, anorexia, jaundice, fever, elevated enzymes, etc.
- **Cirrhosis:** end-stage of chronic liver disease
- Signs and symptoms (by etiology)
    - Hyperestrogenism: hair distribution (frontal balding), gynecomastia, spider nevi, altered pectoral alopecia, palmar erythema, and testicular atrophy
    - Portal hypertension (increasing congestion on various organs): splenomegaly (sometimes with petechiae secondary to splenomegaly-associated thrombocytopenia), encephalopathy, ankle edema, esophageal variceal bleeding, caput medusae, hemorrhoids, and ascites
    - Liver failure (i.e. decreased nitrogenous ammonia/toxin removal, decreased albumin production, decreased bilirubin metabolism, decreased clotting factor production) leading to encephalopathy, edema, jaundice, GI bleeding, respectively
    - Systemic/nonspecific: anorexia, clubbing, fatigue, and fever

7.4. Appendicitis

- Fever, typically low grade, unless there is a perforation
- Worsening of symptoms is the most reliable feature
- Typical presentation includes vague, dull, constant periumbilical pain initially which gradually localizes to McBurney's point
- Positive Rovsing's sign
- May also have a positive psoas sign or a positive obturator sign (depending on location of appendix)
- Peritonitis if there is a perforation
- U/S and CT scan considered to have high positive and negative predictive values

ABDOMINAL

7.5 Celiac Disease

- Most common presentation is mimicker of irritable bowel syndrome
- Anemia and osteopenia are key presentations[3]
- Tissue transglutaminase (tTG) antibodies have high sensitivity, low specificity
- Prevalence varies according to geographic location (more prevalent in Europe and North America with a caucasian predilection)
- IgA levels must be checked to exclude a false negative tTG related to selective IgA deficiency; 1-2% of people with celiac disease have selective IgA deficiency
- Small bowel biopsy required to confirm diagnosis

7.6 Cirrhosis and its Complications

Ascites

- Suspect free fluid in the peritoneal cavity when there has been an increase in abdominal girth
- Causes can be grouped as hepatic and non-hepatic
  - o Hepatic causes (portal hypertension):
    - » Cirrhosis (most common)
  - o Non-hepatic causes:
    - » Fluid retention due to CHF
    - » Cancer: second most common cause of ascites after portal hypertension
    - » Constrictive pericarditis, tricuspid regurgitation
    - » Infection: TB, fungus
    - » Nephrotic syndrome
- Ascites can be detected clinically by:
  - o Detection of shifting dullness on abdominal percussion (most reliable physical exam maneuver)
  - o Elicitation of a fluid wave (with larger collections of fluid)
  - o Examination for bulging or fullness of the flanks
  - o Abdominal U/S (not CT) (gold standard; recommended in all cases but especially for detection of smaller fluid volumes)

Encephalopathy

- Increased amount of toxins (particularly ammonia) in blood due to shunting of portal blood into systemic circulation
- Four stages:
  1. Reversal of sleep rhythm (earliest sign)
  2. Asterixis, lethargy ± disorientation
  3. Stupor (rousable only by pain), hyperreflexic
  4. Coma
- Can be precipitated by an increase in nitrogen load, medications, electrolyte disturbance, infection, constipation, narcotics, sedatives or a worsening of hepatic function (any change in steady state)

EBM: Ascites

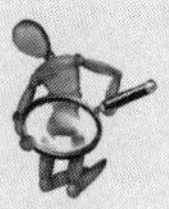

		Sens (%)	Spec (%)	LR+	LR-
History	↑ abdominal girth	87	77	4.16	
	Hepatitis	27	92		
	Ankle swelling	93	66		
Physical Exam	Bulging flanks	81	59	2.0	0.3
	Flank dullness	84	59	2.0	0.3
	Shifting dullness	77	72	2.7	0.3
	Fluid wave	62	90	6.0	0.4

- Useful in ruling out ascites:
  - o History negative for ankle swelling and negative for increased abdominal girth
  - o Physical exam negative for bulging flanks, flank dullness, or shifting dullness
- Useful for ruling in ascites:
  - o Presence of a fluid wave, shifting dullness, or peripheral edema

Williams Jr. JW, Simel DL. 1992. *JAMA* 267(19):2645-2648.

Variceal Bleeding

- Due to portal hypertension; often fatal complication of cirrhosis
- Often worsened by hypocoagulability (as all clotting factors except for VIII are exclusively made in the liver) and thrombocytopenia (see **Gastrointestinal Bleeding**, p.33)

Spontaneous Bacterial Peritonitis

- Consider in a patient with increasing abdominal discomfort and ascites, and worsening liver or renal function even if afebrile, WBC normal
- Any unexplained change in clinical status in a patient with ascites should raise suspicion for spontaneous bacterial peritonitis (SBP)
- Diagnosis made by diagnostic paracentesis (look for neutrophil count >250 x 10^6/L in ascitic fluid)

Note: Liver transplantation is only definitive therapy for end-stage liver disease. Appropriate transplant candidates should be referred for assessment at signs of early decompensation since wait times are long and mortality rates for advanced disease with late features are high.

7.7 Colorectal Cancer

- Primarily a disease of middle aged, older adults: 99% >40 yr and 85% >60 yr[4]
- Primary symptoms
  - o Rectal bleeding persistently without anal symptoms
  - o Change in bowel habit persistently over six wk: most commonly increased frequency and/or looser stools
  - o Abdominal pain characteristically with weight loss
- Secondary effects
  - o Iron deficiency anemia
  - o Intestinal obstruction
  - o Clinical examination may show an abdominal mass or rectal mass
- In work-up, use colonoscopy or CT colonography

7.8 Gallstones

- Ultrasound best test to visualize gallstones
- Gallstones are often an incidental finding on an ultrasound done to investigate non-biliary symptoms, such as dyspepsia
- Can cause: biliary colic, cholecystitis, cholangitis, pancreatitis, gallstone ileus – but do not cause dyspepsia
- Biliary colic: a "set piece": pain starts suddenly, most often late afternoon/evening, RUQ or epigastrium, radiates to back, associated with vomiting, lasts ~3-6 h
- If unsure whether gallstones seen on ultrasound are the cause of the pain, perform hepatobiliary iminodiacetic acid (HIDA) scan: presence of nucleotide in gallbladder on this scan indicates that the cystic duct is patent, virtually ruling out biliary colic/cholecystitis
- Cholecystitis: upper abdominal pain, usually but not always associated with vomiting and fever, liver enzymes only slightly elevated, ultrasound shows stones in the gallbladder and also a thickened gallbladder wall, fluid around gallbladder
- Cholangitis: fever, RUQ pain, jaundice (Charcot's triad); Raynaud's pentad (Charcot's triad + hypotension and confusion) requires urgent ERCP and sphincterotomy

EBM: Acute Cholecystitis

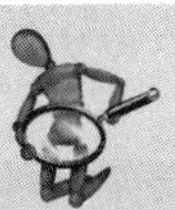

History: RUQ pain, N/V, anorexia, fever
Physical Exam: Murphy's sign, RUQ mass, guarding, rigidity, rebound tenderness

	Sens (%)	Spec (%)	LR+	LR-
Murphy's Sign	65	87	2.8	0.5
RUQ Tenderness	77	54	1.6	0.4

Trowbridge RL, Rutkowski NK, Shojania KG. 2003. *JAMA* 289(1):80-86.

7.9 Gastrointestinal Bleeding

- 3 factors that determine stool color: bleed location, bleed rate, stool/blood transit time
- In an upper GI bleed, the presentation can be a clue to the severity of the bleeding: hematochezia indicates fastest bleeding, melena the slowest bleeding; hence, upper GI source can cause hematochezia if bleeding massive and transit time rapid
- Resuscitation: ABCs, two large bore (16-18g) IV inserted into antecubital fossae; run IV fluids wide open as appropriate
- Octreotide infusion: if suspicious for variceal bleed
- Proton pump inhibitor infusion for active upper GI bleed
- Urgent gastroscopy for significant upper GI bleed
- If lower GI bleed: consider sigmoidoscopy without preparation to rule out mucosal disease/anal source. However, colonoscopy without preparing the colon by lavage is likely to reveal nothing but blood, hence colonic lavage before colonoscopy
- If lower GI bleed does not stop spontaneously, consider angiography

7.10 Inflammatory Bowel Disease (IBD)

- Chronic, relapsing inflammatory disorders of unknown etiology
- Rectal exam and colonoscopy are indicated
- Stool culture and microscopy required to rule out enteric infection
- Divided into two primary diseases (Crohn's and ulcerative colitis)

ABDOMINAL

- **Crohn's (Granulomatous) Disease**
  - Affects any portion of GI tract, but most often in small intestine and colon
- **Ulcerative (Non-Granulomatous) Colitis**
  - Limited to colon (mucosal inflammation)
  - Rectum always involved and disease progresses proximally
  - Symptoms: bloody diarrhea, lower abdominal cramps, urgency
  - Signs: anemia, low serum albumin, negative stool cultures

7.11 Irritable Bowel Syndrome (IBS)

- 15% of U.S. adults report symptoms that are consistent with IBS[5]
  - 3:1 female to male (in countries such as India the ratio is reversed)
- Rome III Criteria[5-7]
  - Recurrent abdominal pain or discomfort for at least 3 d/mo in last 3 mo (not necessarily consecutive) with two or more of the following:
    - Improvement with defecation
    - Onset associated with a change of frequency of stool
    - Onset associated with a change in appearance of stool
- Diagnosis
  - After complete history and physical exam, the following tests should be ordered: CBC, electrolytes, creatinine, BUN, liver function, thyrotropin, albumin, C-reactive protein, transglutaminase serology with protein electrophoresis, stool microscopy, and culture (if diarrhea)
  - Consider endoscopy if worrisome symptoms or blood work abnormal; ESR is of limited use

7.12 Peptic Ulcer Disease (PUD)

- Burning, epigastric pain
- Onset: 1-3 h after meal
- 1/3 of patients awakened at night by pain
- Pain relieved by food or antacid
- Intermittent and may return in several mo
- May present with complications: bleeding, perforation
- *H. pylori* and ASA/NSAID use are the major risk factors
- Cannot distinguish by history from functional dyspepsia[8]

7.13 Primary Biliary Cirrhosis

- Predominantly middle-aged women (mean age at diagnosis 51 yr). Up to 10% are male and 10% are <35 yr. Males and females follow similar clinical course, characterized by elevated serum alkaline phosphatase, positive antimitochondrial antibody[9]
  - Transmural inflammation
  - Symptoms: fever, malaise, abdominal pain, diarrhea, vomiting
  - Signs: fever/temperature increase, weight loss, nutritional problems, anemia, lower-right abdominal mass and/or tenderness, extraintestinal manifestations (eye, mucosal, MSK, hepatobiliary, skin)

Table 7. Symptoms and Frequency of Occurrence in Primary Biliary Cirrhosis

Symptom	Frequency of Occurrence
Pruritus (severe itching)	47%; usually first symptom
Nonspecific Symptoms: fatigue, right upper quadrant pain and dyspepsia	22%
Typical Late Features (though may appear earlier): jaundice, GI bleeding or ascites	19%

ABDOMINAL

REFERENCES

1. Grover SA, Barkun AN, Sackett DL. 1993. The rational clinical examination. Does this patient have splenomegaly? *JAMA* 270(18):2218-2221.
2. Castell DO, Frank BB. 1977. Abdominal exam: Role of percussion and auscultation. *Postgrad Med* 62(6):131-134.
3. Feighery C. 1999. Fortnightly review: Coeliac disease. *BMJ* 319(7204):236-239.
4. Hobbs FD. 2000. ABC of colorectal cancer: The role of primary care. *BMJ* 321(7268):1068-1070.
5. Horwitz BJ, Fisher RS. 2001. The irritable bowel syndrome. *N Engl J Med* 344(24):1846-1850.
6. Longstreth GF, Thompson WG, Chey WD, Houghton LA, Mearin F, Spiller RC. 2006. Functional bowel disorders. *Gastroenterology* 130(5):1480-1491.
7. Moayyedi P, Talley NJ, Fennerty MB, Vakil N. 2006. Can the clinical history distinguish between organic and functional dyspepsia? *JAMA* 295(13):1566-1576.
8. O'Donohue J, Williams R. 1996. Primary biliary cirrhosis. *QJM* 89(1):5-13.
9. Bickley LS, Szilagyi PG, Bates B. *Bates' Guide to Physical Examination and History Taking.* Philadelphia: Lippincott Williams & Wilkins; 2007.
10. Canadian Hypertension Education Program. 2008. The 2008 Canadian Hypertension Education Program recommendations: The scientific summary – an annual update. *Can J Cardiol* 24(6):447-452.

The Breast Exam

Editors:
Maria Jogova
Waed Mallah
Ashna Patel

Faculty Reviewers:
Jaime Escallon, MD, FACS, FRCS(C)
Ruth Heisey, MD, CCFP, FCFP

BREAST

TABLE OF CONTENTS

1. ESSENTIAL ANATOMY

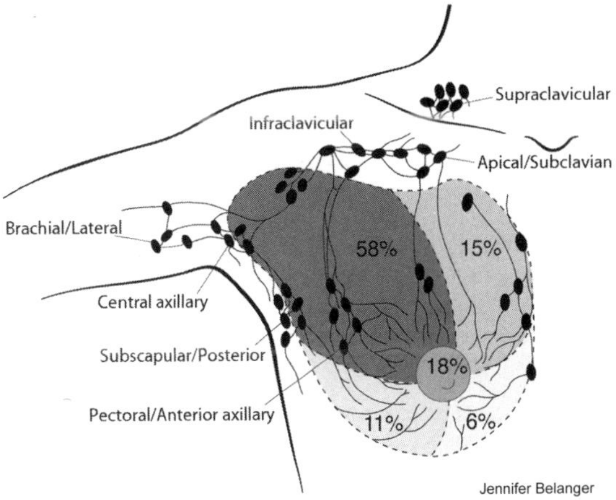

Figure 1. Lymph Nodes of the Breast and Frequency of Disease by Quadrant[1]

BREAST

2. COMMON CHIEF COMPLAINTS

- Breast pain/tenderness
- Breast mass
- Nipple changes (retraction, ulceration, scaling)
- Nipple discharge (spontaneous, upon compression)
- Change in skin of breast (color, induration)
- Change in size of breast

3. FOCUSED HISTORY

In addition to general history taking, important aspects of the breast history include:

- History of the chief complaint (breast pain/tenderness, breast mass, nipple changes/discharge, skin changes)
- Past breast history (surgeries, breast diseases, etc.)
- Assessment of risk factors (age, family history, obstetrical history, gynecological history)

3.1 Chief Complaint and History of Present Illness

- Breast pain (mastalgia): onset, bilateral or unilateral, intermittent or constant, changes with menstrual cycle, recent trauma
- Breast mass: onset, location, progression (worse, better, same), changes with menstrual cycle, recent trauma
- Unilateral breast change: asymmetric induration, breast retraction (often exaggerated on arm elevation)
- Nipple changes:
  - Changes since first noticed (larger, smaller, same)
  - Nipple retraction
  - Ulceration/scaling: may be Paget's disease
- Nipple discharge:
  - Bilateral vs. unilateral
  - Bloody vs. non-bloody
  - Uniductal vs. multiductal
  - Spontaneous vs. with expression

3.2 Risk Factor Assessment (Past Medical History, Family History)

Major Risk Factors for Breast Cancer

- Age >50 yr
- Female
- Personal history of breast or ovarian cancer
- Maternal or paternal family history of breast and/or ovarian cancer in 1st or 2nd degree relatives, especially if early onset (<50 yr)
- Genetics: mutations in the tumor suppressor genes BRCA1, BRCA2
- History of atypical hyperplasia or lobular carcinoma *in situ* (LCIS)
- History of high-dose radiation (e.g. mantle radiation for Hodgkin's)

Minor Risk Factors for Breast Cancer

- Nulliparity
- Menarche <12 yr
- Menopause >55 yr
- Hormone replacement therapy
- Obesity in postmenopausal women
- Excessive alcohol intake (>2 drinks/d)
- Previous history of breast biopsy regardless of findings

> **Clinical Pearl: Breast Cancer Risk**
> Validated tools of estimating breast cancer risk:
> 1) "Breast Cancer Risk Assessment Tool" www.cancer.gov/bcrisktool
> 2) "IBIS Breast Cancer Risk Evaluation Tool"
> www.ems-trials.org/riskevaluator.

4. FOCUSED PHYSICAL EXAM

- Purpose: identify features that distinguish malignant vs. benign lumps (see **Table 1**)
- The patient must be draped appropriately
- Male doctors should have a female witness in the room when possible
- Always examine both breasts, even if complaints are localized to one side
- Clinical breast examination (CBE) can detect up to 50% of cancers not detected by mammography alone
- Cancer cannot be ruled out on the basis of clinical exam alone; other diagnostic tests must be performed (see **Common Investigations**, p.42)[2]
- Increase in breast size, density, nodularity, and tenderness occur 3-5 d prior to menses: the most appropriate time for a breast exam is 7-10 d post menses
- Breasts normally involute and are less dense following menopause
- Document breast, quadrant, location (o'clock position on face of a clock with nipple at center), and distance from nipple
- Document qualities of mass: size, shape, consistency, delineation of borders, tenderness, mobility, and if impacted by menstrual changes (see **Table 1**)

EBM: Breast Cancer and CBE

Four recent studies have been conducted to determine the percentage of breast cancers identified by the CBE but not by mammography. Three showed that 4.6-5.7% of cancers were identified by the clinical breast exam, while one showed that 10.7% of cancers were identified by this exam alone.

Six human studies with women ages 35-74 were considered strong enough for pooling sensitivity and specificity results of the CBE in detecting breast cancer. The gold standard used was clinical follow-up. The National Breast and Cervical Cancer Early Detection Program (NBCCEDP) study conducted by the CDC in 2000 found similar sensitivity and specificity results, indicated in brackets.

Sensitivity: 54.1% (58.8%)   Specificity: 94.0% (93.4%)

Moreover, in a retrospective study of 1752 women with stage I/II breast cancer, physical exam was the sole means of detecting the malignancy in 15% of the cases. In women less than 40, physical exam was the sole means of detection in 40% of the cases.

Spending adequate time on the CBE (3 min per breast) and using proper technique improve breast lump detection.

McDonald S, Saslow D, Alciati MH. 2004. *CA Cancer J Clin* 54(6):345-361.
Diratzouian H, et al. 2005. *Clin Breast Cancer* 6(4):330-333.

Table 1. Interpretation of Findings

	Carcinoma	Fibroadenoma	Fibrocystic Condition
Location of Mass	Usually unilateral and solitary	Usually unilateral and solitary (85%)	Bilateral and multiple
Size	Variable	1-3 cm (may be larger)	Variable
Shape	Irregular	Round	Variable (may have regions of thickening or discrete mass)
Consistency	Firm or hard	Firm and rubbery	Nodular (may be firm)
Delineation	Ill-defined	Discrete	Region of nodular thickening
Tenderness	Nontender	Nontender	Tender
Mobility	May be tethered	Mobile	Mobile
Menstrual Changes	No	May change in size with menstrual cycle	Increased tenderness premenstrually
Age Group	80% ≥40 yr	Usually <30 yr	30-50 yr
Investigations	Mammography, U/S for palpable findings or to evaluate mammography findings further, core biopsy for definitive diagnosis	U/S, mammography if ≥30 yr, core biopsy or FNAB to confirm benign	Mammography if ≥30 yr, U/S for discrete masses, aspirate dominant or symptomatic cysts

FNAB = fine needle aspiration biopsy
Morrow M. 2000. *Am Fam Physician* 61(8):2371-2378.

4.1 Inspection

- Inspect both breasts with the patient in each of the following positions:
  - Patient sitting with hands resting on thighs
  - Patient sitting with arms raised above head
  - Patient sitting with hands pressed against hips
  - Patient sitting and leaning forward

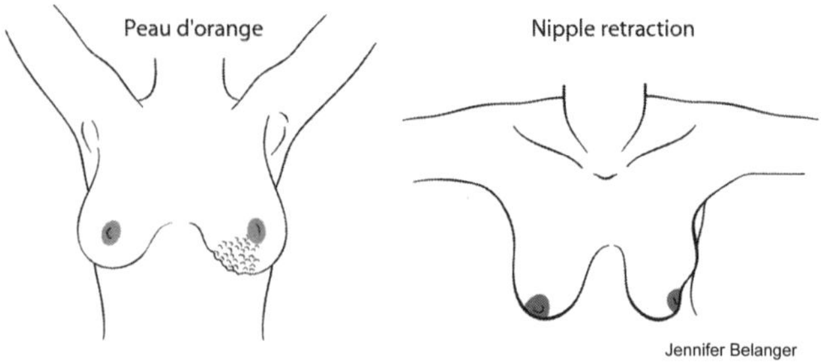

Figure 2. Breast Inspecton

- Inspection of the breast: **4 S**'s
  1. **Size** of each breast
  2. **Symmetry** of two breasts (some variability is normal)
  3. **Shape** and contour: bulges, flattening, skin dimpling, retraction
  4. **Skin** changes:
     » Inflammation
     » Erythema
     » Peau d'orange (edema in skin: may be indicative of advanced cancer or postoperative/postradiation edema) (see **Figure 2**)
     » Abnormal vascularity (increased visibility of blood vessels)
     » Thickening
- Inspection of nipple: **5 S**'s (see **Figure 3**)
  1. **Size**
  2. **Symmetry**
     » Ask patient to raise arms: one nipple may be retracted due to a small cancer in breast (caused by tethering) (see **Figure 2**)
  3. **Skin** changes: eczema or ulceration/scaling
  4. **Spontaneous nipple discharge:** serous, bloody, or colored, from one or more ducts (discharge with expression only is usually benign)
  5. **Supernumerary nipple:** rare, insignificant finding along milk line

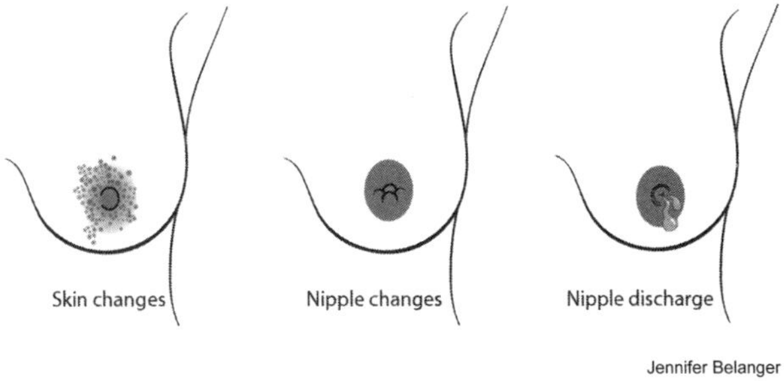

Figure 3. Visible Signs of Breast Disease

> **Clinical Pearl: Palpation**
> Always palpate both breasts.
>
> Palpation in supine position allows breast tissue to stretch more evenly across the chest wall for easier deep palpation. For large breasts or more effective deep palpation, the breast can be palpated in oblique position.

4.2 Palpation

Axillae and Supraclavicular Area

- Three key groups of lymph nodes: axillary, supraclavicular, and infraclavicular (see **Figure 1**)
  - Check for size, location, consistency, and mobility
  - Palpate above and below clavicle with patient's arms resting on thighs
  - Partially abduct patient's arm and support it on your arm to assess axilla
  - Palpate deeply into axilla, along posterior surface of pectoralis muscles, and up along inferior surface of upper arm

BREAST

BREAST

Palpation of Breasts

- Use fleshy pads of three middle fingertips
  - o Systematically cover entire breast area: from 2nd to 6th rib, sternum to midaxillary line
  - o At each new point of contact, first use light, then increasingly stronger pressure
- Two possible patterns of palpation (see **Figure 4**):
  1. Radial vector pattern
     - » Palpation at each location in small circular motion
     - » Begin at "12 o'clock" position at outer edge of breast and move inwards along all "spokes of wheel" with nipple as central point; end with palpation of areolar area and nipple
     - » Continue with next vector, partially overlapping with previous one, and work inwards to nipple
  2. Vertical strip pattern
     - » Palpate each location with small circular motions
     - » Mentally divide breast area into a series of vertical regions, and palpate each one thoroughly from top to bottom
     - » Begin at axilla and palpate downward along midaxillary line to 6th rib
     - » For next strip, work upward from 6th rib to top of breast and partially overlap with first strip
     - » Continue in this antiparallel fashion until the entire breast is examined

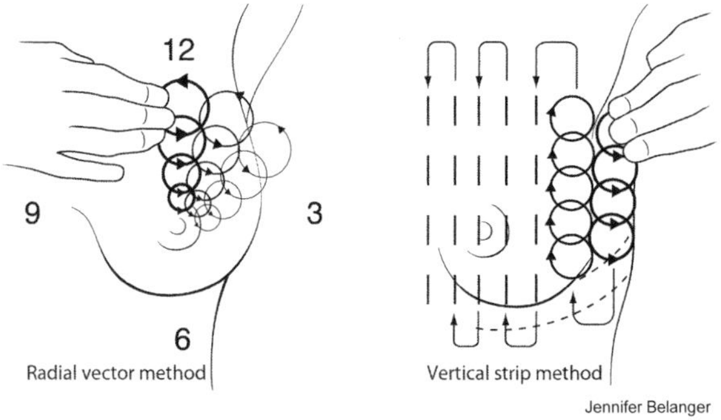

Figure 4. Common Approaches to Breast Palpation

- Distinguish between abnormal mass and normal compressed tissue ridge (inframammary fold) which may be found along lower border of breast, particularly with large breasts
- If a mass is detected:
  - o Determine distance from nipple
  - o Gently elevate breast near the mass and watch for dimpling (suggests an underlying cancer)
- Nipple distortion may be a sign of underlying cancer

5. COMMON INVESTIGATIONS

- Refer to **Figure 5** on p.44 for application and summary

5.1 Screening

- Clinical breast exam (CBE)
- Mammogram

5.2 Diagnosis

Mammogram

- Low dose X-ray to examine breast
- Indication:
  - Evaluation of new or worrisome palpable mass in any woman ≥30 yr
  - Best modality for picking up ductal carcinoma *in situ* (DCIS, earliest stage of breast cancer), often before a mass is palpable (usually presents with microcalcifications)[3]
- Nonpalpable malignancies <1 cm in size may be detected
  - 1/3 of all malignancies detected by mammography are nonpalpable

Note: negative mammogram does not rule out breast cancer

MRI

- For high-risk women (see **Clinical Pearl Box**, below)
- For further evaluation of undifferentiated abnormalities on mammogram/ U/S

Clinical Pearl: Risk Stratification for Screening[4]

Average risk: no personal or family history of breast cancer, known BRCA1 or BRCA2 mutation, or history of chest wall irradiation

Moderate risk: personal or family history of breast cancer or past premalignant biopsy (atypical hyperplasia, lobular carcinoma *in situ* [LCIS])

High risk: BRCA mutation carriers, family history of breast cancer or BRCA mutation, history of chest wall irradiation, multiple major risk factors for breast cancer

Risk Category	Recommended Screening Test		
	CBE	**Mammography**	**MRI**
Average	No (consider in <40 yr, see **EBM** box, p.39)	q2 yr starting at age 50 *discuss harms/ benefits at age 40	No
Moderate	Yes	q1 yr at age 40	No
High	Yes	q1 yr at age 30	q1 yr at age 30

EBM: MRI as Screening Tool

1275 women with BRCA1 or BRCA2 mutations were followed for several years and the incidence of advanced stage breast cancers in a cohort assigned to MRI for screening and a cohort assigned to conventional screening techniques (CBE, mammography) were compared. A similar incidence of breast cancer was found in both groups (9.2% in both). The MRI screened cohort had an incidence of advanced stage breast cancer (II-IV) of 1.9% (95% CI, 02%-3.7%) at 6 years, which was significantly less than the comparison group whose incidence was 6.6% (95%, CI 3.8%-9.3%). The mean size of invasive tumors detected in the MRI screened cohort was 0.9 cm compared to 1.8 cm in the comparison group. This study demonstrated a significant reduction in the incidence of advanced stage breast cancer in women with BRCA1, BRCA2 mutations undergoing annual screening with MRI.

Warner E, et al. 2011. *J Clin Oncol* 29(13):1665-1669.

BREAST

Ultrasound

- Indication:
  - Evaluate palpable/nonpalpable masses or mammographic abnormalities
  - Differentiate cystic masses from solid masses
  - Highly operator-dependent, requires special breast expertise[3]
    - False positives can generate significant anxiety
    - False negatives can miss malignancy
    - Most solid-dominant palpable masses need a biopsy

Fine Needle Aspiration Biopsy (FNAB)

- Smears prepared from aspirate for cytologic evaluation
- If aspirated fluid is bloody or if lesion biopsied was solid, send aspirate for cytology
- Simple cyst: non-bloody aspirate followed by resolution of mass, no cytological evaluation required (follow-up in 4-6 wk to ensure no reoccurrence; if reoccurs, re-aspirate and send fluid to cytology)[3]
- A negative FNAB does NOT rule out cancer[3]

Core Needle Biopsy

- Preferred method for tissue diagnosis[3]
- Better sample and pathology (tissue architecture, staining, hormone receptor status)
- Provides more information for planning surgery (DCIS vs. invasive cancer)
- Results MUST be concordant with imaging findings (radiologist should dictate addendum after reviewing pathology results)

Excisional Biopsy/Lumpectomy

- When core biopsy is not concordant or clinical suspicion is high, even if core biopsy is negative
- When core biopsy is not possible or available
- To treat/rule out cancer

6. COMMON DISORDERS

Disorders marked with (✓) are discussed in **Common Clinical Scenarios**

✓ Breast cyst
✓ Fibroadenoma (benign; accounts for 75% of solitary breast lumps in younger women)
✓ Mastitis (common during breast feeding)
✓ Mastalgia
- Breast abscess
- Breast carcinoma
- Fat necrosis
- Fibrocystic condition (benign; occurs to some extent in 50% of women)
- Intraductal papilloma
- Gynecomastia (breast enlargement in males)

7. COMMON CLINICAL SCENARIOS

7.1 Fibroadenoma (Most Common Benign Solid Breast Mass)

History

- Single nontender lump, 15% are multiple, especially on U/S[6]
- Lump more noticeable in the 2nd half of menstrual cycle
- Usually develop in young women (<30 yr)
- About 1/3 get smaller, 1/3 stay the same, 1/3 grow
- May regress with menopause
- New mass at an older age requires work-up to rule out malignancy

Clinical Presentation of Breast Disease

- 50% — **Symptomatic**
  - Palpable lump
  - Skin change
  - Nipple discharge
- 50% — **Screen detected (Mammography)**
  - Mass
    - 1/3 detected not palpable
  - Calcification
    - Ductal carcinoma *in situ* – earliest stage of breast cancer, "microcalcifications"
  - Density
  - Asymmetry
  - Architectural distortion

Who is Screened
- All women >50, every 2 yr
- Women ≥30 who fall in high-risk group
- Discussion of harms/benefits with women 40-49

Further Investigation of Palpable Finding

1. Mammography in women ≥30 yr with palpable breast mass
2. Ultrasound

Diagnostic Modalities

If Biopsy Shows Cancer

1. Fine needle aspiration biopsy (FNAB)*
- Cytology
  - If fluid non-bloody and mass disappears on aspiration → cyst, no cytology needed
  - If solid → cytology
  - If bloody → cytology
  - Negative FNA does not rule out cancer
2. Core needle biopsy*
- Pathology
- Radiologically assisted
- Distinguishes between noninvasive and invasive disease

*important to know laboratory results before surgery to plan treatment

Possible Assessment of Disease Extent by MRI

- Especially in young women with dense breasts

Develop Treatment Plan

1. Surgery
- Treat local and regional disease
- Staging
2. Radiotherapy
- Minimize local and regional recurrence
- Breast, chest wall
3. Systemic therapy
- Minimize distant recurrence
- Chemotherapy, endocrine, others

Clinical Pearl: Common Outcomes
- Breast radiation almost always after lumpectomy
- Large extent of disease indicative for mastectomy
- For invasive disease, sentinel lymph node biopsy done with lumpectomy

Figure 5. Breast Screening Flow Chart[4-6]

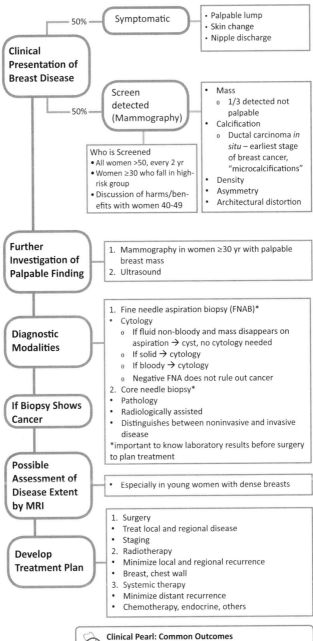

BREAST

Physical Exam
- Palpable breast lump 1-2 cm in size
- Well-defined, nontender, round or lobulated, with firm or rubbery consistency
- No tethering to underlying tissue, very mobile

Investigations
- Mammography, U/S + FNAB or core needle biopsy for tissue diagnosis

Management
- Consider excision if >3 cm, if enlarging (pathology required to rule out Phyllodes tumor) or if diagnosis not conclusive from FNAB/core biopsy
- Repeat U/S q6 mo x 2 yr and if no change, clinically thereafter

7.2 Breast Cyst

History
- Cysts may increase in size rapidly, may decrease or disappear
- Bilateral, with occasional non-spontaneous multi-ductal nipple discharge, color can be murky or greenish-black[6]
- Affected females often 30-50 yr
- Estrogen therapy may cause cyst development in menopausal women

Physical Exam
- Firm, smooth, tender, mobile, and well-defined mass

Investigations
- Mammography, U/S ± FNAB ± cytological studies
- U/S or FNAB are the best ways to differentiate cystic from solid masses[6]

Management
- Aspirate dominant or bothersome cysts
- Simple cysts require one follow-up visit in 6-8 wk to ensure no recurrence
- Cysts determined to be complicated cysts on U/S followed with repeat U/S at 6 mo
- Those determined to be complex cysts require FNAB and tissue diagnosis (identified as complex on U/S or clinically by not resolving completely with aspiration)[6]

7.3 Mastalgia[5]

History
- Common in premenopausal females
- Note type of pain, location, and relationship to menstrual cycle
- Cyclic mastalgia[5]:
  - More common in younger women, bilateral, poorly localized, variable duration, heaviness or soreness that radiates to axilla and arm, etiology unknown, relieved with menses, and resolves spontaneously
- Noncyclic mastalgia[5]:
  - More common in women between 40-50 yr, unilateral, described as sharp, burning pain localized in breast, usually caused by cyst or costochondritis

Physical Exam
- Nonspecific, look for mass
- Check for pain with palpation over the ribs secondary to costochondritis

Investigations
- If normal physical exam, mammography (unless done in past yr) for women ≥30 yr to rule out cancer
- U/S or FNAB is the best way to differentiate cystic from solid masses[6]

Management
- If physical exam and investigations are negative, then reassure given high rate of spontaneous remission (60-80%)[6]
- Other non-pharmacological treatments: evening primrose oil, sports bra, Tylenol™, reassurance

7.4 Mastitis/Superficial Cellulitis of the Breast
History
- Occurs around the time of childbirth, in nursing mothers, or after injury
- Fever, malaise

Physical Exam
- Unilateral erythema, swelling, tenderness, and warmth

Investigations
- *S. aureus* almost always the etiologic agent[5]
- In non-lactating women, need imaging to rule out cancer

Management
- Drain and incise abscess if present
- Antibiotics
- Continue breast feeding
  - If no resolution, investigate further

BREAST

REFERENCES

1. Bickley LS, Szilagyi PG, Bates B. *Bates' Guide to Physical Examination and History Taking,* 10th ed. Philadelphia: Lippincott Williams & Wilkins; 2009.
2. Barton MB, Harris R, Fletcher SW. 1999. The rational clinical examination. Does this patient have breast cancer? The screening clinical breast examination: should it be done? How? *JAMA* 282(13):1270-1280.
3. Klein S. 2005. Evaluation of palpable breast masses. *Am Fam Physician* 71(9):1731-1738.
4. Warner E, Heisey R, Carroll J. 2012. Primer: Applying the 2011 Canadian guidelines for breast cancer screening in practice. *CMAJ* 184(16):1803-1807.
5. Morrow M. 2000. The evaluation of common breast problems. *Am Fam Physician* 61(8):2371-2378.
6. Pruthi S. 2001. Detection and evaluation of a palpable breast mass. *Mayo Clin Proc* 76(6):641-648.
7. Baxter N. 2001. Preventive health care, 2001 update: Should women be routinely taught breast self-examination to screen for breast cancer? *CMAJ* 164(13):1837-1846.
8. Bilimoria MM, Morrow M. 1995. The woman at increased risk for breast cancer: Evaluation and management strategies. *CA Cancer J Clin* 45(5):263-278.
9. Horn-Ross PL, Canchola AJ, West DL, Stewart SL, Bernstein L, Deapen D, et al. 2004. Patterns of alcohol consumption and breast cancer risk in the California Teachers Study cohort. *Cancer Epidemiol Biomarkers Prevent* 13(405):405-411.
10. Humphrey LL, Helfand M, Chan BK, Woolf SH. 2002. Breast cancer screening: A summary of the evidence for the U.S. Preventive Services Task Force. *Ann Intern Med* 137(5 Part 1):347-360.
11. Kösters JP, Gøtzsche PC. Regular self-examination or clinical examination for early detection of breast cancer [CD-ROM]. Copenhagen (DM): Nordic Cochrane Centre; 2003. Cochrane Database Syst Rev 2: CD003373.
12. Lehman CD, Blume JD, Weatherall P, Thickman D, Hylton N, Warner E, et al. 2005. Screening women at high risk for breast cancer with mammography and magnetic resonance imaging. *Cancer* 108(9):1898-1905.
13. Lehman CD, Gatsonis C, Kuhl CK, Hendrick RE, Pisano ED, Hanna L, et al. 2007. MRI evaluation of the contralateral breast in women with recently diagnosed breast cancer. *NEJM* 356(13):1295-1303.
14. Tonelli M, Gorber SC, Joffres M. 2011. The Canadian Task Force on Preventive Health Care. Recommendations on screening for breast cancer in average-risk women aged 40-74 years. *CMAJ* 183(17):1991-2001.

The Cardiovascular Exam

Editors:
Eric Kaplovitch
Kimberly Cai

Faculty Reviewers:
Jeremy Edwards, MD, FRCP(C)
Chi-Ming Chow, MD, CM, MSc, FACC, FASE, FRCP(C)

TABLE OF CONTENTS

1. ESSENTIAL ANATOMY

Chambers of the Heart

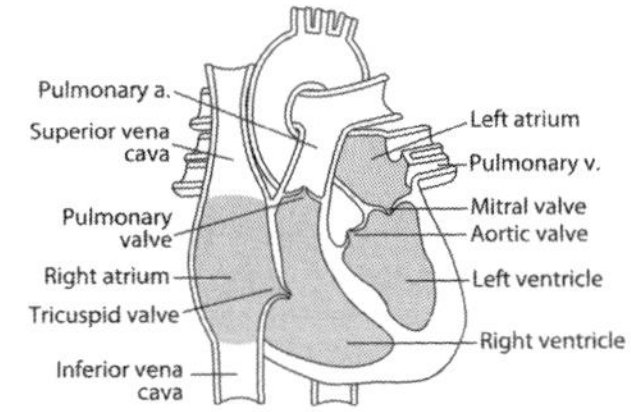

Path of Electrical Impulses

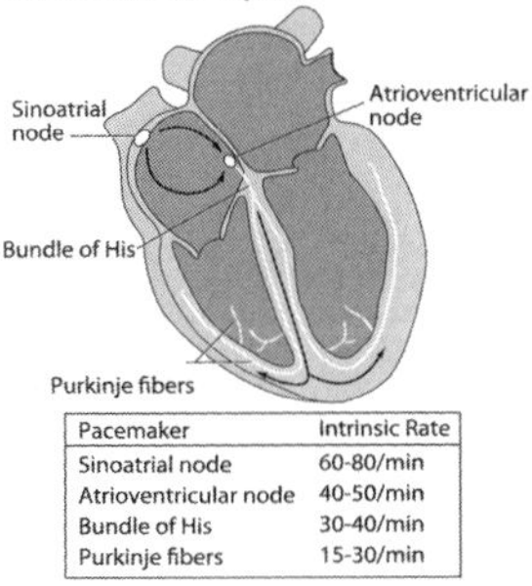

Pacemaker	Intrinsic Rate
Sinoatrial node	60-80/min
Atrioventricular node	40-50/min
Bundle of His	30-40/min
Purkinje fibers	15-30/min

Pina Kingman

Figure 1. Anatomy of the Heart

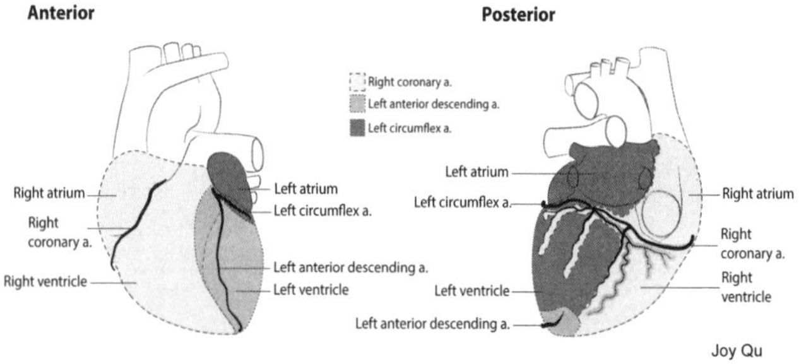

Figure 2. Coronary Vessels and Vascular Territories (shaded)

Review of Physiology

- Circulatory pathway has two components:
  1. Pulmonary (low pressure) system (right ventricle [RV] → pulmonary arteries → lungs for oxygenation → pulmonary veins → left atrium [LA])
  2. Systemic (high pressure) system (left ventricle [LV] → aorta → body tissues for oxygen delivery → caval system → right atrium [rA])
- **Blood supply** to the heart is regulated by the right and left coronary arteries (RCA and LCA) which are the first branches of the aorta
  - Left coronary system is comprised of a short left main artery (LMA), which bifurcates into the left anterior descending artery (LAD) and left circumflex artery (CFX)
  - The RCA bifurcates into the posterior descending artery (PDA) and the posterior lateral artery (PLA)
- The venous drainage occurs through the coronary sinus, which empties into the rA and enters the pulmonary circulation
  - Anatomic variants of the coronary system are common
  - The dominant vessel is the one that supplies the posterior descending artery. Right-dominant circulation occurs 85% of the time (left-dominant 8% and co-dominant 7%)
- **Electrical conduction system** begins at the sinoatrial (SA) node located between the SVC and right atrial appendage → depolarizes both atria (LA via Bachmann's bundle) → internodal branches → atrio-ventricular (AV) node located between the coronary sinus and septal leaflet of tricuspid valve → His-Purkinje system → right bundle branch (RBB) and left bundle branch (LBB) → Purkinje fibers (see **Figure 1**)
- Neural innervation of heart from both sympathetic and parasympathetic nervous systems (SNS and PSNS)
  - SNS causes ↑HR and ↑AV node conduction rate
  - PSNS causes to ↓HR and ↓AV node conduction rate

2. COMMON CHIEF COMPLAINTS

- Chest pain (angina)
- Shortness of breath (dyspnea) at rest, on exertion, when supine (orthopnea), upon waking up at night (paroxysmal nocturnal dyspnea [PND])
- Heart pounding (palpitations)
- Swelling (edema), especially in lower extremities
- Fainting/light-headedness (syncope/presyncope)
- Fatigue, exercise intolerance
- Coughing up blood (hemoptysis)
- Blue lips/fingers/toes (cyanosis)

3. FOCUSED HISTORY

Risk Factors for Cardiac Disease

- Nonmodifiable risk factors:
  - Age (male >45 yr, female >55 yr)
  - Gender (male 10 yr earlier than female)
  - Family history (MI <55 yr in male relatives, <65 yr in female relatives; or <60 yr in first-degree relatives)
  - Ethnic groups (South Asians and African-Caribbeans are at higher risk than the general population)
- Modifiable risk factors:
  - HTN (BP >140/90 mmHg or taking antihypertensive medications)
  - DM
  - Hypercholesterolemia
  - Smoking (or recent ex-smoker)
  - Postmenopausal
  - Obesity
  - Sedentary lifestyle
  - Stress
  - Alcoholism
  - Depression
  - Hyperhomocysteinemia

CARDIOVASCULAR

Chief Complaint and History of Present Illness

Chest Pain (OPQRST)

- Onset/duration: sudden vs. gradual, hours vs. days, previous similar symptoms, frequency, progression, course (constant vs. intermittent), pleuritic, after meals (postprandial)
- Precipitating and relieving factors: better or worse with exercise/rest/sleep/position
- Quality: crushing, pressing, squeezing, burning, stabbing, tightening
- Location: epigastric, periumbilical, flank, back
- Radiation: to neck, jaw, axilla, back, arm (either or both arms can be involved)
- Associated symptoms: fatigue, palpitations, diaphoresis, peripheral edema, N/V, dyspnea
- Stable vs. unstable angina:
  - **Stable angina** is intermittent chest pain during exertion or emotional stress, relieved by rest
  - **Unstable angina** is characterized by:
    - New onset (<2 mo) that is severe (CCS III or IV) and/or frequent
    - Progression of symptoms
    - At rest or nocturnal
    - Post-MI
  - ***Note:*** always assess functional class of angina (see **Table 1** and **Table 2**)
- Risk factors for cardiovascular disease
- Medications: prescribed vs. OTC, antiplatelets, antithrombin therapies, β-blockers, ACE inhibitors, angiotensin receptor blockers (ARBs), calcium channel blockers (CCBs), diuretics, antiarrhythmics, lipid-modifying agents
- See **Essentials of Emergency Medicine**, p.433, for differential diagnosis of chest pain

Table 1. Canadian Cardiovascular Society (CCS) Functional Classification of Angina

Class	Activity Evoking Angina	Limits to Physical Activity
0	Asymptomatic	None
I	Prolonged exertion	None
II	Walking >2 blocks or >1 flight of stairs	Slight
III	Walking <2 blocks or <1 flight of stairs	Marked
IV	Minimal activity or at rest	Severe

CARDIOVASCULAR

Table 2. New York Heart Association (NYHA) Functional Classification of Congestive Heart Failure

Class	Activity Evoking Angina	Limits to Physical Activity
I	None	None
II	Ordinary physical activity	Slight
III	Walking <2 blocks or <1 flight of stairs	Marked
IV	Minimal or at rest	Severe

Dyspnea

- See **Respiratory Exam**, p.350

Peripheral Vascular Disease

- Peripheral edema
- See **Peripheral Vascular Exam**, p.296

4. FOCUSED PHYSICAL EXAM

General

- Patient's level of comfort or distress
- Skin color (pale vs. pink)
- Cyanosis: central (blue mucous membranes) vs. peripheral (blue fingers/toes)
- Respiratory distress: tachypnea, accessory muscle use, intercostal indrawing, position
- Presence of edema in lower limbs
- Extracardiac features: xanthomata, rash, petechiae, nail splinter hemorrhages

Vitals

- HR: rate, rhythm (regular vs. regularly irregular vs. irregularly irregular), amplitude (strong vs. soft)
- BP: both arms
- RR, O_2 saturation
- Temperature
- Orthostatic vitals (HR, BP)

JVP

- Direct assessment of the pressure in the right atrium (i.e. central venous pressure)
- Assessment includes four parameters: height, waveform, Kussmaul's sign, hepatojugular/abdominojugular reflux
- Differentiate internal jugular pulse from carotid pulse (see **Table 3**)

Table 3. Characteristics of Internal Jugular vs. Carotid Pulse

Feature	Internal Jugular Pulse	Carotid
Palpable	No	Yes
Number of Waveforms	Multiple	Single
Finger Pressure above Clavicle	Disappears	Persists
Inspiration/Elevation of the Head of the Bed*	↓	No change
Hepatojugular Reflux/Lowering of the Head of the Bed*	↑	No change

*Change in bed position causes positional change of jugular vein

JVP Height (see **Figure 3**)

- Position the patient at 30° elevation and turn the patient's head slightly to the left, then adjust the angle of elevation until jugular pulsations are observed
- Look between the two heads of the sternocleidomastoid for pulsations: if difficult to observe, shine a light tangentially across the right side of the patient's neck, and look for shadows of pulsations
  - o The JVP is more of an inward, multiple waveform movement and will cast a shadow with tangential light
- Determine JVP by measuring the vertical distance from the sternal angle to a horizontal line drawn from the top of the jugular pulsation
  - o Normal JVP: ≤4 cm
- Elevated JVP suggests increased pressure in the right atrium due to:
  - o Right heart failure (may be secondary to left heart failure)
  - o Constrictive pericarditis or tamponade physiology
  - o ***Note:*** other causes of high blood pressure can occur irrespective of right atrium changes; e.g. superior vena cava (SVC) obstruction

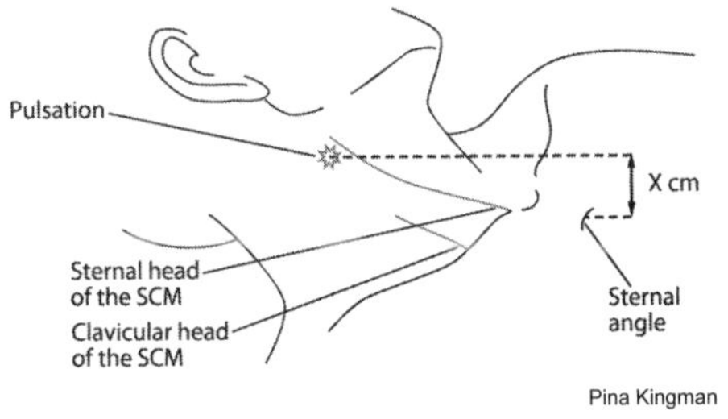

Figure 3. Measuring JVP Height

Kussmaul's Sign

- Rising of JVP with inspiration (paradoxical) suggests that the blood flow into the right heart is impaired. This could result from:
  - o Constrictive pericarditis
  - o Right heart failure
  - o SVC obstruction
  - o Tricuspid stenosis
  - o Restrictive cardiomyopathy

CARDIOVASCULAR

Hepatojugular/Abdominojugular Reflux (HJR/AJR)

- To assess high JVP and RV function:
  - Position the patient so that the top of the JVP is visible
  - Place the right hand over the liver in the right upper quadrant or anywhere in the abdomen
  - Apply moderate pressure (25-30 mmHg) and maintain compression for 10 s
  - The JVP may rise or remain unchanged; a sustained elevation of the JVP height (>4 cm) after 2 spontaneous breaths (to ensure patient is not having a Valsalva maneuver) is pathological

Waveforms

- The JVP is a multiple waveform entity, and an understanding of each of the wave components is essential to conceptualizing how certain diseases are reflected by changes in the JVP:
  - a-wave: atrial contraction
  - x-descent: atrial relaxation following contraction
  - c-wave: closing of the tricuspid valve increases atrial pressure during
  - relaxation
  - v-wave: increasing atrial pressure with venous return
  - y-descent: opening of the tricuspid valve decreases atrial pressure

Precordial Exam

- Divide the precordium into 4 areas where sounds and murmurs from the heart valves are best auscultated. Please note that the classic area of auscultation is not representative of actual valvular location, but radiation of the murmur (see **Figure 4**)

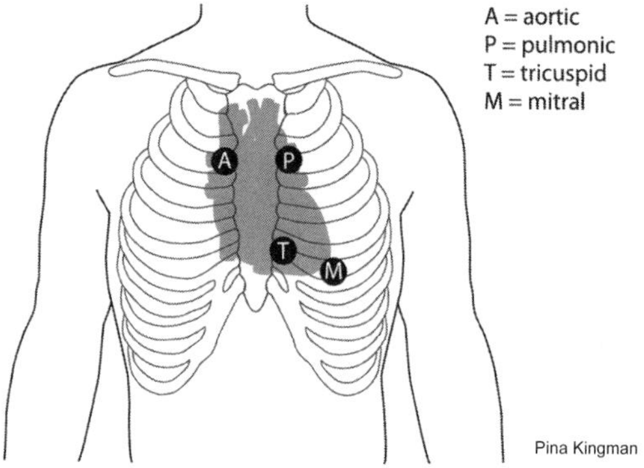

Figure 4. Classic Auscultation Areas of Heart Sounds and Murmurs

Inspection

- Chest shape: normal vs. excavatum (hollow) vs. carinatum (pigeon-like)
- Apex beat (5th intercostal space, mid-clavicular line)
- Abnormal motions (heaves, lifts)
- Scars

Palpation

- Palpate over the 4 auscultation areas and along the sternum
- Palpate for heaves (sustained outward motion), palpable murmur (vibration over area of turbulent blood flow) and impulses (systolic vs. diastolic)
- Palpate over the apex beat and describe it in terms of LADS (location, amplitude, duration, size)

Table 4. Palpable Findings in Precordial Exam

Auscultation Area	Abnormal Findings	Possible Pathology
A	Systolic impulse	Systemic HTN Dilated aortic aneurysm
P	Systolic impulse	Pulmonary HTN
T	Heave, thrill	RV enlargement (2° to pulmonary HTN or left-sided heart disease)
M	Thrill	Mitral regurgitation (MR)

Auscultation

- Auscultate over the 4 auscultation areas for heart sounds and murmurs
- Focus on identifying S1 and S2 first, then listen during systole and during diastole

Table 5. Heart Sounds

	Auscultation	Physiologic Significance	Physiologic Significance Possible Pathologies
S1	Diaphragm over left lower sternal border (T), apex (M)	Closing of the mitral and tricuspid valves	**Loud S1:** mitral stenosis, increased contractility, short PR interval **Soft S1:** first degree AV block, LV failure, LBBB **Variable S1:** AF, AV dissociation, ventricular pacing, Mobitz I 2nd degree block **Split S1:** RBBB
S2	Diaphragm over left 2nd intercostal space	Closing of the aortic and pulmonic valves	**Loud S2:** Loud A2: systemic HTN, hyperdynamic circulation, dilated aorta Loud P2: pulmonary HTN, **Soft S2:** AS or PS **Split S2:** Wide: RBBB, WPW, PS, pulmonary HTN, MR Fixed: ASD Paradoxical: LBBB, AS, WPW, HCM
Mid-Systolic Click	Diaphragm over apex and LLSB while asking patient to squat from standing	Not physiologic	Mitral Valve Prolapse
Opening Snap	Diaphragm at apex and LLSB	Not physiologic	Mitral stenosis
S3	Bell at apex with patient in left lateral decubitus	**Children and Young Adults:** physiologic **Adults:** pathologic	CHF **Left-sided:** MR, AI **Right-sided:** TR, PI

Table 5. Heart Sounds (continued)

	Auscultation	Physiologic Significance	Physiologic Significance Possible Pathologies
S4	Bell over apex	Not physiologic: (atria contracting against stiffened ventricle)	**Left-sided:** LVH, AS, systemic HTN, CAD, cardiomyopathy **Right-sided:** RVH, PS, pulmonary hypertension

AF = atrial fibrillation, AI = aortic insufficiency, AS = aortic stenosis, ASD = atrial septal defect, AV = atrioventricular, HCM = hypertrophic cardiomyopathy, LLSB = left lower sternal border, L/RBBB = left/right bundle branch block, L/RVH = left/right ventricular hypertrophy, LV = left ventricle, MR = mitral regurgitation, PI = pulmonary insufficiency, PS = pulmonic stenosis, TR = tricuspid regurgitation, WPW = Wolff-Parkinson-White

Murmurs

- Describe murmurs in terms of:
  - Timing: systolic, diastolic, continuous
  - Shape: crescendo, decrescendo, crescendo-decrescendo, plateau
  - Location of maximal intensity
  - Radiation: axilla, back, neck
  - Duration
  - Intensity
    - 6-point scale (see **Table 6**)
    - Intensity of murmur not necessarily related to clinical severity
  - Pitch: high, medium, low
  - Quality: blowing, harsh, rumbling, musical, machine-like or scratchy
  - Relationship to respiration
  - Relationship to body position
  - Effect of special maneuvers

Table 6. Intensity Scale

Grade	
I	Softer than S1 and S2
II	Intensity of murmur same as S1 and S2
III	Intensity of murmur louder than S1 and S2 but no palpable thrill
IV	Loud murmur with a palpable thrill
V	Loud murmur with palpable thrill, audible with only one rim of stethoscope touching chest
VI	Loud murmur with palpable thrill and audible with stethoscope lifted off chest

- Murmur is likely nonpathological if:
  - Early systolic, short duration, and low intensity (usually grade 1-2/6)
  - Nonradiating, not associated with other CV abnormalities/murmurs
  - Found in otherwise healthy children, especially in states of hyperdynamic blood flow (e.g. exercise, fever, anxiety)
  - Decreases or disappears upon sitting
- Special maneuvers for auscultation (see **Table 7**)

Table 7. Special Positions and Maneuvers for Auscultation of Heart Sounds

Position	Effect on Heart Sounds	
Sitting upright, leaning forward, holding exhalation	↑ AS, AR, pericardial rubs	
Left lateral decubitus (LLD) (use bell of stethoscope)	S3, S4, MS	
Maneuver	**Physiological**	**Effect on Heart**
Quiet inspiration-sustained abdominal pressure, leg elevation	↑ venous return	↑ right-sided murmurs, TR, PS
Fist-clenching (isometrics)	↑ systemic arterial resistance	↑ some left-sided murmurs (MR, AR, VSD) ↓ AS
Standing (Valsalva strain)	↓ venous return ↓ vascular tone	↑ MVP, HCM ↓ AS
Squatting (Valsalva release)	↑ venous return ↑ vascular tone	↓ MVP, HCM ↑ AS

AR = aortic regurgitation, AS = aortic stenosis, HCM = hypertrophic cardiomyopathy, MR = mitral regurgitation, MS = mitral stenosis, MVP = mitral valve prolapse, PS = pulmonic stenosis, TR = tricuspid regurgitation, VSD = ventricular septal defect

Common Murmurs and Heart Sounds

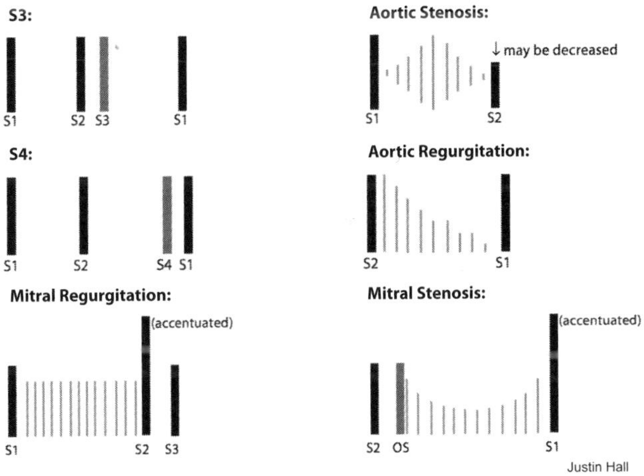

Figure 5. Common Murmurs and Heart Sounds

Respiratory Exam

- See **Respiratory Exam,** p.351

Peripheral Vascular Exam

- See **Peripheral Vascular Exam**, p.297

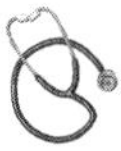

Clinical Pearl: Pediatrics Corner

- Benign heart murmers are common, especially in the pediatric population, and can be exacerbated by high output states.
- Characteristics of benign murmurs are often: harmonic/musical, systolic, and low grade.

5. COMMON INVESTIGATIONS

Table 8. Cardiac Investigations

Study Type	Test	Description	Indication
Stress Tests	Exercise Stress Test	Echocardiogram or ECG monitoring while patient exercises on treadmill at increasing speed until chest discomfort, inordinate dyspnea, abnormal ECG changes or target HR is observed	Suspected CAD Post MI
	Pharmacologic stress	In patients who are unable to exercise maximally, medications such as dobutamine, dipyridamole, and adenosine can be used	
Perfusion	Cardiac Perfusion Test[1]	Radiographic visualization of coronary territory following introduction of contrast material	Assessment of CAD, heart failure
Enyzmes	Creatine phosphokinase MB isoenzyme (CK-MB), Troponins	Enzymes released into circulation following damage to cardiac muscle; used to diagnose myocardial injury/ infarctions	Suspected MI

CARDIOVASCULAR

6. COMMON CLINICAL SCENARIOS

6.1 Acute Myocardial Infarction (AMI)

Symptoms

- **Pain:** classically retrosternal, heavy, squeezing or crushing pain, radiating to arm, abdomen, back, neck, jaw, prolonged (often lasting >30 min)
- **Atypical Pain:** "silent" AMI (more often in patients with DM, hypertension, increased age)
- **Associated Symptoms:** diaphoresis, N/V, weakness, pallor, dizziness, palpitations, cerebral symptoms, sense of impending doom

Physical Exam

- **JVP:** normal, ↑ with RV infarct
- **Pulse:** variable, most commonly rapid and regular, may be normal, ↓ pulse volume, variable BP
- **Palpation:** ↓ point of maximum impulse (PMI), abnormal systolic pulsation 3rd-5th left intercostal space
- **Auscultation:** S3, S4, ↓ intensity of heart sounds, paradoxical split S2, transient apical systolic murmur, mitral regurgitation, pericardial rub
- **Extracardiac Findings:** ↑ RR, pulmonary crackles, signs of arteriosclerosis

6.2 Congestive Heart Failure: Left and Right Heart

Symptoms

- Dyspnea, orthopnea, PND, cough, Cheyne-Stokes respiration, fatigue, weakness, abdominal symptoms (anorexia, nausea, abdominal pain), cerebral symptoms, nocturia, peripheral edema, weight gain

Physical Exam

- **JVP:** ↑, positive hepatojugular reflux
- **Pulse:** ↓ pulse volume, ± pulsus alternans (alternating stronger and weaker beats), sinus tachycardia
- **Palpation:** PMI may be sustained, diffuse and displaced, S3 may be palpable, ± left parasternal lift
- **Auscultation:** S3, S4; S2 may be paradoxically split (often associated with LBBB), murmurs often associated with mitral regurgitation, and tricuspid regurgitation
- **Extracardiac:** systemic hypotension, diastolic pressure may be ↑, pulmonary HTN, peripheral cyanosis, pulmonary crackles, hepatomegaly, ascites, edema, pleural effusion, cachexia

EBM: Congestive Heart Failure

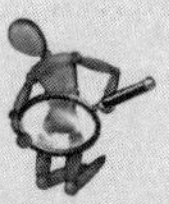

Features most suggestive of diagnosis of congestive heart failure are the overall clinical judgment, history of heart failure, a third heart sound, jugular venous distension, radiographic pulmonary venous congestion or interstitial edema, and electrocardiographic atrial fibrillation.

The single finding that most decreases the likelihood of heart failure is a brain natriuretic peptide (BNP) <100 pg/mL.

Wang CS, et al. 2005. *JAMA* 294(15):1944-1956.

6.3 Mitral Stenosis

Symptoms

- Pulmonary edema, atrial arrhythmias, fatigue, abdominal discomfort, edema, hemoptysis, recurrent pulmonary emboli, pulmonary infection, systemic embolization

Physical Exam

- **JVP:** elevated if RHF, no "a" wave if atrial fibrillation (AF)
- **Pulse:** normal contour, normal volume, may be irregularly irregular as in AF
- **Palpation:** PMI normal, S1 may be palpable, loud S2 suggests pulmonary HTN
- **Auscultation:** loud S1, opening snap, mid-diastolic decrescendo murmur with presystolic accentuation (lost in AF), possible PR (Graham Steell's murmur)
- **Extracardiac:** ± evidence of pulmonary HTN

6.4 Aortic Stenosis

Symptoms

- Dyspnea, angina pectoris, exertional syncope, CHF signs and symptoms in later course

Physical Exam

- **JVP:** normal or prominent "a" wave (septal hypertrophy)
- **Pulse:** pulsus parvus et tardus (slow-rising and small volume pulse), apical-carotid delay, brachial-radial delay
- **Palpation:** sustained apical beat, systolic thrill may be palpable over aortic area
- **Auscultation:** soft S2, delayed A2, S2 splitting may be lost or paradoxical, systolic crescendo-decrescendo ejection murmur radiating to neck/sternal border, S4 (late peaking correlates with severe AS)

EBM: Aortic Stenosis

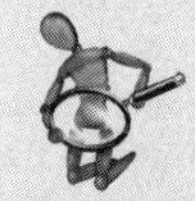

Effort syncope, slow rate of rise of the carotid artery pulsation, timing of peak murmur intensity in mid or late systole, and decreased intensity of S2 are all associated with an increased likelihood for aortic stenosis.

Absence of a systolic murmur or murmur radiating to the right common carotid artery is associated with a decreased likelihood of aortic stenosis.

Etchells E, Bell C, Robb K. 1997. *JAMA* 277(7):564-571.

6.5 Atrial Fibrillation (AF)

Symptoms

- Pulmonary congestion, angina pectoris, syncope, fatigue, anxiety, dyspnea, cardiomyopathy, signs of pulmonary emboli

Physical Exam

- **JVP:** absent “a” wave
- **Pulse:** irregularly irregular pulse, often tachycardic, variable pulse pressure in the carotid arterial pulse
- **Auscultation:** S1 usually varies in intensity

Investigations

- **ECG:** P waves not discernable, undulating baseline or sharply inscribed atrial deflections with varying amplitude and frequency (350-600 bpm)
- **Echocardiogram:** LA size helps to determine the likelihood of successful cardioversion and maintenance of sinus rhythm thereafter; also helps to identify underlying cardiac cause of AF (valvular heart disease or cardiomyopathy)

6.6 Mitral Regurgitation (MR)

Symptoms

- Fatigue, exertional dyspnea, orthopnea, symptoms of right-sided heart failure and LV failure

Physical Exam

- **JVP:** abnormally prominent “a” waves in patients with sinus rhythm and marked pulmonary hypertension and prominent “v” waves in those with accompanying severe TR
- **Pulse:** usually normal, arterial pulse may show a sharp upstroke in patients with severe MR
- **Palpation:** systolic thrill often palpable at cardiac apex, brisk systolic impulse and a palpable rapid-filling wave, apex beat often displaced laterally, RV heave palpable in patients with marked pulmonary hypertension
- **Auscultation:** systolic murmur of at least grade 3/6 intensity, may be holosystolic or decrescendo, S1 generally absent, soft or buried in the systolic murmur, wide splitting of S2, a low-pitched S3 occurring 0.12 to 0.17 s after the aortic valve closure sound, S4 often audible[2]
- **Extracardiac:** pulmonary edema, hepatic congestion, ankle edema, distended neck veins, ascites

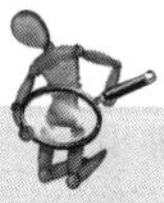

EBM: Mitral Regurgitation

Absence of a mitral area murmur or a late systolic/holosystolic murmur significantly reduces the likelihood of mitral regurgitation.

Etchells E, Bell C, Robb K. 1997. *JAMA* 277(7):564-571.

6.7 Infective Endocarditis (IE)

- Life-threatening infection of the endocardial surface of the heart, usually on the valves
  - Duke's criteria may be helpful in diagnosis

Table 9. Infectious Endocarditis

History	Signs/Symptoms
• Rheumatic fever • Prosthetic valves • Previous IE • IV drug users • Intravascular devices (e.g. arterial lines) • Most congenital heart malformations • Valvular dysfunction • Hypertrophic cardiomyopathy • MVP with MR • Recent surgeries • Indwelling catheters or hemodialysis	• Constitutional: fever, chills, malaise, night sweats, anorexia, arthralgias • Cardiac: murmur, palpitations, heart failure • Pulmonary: septic pulmonary embolism • Neurological: focal deficit, headache, meningitis • Metastatic infection: organ infarction • Embolic manifestations: o Petechiae: conjunctivae, buccal mucosa, palate o Splinter hemorrhages: linear dark red streaks under nails o Janeway lesions: nontender hemorrhagic macules on palm and soles o Osler's nodes: small painful nodules on fingers, toe pads, lasting hours to days o Roth spots: retinal hemorrhage with pale center near optic disc • Immune-mediated phenomena: vasculitis, glomerulonephritis, splenomegaly, synovitis

CARDIOVASCULAR

7. ECG INTERPRETATION

ECG Leads

- Six limb leads record voltages from the heart directed onto the frontal plane of the body (3 bipolar leads I, II, and III; 3 augmented unipolar leads (automated volt left, right, and foot [aVL, aVR, aVF]))[3]
- The six chest leads (V1 to V6) record voltages from the heart directed onto the horizontal plane of the body (6 unipolar leads)
- A wave of depolarization moving toward an electrode will record a positive deflection on an ECG; a negative deflection represents a wave of depolarization moving away from an electrode
- Direction of atrial depolarization: down and right
- Direction of septal depolarization: down and left
- Direction of verticular depolarization: down and right

Table 10. Anatomical Correspondence of the ECG Leads

Leads	Anatomical View
V1-V2	Right ventricle, posterior heart, septum
V3-V4	Interventricular septum, anterior LV wall
V5-V6	Anterior and lateral LV walls
V1-V2	Posterior part of the heart
V1-V4	Anterior part of the heart
R chest leads	Right side of the heart
I, aVL, V5-V6	Lateral part of the heart
II, III, aVF	Inferior part of the heart

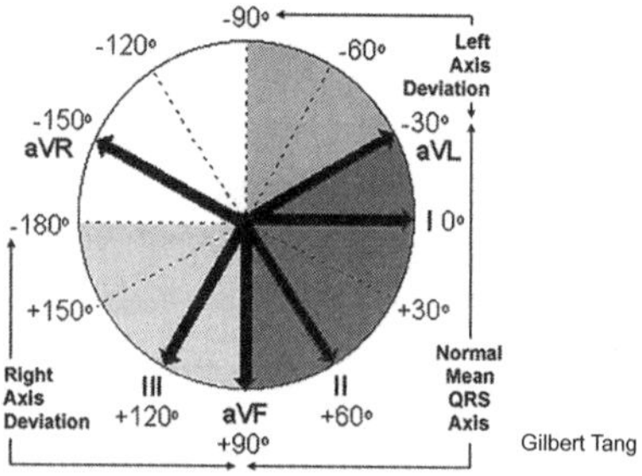

Figure 6. Axial ECG Leads and their Normal Ranges

CARDIOVASCULAR

8. APPROACH TO THE ECG

- Heart rate
- Rhythm
- Mean QRS axis
- Waves and segments
- Hypertrophy and chamber enlargement
- Ischemia/infarction

8.1 Heart Rate

- Each small box is 40 ms; each large box is 200 ms
- If HR is regular, divide 300 by the number of large squares between two consecutive R waves (e.g. HR is 60 if 5 large squares between consecutive R waves since 300/5 = 60)
- If a rough estimate of HR is required, simply count off the number of large boxes between two consecutive QRS complexes, using the sequence 300, 150, 100, 75, 60, 50: this corresponds to the HR in beats/min
- If HR is irregular, multiply the number of complexes in 6 s (30 large squares) by 10 to determine the average ventricular rate
- Normal sinus rhythm = 60-100 bpm; sinus bradycardia <60 bpm; sinus tachycardia >100 bpm

8.2 Rhythm

- Rhythm is considered regular if both RR and PP intervals are equal:
  - Sinus rhythm (i.e. every P wave followed by QRS, and every QRS preceded by P, P wave is positive in leads I or II, and aVF)
  - QRS complex: wide or narrow
  - Relationship between P waves and QRS complexes, prolonged PR intervals
  - Ectopic beats
  - Pattern: regular or irregular
  - If irregular, note if regularly irregular or irregularly irregular

8.3 Mean QRS Axis

- Many methods are available for a fast approximation of the mean QRS axis
- Normal mean QRS axis falls between -30° and +90° (up to +105°)

2-Lead Method (I, II)

1. Is the QRS complex of lead I positive or negative?
2. Is the QRS complex of lead II positive or negative?
3. Determine in which quadrant the mean QRS axis lies (e.g. if I is positive and II is positive, then the mean QRS lies between -30° and +90°, which is normal)

Isoelectric Lead Method (more precise)

1. Look for the most isoelectric lead (i.e. the net area under the curve for the QRS complex is 0): between the baseline and the curve
2. Find the perpendicular lead: is it positive or negative?
3. If positive, the mean QRS complex lies in the positive direction of that lead
   - **Left Axis Deviation:** mean axis between -30° and -90°
     - Common causes: left anterior hemiblock, inferior MI, LBBB, WPW
     - Associated causes: heart movement during respiration or an elevated left diaphragm associated with pregnancy, ascites or abdominal tumors
   - **Right Axis Deviation:** mean axis between +90° and 180°
     - Common causes: RVH, RBBB, dextrocardia, acute heart strain (e.g. massive pulmonary embolism), may also be seen in thin individuals, left posterior hemiblock (diagnosis of exclusion)

Table 11. Important ECG Characteristics

	Significance	Parameters
P Wave	Represents atrial depolarization Rhythm is sinus if P wave is positive in leads I, II, and aVF	<2.5 mm in height and <120 ms
PR Interval	Represents time taken for impulse to travel from SA node to ventricles	Measured from beginning of P wave to beginning of QRS (120-200 ms)
QRS Complex	Represents ventricular depolarization	• Narrow QRS complex (<120 ms) • Normal (120 ms) • Wide QRS (>120 ms) represents abnormally slow ventricular activation
QT Interval	Represents time taken for ventricles to depolarize and then repolarize	• Measured from the beginning of QRS complex to end of T wave • Normal is ½ of the preceding RR interval (HR between 60-90 bpm) • QTc = QT Corrected: o Male <450 ms o Female <460 ms
ST Segment	Represents time interval between depolarization and repolarization	Shorter ST segment with higher heart rate
T Wave	Represents ventricular repolarization	• Usually positive in all leads except aVR • An inverted T wave in leads V3-V6 is usually abnormal

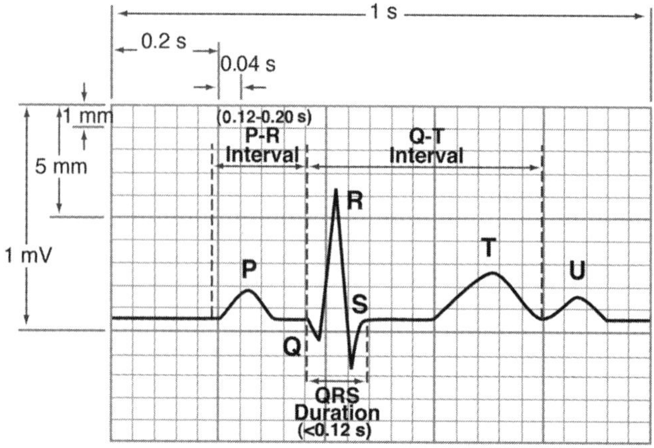

Pina Kingman

Figure 7. ECG and Normal Values

Table 12. Common Arrhythmias (Not Inclusive)

Location	Example	
Atrium		
Premature Atrial Contractions (PAC)	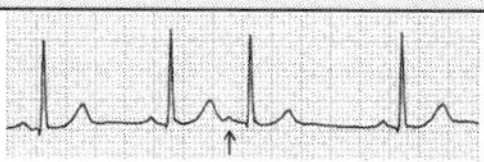	*
Atrial Flutter	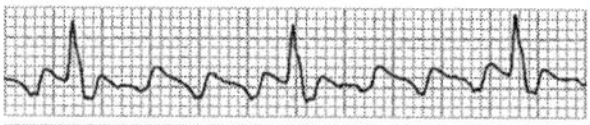	†
Atrial Fibrillation (AF)	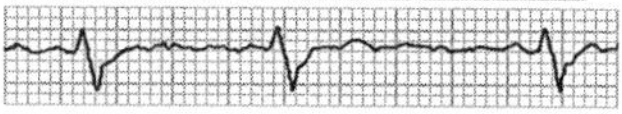	†
Supraventricular Tachycardia (SVT)	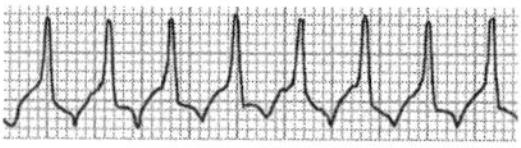	†
AV Node		
Conduction Blocks: **1° Atrioventricular Block** (↑ PR interval)	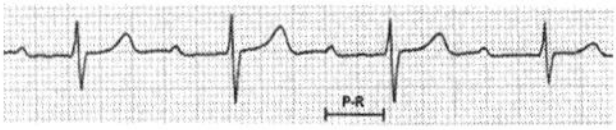	*
2° Atrioventricular Block (Wenckebach shown to the right) – Mobitz Type 1 (Wenckebach) – Mobitz Type 2 (Classic)	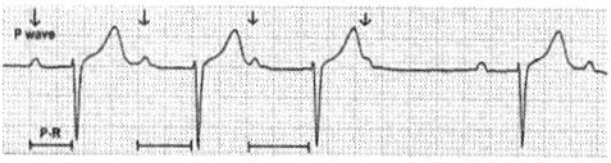	*
3° Atrioventricular Block (complete heart block)	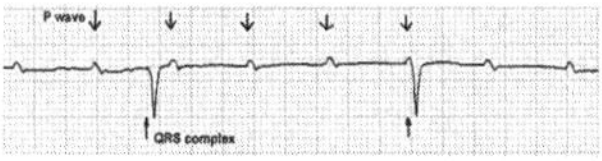	*
Ventricle		
Premature Ventricular Contractions (PVC)	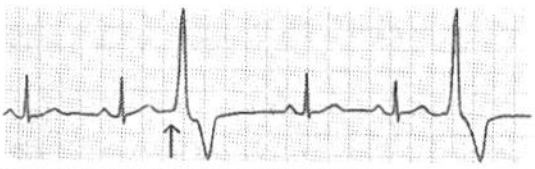	*
Ventricular Tachycardia (VTach)	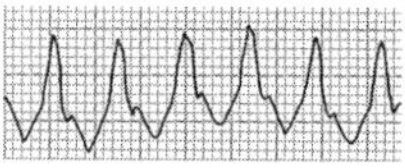	†

Table 12. Common Arrhythmias (continued)

Location	Example
Ventricle	
Torsades de Pointes	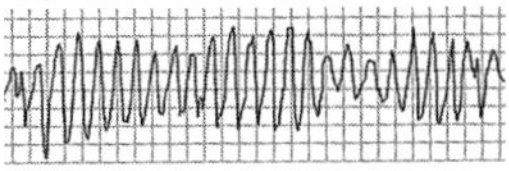 †
Ventricular Fibrillation (VF)	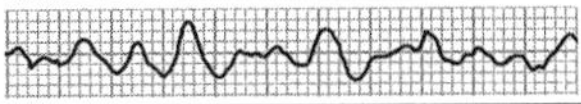 †

*GE Marquette, 2000
†Patient samples

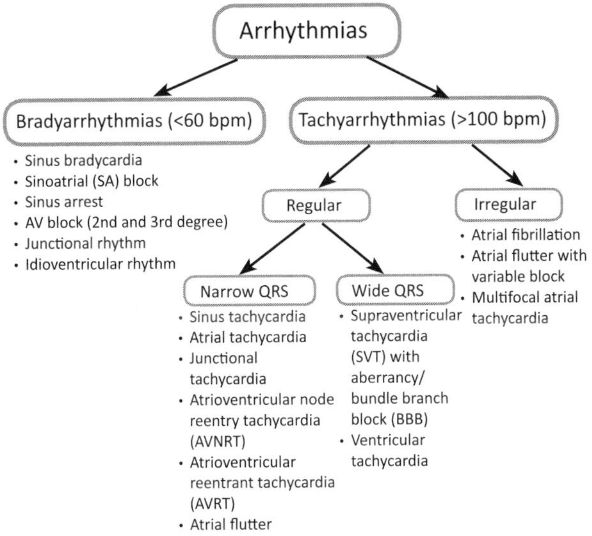

Figure 8. General Approach to Arrhythmias

8.4 Waves and Segments (P Wave Abnormality)

- Left Atrial Enlargement
  - LA enlarges posteriorly (downward deflection in V1)
  - In V1 a deep terminal component that is ≥40 ms and ≥1 mm deep
  - P wave has double peaks and P wave >120 ms (P mitrale) in lead II
- Right Atrial Enlargement
  - rA enlarges vertically (tall P wave in inferior leads)
  - Large P wave >2.5 mm (height) in leads II, III or aVF
  - In V1 a large positive wave >1.5 mm may be seen

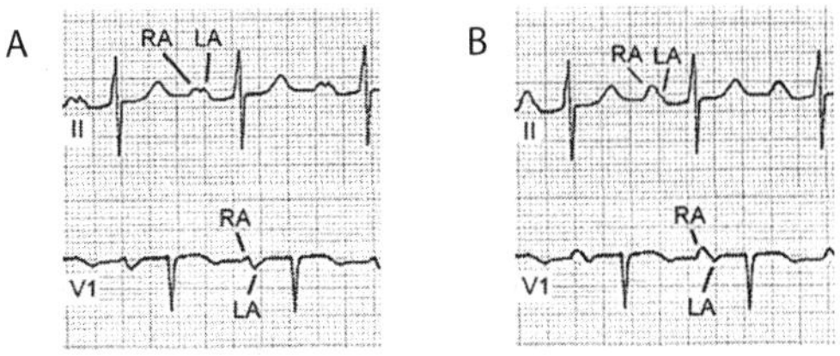

Figure 9. (A) Left and (B) Right Atrial Enlargement ECG Tracing
Dr. F. Yanowitz, 1999.

8.5 Hypertrophy and Chamber Enlargement

- Left Ventricular Hypertrophy (LVH):
  - Leads I, aVL, V5, and V6 show taller R waves
  - Leads V1 and V2 show deeper than normal S waves
  - Criteria for the diagnosis of LVH:
    - » S in V1 + R in V5 or V6 >35 mm above 40 yr (>40 mm for age 31-40 yr, >45 mm for age 21-30 yr)
    - » R in aVL >11 mm
    - » R in I + S in III >25 mm
  - Additional criteria: left atrial enlargement, ventricular strain (asymmetric ST depression in leads I, aVL, V4-V6)
  - Associated features: delayed intrinsicoid deflection (longer QR interval, >0.05 s)
- Right Ventricular Hypertrophy (RVH):
  - Results in a large R wave in V1 and a large S wave in V6
  - Criteria for the diagnosis of RVH:
    - » Right axis deviation
    - » R/S ratio >1 or qR in lead V1
    - » RV strain pattern: ST segment depression and T wave inversion in leads V1-V2
- Bundle Branch Blocks:
  - Left bundle branch block (LBBB)
    - » Right ventricle depolarizes first due to LBBB
    - » QRS >120 ms
    - » Broad-notched R wave in V5, V6, I, aVL
  - Right bundle branch block (RBBB)
    - » QRS >120 ms
    - » QRS positive in lead V1 (rSR')
    - » Broad S wave in leads I, V5-V6 (>40 ms)
    - » Use first 60 ms of the QRS complex to determine mean QRS axis

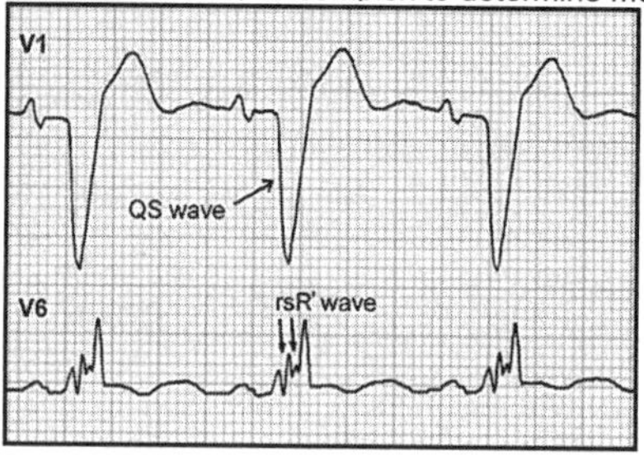

Figure 10. LBBB ECG Tracing
GE Marquette, 2000.

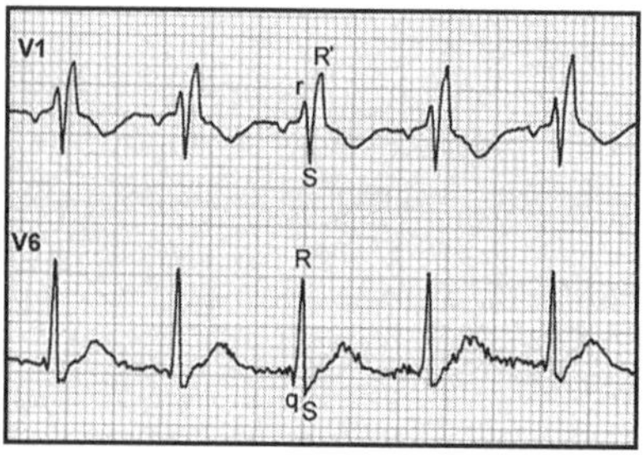

Figure 11. RBBB ECG Tracing
GE Marquette, 2000.

8.6 Ischemia/Infarction

Transmural MI

- Q waves are possible evidence of a prior transmural MI
- A significant Q wave must be either 40 ms wide (1 small box or greater) or one-third the height of the R wave
- For the Q waves to be suggestive of prior infarction, Q waves should be present in at least 2 leads in the same territory

Table 13. Localization of the Acute MI

Anatomical Location	Leads with Abnormal ECG Complexes	Associated Coronary Artery
Posterior	V1, V2 (tall R, not Q)	RCA or CFX (distal)
Inferior	II, III, aVF	RCA
Anterior Septal	V1, V2	LAD
Anterior Apical	V3, V4	LAD (distal)
Lateral	I, aVL, V5, V6	CFX
Anterior	V2-V5	LAD (proximal)
Right Ventricle	R chest leads V3, V4	RCA

CFX = left circumflex artery, LAD = left anterior descending artery, RCA = right coronary artery

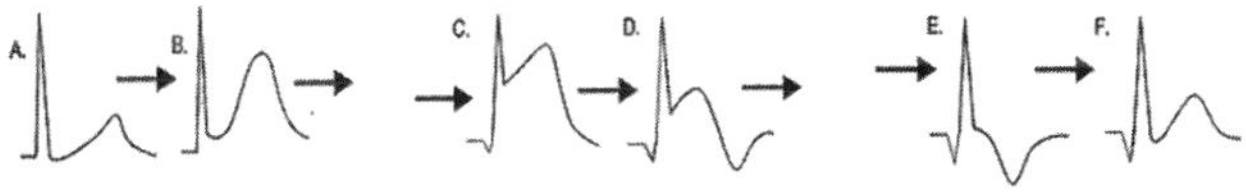

Figure 12. ECG Evolution during Acute Q-Wave MI
Dr. F. Yanowitz, 1999.

Table 14. Legend Corresponding to Figure 12

Time Frame	ECG Changes
A. Normal	None
B. Acute	ST elevation
C. Hours	ST elevation, depressed R wave, Q wave begins
D. 1-2 Days	T wave inversion, increased Q wave
E. Days	ST normalizes, T wave inverted
F. Weeks	ST and T normal, Q wave remains

8.7 ST Segment and T Wave Abnormalities

- Non-Q wave MI involves only the subendocardial layers of the myocardium (not transmural)
- Results in ECG changes, such as T wave inversion and ST segment depression
- Causes of ST segment depression[4]:
  - Angina (ischemia)
  - Subendocardial infarction
  - Acute posterior wall MI (V1 and V2)
  - LVH strain
  - LBBB

- Causes of ST segment elevation[4]:
  - Acute MI
  - Post MI
  - Acute pericarditis
  - Ventricular aneurysm
  - Early repolarization

REFERENCES

1. Braunwald E, Zipes DP, Libby P. *Heart Disease: A Textbook of Cardiovascular Medicine.* Philadelphia: Saunders; 2011.
2. Lilly LS (Editor). *Pathophysiology of Heart Disease: A Collaborative Project of Medical Students and Faculty*, 5th ed. Philadelphia: Wolters Kluwer/Lippincott Williams & Wilkins; 2011.
3. Casella L, Nader A. *ECG Made Simple*. 2012. Available from: http://www.ecgmadesimple.com.
4. Wesley K. *Basic Dysrhythmias and Acute Coronary Syndromes: Interpretation and Management*. St. Louis: Mosby Jems; 2011.
5. Bickley LS, Szilagyi PG, Bates B. *Bates' Guide to Physical Examination and History Taking*, 10th ed. Philadelphia: Lippincott Williams & Wilkins; 2009.
6. Dugani S, Lam D (Editors). *The Toronto Notes 2009: Comprehensive Medical Reference. Toronto*: Toronto Notes for Medical Students, Inc; 2009.
7. Fauci AS. *Harrison's Principles of Internal Medicine*. New York: McGraw-Hill; 2008.
8. Swartz MH. *Textbook of Physical Diagnosis: History and Examination*, 6th ed. Philadelphia: Saunders Elsevier; 2010.

The Geriatric Exam

Editors:
Holly Delaney
Aneta Krakowski

Faculty Reviewers:
Camilla Wong, MD, FRCP(C)
Samir Sinha, MD, DPhil, FRCP(C)

TABLE OF CONTENTS

GERIATRIC

1. COMMON CHIEF COMPLAINTS

- Memory concerns
- Medication issues
- Fatigue
- Dizziness
- Chest pain
- Constipation
- Acute and chronic pain
- Mobility concerns
- Vision or hearing problems
- Urinary and fecal incontinence
- Functional decline
- Elder abuse and neglect
- Falls

2. FOCUSED HISTORY

The geriatric history is similar to a complete, general medical history. However, there are a few specific issues that must be addressed when assessing a geriatric patient.

As early as possible during the interview, evaluate the patient's ability to hear, see, understand, and give an accurate historical account in the language you speak or understand. Consider using sensory aids to assist in history taking.

Identification Data

- Age, gender, and handedness
- Marital status, past/current occupation, and current living status (i.e. living alone at home vs. retirement home)

Chief Complaint

- Illness often presents as a change in function with atypical symptoms
- To elicit a vague CC, use questions such as "What has changed recently?" and "What is your most concerning issue today?"

History of Present Illness

- Patients may present with multiple issues and nonspecific symptoms without a definite organ system involved
- Making a comprehensive problem list is helpful in addressing all complaints in order of functional importance

Past Medical, Surgical, and Psychiatric History

- Often long, complicated, and difficult to remember for many patients
  - The use of collateral history from family doctors, family members, caregivers, and prior patient records is often helpful
- Use of more specific questions can be of assistance: "Have you ever had a heart attack?" or "Have you ever had heart surgery?" instead of "Do you have any medical problems?"

Medications

- Polypharmacy is prevalent in the elderly and you must ask, in detail, about drugs they are taking, drugs they may have recently stopped taking, route of administration (blister pack, dosette, orally), OTC medications, herbal remedies/teas, supplements, and vitamins
  - It may be useful to have the patient or caregiver bring in everything they are taking
- Note that polypharmacy is one of the risk factors of nonadherence: ask to see if they are taking all medications as directed
- The risk of drug-drug interactions and adverse drug reactions increases with the number of prescriptions
- Ask about pneumococcal, influenza, shingles, and tetanus vaccinations

GERIATRIC

Social History

- Determine living arrangements, marital status, presence and willingness to accept help, family support and community resources available. Document existence of directives such as power of attorney for personal care and finances or a living will
- Do not forget that some elders are lesbian, gay, bisexual or transgendered; therefore, use of inclusive language such as 'partner' will help build a better rapport
- Ask about the content of a typical day for the patient, extent of social relationships, suitability and safety of home, occupational history, cultural background, interests, sources of income, and veteran status
- Substance use/abuse (includes smoking, alcohol intake, use of sleep aids, and daily caffeine consumption) is an important and often overlooked aspect of the geriatric history[1]
- Ask if plans exist for times of illness or functional decline
- Ask caregivers whether a back-up plan of care exists for the patient in case of caregiver misfortune or ill-health
- Enquire about availability and attitude of caregivers and neighbors, as well as availability of emergency help
- For inpatients, enquire about their discharge plans

Mental Status Examination

- The Folstein MMSE is a screen for assessing cognitive impairment (see **Psychiatric Exam**, p.322)
- Some patients may be upset or offended by the nature of the questions. Avoid using the word "test" or "exam". One approach is to introduce the MMSE by saying, "I have a few questions and tasks that will allow me to see how your memory and concentration are functioning today." Also telling them in advance that a memory screen is a standard part of your exam allows them to expect it
- If the score is <24/30, suspect cognitive impairment

- Note that MMSE scores may also be low in patients with sensory impairment, dysphasia, depression, poor English or low education level[2]
- The MoCA (Montreal Cognitive Assessment) is a more sensitive tool for detecting mild cognitive impairment compared to MMSE[3]

The Functional Assessment

- Used as a screen to identify any impairments and dependence on others

*Activities of Daily Living (ADLs) (**TEACHD**: **T**oileting, **E**ating, **A**mbulating, **C**leaning, **H**ygiene, **D**ressing)*

- Are you able to get out of bed by yourself in the morning?
- Can you use the bathroom by yourself?
- Do you bathe yourself and do your own grooming?
- Are you able to dress yourself?
- Are you able to walk without any assistance (person, cane, walker)?
- Do you experience difficulty going up or down stairs?

Hint: These are the six things you do every morning!

*Instrumental Activities of Daily Living (IADLs) (**SHAFT**: **S**hopping, **H**ousework, **A**ccounting, **F**ood preparation, **T**ransport, **T**elephoning, **T**aking medications)*

- Do you do the cooking, cleaning, laundry or shopping?
- Are you able to take care of banking, paying the bills, and making financial decisions?
- Does anyone help you to make or get to your appointments?
- Are you driving at the moment? If yes, are you experiencing any difficulties with your driving? (see **Driving Competency and Safety**, p.76)

GERIATRIC

Review of Systems

Remember to ask about these systems in particular:

- **General:** fatigue, sleep patterns, constitutional symptoms
- **H&N:** visual changes, hearing loss
- **GI:** constipation, incontinence
- **GU:** incontinence, frequency, nocturia, sexual function
- **Cognition:** memory, visuo-spatial, language or time/place orientation concerns, executive function
- **CNS/MSK:** gait, balance, falls, and other injuries
- **Psychiatric:** mood changes, isolation, recent loss of loved ones
- **Nutrition:** weight loss, appetite
- **Derm:** skin integrity, wounds, skin changes

Hints and Tips for the Geriatric History

When taking a geriatric history, remember to ask about the geriatric giants and the **5 I**'s:

Geriatric Giants	5 I's
Falls	**I**mmobility
Confusion	**I**ntellect
Incontinence	**I**ncontinence
Polypharmacy	**I**atrogenesis **I**mpaired homeostasis

- Due to communication difficulties or multiplicity of complaints, history taking can be lengthy. If the patient is medically stable, the history need not be completed at once and can be broken down into several sessions. Setting priorities is important for efficient management

- Underreporting of symptoms is a common occurrence in the elderly due to health beliefs, fear, depression, cognitive impairment or cultural barriers. Ask specific questions in a thorough review of systems to uncover medical problems
- A corroborative history, from a family member or caregiver, is often important

3. FOCUSED PHYSICAL EXAM

GERIATRIC

Vital Signs

- **Weight:** acute weight loss (>3%) may be a sign of dehydration in the elderly
- **Height:** reduction may indicate osteoporosis, vertebral compression fractures
- **Orthostatic Hypotension** (see **General History and Physical Exam**, p.12)
  - Could be a normal consequence of aging, medication side effect, or a disease state
  - Check supine vs. standing with a two minute pause in between positions (recommended); if unable, check supine vs. sitting or sitting vs. standing
  - Do not miss auscultatory gap in elderly hypertensive patients (see **General History and Physical Exam**, p.11)

Head and Neck

- **Eyes** (see **Ophthalmological Exam**, p.235)
  - Visual acuity and fields
  - Screen for cataracts, macular degeneration, glaucoma
  - ***Note:*** previous cataract surgery can cause unequal and less reactive pupils but not RAPD (RAPD is always due to optic neuropathy)
- **Ears** (see **Head and Neck Exam**, p.101)
  - Hearing impairment can be caused by wax impaction (can result in a 30% conductive hearing loss)
  - High frequency hearing loss is common with aging
  - Assess for presbycusis and tinnitus
- **Dentition**
  - Ask patient to remove dentures when examining the mouth
  - Check for dryness, odor, dental, and periodontal problems
  - Lack of dental work and ill-fitting dentures may lead to difficulty eating, weight loss, and malnutrition
  - Look for signs of oral cancers
- **Neck** (see **Head and Neck Exam**, p.113)
  - Auscultate for carotid bruits (carotid bruits can indicate diffuse vascular disease and should lead to detailed questioning about symptoms of CAD, and past TIAs/strokes)
  - Thyroid exam (***Note:*** patients can have subclinical hypothyroidism)
  - Assess for neck masses (malignancy, infection, inflammation)
- **Lymph Nodes** (see **Lymphatic System and Lymph Node Exam**, p.125)
  - With advanced age, lymph nodes usually become smaller, decrease in number, and become more fibrotic and fatty

Chest

- Examine for arrhythmias, murmurs, and extra heart sounds (see **Cardiovascular Exam**, p.55)
  - Aortic stenosis, aortic sclerosis, and mitral regurgitation are common in the elderly
  - Although irregular rhythms are common, they should not be considered "normal"
  - A fourth heart sound is often associated with HTN

- Examine for cyanosis, signs of pneumonia, COPD exacerbation, and airway pathology (see **Respiratory Exam**, p.351, 360)
- **Posterior Chest:** Dorsal kyphosis may indicate vertebral compression fractures and osteoporosis

Peripheral Vascular System
- Peripheral pulses, edema (see **Peripheral Vascular Exam**, p.300)
- Arterial or venous insufficiency and complications (especially in diabetics)
- Auscultate for aortic, renal, and femoral artery bruits

Gastrointestinal
- Auscultate and palpate for abdominal aortic aneurysm (see **Peripheral Vascular Exam**, p.307)
- Hernial orifices (abdominal, umbilical) (see **Urological Exam**, p.373)

Genitourinary
- Examine for the following in particular: cystocele, rectocele, atrophic vaginitis (see **Gynecological Exam**, p.84 and **Urological Exam**, p.369)
- Urinary retention
- Hernial orifices (inguinal, femoral) (see **Urological Exam**, p.367)
- Rectal examination (see **Urological Exam**, p.368)

Dermatological
- Cancers are common, especially on the hands and face where sun exposure is greatest; actinic keratoses are precursor lesions and should be treated (see **Essentials of Dermatology**, p.413)
- Investigate for any pressure sores, especially in immobile patients (e.g. sacrum, heel, bony occipital prominence)
- Ulcerations/edema in the lower extremities signal vascular or neuropathic impairments which must be investigated further

Musculoskeletal
- Determine range of motion of all joints
- Pay special attention to the hip and shoulder; impairment in the upper extremities could interfere with ADLs
- Check foot hygiene, deformity, and assess need for chiropody
  - If appropriate, check footwear
- Joint abnormalities in the hips, knees, and feet may lead to gait abnormalities

Neurological
- Diminished vibration sense and an absent ankle jerk reflex are common in elderly patients

Gait Assessment
- Observe the patient:
  - Rising from the bed or chair (note use of arms and foot stance)
  - Note gait initiation, velocity, trajectory, and cadence
    - Parkinsonian patients exhibit delayed gait initiation and reduced gait velocity
    - Abnormal trajectory may be indicative of vestibular disease
  - Note posture, ataxia, and use of hands while walking
    - Kyphosis may indicate osteoporosis
    - Sway and/or use of walking aid may indicate cerebellar dysfunction
  - Step height and step length usually decreased in elderly
    - Asymmetry in step height or length may result from stroke

- Turning (one-step turn vs. multi-step) and balance
  - Parkinsonian patients exhibit a multi-step turn
- Double-stance time increase (where both feet are on the ground for a prolonged time)
  - Parkinsonian shuffle: Patient's feet never leave the ground, stance is narrow, and stride length is decreased

4. COMMON DISORDERS

Disorders marked with (✓) are discussed in **Common Clinical Scenarios**

✓ Falls
✓ Urinary incontinence
- Dizziness
- Memory loss/confusion
- Constipation
- Depression/anxiety
- Shortness of breath (dyspnea)
- Chest pain
- Joint pain
- Intermittent claudication
- Weight loss/poor appetite
- Functional decline

5. COMMON CLINICAL SCENARIOS

GERIATRIC

5.1 Falls

History (SPLATT)

- **S**ymptoms: dizziness, palpitations, dyspnea, chest pain, weakness, loss of consciousness
- **P**revious falls (frequency, time of day)
- **L**ocation, witnesses
- **A**ctivity
- **T**ime of fall
- **T**rauma: physical, psychological (fear of falls)
- Other: recent medication changes, availability of gait aids or Life Line

Physical Exam

- Complete physical exam with emphasis on:
  - **CVS:** orthostatic changes in blood pressure and pulse, arrhythmias
  - **MSK:** injury secondary to fall, lower extremity function, podiatric problems, poorly fitting shoes
  - **CNS:** vision, muscle power and symmetry, lower extremity peripheral nerve sensation, reflexes, gait (turning, getting in/out of a chair) and balance (Romberg test and sternal push), cognitive screen

5.2 Urinary Incontinence

- Transient incontinence
  - Due to factors outside urinary tract
  - Etiology of transient incontinence (**DIAPPERS**):
    - **D**elirium or confusional state
    - **I**nfection, urinary (symptomatic)
    - **A**trophic urethritis, vaginitis
    - **P**harmaceuticals (drugs)
    - **P**sychological disorder, depression
    - **E**xcessive urine output (e.g. due to hypercalcemia)
    - **R**estricted mobility (e.g. Foley catheter, IV line)
    - **S**tool impaction
- Established incontinence
  - If leakage persists after transient causes of incontinence have been addressed, lower urinary tract causes must be considered
- Overactive bladder (OAB or urge incontinence) and stress incontinence are common in the elderly
- For details on classification and pathogenesis, see **Urological Exam**, p.366

History

- Characterize the voiding pattern and determine whether the patient has symptoms of abnormal voiding
  - Voiding record: record of volume and time of each void or incontinent episode; kept by the patient or caregiver during a 48 to 72 h period
  - Type: urge, reflex, stress, overflow or mixed
  - Frequency, hesitancy, duration
  - Pattern: diurnal, nocturnal or both; after taking medications
  - Precipitants (i.e. cough, medication use)
  - Palliating features
  - Associated symptoms, e.g. straining to void, incomplete emptying, dysuria, hematuria, suprapubic or perineal discomfort, prolonged voiding
  - Alteration in bowel habit or sexual function
  - Medications, including nonprescription drugs
  - Assess fluid intake (excessive volume or diuretics e.g. caffeine)
- "Storage" symptoms: ask about **FUND**
  - **F**requency
  - **U**rgency
  - **N**octuria
  - **D**ysuria
- ***Note:*** the effects of the incontinence should be ascertained (e.g. emotional and social factors)

GERIATRIC

Physical Exam

- Identify other medical conditions, e.g. heart failure, peripheral edema
- Test for stress-induced leakage when bladder is full
- **Pelvic:** look for atrophic vaginitis, pelvic muscle laxity, pelvic mass
- **Rectal:** look for irritation, resting tone, and voluntary control of anal sphincter, prostate nodules, fecal impaction
- **Neurological:** mental status and sensory/motor examination, including sacral reflexes, and perineal sensation

5.3 Other Clinical Scenarios

- Delirium, dementia (see **Psychiatric Exam**, p.341)
- Depression (see **Psychiatric Exam**, p.329)
- Heart diseases (see **Cardiovascular Exam**, p.58)

6. ELDER ABUSE

6.1 Definition

- Mistreatment or neglect that a senior experiences at the hands of their spouses, children, other family members, caregivers, service providers or other individuals in positions of power or trust; elder abuse is violence
- Abuse and neglect of older adults occurs in both domestic and institutional settings
- Abused elderly have a significantly increased risk of death

6.2 Types of Elder Abuse

- Physical abuse
- Sexual abuse
- Psychological/emotional abuse
- Social isolation
- Financial exploitation
- Neglect

6.3 Prevalence

- An estimated 2-10% of people over age 65 experience some form of elder abuse[4]

6.4 Risk Factors

- Family history of violence
- Caregiver stress

6.5 Signs of Elder Abuse

- Overall appearance and signs of neglect
- Injuries inconsistent with explanation
- Discrepancies between patient and caregiver account of illness or injury
- Behavior: withdrawn, depressed, fearful, anxious
- Malnourishment
- Pressure ulcers
- Welts, scars, abrasions, lacerations, burns
- Alopecia
- Fractures and bruises
- Multiple injuries in different stages of healing
- Recurrent injuries
- Signs of sexual abuse

GERIATRIC

7. DRIVING COMPETENCY AND SAFETY

Assessing an elderly patient's ability to operate a motor vehicle is a common task in many geriatric settings. In Ontario, the Ministry of Transportation requires everyone over 80 yr of age to pass a vision test as well as a multiple choice exam on road safety.

Some points to keep in mind when assessing such patients:

- **Alcohol**
  - Alcohol dependence: should not be allowed to drive, must complete a rehabilitation program and remain abstinent and seizure-free for 12 mo before driving
  - Drinking and driving: must not drive for 12 mo
- **Blood Pressure Abnormalities**
  - Hypertension: sustained BP >170/110 should be evaluated carefully
  - Hypotension: if syncopal, discontinue until attacks are treated and preventable
- **Cardiovascular Disease**
  - Suspected asymptomatic CAD: no restrictions
  - ST segment elevation myocardial infarction (STEMI), non-ST segment elevation myocardial infarction (NSTEMI, with significant LV damage), coronary bypass: wait 1 mo
  - NSTEMI (no significant LV damage), unstable angina: wait 7 d
  - Percutaneous coronary intervention (PCI): wait 48 h
- **Cerebrovascular Conditions**
  - TIA: should not be allowed to drive until a medical assessment is completed
  - Stroke: should not drive for at least 1 mo; may resume driving if functionally able, no obvious risk for recurrence, and if on medication
- **Chronic Obstructive Pulmonary Disease (COPD)**
  - Mild/moderate impairment: no restrictions
  - Moderate impairment requiring supplemental oxygen: road test with supplemental oxygen
- **Cognitive Impairment**
  - Moderate or severe dementia: ineligible for license pending complete neurologic assessment

- Mild dementia: if unsure of driving safety refer for on-road driving assessment, if sure of driving safety reassess driving ability every 6-12 mo
- **Diabetes**
  - Diet controlled, oral hypoglycemics: no restrictions
  - Insulin use: may drive if no history of impairment due to alcohol or drug abuse and no severe hypoglycemic episode in the last 6 months
- **Drugs**
  - Be aware of: analgesics, anticholinergics, anticonvulsants, antidepressants, antipsychotics, opiates, sedatives, stimulants
  - Degree of impairment varies: patients should be warned about the effect of the medication on driving
- **Hearing Loss**
  - Acute labyrinthitis, positional vertigo with horizontal head movement, recurrent vertigo: advise not to drive until condition resolves
  - Effect of impaired hearing on ability to drive safely is controversial
- **Musculoskeletal Disorders**
  - Physician's role is to report etiology, prognosis, and extent of disability (pain, range of motion, coordination, muscle strength)
- **Postoperative**
  - Outpatient, conscious sedation: no driving up to 24 h
  - Outpatient, general anesthesia: no driving for >24 h
- **Seizures**
  - First, single, unprovoked: no driving for 3 mo until complete neurologic assessment, EEG, CT head
  - Epilepsy: can drive if seizure-free on medication and compliant for 12 mo
- **Visual Impairment**
  - Acuity: should not be <20/50 with adequate continuous field of vision when both eyes are examined simultaneously

Summary: Evaluate SAFE DRIVE

- **S**afety and record (from Ministry of Transportation)
- **A**ttention skills
- **F**amily report
- **E**thanol
- **D**rugs
- **R**eaction time
- **I**ntellectual impairment
- **V**ision and visuospatial ability
- **E**xecutive functions

Clinical Pearl: Tips for Management of Geriatric Patients

1. Fecal or urinary retention: rule out fecal impaction
2. Driving: always consider assessment of fitness to drive in management of any condition in the elderly
3. Renal function: creatinine clearance is a more accurate way to assess renal function than serum creatinine level due to the decline in renal clearance and lean muscle mass that may make serum creatinine normal in the elderly
4. Advance care directives: make sure these are known to the team during routine visits. Such discussions are preferably held during normal outpatient visits rather than when an acute life-threatening event is imminent or occurring
5. For pain control, a good trial of acetaminophen should be attempted first. If a narcotic is needed, hydromorphone is generally better tolerated than morphine in the elderly[5]

GERIATRIC

REFERENCES

1. Blazer DG, Wu LT. 2009. The epidemiology of at-risk and binge drinking among middle-aged and elderly community adults: National Survey on Drug Use and Health. *Am J Psychiatry* 166(10):1162-1169.
2. Crum RM, Anthony JC, Bassett SS, Folstein MF. 1993. Population-based norms for the Mini-Mental State Examination by age and educational level. *JAMA* 269(18):2386-2391.
3. Nasreddine ZS, Phillips NA, Bédirian V, Charbonneau S, Whitehead V, Collin I, et al. 2005. The Montreal Cognitive Assessment, MoCA: A brief screening tool for mild cognitive impairment. *J Am Geriatr Soc* 53(4):695-699.
4. Lachs MS, Pillemer K. 2004. Elder abuse. *Lancet* 364(9441):1263-1272.
5. Pergolizzi J, Böger RH, Budd K, Dahan A, Erdine S, Hans G, et al. 2008. Opioids and the management of chronic severe pain in the elderly: Consensus statement of an International Expert Panel with focus on the six clinically most often used World Health Organization Step III opioids (buprenorphine, fentanyl, hydromorphone, methadone morphine, oxycodone). *Pain Pract* 8(4):287-313.
6. American Geriatrics Society. *American Geriatrics Society/British Geriatrics Society Clinical Practice Guideline for Prevention of Falls in Older Persons*. New York: American Geriatrics Society; 2010.
7. Bickley LS, Szilagyi PG, Bates B. *Bates' Guide to Physical Examination and History Taking*, 10th ed. Philadelphia: Lippincott Williams & Wilkins; 2009.
8. Canadian Medical Association. Determining medical fitness to operate motor vehicles. *CMA Driver's Guide*, 7th ed. Ottawa: Canadian Medical Association; 2006.
9. Frank C, Szlanta A. 2010. Office management of urinary incontinence among older patients. *Can Fam Physician* 56(11):1115-1120.
10. Ganz DA, Bao Y, Shekelle PG, Rubenstein LZ. 2007. Will my patient fall? *JAMA* 297(1):77-86.
11. McDonald L, Collins A. *Abuse and Neglect of Older Adults: A Discussion Paper*. Ottawa: Family Violence Prevention Unit, Health Canada; 2000.
12. Tideiksaar R. 1996. Preventing falls: How to identify risk factors and reduce complications. *Geriatrics* 51(2):43-53.

The Gynecological Exam

Editors:
Cassandra Greenberg
Fanyu Yang

Faculty Reviewers:
Richard Pittini, MD, MEd, FACOG, FRCS(C)
Donna Steele, MD, MA, FRCS(C)

TABLE OF CONTENTS

GYNECOLOGICAL

1. ESSENTIAL ANATOMY

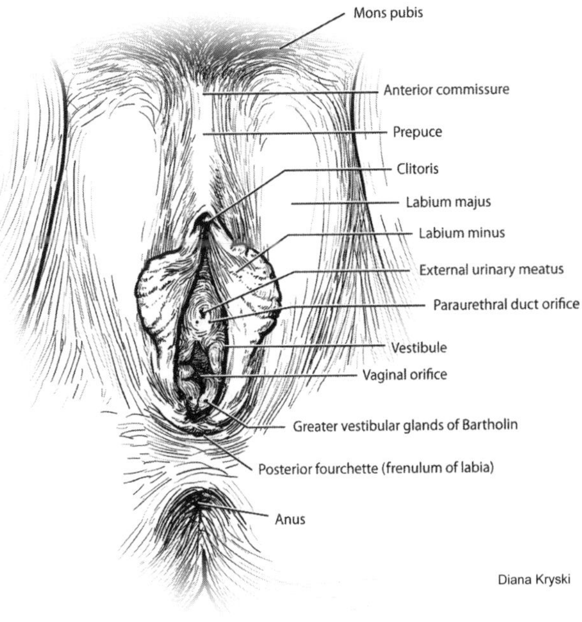

Figure 1. External Female Genitalia

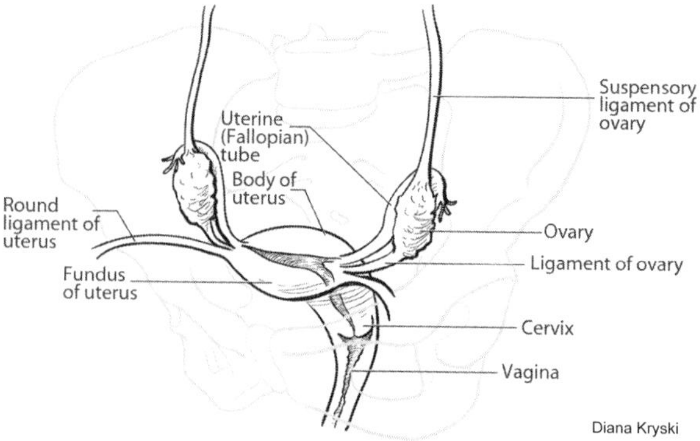

Figure 2. Female Reproductive Tract

2. COMMON CHIEF COMPLAINTS

- Abdominal or pelvic pain
- Abnormal vaginal bleeding (between or during menses, postmenopausal)
- Absence/cessation of menses (amenorrhea)
- Painful menses (dysmenorrhea)
- Decreased libido
- Difficulty getting pregnant (infertility)
- Painful intercourse (dyspareunia)
- Pelvic/abdominal mass
- Symptoms of menopause
- Vaginal discharge
- Vulvovaginal itchiness

GYNECOLOGICAL

3. FOCUSED GYNECOLOGICAL HISTORY

Menstrual History

- Last menstrual period (LMP): specify first day of last menses
- Onset of menopause (normally between 44-55 yr, mean 51.2 yr)
- Duration of menses (normally between 3-7 d)
- Cycle regularity
- Cycle length (measured as interval between first day of menses to first day of menses in subsequent month; normally 21 to 35 d)
- Flow: normal = dark red discharge; bright red blood ± clots may be excessive
  - Pad/tampon count and saturation can help quantify
- Symptoms of premenstrual syndrome (PMS) (4-10 d before menses):
  - Anxiety, nervousness, mood swings, irritability, food cravings, change in libido, difficulty sleeping, breast tenderness, headaches, and fluid retention
- Dysmenorrhea: age of onset, severity of pain (and PQRST), amount of disability, current treatment
- Abnormal menstrual bleeding (see **Table 1**)
- Menopause
  - Symptoms: hot flashes, flushing, sweating, sleep disturbances, vaginal dryness, vulvovaginal atrophy, mood changes, dysuria/frequency
  - Hormonal therapy
  - Postmenopausal bleeding (bleeding after 6 mo without periods warrants further investigation)

Table 1. Types of Abnormal Uterine Bleeding (AUB)

Type	Definition
Amenorrhea	Absence of periods (primary vs. secondary)
Polymenorrhea	Increased frequency
Oligomenorrhea	Decreased frequency (menstrual cycle >35 d)
Menorrhagia	Increased duration or flow
Metrorrhagia	Inter-menstrual bleeding
Contact Bleeding	Postcoital, post-douching

Sexual and Contraceptive History (5 P's)

Table 2. 5 P's of Sexual and Contraceptive History

Component of History Taking	Questions to Consider
Partners	• Current sexual activity, number and gender of partners (men/women/both), duration of marriage(s)/significant relationship(s)
Practices	• Type(s) of sexual practices (vaginal, oral, anal sex), satisfaction (desire, arousal, orgasm)
Protection	• Type and frequency of protection against sexually transmitted infections (STIs)
Past History	• Age of first sexual activity • STIs (type and duration) • History of sexual assault or abuse
Plans for Pregnancy	• Plans for pregnancy; if not, type and duration of contraceptive methods • Compliance, side effects, contraceptive failure, reasons for any discontinuation

Medications and Substance Use

- Use of prescription/OTC medications and herbal remedies
  - Note exogenous hormones
- Use of cigarettes, alcohol, or recreational drugs

Gynecological History

- Symptoms
  - Suggestive of endometriosis: dysmenorrhea, deep dyspareunia, infertility, chronic pelvic pain, menstrual irregularities, hematochezia/hematuria, dyschezia/dysuria
  - Vulvovaginal symptoms: sores, lumps, itching, discharge quantity, color, consistency, odor, and presence of blood
- Patterns
  - Micturition: day/night frequency, pain, urge/stress incontinence, hematuria
  - Bowel Movements: regularity, laxative use, history of pain or bleeding
- Previous Diagnoses
  - Infection history: STIs, pelvic inflammatory disease (PID), vaginitis, vulvitis, UTI; include treatment and complications
  - History of infertility: duration, cause (if known), treatments sought
- Investigations and Procedures
  - Last Pap smear, history/follow-up/treatment of abnormal smear
  - Gynecological or abdominal surgery (e.g. laparoscopy, hysteroscopy, hysterectomy)

Breast Disease History (see **Breast Exam**, p.38)

Obstetrical History (see **Obstetric Exam**, p.208)

Family History
- History of breast cancer, ovarian cancer, endometrial cancer, or colon cancer

4. FOCUSED GYNECOLOGICAL EXAM[1]

4.1 Breast Examination (see **Breast Exam**, p.39)

4.2 Pelvic Examination

Preparing for the Examination
- Explain each step in advance
- Encourage questions and feedback about comfort and pain
- Advise patient to avoid intercourse, douching, or use of vaginal suppositories for 24 to 48 h prior to examination
- Ask patient to empty bladder and remove all clothing below waist
- Avoid terminology that can be mistaken as sexual
  - "Let your knees fall apart" not "spread your legs"
  - "Removing the speculum" not "pulling out"
- Monitor comfort of examination by watching patient's face

GYNECOLOGICAL

Lithotomy Positioning
- Drape cover sheet from lower abdomen to knees; depress drape between knees to provide eye contact
- Patient lies supine, with head and shoulders elevated, arms at sides or folded across chest to enhance eye contact and reduce tightening of abdominal muscles
- Ask patient to place heels in foot rests and slide down table until buttocks flush with table edge
- Ensure hips flexed, abducted, and externally rotated

Inspection of External Genitalia
- **Mons Pubis, Labia, Perineum, and Perianal Area**
  - Inspect for masses, nodules, pubic lice, lesions, scars, fistulas, blisters, ulcers, hemorrhoids, inflammation, discharge, pigmentation, asymmetry, varicosities
- **Vagina and Vulva**
  - Note masses and lesions for signs of vaginal carcinoma and vulvar intraepithelia neoplasia

Speculum Examination
- **Preparation**
  - Place smear and culture material within reach (Pap smear kit, endocervical brush, vaginal culture medium, glass slide, gonococcal or chlamydia sterile cotton swab, and collection tube)
  - Warm speculum under running water, test temperature on inside of patient's thigh
  - Use water to lubricate the speculum if necessary, not gel (interferes with Pap smear and culture test results)
- **Insertion of Speculum**
  - Use index and middle finger to separate labia and expose vaginal opening
  - Insert speculum aiming for posterior fornix, avoiding contact with urethra

- Slide speculum inward along posterior wall of vagina, applying downward pressure to keep the vaginal introitus relaxed
- Open blades slowly
- Locate cervix by adjusting the angle of the speculum; lock speculum in open position once it is well exposed

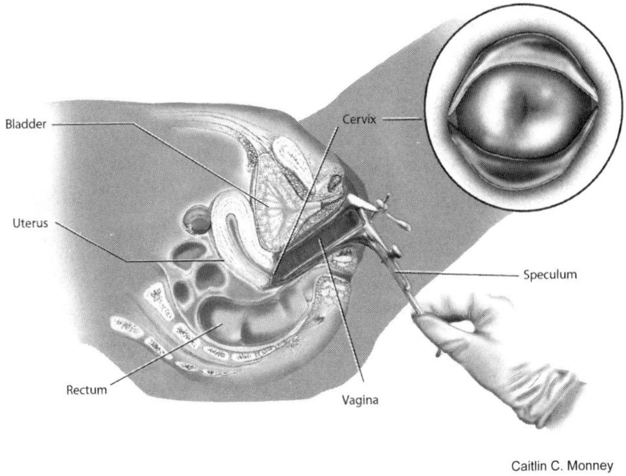

Figure 3. Insertion of the Speculum in Lithotomy Positioning

- **Inspection of Cervix**
  - Note cervical color, shape of os, discharge, polyps, lesions, ulcerations, or inflammation
  - Deviation of cervix from midline may indicate pelvic mass, uterine adhesions, or pregnancy
  - Note position of cervix
    - Anterior cervix: retroverted uterus
    - Posterior cervix: anteverted uterus
- **± Gonococcal (GC) or Chlamydial Culture**
  - Introduce sterile cotton swab through open speculum and insert into os
  - Hold in place for 10-30 s (45 s for chlamydia)
  - Remove swab and insert into collection tube (PCR media for both GC and chlamydia)
- **± Pap Smear**
  - For best results, patient should not be menstruating
  - Inform patient she may feel an uncomfortable scraping sensation

Pap Smear

- **Exocervical/Endocervical Sample**
  - Most centers use the liquid based ThinPrep® technology that provides an improvement in detection over other methods[2]
    - Insert the central bristles of the broom into the endocervical canal
    - Maintaining gentle pressure, rotate the brush five revolutions in a clockwise direction
    - Twirl brush in ThinPrep® solution to loosen cells from broom and discard broom or detach tip of broom into solution
- **± Vaginal Culture**
  - Introduce sterile cotton swab through open speculum
  - Collect any obvious secretions
  - Remove swab and insert into collection container or perform a wet mount where vaginal discharge is placed on a glass slide, mixed with salt solution and viewed under microscope

- **Removal of Speculum and Inspection of Vaginal Walls**
  - Unlock speculum and remove slowly, rotating to inspect vaginal walls (careful not to pinch mucosa)
  - Gradually bring blades together while simultaneously withdrawing speculum; blades should be completely closed by the time the tip of the speculum is removed
  - Maintain downward pressure of speculum to avoid injuring urethra
  - Assess support of vaginal walls. Separate labia with middle and index fingers, ask patient to bear down. Look for any bulging of vaginal walls (cystocele or rectocele)
    - Cystocele: bulging of upper two-thirds of anterior vaginal wall
    - Rectocele: herniation of rectum into posterior wall of vagina

Palpation of External Genitalia

- **Labia**
  - Spread labia majora laterally to see labia minora, introitus, and outer vagina[1]
  - Palpate labia majora between thumb and second finger to feel for masses or tenderness
  - Separate labia minora and palpate as above; palpate introitus and perineum
  - Note any fusion of minora to majora, or other distortion of anatomy
- **Vagina**
  - Place forefinger 2-3 cm into vagina, gently milk urethra and Skene's glands (female paraurethral ducts) with upward pressure (warn patient about sensation of having to urinate)[1]
  - Rotate forefinger posteriorly, palpate Bartholin's glands (greater vestibular gland) between the forefinger and thumb of opposite hand[1]
  - Note color, consistency, and odor of any gland discharge, obtain culture
  - Assess vaginal muscles by asking patient to squeeze vaginal opening around your finger (usually better in nulliparous women)

GYNECOLOGICAL

Palpation of Internal Genitalia (Bimanual Examination)

- Lubricate index and middle finger of gloved examining hand
- Separate labia with non-examining hand and insert examining fingers into vaginal opening, pressing downward against perineum to help muscles relax
- Keep fourth and fifth fingers flexed into palm, thumb extended
- Palpate vaginal walls and fornices as fingers are inserted[1]
  - Normally smooth, homogenous, and nontender with no masses/growths
- **Examination of the Cervix**
  - Locate cervix with palmar surface of fingers
  - Feel its end and circumference for size, length, and shape
  - Consistency: hard suggests nonpregnant, soft suggests pregnant
  - Position: anterior/posterior as discussed in speculum exam
  - Gently move cervix side-to-side between fingers
    - Should move 1-2 cm each way without discomfort (watch for grimace)
    - Cervical motion tenderness suggests inflammatory process
  - Evaluate os patency by trying to insert fingertip 0.5 cm

Table 3. Methods for Examination of the Uterus: Positions of the Uterus

Position	Examination Method
Anteverted (most common)	• Press down with palmar surface of free hand on abdomen, between umbilicus and pubic symphysis • Place intravaginal fingers in posterior fornix and elevate cervix and uterus to abdominal wall • If fundus is felt by abdominal hand, uterus is anteverted
Retroverted	• As above; if fundus is best felt by intravaginal fingers as opposed to abdominal hand, uterus is retroverted
Midposition	• As above; if fundus not felt well by either hand, uterus is midposition

- **Examination of the Uterus**
  - Once position established, assess:
    - Size (normal is approximately that of a closed fist; larger in multiparous women and those with fibroids)
    - Shape (usually pear-shaped; globular with adenomyosis)
    - Contour (rounded and smooth if nulliparous; irregular with fibroids)
    - Mobility in AP plane (absence indicates adhesions)
    - Mobility tenderness (pelvic inflammatory process, ruptured tubal pregnancy, endometriosis)
    - Consistency (soft if pregnant; firm with fibroids)
- **Examination of the Adnexa**
  - Shift abdominal hand to right lower quadrant (RLQ) and press inward and obliquely downward toward pubic symphysis
  - With intravaginal fingers in the right lateral fornix, elevate lateral fornix up toward abdominal hand
  - Assess if ovaries are palpable
  - If ovaries palpable, assess:
    - Size (normally 3 x 2 x 1 cm)
    - Shape (normally ovoid)
    - Consistency (normally firm, smooth)
    - Tenderness (moderately sensitive to compression)
    - Mobility
  - Normal fallopian tube not palpable
  - Repeat on left; exam more difficult due to sigmoid colon

4.3 Rectovaginal Examination

> **Clinical Pearl: Rectovaginal Exam**
> Never do the rectovaginal exam before the vaginal exam.

- Warn patient of possible sensation of having a bowel movement
- Inspect anus for lesions, hemorrhoids, or inflammation
- Insert lubricated index finger in vagina and lubricated middle finger of same hand against anus (insert fingertip into rectum just past sphincter)
- Note sphincter tone
  - Tight: anxiety, scarring, fissures, lesions, inflammation
  - Lax: neurological deficit
  - Absent: improper repair of childbirth tear or trauma
- Slide both fingers forward; rotate rectal finger to assess rectovaginal septum and posterior vaginal wall
  - Note any tenderness, thickening, nodules, polyps, or masses
- Body of a retroflexed uterus may be palpable with rectal finger
  - Assess with intravaginal finger in posterior fornix; push up against cervix and press down with abdominal hand just above pubic symphysis

- Assess cul-de-sac and uterosacral ligaments for nodularity or tenderness
  - Possible endometriosis, PID, or metastatic carcinoma
- Repeat adnexal exam (using same maneuvers as above) if palpation difficult or questionable on bimanual examination
- Gently withdraw fingers and note any blood, secretions, or stool

5. COMMON INVESTIGATIONS

Blood Work

- CBC: preoperation or to evaluate abnormal uterine bleeding, anemia, or infection
- β-hCG: to investigate possible pregnancy/ectopic pregnancy
- LH, FSH, TSH, prolactin (PRL), DHEAS, testosterone, estradiol: to investigate menstrual irregularities, menopause, infertility

Imaging

- U/S: transvaginal and transabdominal examination of pelvic structures
- Sonohysterogram: U/S of saline-infused, expanded uterus; visualizes uterine mass, abnormalities, tubal patency
- Hysterosalpingography (HSG): X-ray of contrast-injected uterus and tubes (rarely done now with availability of sonohysterography)

GYNECOLOGICAL

Colposcopy

- Endoscopic exam of vagina and cervix
- Acetic acid allows visualization of areas to biopsy for identification of dysplasia and/or neoplasia

Genital Tract Biopsy

- Vulvar, vaginal, cervical, endometrial

6. COMMON DISORDERS

Disorders marked with (✓) are discussed in **Common Clinical Scenarios**

✓ Endometriosis
✓ STIs
✓ Infertility
✓ Pelvic inflammatory disease (PID)
- Polycystic ovarian syndrome (PCOS)
- Ectopic pregnancy
- Miscarriage/abortion
- Vaginitis/vulvitis
- Ovarian cysts
- Endometrial/ovarian/cervical cancer
- Uterine fibroids (leiomyomata)

7. COMMON CLINICAL SCENARIOS

7.1 Physiological

The Menstrual Cycle

- The average adult menstrual cycle lasts 28-35 d
  - By convention, the first day of menses represents the first day of the cycle (Day 1)
  - The proliferative phase begins following menses and ends on the day of the luteinizing hormone (LH) surge (Days 5-14)
  - The secretory phase begins on the day of the LH surge and ends at the onset of the next menses (Days 14-28)

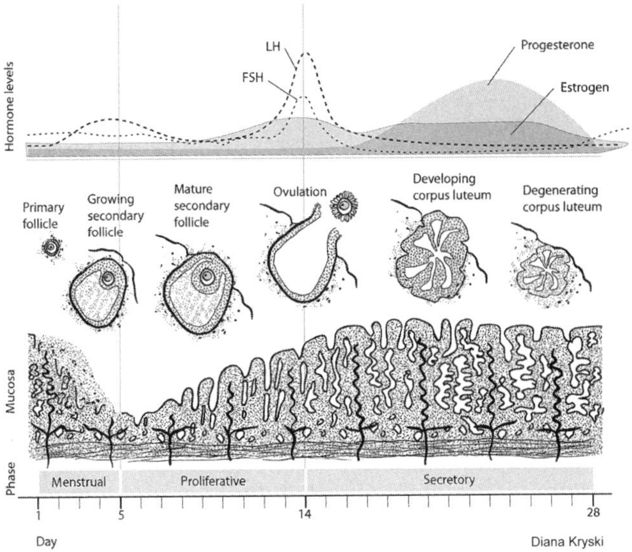

Figure 4. Normal Menstrual Cycle

Menarche

- Onset of menarche (normally between 9-16 yr, mean 12.5 yr)
- Refer to the Tanner stages of development for males and females (see **Pediatrics Exam**, p.274)

Menopause

- Retrospective diagnosis based on the lack of menses for 12 mo, age >40 yr
- Average age for menopause is 51 yr, with 95% of women experiencing it between the ages of 44 and 55 yr
- 60% of menopausal women are relatively asymptomatic, while 15% experience moderate or severe symptoms
- Symptoms (mainly associated with estrogen deficiency)
    - Menstrual cycle alteration: cessation of menses for >12 mo due to ovarian failure
    - Vasomotor instability (aka “hot flushes”)
    - Sleep disturbances (night sweats)
    - Dyspareunia, vaginal dryness/pruritus, genital tract atrophy, vaginal bleeding
    - Increased frequency of urination, urgency, incontinence
    - Fatigue, irritability, mood changes, memory loss, decreased libido
- Signs
    - Skin thinning, decreased elasticity, increased facial hair, thin and brittle nails, vaginal dryness, pale tissues, loss of rugae, less distensible
    - Loss of height secondary to osteoporosis; joint, muscle, and back pain
- Diagnosis
    - Increased levels of FSH (>40 IU/L)
    - Decreased levels of estradiol (15-350 pg/mL)
- Treatment
    - Hormone replacement therapy (HRT): estrogen, progestin
    - Selective estrogen receptor modulators (SERMs)
    - Calcium, vitamin D supplements (to decrease bone loss)

GYNECOLOGICAL

- Bisphosphonates (if osteoporotic or osteopenic)
- Local estrogen cream/vaginal suppository/ring, lubricants (for vaginal atrophy)
- Nonmedical (complementary medicine, exercise, counseling, healthy diet, other lifestyle modifications)

Contraception

Table 4. Contraceptive Methods[3-6,8]

Type	Effectiveness* (perfect use, typical use)	Side Effects	Contraindications
Barrier Methods			
Male Condom Alone	98%, 85%	–	Latex allergy, past expiry date
Spermicide Alone	82%, 71%	Vaginal irritation, may promote HIV transmission, messy, tastes bad, costly	–
Sponge • Parous • Nulliparous	 80%, 68% 91%, 84%	–	–
Diaphragm with Spermicide	94%, 84%	Diaphragm: UTI, vaginal irritation, toxic shock syndrome	Latex allergy
Female Condom	95%, 79%	–	–
Cervical Cap • Parous • Nulliparous	 74%, 68% 91%, 84%	–	–
Hormonal Methods			
Oral Contraceptive Pill (OCP)	99.7%, 92%	Breakthrough bleeding, nausea, headache, depression, bloating, decreased libido, increased venous thromboembolism (VTE) risk, increased stroke or MI risk in smokers and those with other risk factors	Known/suspected pregnancy, undiagnosed abnormal vaginal bleeding, thromboembolic disorders, cerebrovascular or coronary artery disease[7], estrogen dependent tumors, impaired liver function with acute liver disease, smoker >35 yr, migraines with focal neurological symptoms, uncontrolled HTN

GYNECOLOGICAL

Table 4. Contraceptive Methods (continued)

Type	Effectiveness* (perfect use, typical use)	Side Effects	Contraindications
Hormonal Methods			
Progestin-Only Pill (Micronor®)	90-99%	Irregular menstrual bleeding, weight gain, headache, breast tenderness, mood changes, functional ovarian cysts, acne/oily skin, hirsutism	–
Nuva Ring®	99.7%, 92%	Vaginal infections/ irritation, vaginal discharge	–
Transdermal (Ortho Evra®)	99.7%, 92%	–	–
Depo Provera®	99.7%, 97%	Irregular bleeding, weight gain, mood changes, decreased bone density, delay in return of fertility (average 9 mo)	–
Implant Methods			
Copper IUD **Mirena® IUD**	99.3% 99.9%	**All IUDs**: intermenstrual bleeding, expulsion, uterine wall perforation possible, greater chance of ectopic if pregnancy does occur, increased risk of PID in first 10 d **Copper IUD**: increased blood loss and duration of menses, dysmenorrhea **Mirena®**: Bloating, headache, unpredictable bleeding especially in first 4-6 mo	**All IUDs**: Known or suspected pregnancy, undiagnosed genital tract bleeding, acute or chronic PID, lifestyle risk for STIs **Copper IUD**: Known allergy to copper, Wilson's disease
Surgical Methods			
Tubal Ligation **Vasectomy**	99.7% 99.9%	Invasive, generally permanent, surgical risk	

Table 4. Contraceptive Methods (continued)

Type	Effectiveness* (perfect use, typical use)	Side Effects	Contraindications
Emergency Contraception			
Yuzpe® Method (OCP 2 tabs 12 h apart)	98% (in 24 h), decreases by 30% at 72 h	Nausea, spotting	Pre-existing pregnancy, caution in women with contraindications to OCP
"Plan B" Levonorgestrel Only	98% (in 24 h), decreases by 70% at 72 h		
Postcoital IUD	99.9%	See above	See above
Physiological Methods			
Withdrawal/ Coitus Interruptus	77%	–	–
Rhythm Method/ Calendar/ Mucus/Sympt-othermal	98%, 76%	–	–
Lactational Amenorrhea	98% (first 6 mo postpartum)	–	–
No Method Used	10%	–	–
Abstinence of All Sexual Activity	100%	–	–

*Effectiveness: percentage of women reporting no pregnancy after 1 yr of use

7.2 Pathological

Infectious

Sexually Transmitted Infections

- See **Essentials of Infectious Diseases**, p.493

Clinical Pearl: STI Co-Infection
If one STI is detected, other pathology or diseases may co-exist. Both partners must be treated for an STI to prevent recurrence. If gonococcal infection is suspected, simultaneous treatment for chlamydia should be given.

Clinical Pearl: Reportable Infections
Chlamydia trachomatis and *Neisseria gonorrhoeae* infections are reportable according to certain provincial/territorial public health acts. Contact tracing, the process of informing all sexual partners within 60 d of onset of symptoms, is recommended by the Canadian Guidelines on Sexually Transmitted Infections. Contact tracing may be done by the patient or confidentially by a healthcare provider or public health officials without naming the index case.

EBM: HPV Vaccination

A recent systematic review of seven independent randomized controlled trials (RCTs) comparing prophylactic HPV vaccination vs. placebo showed that vaccination is highly efficacious in preventing oncogenic HPV infection types (HPV-16, HPV-18) and high-grade cervical lesions. Efficacy ranges were 75-85% against persistent HPV infections, and 57-78% against high-grade cervical lesions, with no significant difference in risk of adverse events between vaccine and control groups (RR: 1.82; 95% CI: 0.79-4.20). Currently, HPV-2 or HPV-4 vaccine is recommended for females aged 9-26 yr (Canada) and 11-26 yr (US). The HPV-4 vaccine is also recommended for males aged 9-26 yr (Canada) and for men who have sex with men who are younger than 26 yr (US).

Lu B, et al. 2011. *BMC Infect Dis* 11(1):13.
National Advisory Committee on Immunization (NACI). 2012. *Can Commun Dis Rep* 39(ACS-2):1.
Bridges CB, Woods L, Coyne-Beasley T. 2013. *MMWR* 62(1):9-19.

Pelvic Inflammatory Disease[9]

- Inflammatory disorder of the uterus, fallopian tubes, and adjacent pelvic structures caused by direct spread of microorganisms ascending from the vagina and cervix
- Common organisms: *Neisseria gonorrhoeae*, *Chlamydia trachomatis*, genital mycoplasmas
- Risk Factors: young age at first intercourse, multiple partners, uterine instrumentation, smoking
- Complications: infertility, ectopic pregnancy, chronic pain
- Symptoms
  - Low abdominal or pelvic pain of recent onset that may be bilateral
  - Vaginal discharge
  - Irregular vaginal bleeds (irregular menstrual cycle and/or intermittent bleeds)
  - Deep dyspareunia
- Signs
  - Fever
  - Abdominal tenderness; signs of peritoneal irritation
  - Cervical motion tenderness
  - Cervical discharge
  - Adnexal mass and/or tenderness on bimanual examination
  - Pelvic heat
- Physical Exam and Investigations
  - On abdominal exam: look for focal tenderness/peritoneal signs
  - On speculum: look for mucopurulent discharge
  - On pelvic exam: look for adnexal masses, cervical motion tenderness, adnexal tenderness
- Treatment
  - Outpatient: PO/IM antibiotics (e.g. ceftriaxone IM + doxycycline PO +/- metronidazole PO x 14 d)
  - Inpatient: IV antibiotics with step-down to PO antibiotics 24 h after clinical improvement (e.g. cefoxitin IV + doxycycline IV/PO)

Candidiasis[9]

- Overgrowth of yeast in the vagina
- Common organisms: *Candida albicans* (90%), *Candida tropicalis*, *Candida glabrata*
- Predisposing Factors: immunosuppression, antibiotic use, pregnancy
- Symptoms
  - Asymptomatic (20%)
  - Itching, burning
  - White, lumpy, "cottage cheese" discharge

- Investigations
  - pH test: pH <4.7
  - Wet mount: 50-60% sensitive; can see budding yeast, hyphae, pseudohyphae
  - Culture: higher sensitivity than wet mount; can identify species of yeast
- Treatment
  - Topical azole drugs most effective
    - Available as ovules and creams for 1, 3, or 7 d
  - Oral therapy also available
  - Treat male partner only if yeast balanitis present

Bacterial Vaginosis[9]

- Replacement of normal vaginal flora with other organisms
- Common organisms: *Gardnerella vaginalis*, *Mycoplasma hominis*, certain anaerobes
- Symptoms
  - Malodorous
  - Thin, white/gray adherent discharge
  - Possible itching
- Investigations
  - pH test: pH >4.5
  - Wet mount: clue cells with adherent coccoid bacteria
  - KOH whiff test: fishy odor
- Treatment
  - Metronidazole
  - No treatment for male partner

GYNECOLOGICAL

Inflammatory

Endometriosis[10]

- Affects 5-10% of reproductive-age women and 25-35% of women with infertility
- History of cyclic pelvic pain and dysmenorrhea supports the diagnosis, but needs to be distinguished from chronic pelvic pain
- Symptoms: pelvic pain, dysmenorrhea (worsens with age), infertility, deep dyspareunia, premenstrual and postmenstrual spotting, increased frequency of urination, dysuria, hematuria, diarrhea, constipation, hematochezia
- Signs: tender nodularity of uterine ligaments and cul-de-sac, fixed retroversion of the uterus, firm, fixed adnexal mass (endometrioma)
- Diagnosis: responds to medical treatment (presumptive), laparoscopy ± histology (definitive)
- Treatment:
  - Medical
    - 1st line: NSAIDs, OCP (cyclic/continuous), progestin therapy (oral or injection)
    - 2nd line: antiestrogen agents (e.g. Danazol), gonadotropin releasing hormone agonists
  - Surgical: laparoscopic resection/vaporization/ablation of implants, removal of adhesions
  - Mirena IUD

Infertility

- Failure to conceive after 1 yr of unprotected sexual intercourse
- Approximately 40% due to a male factor, 40% due to a female factor, and 20% due to both male and female contributing causes, 10-15% unexplained
- Symptoms/signs: often asymptomatic; not recognized until pregnancy attempts unsuccessful

Table 5. Infertility Etiology and Diagnosis

Site	Examples	Diagnosis
Ovulatory Dysfunction (20-40% of cases)	Hyperprolactinemia, thyroid disease, PCOS, luteal phase defects, certain systemic diseases, congenital diseases, poor nutrition, stress, excessive exercise, eating disorder, hypothalamic-pituitary dysfunction	Serum PRL, TSH, LH, FSH, history of cycle patterns, basal body temperature, mucus quality, endometrial biopsy for luteal phase defect, serum progesterone level, karyotype, liver and renal function
Tubal Factors (20-30% of cases)	PID, adhesions, tubal ligation, previous gynecological surgery	Hysterosalpingogram, sonohysterogram, laparoscopy with dye
Cervical Factors (<5% of cases)	Structural abnormalities, antisperm antibodies, hostile acidic cervical mucus, glands unresponsive to estrogen	Postcoital test
Uterine Factors (<5% of cases)	Polyps, infection, intrauterine adhesions, congenital anomalies, leiomyomata	Hysterosalpingogram, sonohysterogram, hysteroscopy

LH = luteinizing hormone, PCOS = polycystic ovary syndrome, PID = pelvic inflammatory disease, PRL = prolactin

GYNECOLOGICAL

Common Neoplasms

Benign

- **Lichen Sclerosus**
  - Site: vulva
  - Description: benign, inflammatory, immune-mediated skin disease
  - Most common in postmenopausal women
  - Clinical Features: pruritus, dyspareunia, burning
  - Diagnosis: silver or ivory white tissue on examination and shiny or crinkly, with areas of purpura or ecchymosis
  - Treatment: topical steroids
- **Cervix: Endocervical Polyps and Uterine Fibroids**
  - Site: cervix, uterus (leiomyomata [fibroids])
  - Description: growth from smooth muscle (monoclonal); can be submucosal, intramural, subserosal, or pedunculated
  - Clinical Features: asymptomatic (60%), abnormal uterine bleeding (30%; most often from submucosal fibroid), pressure/bulk symptoms (20-50%), acute pelvic pain, infertility
  - Diagnosis: bimanual exam, CBC (anemia), ultrasound, sonohysterogram/saline infusion hysterography
  - Treatment
    - Conservative: useful if minimal symptoms, size <8 cm or stable
    - Medical: ibuprofen, tranexamic acid, OCP/Depo-Provera®, GnRH agonists
    - Interventional radiology: uterine artery embolization
    - Surgical: myomectomy (hysteroscopic if intracavitary, laparoscopic, or laparotomy), hysterectomy
- **Benign Ovarian Tumors**
  - Site: ovary
  - Clinical Features: mostly asymptomatic; may present as pain due to rupture or torsion

- **Hydatidiform Mole** (benign form of gestational trophoblastic neoplasm)
  - Complete mole
    - Description: 2 sperm fertilize empty egg or 1 sperm with reduplication
    - Clinical Features: vaginal bleeding, excessive uterine size, theca-lutein cysts >6 cm, preeclampsia, hyperemesis gravidum, hyperthyroidism, β-hCG >100,000, no fetal heart detected
    - Risk Factors: maternal age >40 yr, low beta carotene diet, vitamin A deficiency
    - Treatment: D&C; watch out for thyroid storm and be prepared to treat appropriately (rare complication)
  - Partial mole
    - Description: single ovum fertilized by 2 sperm; often associated with fetus that is growth restricted and has multiple congenital malformations
    - Clinical Features: similar to spontaneous abortion (spontaneous loss of a fetus before the 20th wk)
    - Diagnosis: ultrasound showing abnormal placental features, β-hCG high for early pregnancy; diagnosis often based on pathology from D&C
    - Treatment: D&C with sharp curettage and oxytocin, hysterectomy if future fertility not desired, prophylactic chemotherapy (controversial); RhoGAM® if patient is Rh negative
    - Avoid pregnancy for 6-12 mo

GYNECOLOGICAL

Malignant

- **Vulva**
  - Description: 90% squamous cell carcinoma
  - Clinical Features: asymptomatic, localized pruritus, lump, or mass, raised red, white or pigmented plaque, ulcer, bleeding, discharge, pain, dysuria
  - Risk Factors: HPV infection (HPV-16, HPV-18), vulvar intraepithelial neoplasia
- **Cervix**
  - Description: 95% squamous cell carcinoma
  - Clinical Features:
    - Early: asymptomatic, discharge (watery, becoming brown or red), postcoital bleeding
    - Late: bleeding (postcoital, postmenopausal, irregular), pelvic or back pain, bladder/bowel symptoms
  - Risk Factors: HPV infection (HPV-16, HPV-18), smoking, high risk sexual behavior
  - Prevention (secondary): regular Pap smears
  - Diagnosis: Pap screening, colposcopy, endocervical curettage, cervical biopsy, cone biopsy
- **Uterus: Endometrial Carcinoma**
  - Description: most common gynecological malignancy
  - Clinical Features: postmenopausal bleeding, abnormal uterine bleeding
  - Diagnosis: endometrial biopsy, D&C ± hysteroscopy
  - Treatment:
    - Stage 1: total abdominal hysterectomy (TAH)/bilateral salpingo-oophorectomy (BSO) and washings
    - Stages 2 and 3: TAH/BSO, washings, and nodal dissection
    - Stage 4: nonsurgical
      - Adjuvant radiotherapy: based on myometrial penetration, tumor grade, lymph node involvement
      - Hormonal therapy: progestins for distant or recurrent disease
      - Adjuvant chemotherapy: based on disease progression

Clinical Pearl: Vaginal Bleeding
Vaginal bleeding in postmenopausal women is endometrial cancer until proven otherwise.

- **Ovary**
  - Description: 3 types: epithelial (80-85%), germ cell (10-15%), and stromal cell (3-5%); 4th leading cause of cancer death in women
  - Clinical Features: usually asymptomatic until advanced (Stage III)
    - Early: vague abdominal symptoms (nausea, bloating, dyspepsia, anorexia, early satiety), postmenopausal or irregular bleeding (rare)
    - Late: increased abdominal girth, urinary frequency, constipation, ascites
  - Risk Factors: white race, late age at menopause, family history of ovarian, breast or bowel cancer, prolonged intervals of ovulation uninterrupted by pregnancy
  - Diagnosis: bimanual exam, CBC, LFTs, electrolytes, creatinine, CA-125, CXR, abdominal/pelvic U/S ± transvaginal U/S
  - Treatment:
    - Early: TAH/BSO, infracolic omentectomy, and thorough surgical staging
    - Late: cytoreductive surgery ("debulking") and chemotherapy
- **Gestational Trophoblastic Neoplasms**
  - Description: includes invasive mole (a locally invasive lesion) and choriocarcinoma (a frankly malignant form)
  - Clinical Features: symptoms of metastatic disease, vaginal bleeding, hemoptysis, cough or dyspnea, headaches, dizzy spells, "blacking out" or rectal bleeding
  - Risk Factors: preceding molar pregnancy
  - Diagnosis: increase or plateau in β-hCG following treatment of molar pregnancy, molar tissue on histology
  - Treatment: chemotherapy (single agent or combination), radiation for metastases to brain or liver
  - Choriocarcinoma: may follow any type of pregnancy, highly anaplastic
    - Diagnosis: CBC, electrolytes, creatinine, β-hCG, TSH, LFTs, CXR, pelvic U/S, CT abdomen/pelvis, CT head
    - Treatment: chemotherapy

REFERENCES

1. Edelman A, Anderson J, Lai S, Braner DAV, Tegtmeyer K. 2007. Pelvic examination. *N Engl J Med* 356(26):e26.
2. Dawson AE. 2004. Can we change the way we screen?: The ThinPrep Imaging System. *Cancer* 102(6):340-344.
3. Black A, Francoeur D, Rowe T, Collins J, Miller D, Brown T, et al. 2004. SOGC clinical practice guidelines: Canadian contraception consensus. Part 1. *J Obstet Gynaecol Can* 26(2):143-156.
4. Black A, Francoeur D, Rowe T, Collins J, Miller D, Brown T, et al. 2004. SOGC clinical practice guidelines: Canadian contraception consensus. Part 2. *J Obstet Gynaecol Can* 26(3):219-296.
5. Black A, Francoeur D, Rowe T, Collins J, Miller D, Brown T, et al. 2004. SOGC clinical practice guidelines: Canadian contraception consensus. Part 3. *J Obstet Gynaecol Can* 26(4):347-387.
6. Boroditsky R, Fisher WA, Sand M. 1995. The Canadian contraception study. *J Obstet Gynaecol Can* 17(Suppl):S1-28.
7. Manson JE, Hsia J, Johnson KC, Rossouw JE, Assaf AR, Lasser NL, et al, 2003. Estrogen plus progestin and the risk of coronary heart disease. *N Engl J Med* 349(6):523-534.
8. Woodford C, Yao C. *Toronto Notes 2013*. Toronto: Toronto Notes for Medical Students, Inc; 2013.
9. MacDonald N, Wong T. 2007. Canadian guidelines on sexually transmitted infections, 2006. *CMAJ* 176(2):175-176.
10. Leyland N, Casper R, Laberge P, Singh SS, SOGC. 2010. Endometriosis: Diagnosis and management. *J Obstet Gynaecol Can* 32(7 Suppl 2):S1-32.
11. DeCherney AH, Nathan L, Laufer N, Roman AS. *Current Diagnosis & Treatment Obstetrics & Gynecology*, 11th ed. McGraw-Hill Medical; 2013.

The Head and Neck Exam

Editors:
James England
Sheron Perera

Faculty Reviewers:
Kevin M. Higgins, MD, FRCS(C)
Allan D. Vescan, MD, FRCS(C)

TABLE OF CONTENTS

1. EAR

1.1 Essential Anatomy

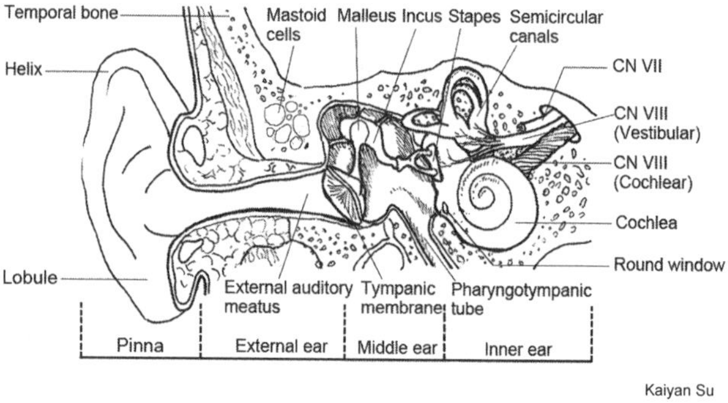

Figure 1. Cross Section of the Right Ear

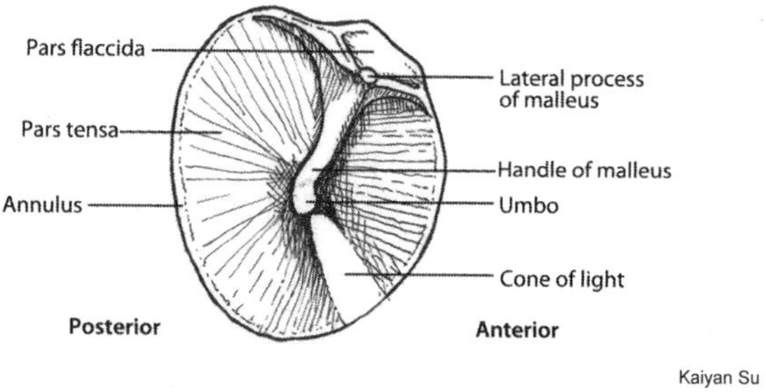

Figure 2. Tympanic Membrane of the Right Ear

HEAD & NECK

1.2 Common Chief Complaints

- Ear pain (otalgia)
- Ear discharge (otorrhea)
- Ringing, whistling, blowing, or humming in the ears (tinnitus)
- Dizziness
- Hearing loss

1.3 Focused History

- For all otological complaints: see **Table 1**
- Unilateral vs. bilateral (***Note:*** be cautious of unilateral concerns)
- Onset, duration, progression, frequency
- Accompanying vestibular symptoms
- Previous surgery
- Recent or past head/ear trauma
- Noise exposure
- Family history
- Medications (especially ototoxic meds, see **Table 4**)
- Systemic diseases (e.g. MS, SLE, DM)
- Infection (local, systemic)

Table 1. Focused History for Specific Otological Complaints

Complaint	Focused History	Differential Diagnosis
Otalgia	• OPQRSTUVW • Hyperacusis (painful sensitivity to ordinary sound levels) • Otorrhea (see below) • Dizziness/imbalance (see below)	**Local Causes:** • Acute otitis media (AOM) (recent history of URTI) • Acute mastoiditis (>2 wk after untreated AOM) • Otitis externa (Swimmer's ear) • Foreign body or impacted cerumen in canal **Referred from CN V, VII, IX, X (Ten Ts+2)[1]:** • Eus**t**achian Tube • **T**MJ syndrome (pain in front of the ears) • **T**rismus (spasm of masticator muscles, early symptom of tetanus) • **T**eeth • **T**ongue • **T**onsils (tonsillitis, tonsillar cancer, post-tonsillectomy) • **T**ic (glossopharyngeal neuralgia) • **T**hroat (cancer of larynx) • **T**rachea (foreign body, tracheitis) • **T**hyroiditis • Geniculate herpes and Ramsay Hunt syndrome type 2 ± CN VII palsy (Bell's palsy)
Otorrhea	• Quality (color, smell, quantity, consistency) • DM, elderly, immunocompromised (suspect necrotizing otitis externa) • Recent ear or throat infection • Recent otalgia • Headache ± fever • Pruritus in the ear • Hearing loss • Duration of symptoms • Any recent above-shoulder body trauma • Swimming injury	**Purulent Discharge:** mastoiditis with tympanic membrane perforation, otitis externa with tympanic membrane perforation, cholesteatoma with tympanic membrane, acute and chronic suppurative otitis media, necrotizing otitis externa (medical emergency) **Nonpurulent Discharge:** CSF leakage (head trauma), foreign body, invasive otitis externa **Bloody Discharge:** hemorrhage (head trauma), barotrauma, foreign body, external trauma
Tinnitus (ear ringing)	• Subjective vs. objective ear ringing • Characteristic of ear sound (ringing, buzzing or hissing) • Constant vs. intermittent • Duration • Unilateral vs. bilateral • Hx of head trauma • Hx of anxiety • Medication Hx • Presence/absence of vertigo • Presence/absence of hearing loss • Presence/absence of other neurological signs/symptoms	**Subjective** (heard by patient; common) • Otologic: otitis media with effusion (OME), otosclerosis, presbycusis, Ménière's disease, cerumen, noise-induced hearing loss • Drugs (see **Table 4**) • Metabolic: hyperlipidemia, vitamin A deficiency, vitamin B deficiency • Neurologic: head trauma, MS, meningitis, temporal lobe tumor, acoustic neuroma • Psychiatric: anxiety, depression **Objective** (heard by others; rare) • Muscular: stapedius spasm, palatal myoclonus • Vascular: arterial bruits, venous hums, arteriovenous malformation

Table 1. Focused History for Specific Otological Complaints (continued)

Complaint	Focused History	Differential Diagnosis
Hearing Loss	See **Table 2** (Conductive) and **Table 3** (Sensorineural)	
Dizziness/ Imbalance	See **Common Clinical Scenarios**, p.115	

Table 2. Conductive Hearing Loss

Differential Diagnosis	History	Otoscopic Examination
Physical Obstruction (cerumen, foreign body)	Sudden (foreign body) or gradual (cerumen) painless loss	Obstruction visible in canal
Congenital (atresia of auditory canal, ossicular abnormalities)	Hearing loss present since birth	Various abnormalities
Tympanic Membrane Perforation (cholesteatoma, trauma, untreated infection)	Painless hearing loss (± pain prior to membrane perforation) History of ear infections/trauma Chronic drainage	Perforation is usually visible (check periphery)
Otitis Externa (bacterial or fungal infection of the external auditory canal)	Sudden painful hearing loss Moisture (swimming) Trauma (foreign bodies)	Narrow canal with debris Canal erythema Variable discharge Pain on moving pinna
Otitis Media with Effusion (OME), Acute Otitis Media (AOM) – viral, bacterial infection	Sudden painful loss	Tympanic membrane: decreased mobility, red or yellow, bulging, injected or cloudy
Otosclerosis	Gradual painless loss	Normal otoscopy Audiogram: Carhart's notch (sensorineural loss at 2 kHz)[2]
Glomus Tumor/Vascular Abnormality	Gradual painless loss	Intact tympanic membrane Red-blue, pulsating mass behind tympanic membrane

Table 3. Sensorineural Hearing Loss

Differential Diagnosis	History/Physical Findings	Audiogram
Acoustic Neuroma (CN VIII schwannoma)	• Gradual unilateral hearing loss • Tinnitus is common • Unsteadiness (vertigo uncommon) • Facial nerve palsy (late finding)	• Gradual, asymmetric, sensorineural loss • Unilateral
Congenital (e.g. genetic, ischemia, prenatal infection – TORCH, toxins)	Present at birth	U-shaped or "cookie-bite" audiogram (hearing is better in low and high frequencies than in middle frequencies)

HEAD & NECK

Table 3. Sensorineural Hearing Loss (continued)

Differential Diagnosis	History/Physical Findings	Audiogram
Ménière's Disease (idiopathic endolymphatic hydrops)	• Unilateral, sudden, fluctuating, progressive loss • Episodic tinnitus • Episodic aural fullness • Episodic vertigo ± N/V	• Low-frequency loss "peaking" (tent-shaped) or flat audiogram • Unilateral
Noise-Induced	• Gradual onset of hearing loss • Tinnitus common • History of noise exposure (occupational, recreational)	• Boiler maker's notch (loss centered at 4 kHz) • Bilateral and symmetric
Ototoxic Medications (see **Table 4**)	± tinnitus ± vertigo	• High frequency loss • Typically bilateral
Presbycusis (age-related hearing loss)	• Gradual onset of hearing loss • Noise exposure • Tobacco use	• High frequency loss • Bilateral
Sudden Sensorineural Hearing Loss* (e.g. idiopathic, viral, autoimmune, vascular, trauma)	• Sudden onset (<3 d) of hearing loss, 65% of patients recover hearing spontaneously[3]	• Loss >30 dB in three contiguous frequencies[3]

*Medical emergency
TORCH = toxoplasmosis, others (e.g. HIV), rubella, cytomegalovirus, herpes simplex

Table 4. Ototoxic Compounds

Class	Examples
Aminoglycosides[4]	Gentamicin, tobramycin, amikacin, neomycin
NSAIDs[5]	Aspirin, acetaminophen
Antimalarials[6]	Quinine, chloroquine
Heavy Metals[7]	Lead, mercury, cadmium, arsenic
Loop Diuretics[6]	Furosemide, ethacrynic acid
Chemotherapy Agents[8]	Cisplatin, 5-fluorouracil, bleomycin
Antibiotics[6]	Erythromycin, tetracycline
Phosphodiesterase-5 Inhibitors[9]	Sildenafil, tadalafil, vardenafil

1.4 Focused Physical Exam

External Exam

- Inspection
  - Pinna for size, position, deformity, inflammation, symmetry, nodules, scars or lesions
    - e.g. microtia, macrotia, cauliflower ear
  - External auditory canal
  - Look for presence of ear discharge: color, consistency, clarity, presence or absence of an odor

- Palpation
  - Pinna, periauricular area, and mastoid process for tenderness, nodules
    - Pain elicited by tugging on pinna/tragus is associated with otitis externa
    - Pain over the mastoid process with an outward and inferior protrusion of the pinna and discharge is found in acute mastoiditis

Table 5. Auditory Acuity Testing

Procedure	Results
Whisper Test[10]: assessment of hearing impairment • Lightly rub your fingers together next to the ear not being tested and ask the patient to repeat what you whisper into tested ear • Repeat on other ear	• If the patient cannot hear, continue to increase the volume of your voice until it is heard by the patient • 90-100% sensitivity • 70-87% specificity
Weber Test: assessment of sound lateralization • Place the base of the tuning fork on the center of the patient's forehead • Ask the patient if he/she hears the sound louder on one side or if it is equal on both sides	• Normal hearing = no sound lateralization (patient hears sound or feels vibration in middle) • Conductive hearing loss = sound lateralization to AFFECTED ear • Sensorineural hearing loss = sound lateralization to NON-AFFECTED ear
Rinne Test: assessment of air vs. bone conduction • Apply tuning fork against the patient's mastoid process, then place it still vibrating next to the patient's ear (abbreviated version) • Ask the patient to identify which placement sounds louder • Repeat with opposite ear	• Rinne positive (normal) = air > bone conduction • Rinne negative* (conductive hearing loss) = bone > air conduction • Partial sensorineural hearing loss = air > bone conduction (but both decreased) • *Complete hearing loss in one ear in which patient may still process bone conduction that is picked up by contralateral cochlea is known as "false-negative Rinne"

*For Weber and Rinne testing, strike a 512 Hz tuning fork on bony prominence (e.g. patella/styloid process of radius). Do not place tuning fork over hair.
Bickley LS, Szilagyi PG, Bates B. *Bates' Guide to Physical Examination and History Taking*, 10th ed. Philadelphia: Lippincott Williams & Wilkins; 2009.

Otoscopic Exam

- Examine:
  - External auditory meatus (foreign body, cerumen, inflammatory, discharge)
  - Tympanic membrane (see **Table 6**)
- Techniques:
  - Use largest speculum that can be comfortably inserted to maximize visual field and to avoid irritation of bony canal
  - Adults: gently pull the pinna backward and upward
  - Children: gently pull the pinna backward and slightly downward
  - Stabilize otoscope by placing fifth digit against patient's cheek to protect against sudden movements

Table 6. Otoscopic Examination of Tympanic Membrane

Inspect	Normal	Abnormal
Color	Translucent and pearly gray	• Red (hyperemia due to inflammation, fever, Valsalva/crying/screaming) • Yellow (pus in middle ear, suggests otitis media with effusion [OME]) • Blue (glomus jugulare, glomus tympanicum)
Light Reflex	Cone of light directed anteriorly and inferiorly	• Absent/distorted (abnormal geometry due to bulging or retraction, perforation, thickening)
Landmarks	Pars flaccida, malleus (near center), incus (posterior to malleus)	• Obscured landmarks may indicate inflammation, fluid/pus in middle ear or membrane thickening
Abnormal Margins	Clear and tense margins	• Perforation (untreated ear infection, cholesteatoma, trauma [e.g. cotton swab use])
Mobility	Brisk, equal movement with positive and negative pressure using pneumatic otoscopy	• Reduced/absent mobility: increased middle ear pressure (mucoid, serous or purulent effusion) • Increased mobility: negative middle ear pressure (Eustachian tube dysfunction)
Shape	Drawn inwards slightly at center by handle of malleus	• Bulging: suggests pus/fluid in middle ear • Retraction: Eustachian tube dysfunction resulting in negative middle ear pressure

Bickley LS, Szilagyi PG, Bates B. *Bates' Guide to Physical Examination and History Taking*, 10th ed. Philadelphia: Lippincott Williams & Wilkins; 2009.

HEAD & NECK

1.5 Common Investigations

Table 7. Common Auditory Investigations

Test	Description	Results
Pure Tone Audiogram	• Tests for threshold response at generated frequencies • Tests both air and bone conduction	• Audiogram describes hearing deficits across all frequencies
Tympanometry[11]	• Applies positive and negative air pressure to eardrum and measures compliance of tympanic membrane	• Low compliance of tympanic membrane indicates fluid in middle ear or otosclerosis • High compliance occurs in ossicular chain discontinuity • 65-92% sensitivity • 60-91% specificity
Otoacoustic Emissions[12]	• Tests for presence and strength of sound generated by cochlea in response to a sound stimulus • Part of screening for hearing loss in newborns	• Presence of emission suggests inner ear dysfunction • 71% sensitivity • 73% specificity

Clinical Pearl: Degrees of Hearing Loss From Audiogram Testing[13]

Degree of Hearing Loss	Hearing Loss (dB Hearing Level [HL])
Slight	16 to 25
Mild	26 to 40
Moderate	41 to 55
Moderately Severe	56 to 70
Severe	71 to 90
Profound	>90

2. NOSE

2.1 Essential Anatomy

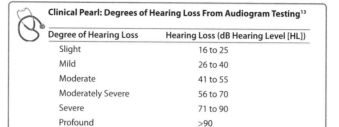

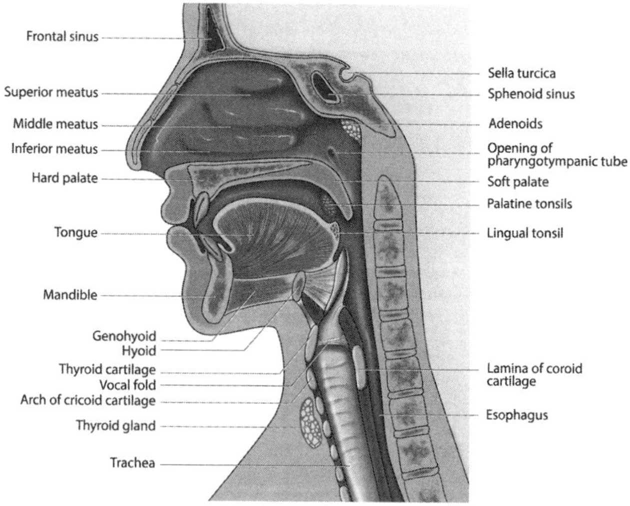

Figure 3. Anatomy of the Right Nasal Cavity, Oropharynx, and Larynx (lateral aspect)

2.2 Common Chief Complaints

- Loss of smell (anosmia)
- Facial pain
- Stuffy nose (congestion)
- Nasal discharge (rhinorrhea)
- Nosebleeds (epistaxis)

2.3 Focused History

- A focused history should be based on the chief complaint (see **Table 8**)

HEAD & NECK

Table 8. Focused History for Nose and Sinuses

Focused History	Differential Diagnosis
Anosmia	
• Unilateral vs. bilateral • Onset • Associated neurological symptoms • Recent head trauma, clear fluid on pillow • Rhinorrhea	• Nasal obstruction/congestion (URTI, polyps, enlarged turbinates, ethmoid tumor, rhinosinusitis) • Head trauma (fracture of cribriform plate) • Kallman's syndrome (congenital anosmia) • Intracranial pathology (meningitis, hydrocephalus, frontal lobe tumor, meningioma of olfactory groove)
Facial/Sinus Pain	
• Rhinorrhea, purulent discolored nasal discharge • Post-nasal drip, cough • Hyposmia/anosmia • Fever • Diabetic • Immunocompromised • Bone marrow recipient	• Acute rhinosinusitis (commonly maxillary and anterior ethmoid sinuses) • Chronic sinusitis (>12 wk, bacterial/fungal) • Frontal, ethmoid, sphenoid acute bacterial rhinosinusitis* • Mucormycosis† (invasive fungal infection common in diabetic, immunocompromised, and bone marrow recipients; rare in normal population)
Nasal Congestion	
• Congestion or stuffiness • Nasal discharge, "runny nose" • Facial tenderness/pain • Noisy breathing, snoring • Pruritus of nose, eyes (allergies)	**Common:** • Acute/chronic allergic, vasomotor rhinitis, rhinitis medicamentosa • Septal deviation • Adenoid/inferior turbinate hypertrophy **Less Common:** • Polyps, foreign bodies, trauma, enlarged turbinates **Rare:** • Neoplasm (nasopharynx, nasal cavity) • Septal hematoma or abscess
Rhinorrhea	
• Duration • Exacerbating and alleviating factors • Allergies • Character and color • Associated facial pain	**Watery/mucoid** (most common): • Allergic, viral or vasomotor rhinitis • CSF (fracture of cribriform plate) **Mucopurulent** (less common): • Bacterial infection • Foreign body **Serosanguinous** (rare): • Neoplasm • Infectious (e.g. mucormycosis) **Bloody** (rare): • Trauma • Coagulopathy • HTN/vascular disease • Neoplasm
Epistaxis	
See **Common Clinical Scenarios**, p.117	

*Requires aggressive management
†Medical emergency

HEAD & NECK

> **Clinical Pearl: Allergic Salute**
> The allergic salute is a horizontal nasal crease below the bridge of the nose in children that results from persistent upward rubbing of the nose secondary to allergic rhinitis.

2.4 Focused Physical Exam

External Exam

- Inspection
  - Note any swelling, trauma, deviation or congenital abnormalities
  - Extend patient's neck and examine the symmetry of the nares
- Palpation
  - Test airway patency: occlude one nostril and ask the patient to sniff then exhale and look for mirror fogging or movement of cotton wisp

Internal Exam (Nasal Speculum)

- Hold speculum in nondominant hand and introduce horizontally, 1 cm into the vestibule. Place index finger of nondominant hand atop nose to anchor speculum
- ***Note:*** any swelling, trauma, deviation, masses, discharge or congenital abnormalities

Inspection

- Septum for deviation or perforation
- Mucous membranes: normally pink, moist and smooth; blue/gray with allergies; red with inflammation
- Little's area for vascular engorgement or crusting (indicates recent epistaxis)
- Turbinates for size and color (black turbinates may indicate mucormycosis)
- Presence of nasal polyps (grayish color)
- Turbinates are rarely symmetric; asymmetry on inspection is frequently normal

Olfactory Exam

- To assess CN I, perform the University of Pennsylvania Smell Identification Test (UPSIT) (standardized scratch and sniff test)

2.5 Common Investigations

- Allergy testing
- IgE levels (for allergic patients)
- Endoscopic guided cultures (for sinusitis)
- β-2 transferrin of nasal fluid (if CSF leak suspected)
- CT (to confirm diagnosis or if complications suspected)

3. ORAL CAVITY AND PHARYNX

3.1 Essential Anatomy

- See **Figure 3**

3.2 Common Chief Complaints

- Cough
- Sore throat (pharyngitis)
- Difficulty swallowing (dysphagia)
- Painful swallowing (odynophagia)
- Lump (globus hystericus)
- Hoarseness

3.3 Focused History

- See **Table 9**
- For all oral cavity and pharynx complaints, ask about:
  - Hemoptysis
  - Constitutional symptoms
  - Lifestyle habits (smoking, alcohol)

Table 9. Focused History for Oral Cavity and Pharynx

Focused History	Differential Diagnosis
Cough (see **Respiratory Exam**, p.349)	
• Onset and duration • Worse day or night • Dry or productive (volume, color, odor, consistency, pus) • Dyspnea and/or chest pain • Environmental/occupational exposures (asbestos, radiation)	• URTI (e.g. pharyngitis, bronchitis) • Pneumonia • COPD • Tuberculosis • Rhinosinusitis, post-nasal drip • Neoplasms (e.g. primary or secondary lung, breast, laryngeal)
Pharyngitis	
• OPQRSTUVW • Signs of infection (e.g. fever, malaise, anorexia, halitosis) • Cough (acute or chronic) • Referred otalgia • Neck lymphadenopathy • Splenomegaly (EBV) • Trismus, "hot potato" voice (peritonsillar abscess)	• Otitis media • Viral pharyngitis (EBV, HSV) • Bacterial pharyngitis (strep throat) • Tonsillitis • Peritonsillar abscess (quinsy) • Radiation-induced
Dysphagia	
• Mass (painful, painless) • Fluctuating pain with meals • Regurgitation • Aspiration • Hoarseness • Noisy breathing, drooling (suspect epiglottitis)	**Pharyngeal causes:** • Neoplasm (oro/naso/hypopharyngeal) • Ranula (salivary pseudocyst from blocked sublingual gland) • Epiglottitis*/supraglottitis • Retropharyngeal or peritonsillar abscess • Ludwig's angina* • Foreign body **Esophageal causes** (see **Abdominal Exam**, p.18)
Globus Hystericus	
• Dysphagia (± odynophagia) • Nocturnal cough • Hoarseness • Referred otalgia	• Reflux laryngitis • Laryngopharyngeal reflux • Neoplasm (naso/oro/hypopharyngeal) • Thyroid mass • Functional • Rhinosinusitis, post-nasal drip (associated with nocturnal cough)

*Medical emergencies – must first ensure secure airway before examination (see **Essentials of Emergency Medicine**, p.421)
EBV = Epstein-Barr virus, HSV = herpes simplex virus

3.4 Focused Physical Exam

- Routine examination of the oral cavity is important as 30% of patients with oral carcinoma are asymptomatic

Inspection (see **Table 10**)

- Adequate lighting is required
- Ask patient to remove dentures if present
- If discharge present, note volume, color, odor, consistency, and presence of blood
- For common signs of the mouth: see **Table 11**

Table 10. Inspection of Oral Cavity and Pharynx

Anatomic Region	Inspection	Features to Assess
Oral Cavity (lips, tongue, inside cheek, teeth, floor of mouth, gingivae, palate)	• Inspect entire oral cavity visually using two tongue depressors	• General (lesions, lumps, ulcers, purulence, blood, gum disease, xerostomia [dry mouth]) • Lips (color, pigmentation, symmetry, lesions, edema, ulcers, sores, lumps, fissures) • Tongue (lesions, size, lumps, atrophy, fasciculations, symmetry) • Teeth (number, size, wasting, pitting) • Palate (perforation, edema, petechiae) • Buccal mucosa (white lesions)
Palatine Tonsils (between anterior and posterior pillars)	• Inspect visually using tongue depressor	• Enlargement, injection, exudate, ulcerations, crypts
Salivary Apparatus (parotid gland, submandibular gland)	• Direct: bimanual with two tongue depressors	• Gland enlargement • Lumps, masses, lesions • Painful or painless mass • Discharge, salivary production • Salivary stones • Ranula
Posterior Nasopharynx (posterior nasal choanae, posterior nasopharyngeal wall, Eustachian tube orifices)	• Indirect laryngoscopy and tongue depressor • Flexible nasopharyngoscopy	• Nasal polyps • Lesions • Ulceration • Inflammation, edema • Purulence, blood
Hypopharynx/ Larynx (posterior tongue, epiglottis, piriform fossa, vocal cords, false cords, posterior and lateral pharyngeal walls)	• Indirect laryngoscopy and tongue depressor • Flexible nasopharyngoscopy	• Lesions, nodules • Inflammation • Ulceration • Leukoplakia

Palpation

- With a gloved hand, palpate inside the mouth using one finger and use the opposite hand to follow alongside on the surface of the face
- Examine for texture, tenderness, masses, and lesions including plaques, vesicles, nodules, and ulcerations
- Follow a systematic approach: palpate the vermilion of lips, the inner mucosa of lips, mandible, cheeks, roof of mouth, floor of mouth, top of tongue, floor of mandible as far as the angle of the jaw, tonsils (ask patient not to bite)
- Salivary Apparatus
    - Parotid and submandibular glands (enlargement, masses, tenderness, salivary stones)
    - Examine the orifice of each gland:
        - Stenson's duct (parotid duct orifice) opposite upper second molar on buccal mucosa
        - Wharton's duct (submandibular duct orifice) lateral to frenulum of tongue on floor of mouth
    - Massage the gland and observe the discharge from each orifice:
        - Clear vs. cloudy
        - Pain on palpation of the gland

> **Clinical Pearl: Parotid Gland Tumor**
> Tumors of the parotid gland are the most common type of salivary gland tumor, which typically presents as a firm, nontender mass anterior to the ear with normal overlying skin.

Motor Exam (see **Neurological Exam**, p.180)

- Gag reflex (CN IX/X)
- Equal palatal elevation (CN X)
- Central tongue protrusion (CN XII)

Table 11. Common Signs of the Mouth

Signs and Symptoms	Possible Causes
Herpetic Lesions	Fever, pneumonia, immunocompromised state
Aphthous Ulcers (oral lesion)	Associated with celiac disease or IBD
Gum Hypertrophy	Leukemia
Leukoplakia	Neoplasms, HIV
Angular Stomatitis	Vitamin B12 or folate deficiency
Tongue Telangiectasias	GI bleeding
Peutz-Jeghers Spots (brown spots on lips and oral mucosa)	Peutz-Jeghers syndrome, associated with intestinal polyps and GI bleeding
Glossitis	Vitamin B12 deficiency

3.5 Common Investigations

Table 12. Investigations for Mouth and Throat Pathology

Indication	Test
Infection	CBC and differential
Sore Throat with fever >38°C Swollen, red tonsils with exudate Peritonsillar abscess	Throat swab and culture (sensitivity for GAS 90-95%)[14]
Suspected Neoplasm (neck mass, salivary gland, thyroid) ***Note:*** diagnosis of follicular adenoma (thyroid) not possible with FNAB	FNAB
Salivary Stone >90% submandibular calculi are radiopaque >90% parotid calculi are radiolucent	Plain film X-ray, U/S, CT
Neoplasm (Hx smoking, smokeless tobacco, alcohol), salivary stone, abscess, branchial cleft cyst/sinus	CT/MRI Bone scan if mandible involved

- McIsaac Modification of the Centor Strep Score (see **Essentials of Infectious Diseases**, EBM: Sore Throat Score, p.487)

4. NECK & THYROID

4.1 Essential Anatomy

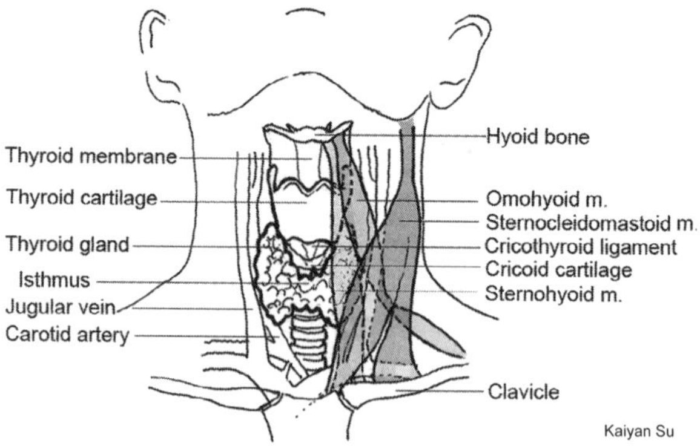

Figure 4. Anatomy of the Neck

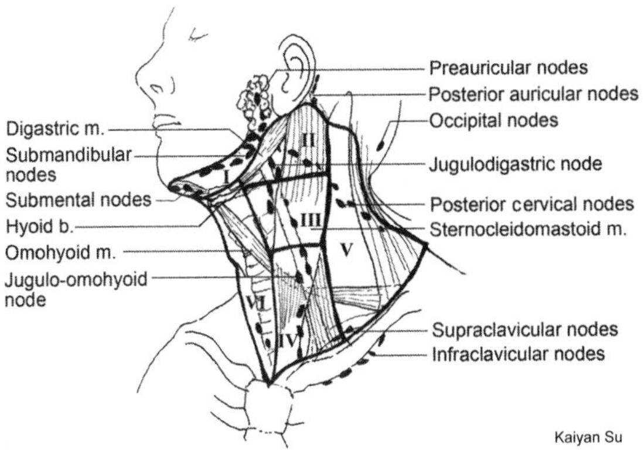

Figure 5. Lymph Node Groups and Levels of the Head and Neck

Table 13. Lymph Node Groups and Levels of the Head and Neck (**see Figure 5**)

Nodal Group/Level	Location	Drainage
Occipital	Base of skull, posterior	Posterior scalp
Posterior Auricular	Superficial to mastoid process	Scalp, temporal region, external auditory meatus, posterior pinna
Preauricular	In front of ear	External auditory meatus, anterior pinna, soft tissues of frontal and temporal regions, roof of nose, eyelids, palpebral conjunctiva
Submental (Level IA)	(Midline) Anterior bellies of digastric muscles, tip of mandible, and hyoid bone	Floor of mouth, anterior oral tongue, anterior mandibular alveolar ridge, lower lip
Submandibular (Level IB)	Anterior belly of digastric muscle, stylohyoid muscle, body of mandible	Oral cavity, anterior nasal cavity, soft tissues of the mid-face, submandibular gland
Upper Jugular (Levels IIA and IIB)	Skull base to inferior border of hyoid bone along sternocleidomastoid (SCM) muscle	Oral cavity, nasal cavity, naso/oro/hypopharynx, larynx, parotid glands
Middle Jugular (Level III)	Inferior border of hyoid bone to inferior border of cricoid cartilage along SCM muscle	Oral cavity, naso/oro/hypopharynx, larynx
Lower Jugular (Level IV)	Inferior border of cricoid cartilage to clavicle along SCM muscle	Hypopharynx, thyroid, cervical esophagus, larynx

Table 13. Lymph Node Groups and Levels of the Head and Neck (continued)

Nodal Group/Level	Location	Drainage
Posterior Triangle* **(Levels VA and VB)**	Posterior border of SCM, anterior border of trapezius, from skull base to clavicle	Nasopharynx and oropharynx, cutaneous structures of the posterior scalp and neck
Anterior Compartment† **(Levels VI)**	(Midline) Hyoid bone to suprasternal notch between the common carotid arteries	Thyroid gland, glottic and subglottic larynx, apex of piriform sinus, cervical esophagus

*Includes some supraclavicular nodes
†Contains Virchow, pretracheal, precricoid paratracheal and perithyroidal nodes
Bickley LS, Szilagyi PG, Bates B. *Bates' Guide to Physical Examination and History Taking*, 10th ed. Philadelphia: Lippincott Williams & Wilkins; 2009.
Robbins KT, et al. 2002. *Arch Otolaryngol Head Neck Surg* 128(7):751-758.

4.2 Common Chief Complaints

- Neck stiffness (nuchal rigidity)
- Neck mass
- Neck swelling
- Neck pain

HEAD & NECK

4.3 Focused History

Neck Stiffness

- Headache (if no other signs/symptoms, suspect tension headache)
- Fever (if present, assess for meningitis, see **Essentials of Infectious Diseases**, p.500)
- Cardiovascular history (referred pain from angina or myocardial infarction)
- If associated with focal neurological symptoms, suspect cerebrovascular accident (CVA)

Neck Mass

- Location: lateral vs. midline (see **Table 14**)
- Age of patient
  - Young (age <40 yr): congenital or inflammatory, neoplasms rare
  - Adult: neck mass malignant until proven otherwise[15]
- Onset, tenderness, and rate of growth
  - A tender mass with rapid onset of swelling is suggestive of an inflammatory, acute infectious etiology or metastasis
  - A nontender, slow-growing mass is suggestive of a malignancy
- Constitutional symptoms (fever, chills, night sweats, weight loss)
- Risk factors for cancer (e.g. tobacco use, alcohol, radiation)
- Presence of recurrent head and neck infection (e.g. HPV, Epstein-Barr virus [EBV])
- Cough, hemoptysis, bone pain
- For thyroid disorders (see **Essentials of Endocrinology**, p.448)

Table 14. Differential Diagnosis of Neck Mass

Focused History	Differential Diagnosis
Lateral Neck Mass	
• Unilateral/bilateral delimitation (borders) • Epistaxis/nasal obstruction • Oral ulcers, persistent sore throat (>3 wk) • Otalgia (referred) • Dysphagia, odynophagia hoarseness, dyspnea • Environmental/occupational exposures (e.g. radiation, asbestos) • Travel history	**Congenital:** • Branchial cleft cyst • Laryngocele • Lymphatic malformation **Benign Neoplastic:** • Salivary gland neoplasm (pleomorphic adenoma, Warthin's tumor) • Vascular lesions (carotid body tumor, aneurysm) • Hemangioma • Lipoma • Fibroma • Nerve or nerve sheath tumor **Malignant Neoplastic:** • Primary: Hodgkin's or non-Hodgkin's lymphoma, salivary gland neoplasm (parotid, submandibular), thyroid, sarcoma • Metastatic: head and neck (usually squamous cell carcinoma), thoracic, abdominal, leukemia **Inflammatory/Infections:** • Reactive adenopathy (abscess, tonsillitis, viral URTI, mononucleosis, HIV, Kawasaki's) • Granulomatous disease (TB, sarcoidosis, syphilis, toxoplasmosis, cat scratch disease) • Salivary glands (sialadentitis, sialolithiasis)
Midline Neck Mass	
• Features of hyper/hypothyroidism • Hoarseness • Environmental/occupational exposures	• Thyroglossal duct cyst* • Thyroid tumor, goiter or pyramidal lobe • Ranula • Dermoid cyst
Diffuse Neck Swelling	
Signs and symptoms of infection, inflammation	Ludwig's angina (neck space infection)† Lymphangioma

*A thyroglossal duct cyst is the most common anterior midline neck mass in children
†Medical emergency: associated swelling may obstruct airway nodes

Clinical Pearl: Neck Masses[15]
90% of pediatric neck masses are inflammatory whereas 90% of adult (>40 yr) neck masses are malignant.

4.4 Focused Physical Exam

General Head and Neck

Inspection

- Position of head, symmetry
- Hair quantity, quality, distribution
- Skin texture, color, moisture, scars
- Skin lesions (location, arrangement, color, size, type)
- Signs of muscle weakness/paralysis of CN VII, X, XII (e.g. facial drooping, flattened nasolabial fold)
- Neck masses (size, location, symmetry)
- Enlarged parotid or submandibular glands
- Trachea (should be in midline)

Palpation

- See **Lymphatic System and Lymph Node Exam**, p.126
- Have the patient sit with head slightly flexed forward and neck relaxed
- Use a consistent order when palpating lymph nodes (e.g. start with occipital nodes, move to posterior auricular and preauricular nodes and then palpate the levels of the neck in order)
- Use bimanual approach to examine Level I (submandibular and submental nodes) with one gloved finger in the floor of the mouth and fingers of other hand following along skin externally
- Note tenderness, size, consistency, mobility, level
- Palpate salivary glands

> **Clinical Pearl: Supraclavicular Lymph Nodes[16]**
> Left-sided enlargement of a supraclavicular node (Virchow's node) may indicate an abdominal malignancy; right-sided enlargement may indicate malignancy of lungs, mediastinum or esophagus. Enlargement of occipital nodes may be a sign of rubella.

Thyroid

Inspection

- Identify the thyroid and cricoid cartilages and the trachea (note any tracheal deviation)
- Visible thyroid is suspicious for enlargement (goiter)
- Look for systemic signs of thyroid disease (see **Essentials of Endocrinology**, p.448)

Palpation

- Patient's neck should be slightly flexed
- Anterior approach: position yourself in front and to the side of the patient
- Posterior approach: position yourself behind the patient's chair
- Examine one side at a time:
    - Relax the right sternocleidomastoid by turning patient's head slightly to right
    - Landmark using thyroid and cricoid cartilages
    - Displace trachea to right while palpating right side
    - Ask patient to swallow some water and feel for glandular tissue on right side rising under fingers
    - Repeat for left side
- The thyroid isthmus is often palpable
- Describe gland:
    - Shape/size: normal ~ size of an adult distal phalanx of thumb
    - Consistency:
        - Rubbery (normal)
        - Hard (associated with cancer or scarring)
        - Soft (associated with toxic goiter)
    - Nodules: size, consistency, number, tenderness (suggests thyroiditis)
- Pemberton's sign: a large goiter extending retrosternally may block the thoracic inlet and compress jugular veins, causing facial plethora when both arms are raised

Auscultation

- Auscultate over the lateral lobes to detect any bruits
- A localized systolic or continuous bruit may be heard in thyrotoxicosis (e.g. Graves' disease)

> **Clinical Pearl: Thyroglossal Duct Cysts**
> A thyroglossal duct cyst will elevate with tongue protrusion while a thyroid nodule will not.

4.5 Common Investigations

Table 15. Investigations for Head and Neck Pathology

Indication/Finding	Test
Infection (acute, chronic) Tumor	CBC and differential
Suspected thyroid disease	T_4 and TSH levels
Hoarseness 1-3 wk of unknown etiology[17] Persistent neck mass of unknown etiology Visualize naso/oro/hypopharynx for neoplasm Suspected laryngocele	Indirect laryngoscopy, laryngoscopy and/or flexible nasopharyngoscopy
Lateral or midline mass (tumors, cysts, salivary stones, abscess) Enhancing wall, contents of mass	CT/MRI
Branchial cleft cyst, ranula, multinodular goiter, thyroid goiter, thyroid nodule	U/S
Persistent neck mass (>4 wk) unknown etiology	FNAB
Suspicious neck mass/primary, difficult biopsy sites	Endoscopy with biopsy

5. COMMON CLINICAL SCENARIOS

5.1 Dizziness

- **Dizziness:** a term used to describe any of a variety of sensations that produce spatial disorientation
- **Vertigo:** illusion that the body or environment is spinning or tumbling (rotational, linear or tilting movement)
- **Lightheadedness:** sense of impending faint, presyncope
- **Oscillopsia:** inability to focus on objects with motion
- **Disequilibrium:** sensation of instability of body positions, "off-balance"
- Differential diagnosis of dizziness complaint[18]:
  - Peripheral: benign paroxysmal positional vertigo (BPPV), Ménière's disease, vestibular neuronitis, cerebellopontine angle tumor (e.g. acoustic neuroma)
  - Central: MS, other neurologic disorders (stroke, seizure, cerebellar lesion)
  - Systemic: metabolic (e.g. hypo/hyperthyroidism, DM)
  - Medications and intoxicants
  - Vascular: basilar migraine syndrome, vertebrobasilar insufficiency

Focused History

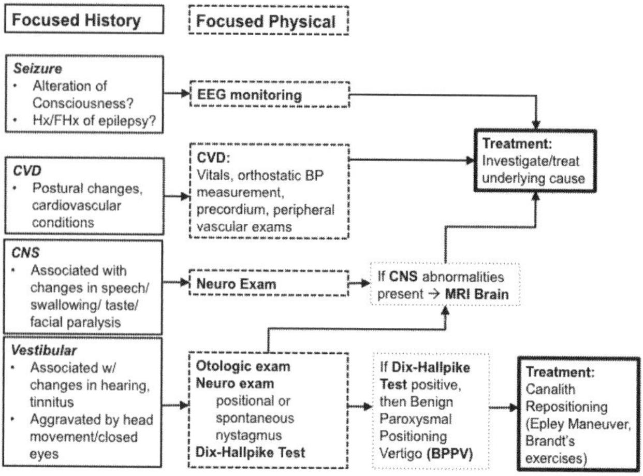

Figure 6. Clinical Evaluation of "Dizziness"
Post RE, Dickerson LM. 2010. Dizziness: A diagnostic approach. *Am Fam Physician* 82(4):361-369.

Focused Physical Exam

- **Dix-Hallpike Maneuver** (test for BPPV)
  - Start in sitting position, turn and support head at 45° to right
  - Swiftly move patient into supine position with head overhanging bed
  - Maintain the head at 45° and watch eyes (i.e. keep them open)
  - Can have latency up to 30 s before nystagmus occurs
  - Crescendo-decrescendo rotatory geotropic nystagmus (subsides within minutes)
  - When present, indicates disease in the ear closest to the ground
  - Upon sitting back up, look for nystagmus (if present, could reverse in direction or in an oblique upbeat direction)
  - Sensitivity 79%, Specificity 75%[19]
- **Dizziness Stimulation Tests:** positional vertigo, orthostatic hypotension, hyperventilation

5.2 Acute Otitis Media (see **Figure 7**)

- Acute inflammation of the middle ear
- 60-70% of children have at least 1 episode before 3 yr of age[20]

5.3 Epistaxis

- Anterior epistaxis (from Kiesselbach's plexus in Little's area) is more common (80%) and is seen more often in children
- Posterior epistaxis is less common (20%) and is seen more often in patients >50 yr

> **Clinical Pearl: Epistaxis**
> Severe, unilateral epistaxis with no history of trauma in an adolescent male is **juvenile nasopharyngeal angiofibroma** until proven otherwise.
>
> Recurrent epistaxis in older males of south-eastern Asian or southern Chinese descent is **nasopharyngeal carcinoma** until proven otherwise.

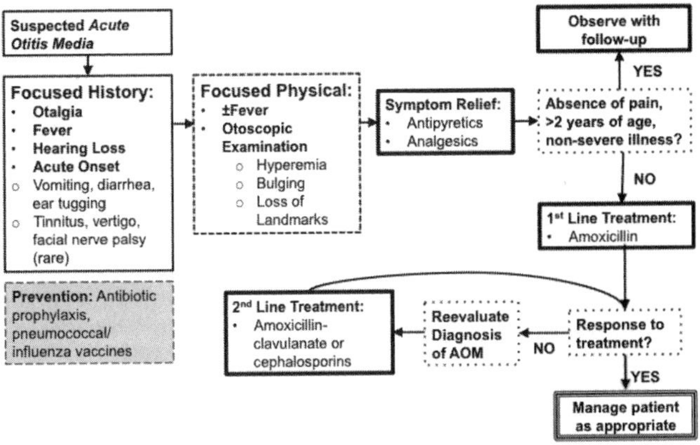

Figure 7. Clinical Evaluation and Management of Acute Otitis Media
American Academy of Pediatrics. 2004. *Pediatrics* 113(5):1451-1465.
Leach AJ, Morris PS. Cochrane Database of Systematic Reviews 2006, Issue 4. Art. No.: CD004401.

Focused History

- Onset/duration of bleeding
- Frequency and past episodes
- Taste of blood in throat
- Medications and street drugs (cocaine)
- Symptoms of local problems and systemic diseases (see **Table 16**)

Focused Physical Exam

- Vitals
- Volume assessment
- Nasal speculum exam (use suction, gloves, face mask, and eye protection)
- Posterior bleeds often reveal little bleeding from the nostrils and more blood along the posterior pharynx
- Flexible nasopharyngoscope for suspicion of posterior epistaxis

Management

- Anterior epistaxis
  - Have the patient pinch his/her nose over cartilaginous portion (not nasal bones) and tilt head forward
  - Most bleeds will respond to local finger compression within 10-12 min
  - If bleeding persists and the patient has no history of heart disease, consider application of topical vasoconstrictor (oxymetazoline, cocaine hydrochloride)
  - If bleeding persists, attempt silver nitrate chemical cautery or anterior pack
  - If bleeding still persists, suspect HTN, inadequate exterior packing, coagulopathy or posterior epistaxis
- Posterior epistaxis
  - Requires a posterior pack and prophylactic antibiotics
  - Treat HTN if present
  - If bleeding persists after 3-5 d, consider endoscopic arterial ligation or embolization
- Correct hypovolemia if present
- If indicated, discontinue NSAIDs, adjust anticoagulant dose, replace clotting factors

Investigations

- If bleeding is minor and does not recur, no investigations needed
- If bleeding is recurrent and/or heavy:
  - Blood type and cross-match
  - CBC, hematocrit
  - aPTT, INR, LFTs (anticoagulant use, suspected liver disease)
  - CT and/or MRI and/or nasopharyngoscopy if foreign body or neoplasm suspected

Table 16. Differential Diagnosis of Epistaxis

Category	Differential Diagnosis
Local Factors	• Trauma (nose-picking, accidental injury) • Mucosal drying secondary to nasal septal deviation, spurs, perforations causing turbulent air flow • Foreign body (unilateral, foul discharge, occasional epistaxis) • Iatrogenic (septal, orbital, turbinate, sinus surgery) • Inflammation (URTI, sinusitis, allergies, chemical irritation) • Chemicals (cocaine, nasal sprays, ammonia, gasoline, phosphorus, chromium salts, sulfuric acid, mercury)
Environmental	• Barotrauma; cold, dry air
Neoplasms	• Adults: melanoma, squamous cell carcinoma, inverted papillomas, adenoid cystic carcinoma • Children: polyps, encephaloceles, gliomas, meningoceles
Systemic	• Coagulopathies: anticoagulant use (coumadin, heparin), liver disease, hemophilia, thrombocytopenia, von Willebrand's disease, NSAIDs, chemotherapy • Malignant tumors • Vascular disorders: HTN, arteriosclerosis, Osler-Weber-Rendu disease (hereditary hemorrhagic telangiectasia) • Granulomatous diseases: Wegener's, SLE, TB, rhinoscleroma, sarcoidosis, leprosy
Complementary and Alternative Medications[21]	• Fish oil, evening primrose, garlic, cranberry juice, aloe, vitamin E, echinacea, ginseng, St. John's wort, ginkgo biloba, valerian, ginger, kava, melatonin, ephedra, saw palmetto

5.4 Hoarseness (Dysphonia)

- Abnormality of the voice affecting one or more of: pitch, volume, resonance, quality
- Often associated with URTI of viral origin in otherwise healthy patients
- Hoarseness lasting more than 1-3 wk must be investigated with a complete head and neck exam including indirect laryngoscopy and/or nasopharyngoscopy to rule out laryngeal cancer[17]
- See **Table 17** for differential diagnosis

Focused History

- Onset and progression, past occurrences
- Timing (A.M./P.M./continuous)
- Associated pharyngitis and/or otalgia (referred via CN IX and CN X)
- Cough, hemoptysis, constitutional symptoms
- Associated dysphagia, odynophagia
- Habits (smoking, alcohol)
- Past history of radiation exposure (treatment of scars, occupational exposure)
- Previous surgery and/or intubations

- History of GERD, past or present lung or breast cancer or lymphoma

Focused Physical Exam

- Palpation of head and neck lymph nodes
- Laryngeal crepitus:
  - Normal: crepitus is felt when larynx is gently moved laterally
  - Absence of crepitus suggests mass in retropharyngeal space or hypopharynx
- Examination of oral and nasal cavities
- Indirect laryngoscopy and/or flexible nasolaryngoscopy:
  - Have the patient say 'eeeee' to assess vocal cord mobility

Investigations

- Indirect laryngoscopy and/or nasopharyngoscopy
- Pneumatic otoscopy
- CXR, CT with contrast
- TSH, CBC, ESR, rheumatoid factor (RF), and biopsy

Table 17. Differential Diagnosis of Hoarseness

History	Physical Findings
Acute Viral Laryngitis	
• Viral URTI preceding aphonia ± history of pharyngitis	• Bilateral vocal cord edema and erythema
GERD-Associated Laryngitis	
History of GERD and its precipitating factors	• Erythema and edema of the mucosa lining the arytenoids ± ulcers or granulomas in same region
Vocal Cord Nodules	
• Singers, females, and children • Aggravated by URTI, sinusitis, smoke, and alcohol	• **Acute:** soft, red • **Chronic:** fibrotic, hard, white • Bilateral (paired) on anterior 1/3 of cords
Vocal Cord Polyp	
• Males, smokers, vocal misuse/abuse or irritant exposure ± dyspnea, cough	• Unilateral or bilateral, asymmetric, broad-based and pedunculated with a smooth, soft appearance
Squamous Papillomas	
• HPV infection • Past episodes	• Anterior commissure and true vocal cord most common location; subglottic and supraglottic areas may be involved • White to reddish verrucous mass
Laryngeal Carcinoma	
Risk Factors: alcohol, smoking, exposure to radiation, juvenile papillomatosis (HPV), nickel exposure, laryngocele Dysphagia, odynophagia Otalgia (referred from CN IX or CN X) Hemoptysis Cough	• Dysplasia or carcinoma *in situ* may appear as leukoplakia • Tumor appears as ulcerated growth on vocal cord membrane ± neck mass • Paralyzed vocal cord

Table 17. Differential Diagnosis of Hoarseness (continued)

History	Physical Findings
Spasmodic Dysphonia	
• Strained, strangled voice associated with facial grimacing • Voice is normal during singing, crying or laughing	• Hyperadduction of the true and false cords
Cord Paralysis	
• Dramatic "breathy" voice due to air escape • Bilateral paralysis may lead to airway compromise • History of recurrent laryngeal nerve damage (surgical, endotracheal tube, breech birth in neonates) • Lung, breast cancer (infiltration of recurrent laryngeal nerve as it loops through thorax)	**Unilateral:** • Cord abducted in resting position and unable to adduct during phonation **Bilateral:** • Cords adducted, unable to abduct with little space between
Trauma	
• History of trauma to the larynx • Trauma-induced lesions of the vocal cord (screaming, singing)	• Severe trauma can result in fracture or dislocation of arytenoids • Vocal abuse results in benign vocal cord polyps, nodules or contact granulomas

REFERENCES

1. Harvey H. 1992. Diagnosing referred otalgia: The ten Ts. *Cranio* 10(4):333-334.
2. Laitakari K, Löppönen H. 1994. Carhart notch and electric bone-conduction audiometry. *Scandinavian Audiology* 23(2):139-141.
3. Schreiber BE, Agrup C, Haskard DO, Luxon LM. 2010. Sudden sensorineural hearing loss. *Lancet* 375(9721):1203-1211.
4. Roland PS, Stewart MG, Hannley M, Friedman R, Manolidis S, Matz G, et al. 2004. *Otolaryngol Head Neck Surg* 130(3 Suppl):S51-56.
5. Curhan SG, Eavey R, Shargorodsky J, Curhan GC. 2010. *Am J Med* 123(3):231-237.
6. Bisht M, Bist SS. 2011. Ototoxicity: The hidden menace. *Indian J Otolaryngol Head Neck Surg* 63(3):255-259.
7. Prasher D. 2009. *Noise Health* 11(44):141-144.
8. Lee CA, Mistry D, Uppal S, Coatesworth AP. 2005. Otologic side effects of drugs. *J Laryngol Otol* 119(4):267-271.
9. McGwin G Jr. 2010. *Arch Otolaryngol Head Neck Surg* 136(5):488-492.
10. Pirozzo S, Papinczak T, Glasziou P. 2003. Whispered voice test for screening for hearing impairment in adults and children: Systematic review. *BMJ* 327(7421):967.
11. MRC Multi-Centre Otitis Media Study Group. 1999. Sensitivity, specificity and predictive value of tympanometry in predicting a hearing impairment in otitis media with effusion. *Clin Otolaryngol Allied Sci* 24(4):294-300.
12. Meyer C, Witte J, Hildmann A, Hennecke KH, Schunck KU, Maul K, et al. 1999. Neonatal screening for hearing disorders in infants at risk: Incidence, risk factors, and follow-up. *Pediatrics* 104(4):900-904.
13. Clark JG. 1989. Uses and abuses of hearing loss classification. *ASHA* 23(7):493-500.
14. Bisno AL, Gerber MA, Gwaltney JM, Kaplan EL, Schwartz RH. 2002. Practice guidelines for the diagnosis and management of group A streptococcal pharyngitis. *Clin Infect Dis* 35(2):113-125.
15. Otto RA, Bowes AK.1990. Neck masses: Benign or malignant? Sorting out the causes by age-group. *Postgrad Med* 88(1):199-204.
16. Chau I, Kelleher MT, Cunningham D, Norman AR, Wotherspoon A, Trott P, et al. 2003. Rapid access multidisciplinary lymph node diagnostic clinic: Analysis of 550 patients. *Br J Cancer* 88(3):354-361.
17. Schwartz SR, Cohen SM, Dailey SH, Rosenfield RM, Deutsch ES, Gillespie MB, et al. 2009. Clinical practice guideline: Hoarseness (dysphonia). *Otolaryngol Head Neck Surg* 141(3 Suppl 2):S1-S31.
18. Post RE, Dickerson LM. 2010. Dizziness: A diagnostic approach. *Am Fam Physician* 82(4): 361-369.
19. Halker RB, Barrs DM, Wellik KE, Wingerchuk DM, Demaerschalk BM. 2008. *Neurologist* 14(3):201-204.
20. Teele DW, Klein JO, Rosner B. 1989. Epidemiology of otitis media during the first seven years of life in children in greater Boston: A prospective, cohort study. *J Infect Dis* 160(1):83-94.
21. Melia L, McGarry GW. 2011. Epistaxis: Update on management. *Curr Opin Otolaryngol Head Neck Surgery* 19(1):30-35.
22. Bickley LS, Szilagyi PG, Bates B. *Bates' Guide to Physical Examination and History Taking*, 10th ed. Philadelphia: Lippincott Williams & Wilkins; 2009.
23. Cummings CW. *Otolaryngology – Head & Neck Surgery*. Philadelphia: Elsevier Mosby; 2005.
24. Dhillon RS, East CA. *Ear, Nose and Throat and Head and Neck Surgery*. Edinburgh: Churchill Livingstone/Elsevier; 2006.
25. Jafek BW, Murrow BW. *ENT Secrets*. Philadelphia: Elsevier/Mosby; 2005.

HEAD & NECK

The Lymphatic System and Lymph Node Exam

Editors:
Neil Dinesh Dattani
Yayi Huang
Alex Zhao

Faculty Reviewers:
Tina Borschel, MD, MSc
Yoo-Joung Ko, MD, MSc, FRCP(C)

TABLE OF CONTENTS

LYMPHATIC

1. ESSENTIALS OF ANATOMY

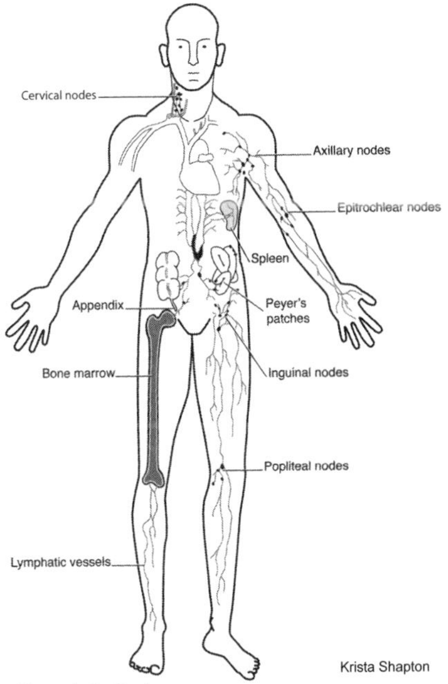

Figure 1. Overview of Lymphatic System

Table 1. Functional Overview of Lymph Tissues

Lymphoid Tissue	Function	Site
Lymph Nodes	Lymphatic drainage of various body areas	Located throughout body (see **Table 2** for details)
Tonsils (lingual, palatine, tubal, adenoids making up Waldeyer's ring)	Protects entrance to respiratory passages	Base of tongue, pharyngeal and nasopharyngeal walls
Spleen	RBC and platelet storage, defective RBC disposal, antibody formation by intrinsic B-cells	Left upper quadrant of abdomen
Peyer's Patch	IgA antibody formation by intrinsic B-lymphocytes	Ileal walls
Appendix	IgA immune response to ingested antigens	Lower cecal outpouching

Moore KL, Dalley AF, Agur AMR. *Clinically Oriented Anatomy*, 7th ed. Philadelphia: Lippincott Williams & Wilkins; 2013.

Table 2. Overview of Lymph Node Drainage

Lymph Node Group	Location	Drainage
Head and Neck Nodes (see **Head and Neck Exam, Table 13**, p.111)		
Supraclavicular	Superior to clavicle	H&N and axillary nodes
Infraclavicular	Inferior to clavicle	H&N and axillary nodes
Scalene	Posterior to clavicle	H&N and axillary nodes
Upper Extremities: Axillary		
Apical Group	At apex of axilla	All other axillary nodes
Central Group	High in axilla, deep to pectoralis minor (often palpable)	Pectoral, lateral, and subscapular nodes
Pectoral (Anterior) Group	Inside anterior axillary fold, along lower border of pectoralis major	Anterior chest wall and breast
Subscapular (Posterior) Group	Deep in posterior axillary fold, along lateral border of scapula	Anterior chest wall and breast
Lateral Group	Along upper humerus	Most of arm
Epitrochlear or Cubital	Above medial epicondyle	Ulnar aspect of hand and forearm
Lower Extremities: Inguinal Nodes		
Superficial Vertical Group	Near upper portion of leg along the proximal portion of the great saphenous vein	Superficial tissue of upper leg
Superficial Horizontal Group	Just below inguinal ligament	Skin of lower abdominal wall, external genitalia (except testes), anal canal, lower third of vagina, gluteal region

Table 2. Overview of Lymph Node Drainage (continued)

Lymph Node Group	Location	Drainage
Lower Extremities: Inguinal Nodes		
Superficial Popliteal	Popliteal fossa (one) node	Heel and lateral aspect of foot
Deep Inguinal	Deep medial aspect of femoral vein	Popliteal and superficial inguinal regions

2. COMMON CHIEF COMPLAINTS

- Enlarged lymph node (e.g. lump or bump with or without pain)
- Swollen extremity (e.g. arm, leg, or ankle as in lymphedema)

3. FOCUSED HISTORY

- **History of Present Illness**
  - Enlarged lymph node: “Do you have any abnormal lumps or bumps?”
    - Character: onset, location, duration, tenderness, number
    - Associated symptoms: pain, fever, erythema, warmth, itchiness, red streaks
    - Predisposing factors: infection, surgery, trauma
  - Swollen extremity: “Do you have any swelling?”
    - Character: unilateral/bilateral, intermittent/continuous, duration
    - Associated symptoms: warmth, erythema, discoloration, ulceration
    - Predisposing factors: cardiac and/or renal disorder, malignancy, surgery, infection, trauma, venous insufficiency
    - Alleviating factors: support stockings, elevation
  - Constitutional symptoms: fever, night sweats, weight loss, fatigue
- **Past Medical History**
  - Past surgeries/injuries (e.g. trauma to regional lymph nodes), medications (e.g. phenytoin, chemoradiation), malignancies, recurrent infections, chronic inflammatory diseases (e.g. SLE, RA), immunosuppression
- **Family History**
  - Malignancy, recurrent infections, TB
- **Social History**
  - Sexual behavior, STIs (e.g. syphilis, chlamydia, HIV), occupational/travel (e.g. infectious or carcinogenic exposures)

4. FOCUSED PHYSICAL EXAM

The lymphatic system is often examined along with other body systems, and consists primarily of inspection and palpation of lymph nodes. Consider the regional drainage patterns of these lymph nodes, and look for any signs of infection or malignancy in those areas. Distinguish between regional and generalized lymphadenopathy by assessing lymph nodes elsewhere.

- **Screening Exam**
  - In a patient who is otherwise asymptomatic or presenting with an unrelated chief complaint: inspect and palpate H&N, axillary and inguinal nodes, liver, and spleen
- **Inspection**
  - In each region, look for visible node enlargement, edema, muscle bulk/symmetry, color changes (e.g. erythema or red streaks) or ulceration
- **Palpation**
  - In each area, using the pads of the index and middle fingers, move in circular motions over the underlying tissues first by applying light pressure, then gradually increasing the pressure

- Note that excess pressure from the start may displace or obscure the nodes into deeper soft tissues before they are recognized
- For comparison, palpate right and left lymph nodes simultaneously and note:
  - Location
  - Size (<1 cm or >1 cm)
  - Shape (regular or irregular borders)
  - Delimitation (discrete or matted together)
  - Mobility (fixed or mobile/tethered to skin or deeper tissues)
  - Consistency (soft, hard, or firm)
  - Tenderness (tender or nontender)

Clinical Pearl: Malignant Lymph Node
Lymph nodes that rapidly increase in size, fixate to skin or soft tissues, become confluent, or are painless may indicate malignancy.

- A normal lymph node should be <1 cm in size, feel soft and nontender, and have regular and discrete borders
- If edema is noted, check for pitting edema to rule out lymphedema, which does not have the characteristic pitting that is associated with other causes of edema
- Approach an unexplained enlarged lymph node by examining **PALS**: **P**rimary site, **A**ll associated nodes, **L**iver, **S**pleen

Clinical Pearl: Inflammatory Lymph Node
Lymph nodes <2 cm in size, regularly bordered, tender to touch, soft, and mobile are likely inflammatory in nature and less worrisome.

Clinical Pearl: Distinguishing Lymph Nodes from Other Structures

Character	Lymph Node	Artery	Cyst	Muscle
Rolls in 2 directions	✓	x	x	x
Pulsates	x	✓	x	x
Transilluminates with direct light	x	x	✓	x

Clinical Pearl: Palpating Lymph Nodes
Palpate lymph nodes in a firm, circular motion with the pads of your fingers and always evaluate for symmetry. Make sure fingernails are trimmed!

4.1 Head and Neck

It is important to develop a systematic approach to palpating lymph nodes in the head and neck to ensure no groups are missed. A suggested practical approach is presented in groups of 3+3+3+1 sets of lymph nodes:

- Above the mandible
  - Preauricular: in front of the ears
  - Posterior auricular: behind the ears and superficial to the mastoid process
  - Occipital: posterior base of the skull
- At the mandible
  - Tonsillar: angle of the mandible
  - Submandibular: under the mandible between the angle and anterior tip
  - Submental: anterior tip of mandible

- Below the mandible
  - Superficial cervical: superficial to sternocleidomastoid (SCM)
  - Posterior cervical: in posterior triangle along the border of trapezius
  - Deep cervical: deep to SCM; accessible by placing thumb on muscle belly of SCM and hooking fingers around the anterior border
- At the clavicle
  - Supraclavicular and infraclavicular: >1cm is significant
- Remember that other structures such as the salivary glands (parotid, sublingual, submandibular), arteries (carotid, temporal), and cysts can be encountered in these areas and may mimic lymph nodes (see **Clinical Pearl: Distinguishing Lymph Nodes from Other Structures**, p.126)

> **Clinical Pearl: Normal vs. Malignant Cervical Lymphadenopathy**
> Cervical lymph node enlargement is common in children and over 90% of cases are caused by either benign enlargement secondary to infection/inflammation, or physiological enlargement. Nodes that are fixed, matted down, present for >3 mo and enlarging, >2 cm, and any supraclavicular enlargement may represent a malignant process.

4.2 Upper Extremities

- **Axillary:** to examine the right axilla, support and slightly abduct the patient's flexed right arm with your right hand and palpate 5 regions with left hand including:
  - Anteriorly: pectoral muscles
  - Posteriorly: latissimus dorsi and subscapularis
  - Medially: rib cage
  - Laterally: upper arm
  - Apically: axilla
- Vice versa for the left axilla
- **Epitrochlear:** support patient's flexed elbow in one hand, and palpate using the other hand in the depression above and posterior to the medial epicondyle of the humerus

4.3 Lower Extremities

- **Inguinal:** ask patient to lie supine with knee slightly flexed, roll fingers above and below inguinal ligament to access only the superficial nodes (small nodes of 0.5 cm are often found; deeper abdominal, pelvic, and para-aortic nodes that drain the testes and internal female genitalia are inaccessible by palpation)
- **Popliteal:** with both hands hooked around knee, place thumbs on tibial tuberosity and palpate deeply in popliteal fossa with 3-4 fingers from each hand (one node is occasionally palpable)

Table 3. Significance of Lymph Node Character and Location

Lymph Node Character	Indication
Hard (often asymmetrical with unremarkable contralateral node), size >2 cm, nontender, fixed	Carcinoma
Firm, Rubbery, Nontender	Lymphoma
Tender	Inflammation
Nonpitting Edema (pitting edema more often associated with other causes)	Lymphedema

Table 3. Significance of Lymph Node Character and Location (continued)

Location of Enlarged Nodes	Indication
Occipital	Scalp infection, rubella
Preauricular	Conjunctival infection, cat scratch disease
Cervical	URTI, oral or dental lesion, infectious mononucleosis (posterior) or other viral illness, metastases from H&N, lung, breast, or thyroid
Supraclavicular and Scalene (always abnormal)	Metastases: • Virchow's (left supraclavicular): from gastrointestinal system, lungs, breast, testes, ovaries • Right-sided Virchow's: from thoracic regions (mediastinal, lung, esophageal) Non-neoplastic causes: TB, sarcoidosis, toxoplasmosis
Axillary	Infection/injury of ipsilateral upper extremity, metastases from breast, melanoma of upper extremity
Epitrochlear	Syphilis, non-Hodgkin's lymphoma
Inguinal	Infection/injury of ipsilateral lower extremity, metastases from rectum/genitalia (penile/scrotal or vulval/lower third of vaginal areas), melanoma of lower extremity, certain STIs (primarily syphilis)

Note: A normal (non-malignant) palpable lymph node is <1 cm in size, soft and nontender, with regular and discrete borders.

Clinical Pearl: Inguinal Lymph Node Biopsies
Inguinal lymphadenopathy is relatively nonspecific and should be avoided for biopsy if there is another appropriate node to biopsy, given the frequency of lower extremity trauma and infection.

5. COMMON INVESTIGATIONS

Laboratory tests should be used to confirm a diagnosis suspected on the basis of history and physical exam findings (e.g. infectious or malignant). If the clinical evaluations are nonconfirmatory, diagnostic work-up should consider if the adenopathy is localized or generalized.

- **Generalized (lymphadenopathy in more than one region):** CBC, electrolytes, CXR (PA/AP and lateral views), urine routine and microscopy (R&M)/culture and sensitivity (C&S), throat and genital swabs
  - If normal, consider infections:
    - Tuberculin purified protein derivative test (PPD)
    - HIV antibody
    - Rapid plasma reagin (RPR) for syphilis
    - Antinuclear antibody (ANA) for autoimmune diseases
    - Heterophile/monospot test for infectious mononucleosis due to Epstein-Barr virus
  - If uncertain, then: excisional biopsy of the most abnormal node (or supraclavicular, neck, axilla or groin in this order if a single node is unattainable) for abnormal cells and architecture using local anesthesia

- **Localized (involving one region of lymph nodes):** observe for 3-4 wk if history is not suggestive of malignancy, but if adenopathy is nonresolving then consider an open biopsy
  - Fine needle aspiration for cytology (especially in HIV+ patients)
  - Core needle biopsy for special studies and architecture
- **Imaging:** CT, U/S, Doppler, or MRI are all modalities to distinguish enlarged lymph nodes from other structures, to define pathological processes, to stage malignancy, and to help guide fine needle aspiration

> **Clinical Pearl: Fluctuant Nodes**
> Incision and drainage of a fluctuant node is useful to help relieve pain and reduce infection, but not useful for diagnosis.

6. COMMON DISORDERS

Disorders marked with (✓) are discussed in **Common Clinical Scenarios**

- ✓ Acute suppurative lymphadenitis
- ✓ Epstein-Barr virus mononucleosis
- ✓ HIV seropositivity
- ✓ Acute lymphangitis
- ✓ Lymphedema
- ✓ Elephantiasis
- ✓ Systemic lupus erythematosus
- ✓ *Mycobacterium* infection
- ✓ Drugs causing generalized lymphadenophathy
- Metastatic carcinoma
- Hodgkin's lymphoma
- Non-Hodgkin's lymphoma

> **Clinical Pearl: Diagnosis of Lymphoma**
> To rule out lymphoma you need a core or excisional lymph node biopsy, as fine needle aspirates are not able to evaluate the lymph node architecture.

7. COMMON CLINICAL SCENARIOS

	Etiology	Character	Associated with...	Notes
Acute Suppurative Lymphadenitis	Group A beta-hemolytic *streptococci* or coagulase-positive *staphylococci* (often young children) causing one-sided pus-forming inflammation of lymph nodes	Firm and tender swollen nodes on palpation, possible erythema on overlying skin and tissue	Sudden onset fever, anorexia, and irritability	
Epstein-Barr Virus Mononucleosis	Viral infection producing abnormally large number of mononuclear leukocytes (mostly B cells) in blood, and leading to bilateral inflammation of any lymph node chains (especially cervical)	Generally discrete and sometimes tender nodes with varying firmness on palpation (cervical nodes are especially affected)	Pharyngitis, often fever, fatigue, malaise, nausea only, and splenomegaly	

Common Clinical Scenarios (Continued)

	Etiology	Character	Associated with...	Notes
HIV Sero-positivity	HIV causing persistent generalized lymphadenopathy for >3 mo and involving 2 or more extra-inguinal sites (may be first sign of initial infection and is part of the asymptomatic phase)	Generally tender, discrete and freely mobile nodes on palpation; presence of small, ill-defined nodes may indicate disease progression, and/or treatment failure	Severe fatigue, malaise, fever, weight loss, weakness, arthralgias, and persistent diarrhea	See **Infectious Diseases Exam**, p.491 for more detail

7.1 Disorders of the Lymphatic Vessels

Acute Lymphangitis

- **Etiology:** infection at a site distal to the lymphatic vessels resulting in inflammation of the lymphatic vessels
- **Character:** fine, red streaks along the lymphatic collecting ducts
  - Tubules may be slightly indurated and palpable by gentle touch
  - Inspect distally for sites of infection, especially in the interdigital spaces for cracks
- **Associated with:** pain in affected extremity, malaise, and possibly fever

Lymphedema

- **Etiology:** swelling of the subcutaneous tissue from accumulation of lymph fluid due to primary (congenital) or secondary (acquired) obstruction of lymph drainage
  - Primary lymphedema: hypoplasia or maldevelopment of the lymphatic system
  - Secondary lymphedema: lymph node dissection or radiation, malignant obstruction or infection
- **Character:** painless, non-pitting swelling of an extremity, usually with involvement of the digits
  - Over time, the skin becomes dry, firm, and fibrous to palpation
- **Associated with:** increased susceptibility to local inflammation from infection or limb injury; should evaluate for cellulitis from staphylococcal or streptococcal skin infections

Lymphatic Filariasis (Elephantiasis)

- **Etiology:** infection with one of three nematodes (*Wuchereria bancrofti*, *Brugia malayi*, or *Brugia timori*) causing lymphatic obstruction through host immune response, direct actions of the parasite or its products
- **Character:** initially similar to lymphedema, over time texture of the skin changes and becomes hyperkeratotic with verrucous and vesicular skin lesions
- **Associated with:** three distinct phases: asymptomatic microfilaremia, acute episodes of adenolymphangitis (ADL), and chronic disease (irreversible lymphedema), which is often superimposed upon repeated episodes of ADL
- Major cause of disfigurement and disability in endemic areas, leading to significant economic and psychosocial impact

7.2 Other Common Scenarios

Systemic Lupus Erythematosus

- **Etiology:** the exact etiology of SLE remains unknown; there is a role for genetic, hormonal, immunologic, and environmental factors. Clinical manifestations of this multisystem disorder are mediated directly or indirectly by antibody formation and the creation of chronic immune complexes
- **Character:** nodes are typically soft, nontender, discrete, variable in size, and usually detected in the cervical, axillary, and inguinal areas
- **Associated with:** the onset of disease or an exacerbation. Lymph node enlargement can also be the result of infection or a lymphoproliferative disease in SLE; when infections are present, the enlarged nodes are more likely to be tender

Mycobacterium Infection

- **Etiology:**
  - Adults: *M. tuberculosis*
  - Children: other mycobacteria (e.g. *M. avium* complex, *M. scrofulaceum*)
  - In patients with generalized lymphadenopathy, miliary tuberculosis should be considered
- **Character:** nodes are typically nontender, enlarge over weeks to months without prominent systemic symptoms, and can progress to matting and fluctuation
- **Associated with:** lymphadenopathy alone, especially in the neck

Drugs Causing Generalized Lymphadenopathy

- Drug Classes
  - Anticonvulsants: carbamazepine, primidone, phenytoin (can cause generalized lymphadenopathy in the absence of a serum sickness reaction)
  - Antimicrobials: cephalosporins, penicillin, sulfonamides, pyrimethamine
  - Antihypertensives: atenolol, captopril, hydralazine
  - Antiarrythmics: quinidine
  - Anti-inflammatories: sulindac, gold
  - Antigout: allopurinol
- Specialty Specific
  - Neurology: carbamazepine, primidone, phenytoin (can cause generalized lymphadenopathy in the absence of a serum sickness reaction)
  - Infectious diseases: cephalosporins, penicillin, sulfonamides, pyrimethamine
  - Cardiology: quinidine, atenolol, captopril, hydralazine
  - Rheumatology: allopurinol, gold, sulindac

REFERENCES

1. Bickley LS, Szilagyi PG, Bates B. *Bates' Guide to Physical Examination and History Taking*, 10th ed. Philadelphia: Lippincott Williams & Wilkins; 2009.
2. Seidel HM, Ball JW, Dains JE, Flynn JA, Solomon BS, Stewart RW. *Mosby's Guide to Physical Examination*, 7th ed. St. Louis: Mosby Elsevier; 2011.
3. Porter RS (Editor). *The Merck Manual of Diagnosis and Therapy*, 19th ed. Whitehouse Station: Merck Research Laboratories; 2011.
4. Longo DL, Fauci AS, Kasper DL, Hauser SL, Jameson JL, Loscalzo J (Editors). *Harrison's Online*, 18th ed. New York: McGraw-Hill; 2012.
5. Swartz MH. *Textbook of Physical Diagnosis: History and Examination*, 6th ed. Philadelphia: Saunders Elsevier; 2010.

The Musculoskeletal Exam

Editors:
Joel Davies
David Tsui

Faculty Reviewers:
Khalid Syed, MD, FRCS(C)
Paul Kuzyk, MD, MASc, FRCS(C)
Anne Agur, PhD, MSc, BSc(OT)

TABLE OF CONTENTS

1. FOCUSED HISTORY

In addition to general history taking, important aspects of the musculoskeletal history include:

Pain: OPQRST

- **O**nset (slow or sudden)
- **P**alliative factors, **P**rovocative factors (pain associated with rest, activity, certain postures, time of day)
- **Q**uality
  - o Nerve pain: sharp, burning, follows distribution of nerve
  - o Bone pain: deep, localized
  - o Vascular pain: diffuse, aching, poorly localized, may be referred to other areas
  - o Muscle pain: dull and aching, poorly localized, may be referred to other areas
- **R**adiation, **R**eferred pain
- **S**ymptoms associated (joint locking, unlocking, instability; changes in color of limb, pins and needles)
- **T**iming (onset, duration, frequency)

Referred Symptoms from other Joints/Organs
- Shoulder pain (from heart or diaphragm)
- Arm pain (from neck)
- Leg pain (from back)
- Knee pain (from hip or back)
- Hip pain (from appendix)

Inflammatory Symptoms
- Pain, erythema, warmth, swelling, morning stiffness (>30 min)
- Improves with activity
- Important to differentiate from mechanical/degenerative manifestations

Mechanical/Degenerative Symptoms
- Pain is worse at end of day, better with rest, worse with exercise
- Ligament or meniscal symptoms (joint collapsing, clicking, locking, instability)

Neoplastic and Infectious Symptoms
- Constant pain, night pain, fever, chills, weight loss, anorexia, fatigue, weakness
- History of prostate, thyroid, breast, lung or kidney cancer

Neurological Symptoms
- Paresthesia, tingling, bowel and bladder complaints, headaches, weakness

Vascular Symptoms
- Exercise-induced pain (usually in calf but can be in buttock, hip, thigh, or foot) that makes the patient stop exertion, no pain at rest, pain disappears within 10 min
- Differentiate vascular from neurologic claudication

2. FOCUSED PHYSICAL EXAM
- Always examine the joint above and below the site of interest
- If lower extremity complaint: examine lower back and perform complete neurological exam of lower limbs
- If upper extremity complaint: examine neck and perform complete neurological exam of upper limbs
- See **Examination of Specific Joints** for site-specific tests

Inspection
In general, inspect each joint for the following: **SEADS**
- **S**welling
- **E**rythema
- **A**trophy of muscle
- **D**eformity (alterations in shape, bony alignment or posture)
- **S**kin changes (bruising, discoloration)

Also, inspect for the following while conducting the physical exam:
- Symmetry of the bony contours, soft tissues, limb positions
- Presence of scars to indicate recent injury/surgery
- Any crepitus or abnormal sound in joints when patient moves them
- Patient's attitude (apprehensiveness, restlessness)
- Patient's facial expression (indicating discomfort)
- Patient's willingness to move; normality of movements

Palpation

In general, palpate skin, soft tissues, bones, and joints while patient is as relaxed as possible. Palpation must be carried out in a systematic fashion to ensure that all structures are examined and any asymmetry is noted. The following should be noted when palpating:

- Identify shapes, structures, tissue type, and detect any abnormalities
- Determine tissue thickness and texture, and determine whether it is pliable, soft, or resilient
- Specifically, feel for tenderness, nodules, warmth, crepitus, effusion
- Determine joint tenderness by applying firm pressure to the joint
- Palpate for variation in temperature, pulses, tremors, and fasciculations
- Palpate for dryness or excessive moisture of the skin

ROM

Active Movements

- Performed voluntarily by patient
- Abnormalities in active ROM result from either neurological problems or mechanical disruption of flexor/extensor mechanisms
- When testing active movements, note the following:
  - Any movements resulting in pain; if present, note quality and amount of pain
  - Amount of observable restriction
  - Any limitation and its nature
  - Willingness of patient to move the joint
  - Quality of movement
  - Crepitus

Passive Movements

- Joint is moved through a range of motion by the examiner while the patient is relaxed
- Detect any limitation of movement (stiffness) or excessive range (hypermobility), and any associated pain
- Hypermobile joints: could be a result of ligament tears, collagen disorders, chronic pain, tendinitis, rheumatoid arthritis
- Hypomobile joints: could be a result of muscle strains, pinched nerve syndromes, tendinitis, osteoarthritis

End Feel

- Defined as the sensation felt in the joint as it reaches the end of its ROM
- In passive movement, the examiner should determine the quality of end feel
- Three normal types of end feel:
  1. Bone to Bone: a "hard" unyielding compression that stops further movement (e.g. elbow extension)
  2. Soft Tissue Approximation: a yielding compression that stops further movement (e.g. elbow and knee flexion where movement is stopped by muscles)
  3. Tissue Stretch: hard or "springy" (firm) movement with a slight give. There is a feeling of elastic resistance toward the end of the ROM with a feeling of "rising tension". Feeling depends on thickness of tissue and may be very elastic (i.e. Achilles tendon stretch) or slightly elastic (i.e. wrist flexion: lateral rotation of shoulder, extension of MCP joint)
- Abnormal end feel indicates pathology

Power Assessment/Isometric Movements

- Type of movement that consists of strong, static, voluntary muscle contraction
- Examiner positions the joint in the resting position and asks the patient to maintain the position against an applied force
- Muscle weakness can be a result of:
  - Upper motor neuron lesion
  - Injury to peripheral nerve
  - Neuromuscular junction pathology
  - Pathology of muscles themselves
  - Disuse atrophy
- In certain anatomic sites (e.g. lumbar spine, cervical spine), isometric contractions are used to test for myotome function

Functional Assessment

- Should always be performed on the joint during examination
- May involve task analysis or simply a history of patient's daily activities
- Assess limitations in activities of daily living (ADLs):
  - Getting up, sitting down, walking up stairs
  - Using bathroom, brushing teeth, combing hair
  - Transferring from shower or bathtub

Reflexes

- Test reflexes to assess the nerve or nerve roots that supply the reflex (see **Neurological Exam**, p.182)

Special Tests

- Refer to specific anatomic sites

Other Considerations

- Gait Assessment
  - Walking: normal, heel-to-toe, heels only, toes only
  - Look for: Trendelenburg gait in hip disorders, high stepping, circumduction, antalgic gait (due to pain)
- Peripheral Vascular Exam
  - Test peripheral pulses (see **Peripheral Vascular Exam**, p.298)
- Neurological Exam
  - Test power, sensation (see **Neurological Exam**, p.184, 191)

MUSCULOSKELETAL

3. EXAMINATION OF SPECIFIC JOINTS

- Each joint should be inspected, palpated, put through the various range of motion maneuvers, have relevant reflexes examined, and put through special tests if appropriate
- Look for the symptoms listed above (see **Focused Physical Exam**, p.134)

3.1 Shoulder

Common Symptoms

- Pain: consider possibility of referral from chest/abdomen or neck
- Weakness
- Muscle atrophy: may point to lesions in cervical nerves

Physical Exam

Inspection

- Compare shoulder contours (anteriorly), alignment of the clavicles, symmetry of sternoclavicular and acromioclavicular joints, and scapulae (posteriorly) (see **Figure 1**)

- Note any scars, masses, lesions, abrasions, bruising, and erythema of the skin at and around the shoulders
- Note any swelling, deformity, muscle atrophy, and asymmetry of the soft tissues and bones
- Note biceps tendon rupture by asking the patient to flex his/her arm and observe for a bulge of tissue ("Popeye sign")

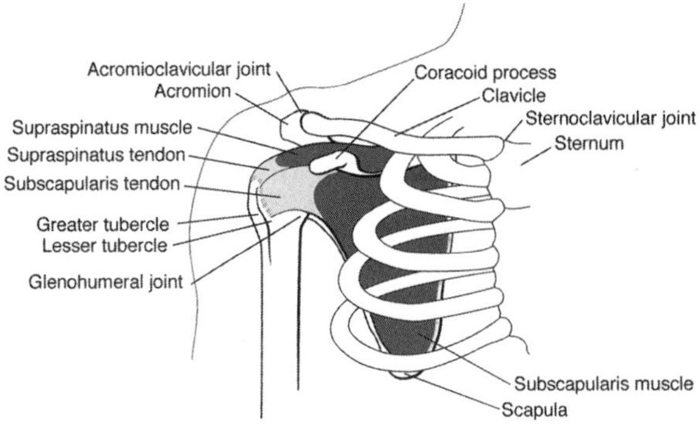

Jennifer Belanger

Figure 1. Anatomy of the Right Shoulder

Palpation

- Palpate the sternoclavicular joint and along the clavicle to the acromioclavicular joint to detect for asymmetry and/or discontinuity
- Palpate the anterior and lateral aspects of the glenohumeral joint assessing the bicipital groove, subdeltoid bursa, and rotator cuff insertion for tenderness
- Palpate the glenohumoral joint for crepitus by placing your hand over the subacromial bursa and passively circumducting the arm
- Palpate over the deltoids to test axillary nerve sensation

Range of Motion

- Perform the following screening test by instructing your patients to do the following, noting any crepitus by cupping your hand over the shoulder joint during these movements (see **Table 1** for normal values):
  - Forward flexion: "Raise both your arms in front of you until they are straight above your head"
  - External rotation and abduction: "Place both your hands behind your neck with your elbows out to the sides"
    - Hands should reach the neck base
  - Abduction and adduction: "Raise both arms from your sides straight over head, palms together; now bring them slowly down to your side again"
  - Extension and internal rotation: "Bring your arms toward your back and place your hands between the shoulder blades"
    - Hands should normally reach the inferior angle of the scapulae; record the level of the scapulae that can be reached
- Pain during motion can be localized
- Both shoulders can be assessed simultaneously
- If the screening tests above demonstrate any limitation of motion, assess the range of motion for passive movements as well

Table 1. Shoulder: Normal Ranges of Motion

Movement	Range of Motion
Forward Flexion	180°
Backward Extension	60°
Abduction	180°
Adduction	50°
External Rotation (with elbows at sides)	90°
Internal Rotation (with shoulder abducted to 90° and elbow flexed)	70°

Gross G, Fetto J, Rosen E. *Musculoskeletal Examination.* Malden: Blackwell; 2002.

Special Tests

Tests for Anterior Shoulder Instability

- **Anterior Apprehension Test:** with patient sitting or standing, patient's arm is passively abducted to 90°, elbow is flexed to 90° and arm is externally rotated 90° (into a "throwing position"); examiner then applies pressure to posterior aspect of humerus
  - Test is "positive" if the patient expresses anxiety that the shoulder will dislocate or be painful
- **Relocation Test:** with patient supine, patient's arm is passively abducted to 90°, elbow is flexed to 90° and arm is externally rotated 90°; examiner then applies downward (posterior) pressure to humeral head
  - Test is "positive" if the apprehension and/or pain is relieved
- **Anterior Release Test:** the relocation test is performed, and the examiner's hand is suddenly removed from the proximal humerus
  - Test is "positive" if the patient has apprehension or pain

Test for Posterior Shoulder Instability (Posterior Apprehension Test)

- With the patient supine, the arm is abducted to 90°, the elbow is flexed to 90°, and the humerus is maximally internally rotated
- Examiner applies downward (posterior) pressure to humeral head
- Test is "positive" if the patient expresses apprehension

Test for Inferior Shoulder Instability (Sulcus Sign)

- The patient stands or sits with the arm by the side and shoulder muscles relaxed
- Arm is pulled vertically downward
- Presence of a sulcus sign (indentation between acromion and humeral head) is suggestive of inferior shoulder instability

EBM: Shoulder Instability or Labrum Lesion Instability

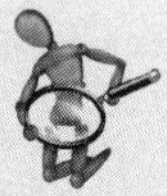

The relocation test and the anterior release test are the most useful in diagnosing anterior instability. The apprehension test is of limited value due to low specificity, but is included as part of the series of tests for anterior stability.

- Relocation Test: LR+ = 6.5, 95%CI = 3.0-14.0; LR- = 0.18, 95%CI = 0.07-0.45
- Anterior Release Test: LR+ = 8.3, 95%CI = 3.6-19; LR- = 0.09, 95%CI = 0.03-0.27
- The sulcus sign for inferior instability has a sensitivity of 31% and a specificity of 89%.

Luime JJ, et al. 2004. *JAMA* 292(16):1989-1999.

Test for Glenoid Labral Pathology

- **O'Brien's Sign:** the patient's arm is flexed to 90° with the elbow in full extension and then the arm is adducted 15° medial to sagittal plane; arm is then internally rotated (thumb pointing downward) and the patient resists the examiner's downward force[1]
- Procedure is then repeated in supination
- Test is "positive" if pain is elicited by the first maneuver and is reduced by the second maneuver
- A false positive result may occur with rotator cuff or AC joint pathology

Test for Impingement Syndrome (Rotator Cuff Tendinitis)

- **Neer's Test:** with patient sitting or standing, the examiner stabilizes the patient's scapula and maximally forward flexes the patient's shoulder with the other hand
  - Reproduction of patient's pain at maximal forward flexion is a positive test; test can be repeated with the patient's elbow flexed and humerus internally rotated to increase the discomfort if no pain is felt (see **Figure 2**)
- **Hawkins-Kennedy Test:** with patient standing, the examiner will raise the patient's arm to 90° forward flexion and then gently internally rotate the arm so that the thumb is turning downward
  - Test is "positive" if internal rotation and shoulder flexion reproduces patient's pain
- **Painful Arc Test[2]:** with patient sitting or standing, the examiner will instruct the patient to abduct his/her shoulder
  - Test is "positive" if active abduction between 60-120° causes pain of the superior shoulder
- **Swim Stroke Test:** with patient sitting or standing, the examiner will instruct the patient to circumduct his/her arm so that he/she is imitating a freestyle swimming stroke
  - Test is "positive" if active abduction between 60-120° causes pain

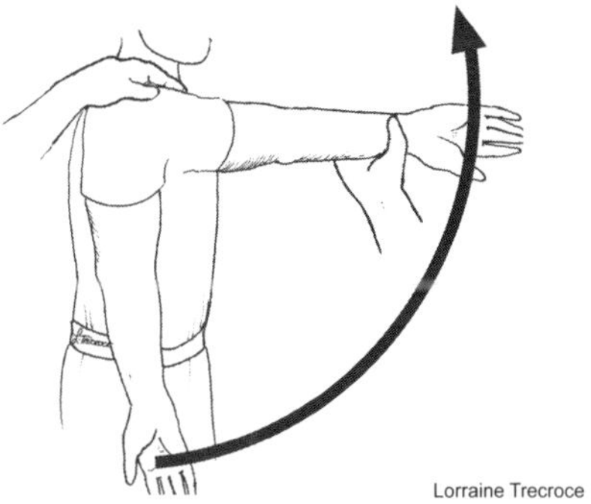

Figure 2. Neer's Test for Shoulder Impingement

Tests for Rotator Cuff Tears

- **Drop Arm Test:** the patient's arm is passively abducted to 90° with the elbow in full extension; the patient is then asked to slowly lower his/her arm back to the side. If arm drops suddenly or if patient has severe pain, this indicates rotator cuff tear
- **Empty Can (Jobe's) Test:** the patient's shoulders are abducted to 45° and with his/her hands turned downward so that the thumbs are pointing down (i.e. emptying a can); patient is then asked to move his/her arm upward as you apply a downward resistance. If the patient has severe pain, this indicates a tear in the supraspinatus muscle (see **Figure 3**)

MUSCULOSKELETAL

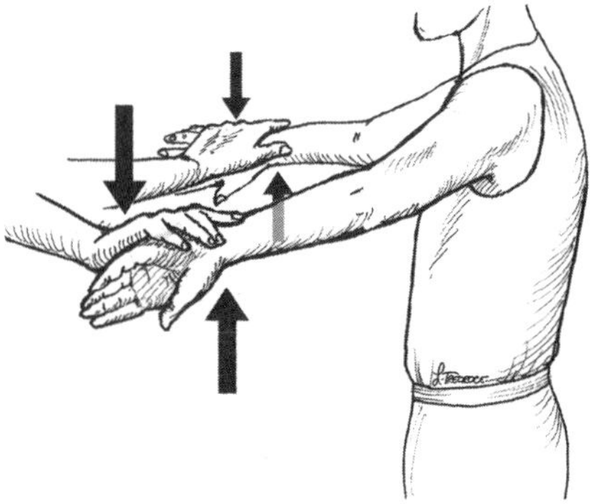

Lorraine Trecroce

Figure 3. Empty Can (Jobe's) Test for Supraspinatus Tear

- **Infraspinatus and Teres Minor Strength Test:** the patient's shoulders are abducted to 25° with elbows bent at 90°; patient is then asked to rotate his/her shoulders externally as you apply a resistance on his/her arms toward the midline of his/her body. If the patient has severe pain, this indicates a tear in the infraspinatus and/or teres minor muscle (see **Figure 4**)

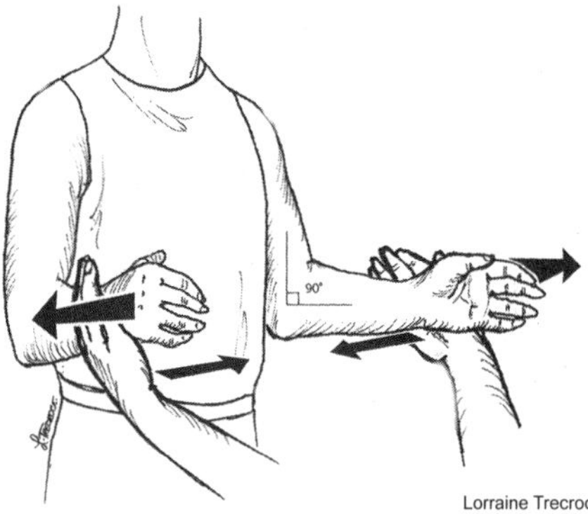

Lorraine Trecroce

Figure 4. Infraspinatus and Teres Minor Strength Test

- **Gerber's Lift Off Test[3]:** the patient's hands are placed behind his/her back with palms facing out, with forearms almost 90° to the length of the spine; patient is then asked to lift his/her hands away from his/her back as you apply a resistance toward his/her body. If the patient has severe pain, this indicates a tear in the subscapularis muscle (see **Figure 5**)

> **Clinical Pearl: Shoulder Pain**
> Shoulder pain (radiating down the arm to the elbow) when combing one's hair, putting on a coat, or reaching into a back pocket indicates supraspinatus inflammation.
> Diffuse shoulder pain upon moving the humerus posteriorly (without radiation to the arm) indicates infraspinatus inflammation.
> Discomfort and weakness of the upper extremity and "winging" of the ipsilateral scapula indicates a dysfunction of the serratus anterior or trapezius muscles often secondary to long thoracic or accessory nerve palsies.

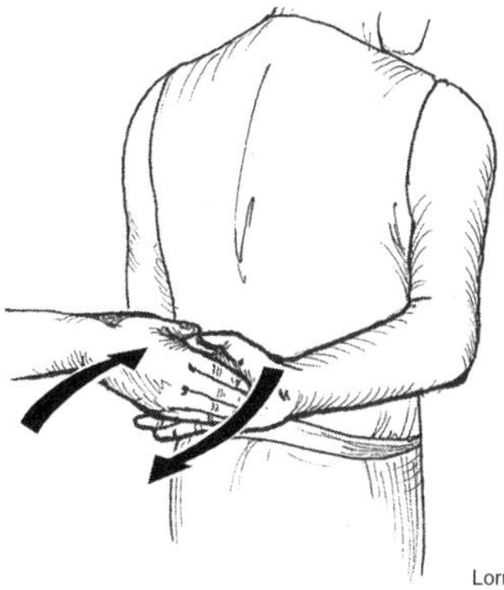

Lorraine Trecroce

Figure 5. Gerber's Lift-Off Test for Subscapularis Tear

Common Clinical Scenarios

- Shoulder pain can be acute or chronic in nature and is commonly caused by soft tissue trauma/inflammation (see **Table 2**)

Table 2. Common Clinical Conditions of Shoulder[4-6]

Condition	Clinical Features
Rotator Cuff Tendinitis	• Shoulder pain on activity • Sharp pain on elevation of arm into overhead position • History of chronic usage (e.g. throwing, swimming) or trauma
Rotator Cuff Tear/Rupture	• Sharp pain after trauma • Pain over greater tubercle • Characteristic shoulder shrug and pain on attempted abduction • Weakness on external rotation
Bicipital Tendinitis	• Generalized anterior tenderness over long head of biceps • Associated with pain, especially at night • Hallmark is reproduction of anterior shoulder pain during resistance to forearm supination
Dislocation	• Feeling of shoulder instability • Poor range of motion • Shoulder pain on activity • Anterior dislocation: present with slight abduction and external rotation • Posterior dislocation: present with slight adduction and internal rotation
Adhesive Capsulitis	• Progression of pain over several weeks from onset at night or with involved movements, to constant pain with any movement • A higher incidence of adhesive capsulitis exists among patients with DM • Pain at end of range of motion may be the only finding early in disease process • Passive range of motion becomes painful; affected motions include (in order of most common to least common): external rotation, abduction, internal rotation, and flexion

Table 2. Common Clinical Conditions of Shoulder[4-6] (continued)

Condition	Clinical Features
Clavicular Fracture	• Mechanism of action: fall onto outstretched upper extremity or shoulder, or direct trauma • Inferior and anterior displacement of shoulder secondary to loss of support • Tenderness, crepitus, edema, and deformity
Acromioclavicular Joint Pathology	• Swelling, bruising, and prominent clavicle depending on severity of sprain • Poor range of motion and moderate pain when raising arm • Reproduction of pain with adduction of elevated affected arm across the body

3.2 Elbow

Common Symptoms

- Pain (well-localized)
- Swelling
- Stiffness

Physical Exam

Inspection

- Inspect for swelling or masses (e.g. olecranon bursitis or rheumatic nodules)
- Ask the patient: "With your palms facing up, bend and then extend your elbow"
  - Note differences in carrying angles, flexion contractures, hyperextension

Palpation

- Palpate olecranon process, medial and lateral epicondyles, and extensor surface of forearm (3-4 cm distal to olecranon) for swelling, masses, tenderness, and nodules
- Grasp the elbow with your fingers under the olecranon and your thumb next to the biceps tendon then passively flex and extend the elbow
  - Note any crepitus, tenderness or restricted movement
  - Palpate for masses on each side of the biceps tendon

MUSCULOSKELETAL

Range of Motion

- Ask the patient: "Bend your elbows until you can touch your shoulders (flexion) and then place your arms back down (extension)"
- With the patient's arms at sides and elbows flexed, ask patient to "Turn your palms up (supination) and down (pronation); hold a pencil in your fist" (may help with estimating the range of motion in degrees)
- Note any limitation of motion (see **Table 3**) or pain

Table 3. Elbow: Normal Ranges of Motion

Movement	Range of Motion
Flexion	150°
Extension	0°
Supination	80-90° from vertical (with pencil grasped in hand)
Pronation	80-90° from vertical (with pencil grasped in hand)

Gross G, Fetto J, Rosen E. *Musculoskeletal Examination.* Malden: Blackwell; 2002.

Interpretation of Findings

Table 4. Clinical Features Differentiating Diseases Affecting the Elbow

Clinical Feature	Rheumatoid Arthritis	Psoriatic Arthritis	Acute Gout	Osteoarthritis	Lateral Epicondylitis
Age	3-80	10-60	30-80	50-80	20-60
Pain Onset	Gradual	Gradual	Abrupt	Gradual	Gradual
Stiffness	Very Common	Common	Absent	Common	Occasional
Swelling	Common	Common	Common	Common	Absent
Redness	Absent	Uncommon	Common	Absent	Absent
Deformity	Flexion contractures, usually bilaterally	Flexion contractures, usually bilaterally	Flexion contractures, only in chronic state	Flexion contractures	None

Swartz MH. *Textbook of Physical Diagnosis: History and Examination,* 6th ed. Philadelphia: Saunders Elsevier; 2010.

Common Clinical Scenarios

Olecranon Bursitis

- Most commonly results from repeated minor injuries to the elbow (e.g. repeated leaning on the point of the elbow on a hard surface)[7]
- Focal swelling at the posterior elbow
- Pain is often exacerbated by pressure
- Onset of bursal inflammation may be sudden if it is secondary to infection or acute trauma, or gradual if secondary to chronic irritation

Epicondylitis

- Characterized by pain in the region of the epicondyle(s) of the humerus, radiating down the surface of the forearm
- Patients often experience pain when attempting to open a door or when lifting a glass

Lateral Epicondylitis (Test for Tennis Elbow)

- While palpating the lateral epicondyle, pronate the patient's forearm, flex the wrist fully, and extend the elbow
- Pain over the lateral epicondyle is diagnostic

Medial Epicondylitis (Test for Golfer's Elbow)

- While palpating the medial epicondyle, the patient's forearm is supinated and the elbow and wrist are extended
- Pain over the medial epicondyle is diagnostic

3.3 Wrist

Common Symptoms

- Pain in the wrist or hand
- Numbness or tingling (paresthesia) in the wrist or fingers
- Loss of movement and stiffness
- Deformities

Physical Exam

Inspection

- Inspect the palmar and dorsal surfaces of the wrist for swelling over the joints or deformities

Palpation

- Palpate the distal radius and ulna on the lateral and medial surfaces
- Palpate the groove of each wrist joint with your thumbs on the dorsum of the wrist, while your fingers support the wrist from beneath
- Note any tenderness, swelling, warmth or redness
- Palpate the anatomical snuffbox (a hollowed depression just distal to the radial styloid process formed by the abductor and extensor tendons of the thumb)
  - Tenderness over the snuffbox suggests a scaphoid fracture or carpal arthritis

Range of Motion

- **Extension:** ask the patient to press the palms of the hands together in the vertical plane and to bring the forearms into the horizontal plane
- **Flexion:** ask the patient to put the backs of the hands in contact and then to bring the forearms into the horizontal plane
- Note any asymmetry and limitation of motion (see **Table 5**)
- Test active ulnar and radial deviation
- Test active pronation and supination (having a patient hold a pencil in his/her fist may help with estimating the range of motion in degrees)

Table 5. Wrist: Normal Ranges of Motion

Movement	Range of Motion
Flexion	80°
Extension	70°
Radial Deviation	20°
Ulnar Deviation	30°
Supination	80-90° from vertical (with pencil grasped in hand)
Pronation	80-90° from vertical (with pencil grasped in hand)

Gross G, Fetto J, Rosen E. *Musculoskeletal Examination.* Malden: Blackwell; 2002.

Common Clinical Scenarios

Carpal Tunnel Syndrome

- Carpal tunnel: a bony trough covered by the flexor retinaculum through which the median nerve and wrist flexors pass
- Usually diagnosed in patients 20-40 yr; ratio of women to men is 3:1
- Entrapment of the nerve produces symptoms of burning, tingling (pins and needles), and numbness in the median nerve distribution (generally worse at night)
- Common causes: fluid retention (common in pregnancy), hypothyroidism, DM, and overuse of the tendons from repeated forceful movements of the wrist (work or recreation)

Tests for Carpal Tunnel Syndrome

- **Tinel's Sign:** a sharp tap is given with the fingers directly over the median nerve (located medial to the flexor carpi radialis tendon at the most proximal aspect of the palm)
  - Test is positive if tingling, paresthesia or pain in the area of the thumb, index finger, middle finger, and radial half of the ring finger is elicited
- **Phalen's Sign:** the patient is asked to put the dorsal aspects of his/her hands in contact so that his/her wrists are maximally flexed
  - Test is positive if the patient notes paresthesia or numbness in the area of the thumb, index finger, middle finger, and radial half of the ring finger after holding this position for 60 s or less

- **Katz Hand Diagram**[8]: ask patient to indicate location of sensory symptoms on a diagram of hand and arm
  - Classic pattern or probable pattern (see **Table 6**) suggests diagnosis
- Compare ability to perceive painful stimuli applied along the palmar aspect of the index finger compared with the ipsilateral little finger
  - Decreased sensitivity to pain (hypoalgesia) in the index finger suggests diagnosis
- Test strength in abductor pollicis brevis (thumb abduction)
  - Weakness suggests diagnosis

Table 6. Katz Hand Diagram

Pattern	Description
Classic Pattern	At least two of the thumb, index finger or middle finger are affected. This pattern permits symptoms in the ring finger and small finger, wrist pain, and radiation of pain proximal to wrist. Symptoms on palm or dorsum of hand are not allowed
Probable Pattern	Same as classic but palmar symptoms allowed unless solely confined to ulnar aspect
Possible Pattern	Symptoms involve only one of thumb, index finger or middle finger
Unlikely Pattern	No symptoms are present in thumb, index finger or middle finger

D'Arcy CA, McGee S. 2000. *JAMA* 283(23):3110-3117.

EBM: Carpal Tunnel Syndrome

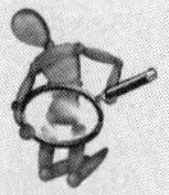

Katz Hand Diagram
- Classic or probable hand diagram has a sensitivity of 64% and a specificity of 73%.
- Hypoalgesia in the median nerve territory:
  - Pooled studies yielded LR+ 3.1, 95%CI = 2.0-5.1; LR- 0.7, 95%CI = 0.5-1.1

Weak Thumb Abduction
- Pooled studies yielded LR+ 1.8, 95%CI = 1.4-2.3; LR- 0.5, 95%CI = 0.4-0.7

D'Arcy CA, McGee S. 2000. *JAMA* 283(23):3110-3117.

3.4 Hand

Common Symptoms
- Pain and swelling of joints

Physical Exam
Inspection
- Carefully inspect for deformities, cuts, scars, and wounds with special emphasis on possible damage to nerves and tendons (see **Table 7** and **Figure 6**)
- Note any tenderness, redness, or swelling

Table 7. Common Deformities of the Hand

Name of Deformity	Interpretation
Mallet Finger/Thumb	Trauma or RA
Swan Neck Deformity	RA, but has many other causes
Boutonnière Deformity	Trauma or RA Occurs when the central slip of the extensor tendon detaches from the middle phalanx

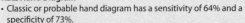

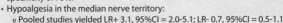

Table 7. Common Deformities of the Hand (continued)

Name of Deformity	Interpretation
Dupuytren's Contracture	Nodular thickening in the palm and fingers Associated with DM, epilepsy, alcoholism, and hereditary tendencies
Heberden's Nodes	OA often associated with a deviation of the DIPs
Bouchard's Nodes	Similar to Heberden's nodes, but affects the PIPs

OA = osteoarthritis, RA = rheumatoid arthritis
Swartz MH. *Textbook of Physical Diagnosis: History and Examination,* 6th ed. Philadelphia: Saunders Elsevier; 2010.

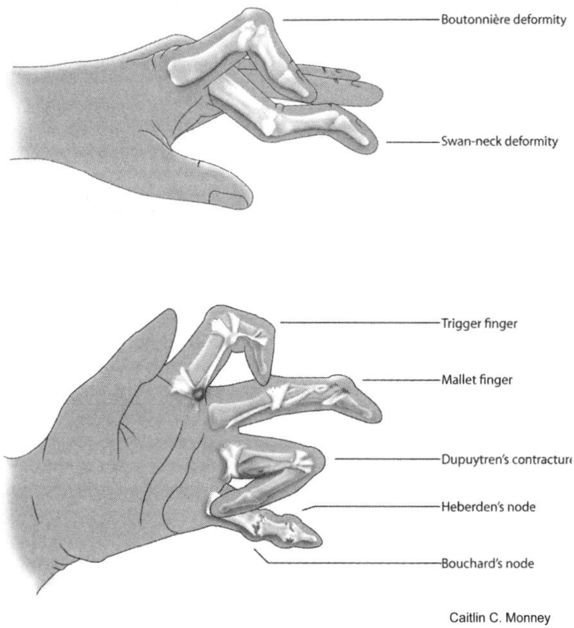

Figure 6. Common Deformities of the Hand

Palpation

- Compress the metacarpophalangeal (MCP) joints by squeezing the patient's hand between your thumb and index finger
  - If this causes pain, use your thumb to palpate the dorsal side of each MCP joint while using your index finger to feel the heads of the MCPs on the palmar side
- Palpate the medial and lateral aspects of each PIP and DIP joint (dorsal and volar surfaces) with your index finger and thumb

Range of Motion

- Check for smooth, coordinated, and easily performed movements (see **Table 8**)
- See **Table 9** for sensory and motor distribution of the radial, ulnar, and median nerves

- Ask the patient: "Make a fist with each hand with your thumb across the knuckles, and then open your hand and spread your fingers" and assess
  - During flexion:
    - Normal fingers should flex to the distal palmar crease
    - Thumb should oppose the DIP joint
  - During extension:
    - Each finger should extend to the zero position in relation to its metacarpal upon opening
- Assess motion of the thumb: flexion, extension, abduction, adduction, opposition (movement of the thumb across the palm)

Table 8. Hand: Normal Ranges of Motion

Movement	Joint	Range of Motion
Fingers	MCPs	80°
	PIPs	110°
	DIPs	90°
Thumb	MCP	0° extension; 50° flexion
	IP	20° extension; 90° flexion

IP = interphalangeal, MCP = metacarpophalangeal
Gross G, Fetto J, Rosen E. *Musculoskeletal Examination.* Malden: Blackwell; 2002.

Table 9. Nerves Supplying the Hand

Nerve	Sensory	Motor
Radial	Dorsum of first web space	Extension of fingers, thumb, and wrist
Posterior Interosseous Branch	None	Extension of fingers, thumb, and wrist
Ulnar	Tip of small finger (dorsum) Small finger/medial ring finger	Finger abduction and adduction, ring and small finger DIP flexion, opposition of small finger, wrist flexion
Median	Tip of index/middle/lateral half of ring finger (dorsum) Index/middle/lateral half of ring finger (palmar)	Thumb IP flexion, index/middle finger flexion, wrist flexion
Anterior Interosseous Branch	None	Flexion of index/middle finger
Recurrent Terminal Branch	None	Thumb opposition

IP = interphalangeal
Gross G, Fetto J, Rosen E. *Musculoskeletal Examination.* Malden: Blackwell; 2002.

Special Tests

- For intact flexor digitorum superficialis: restrict motion of 3 out of 4 fingers by holding down distal phalanges with the dorsum of the patient's hand (palm up) rested on a table; ask the patient to flex the free finger and look for PIP flexion
- For intact flexor digitorum profundus: hold down both the proximal and middle phalanges and ask the patient to flex fingers; look for DIP flexion

Interpretation of Findings

Table 10. Arthritis in the Hand and Wrist

Joint	Osteoarthritis	Rheumatoid
DIP	Very common	Rare
PIP	Common	Very common
MCP	Rare	Very common
Wrist	Rare*	Very common

MCP = metacarpophalangeal
*Osteoarthritis will sometimes affect only the carpometacarpal joint of the thumb
Swartz MH. *Textbook of Physical Diagnosis: History and Examination, 6th ed.* Philadelphia: Saunders Elsevier; 2010.

Common Clinical Scenarios

De Quervain's Disease

- Tenosynovitis involving abductor pollicis longus and extensor pollicis brevis
- Patient complains of weakness of grip and pain at the base of the thumb which is aggravated by certain movements of the wrist
- **Finkelstein Test:** ask the patient to flex thumb and close the fingers over it; then attempt to move the hand into ulnar deviation
  - Excruciating pain with this maneuver occurs in De Quervain's tenosynovitis

3.5 Spine

Common Symptoms

- Pain (most common symptom with characteristic patterns)

Table 11. Common Patterns of Back Pain[9-11]

Etiology	Clinical Features
Intervertebral Discs or Adjacent Ligament Involvement	• Back dominant (back, buttock) • Pain: worse with flexion • Pattern: constant or intermittent
Posterior Joint Complex Involvement	• Back dominant • Pain: worse with extension (never worse with flexion) • Pattern: intermittent
Radiculopathy: L4, L5, S1, S2	• Leg dominant (below buttock) • Pain: worse with back movement • Pattern: previously or currently constant
Neurogenic Claudication due to Nerve Compression	• Leg dominant • Pain: worse with activity and better with rest • Pattern: intermittent (short duration)

Differential Diagnosis of Back Pain (Age-Dependent)

- Degenerative (90% of all back pain)[10]
  - Mechanical problem (degenerative, facet)
  - Spinal stenosis (congenital, osteophyte, central disc)
  - Peripheral nerve compression (disc herniation)
- Other[10]
  - Infection
  - Cauda equina syndrome
  - Neoplastic: primary or metastatic
  - Trauma: fracture (e.g. compression, distraction, translation, rotation)

- Spondyloarthropathies (e.g. ankylosing spondylitis)
- Referred: aorta, renal, ureter, pancreas

Physical Exam for Cervical Spine

Inspection

- May be examined with the patient seated; in general, check for deformity, unusual posture, physical asymmetries, and guarding
- In normal sitting posture, nose should be in line with manubrium and xiphoid process of sternum; from side, ear lobe should be in line with acromion process
- Check for head tilting or lateral rotation; indicates possible torticollis
- Check for Klippel-Feil syndrome (fusion of the cervical vertebrae resulting in a short and relatively immobile neck; congenital)
- Check for venous obstruction in the upper limbs
  - Note any temperature changes, sensory changes, altered coloration of the skin, ulcers, or vein distension

Palpation

- Palpate for any tenderness, trigger points, muscle spasms, skin texture and bony/soft tissue abnormalities on the posterior, lateral, and anterior aspects of the neck
- Posterior aspect: external occipital protuberance, spinous processes and facet joints of cervical vertebrae, mastoid processes
- Lateral aspect: transverse processes of cervical vertebrae, lymph nodes and carotid arteries, temporomandibular joints, mandible, and parotid glands
- Anterior aspect: hyoid bone, thyroid cartilage, supraclavicular fossa

Range of Motion: Active Movements

- Ask the patient to perform the movements in **Table 12**

Table 12. Active Movements of the Cervical Spine: Normal Ranges of Motion

Maneuver	Range of Motion
Flexion ("Touch your chin to your chest")	80-90°
Extension ("Put your head back")	70°
Side Flexion* ("Touch each shoulder with your ear without raising your shoulders")	20-45°
Rotation* ("Turn your head to the left and right")	70-90°

*Look for symmetrical movements
Gross G, Fetto J, Rosen E. *Musculoskeletal Examination*. Malden: Blackwell; 2002.
Magee DJ. *Orthopedic Physical Assessment*. St. Louis: Saunders Elsevier. 2008.

Range of Motion: Passive Movements

- Flexion, extension, side flexion, and rotation should all be tested with passive movements to test the "end feel" of each movement (tissue stretch)

Power Assessment/Isometric Movements

- Flexion, extension, side flexion, and rotation should all be tested with isometric movements
- Determine muscle power and possible neurological weakness originating from the nerve roots in the cervical spine by testing the myotomes with isometric movements (each contraction should be held for ≥5 s) (see **Table 13**)

Table 13. Cervical Spine Movements and their Respective Myotomes

Movement	Myotome
Neck Flexion	C1-C2
Neck Side Flexion	C3
Shoulder Elevation	C4
Shoulder Abduction	C5
Elbow Flexion and/or Wrist Extension	C5-C6
Elbow Extension and/or Wrist Flexion	C7
Thumb Extension and/or Ulnar Deviation	C8
Abduction and/or Adduction of Hand Intrinsics	T1

Magee DJ. *Orthopedic Physical Assessment*. St. Louis: Saunders Elsevier; 2008.

Reflexes

- Biceps (C5, C6), triceps (C6, C7, C8), brachioradialis (C5, C6) need assessment (see **Neurological Exam**, p.189)

Special Tests

Tests for Thoracic Outlet Syndrome (see p.155 for definition)

- Look for evidence of ischemia in one hand (coldness, discoloration, trophic changes)
  - Bilateral changes are more suggestive of Raynaud's disease[10]
- Palpate radial pulse and apply traction to arm; obliteration of pulse is not diagnostic, but a normal pulse present on opposite arm may suggest thoracic outlet syndrome
- Paresthesia in the hand is usually severe
- May have hypothenar wasting; thenar wasting less common

Physical Exam for Thoracic Spine

Inspection

- Examine with the patient standing
- SEADS
- Inspect for
  - Kyphosis, scoliosis (an imaginary line drawn down from T1 should fall through the gluteal cleft)
  - **Adam's Forward Bend Test:** have the patient bend forward to see if there is a rib prominence (rib hump) on one side (an indication of scoliosis)
- Inspect for chest deformities
  - e.g. pectus carinatum, pectus excavatum, barrel chest
  - Note asymmetry
  - Look for symmetrical folds of skin on either side of the spine
- Look for differences in height of shoulders and iliac crests

Palpation

- Palpate for tenderness, muscle spasm, altered temperature, swelling
  - Usually done with patient sitting
- Anterior aspect: sternum, ribs and costal cartilages, clavicles, abdomen
- Posterior aspect: scapulae, spinous processes of the thoracic spine

Percussion

- Percussion of spine performed to examine for tenderness and irritability
- Ask patient to stand and bend forward

- Lightly percuss spine with fist in an orderly progression from root of neck to sacrum
- Significant pain is a feature of TB and other infections, trauma (especially fractures), and neoplasms

Range of Motion: Active Movements

- Ask the patient to perform the movements in **Table 14**

Range of Motion: Passive Movements

- Flexion, extension, side flexion, and rotation should all be tested with passive movements to test the "end feel" (tissue stretch) of each movement

Power Assessment/Isometric Movements

- Performed with patient sitting
- The examiner is positioned behind the patient and instructs the patient to resist movements of forward flexion, extension, side flexion, and rotation of the spine

Reflexes

- Patellar (L3, L4), medial hamstring (L5, S1), and Achilles reflex (S1, S2) need assessment since pathology of thoracic spine can affect these reflexes
- Abdominal reflexes should also be tested to assess the mid-thoracic cord (see **Neurological Exam**, p.190)

Table 14. Thoracic and Lumbar Spine: Normal Ranges of Motion

Maneuver and Instruction to Patient	Range of Motion	
	Thoracic Spine	Lumbar Spine
Forward Flexion: "Bend forward and touch your toes"*	20-45°	40-60°
Extension: Standing behind the patient at an arm's length, stabilize pelvis to prevent patient from falling; then ask: "Arch your back"	25-45°	20-35°
Side Flexion: For each side, ask patient to: "Slide your hand down your leg"**	20-40°	15-20°
Rotation: With the patient seated, ask the patient to: "Rotate toward each side"	35-50°	3-18°
Chest Expansion: Place a tape measure around patient's chest; note difference between rest and full inspiration	Normal is >5 cm	N/A

*With forward flexion, the distance from the fingers to the ground is measured; majority of patients can reach the ground within 7 cm. Other methods are: 1) the examiner first measures the length of the spine from the C7 spinous process to the T12 spinous process with the patient standing. The patient is asked to bend forward, and the spine is measured again: a 2-7 cm difference in tape measure length is considered normal; and 2) the examiner compares the length of the spine from the C7 spinous process to the S1 spinous process with the patient standing and with the patient bent forward: a 10 cm difference in tape measure length is considered normal. This measures thoracic and lumbar movement, but with most movement, 7.5 cm occurs between T12 and S1.
**With side flexion, distance from fingertips to floor is measured and compared with other side – should be same

Gross G, Fetto J, Rosen E. *Musculoskeletal Examination*. Malden: Blackwell; 2002.
Magee DJ. *Orthopedic Physical Assessment*. St. Louis: Saunders Elsevier; 2008.

Special Tests

Slump Test (Sitting Dural Stretch Test)

- The patient sits and is asked to "slump": spine flexes and shoulders sag while head and chin are held erect by examiner
  - If no symptoms (e.g. pain) are produced, examiner flexes the neck and applies a small amount of pressure
  - If no symptoms are produced, one knee is extended passively
  - If no symptoms are produced, the foot on the same side is dorsiflexed
- Process is repeated with other leg
- Positive test: reproduction of patient's symptoms (pain) may indicate possible impingement of the dura, spinal cord or nerve roots[10]

Physical Exam for Lumbar Spine

Inspection

- Deformities or swelling
- Inspect for scoliosis, lumbar lordosis (see **Thoracic Spine**, p.150)
- Check body type of patient (ectomorphic, mesomorphic or endomorphic)
- Inspect gait
- Inspect total spinal posture (waist angles should be equal, "high" points on iliac crest should be the same height, leg length should be equal)
- Inspect for skin markings: café-au-lait spots may indicate neurofibromatosis or collagen disease
- Check for dimples and scars

Palpation

- Tenderness, altered temperature, muscle spasm
- Palpate the paravertebral muscles
- Anterior aspect: with patient supine, palpate umbilicus, inguinal areas (look for hernia, abscess, infection), iliac crests, symphysis pubis
- Posterior aspect: with patient prone, palpate spinous processes of lumbar vertebrae and at the lumbosacral junction, sacrum, sacroiliac joints, coccyx, iliac crests, ischial tuberosities

Percussion

- Same procedure as percussion for thoracic spine (see p.150)

Range of Motion

- See **Table 14** for directions and normal ROM

Power Assessment/Isometric Movements

- As described in thoracic spine isometric movement exam (see p.151)
- Myotomes are tested with the examiner placing the test joint or joints in a neutral or resting position and then applying a resisted isometric pressure that is held for ≥5 s (see **Table 15**)

Table 15. Lower Limb Movements and their Respective Myotomes

Movement	Myotome
Hip Flexion	L2
Knee Extension	L3
Ankle Dorsiflexion	L4
Great Toe Extension	L5
Ankle Plantar Flexion, Ankle Eversion, Hip Extension	S1
Knee Flexion	S2

Magee DJ. *Orthopedic Physical Assessment*. St. Louis: Saunders Elsevier; 2008.

Reflexes

- Patellar (L3, L4), medial hamstring (L5, S1), and Achilles reflex (S1, S2) need assessment since pathology of lumbar spine can affect these reflexes

Special Tests

Straight Leg Raise (Lasègue) Test (see **Figure 7**)

- The patient is in the supine position with the hips in a neutral position
- The examiner, ensuring the patient's knee remains extended, supports and raises the leg until radicular pain (back or leg) is felt
- This maneuver stretches the sciatic nerve
- Note the degree of elevation (pain usually occurs at <60° if there is an abnormality, as well as quality and distribution of the pain)
- Back pain suggests a central disc prolapse while leg pain suggests a lateral protrusion (ensure that pain is not due to hamstring tightness)
- The leg is lowered in increments until pain is relieved
- If dorsiflexion of the ankle results in a return of the pain, it is an indication of nerve root irritation (positive Lasègue sign)
- Paresthesia or radiating pain in the distribution of the sciatic nerve (L4-S3) suggests nerve root irritation/tension
- ***Note:*** the pain must be below the knee if the roots of the sciatic nerve are involved
- Compare with the other leg (with central disc protrusions, crossover pain may occur: e.g. straight leg raising on one side may cause pain down the opposite leg)

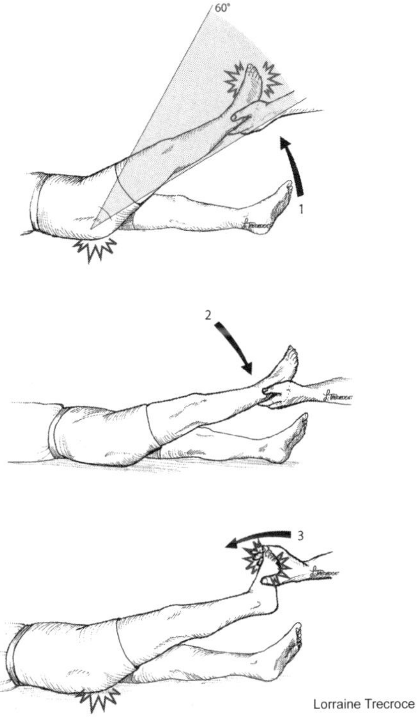

Figure 7. Straight Leg Raise (Lasègue) Test for Nerve Root Irritation

MUSCULOSKELETAL

EBM: Lumbar Disc Herniation

Straight Leg Raise Test
- Sensitivity of 91% and specificity of 26% in a surgical case-series
- Diagnostic value: ruling out lumbar disc herniation

Crossed Straight Leg Raise Test
(Positive result = reproduction of contralateral pain with elevation and abduction of unaffected, well leg)
- Sensitivity of 29% and specificity of 88% in a surgical case-series
- Diagnostic value: ruling in lumbar disc herniation

Devillé WLJM, et al. 2000. *Spine* 25(9):1140-1170.

Femoral Stretch Test (Reverse Lasègue)
- With the patient lying prone, stretch the femoral nerve roots (L2-L4) by extending the hip (lift the thigh with one hand and use the other hand to maintain full extension of the knee)
- Limited hip extension due to pain radiating into the thigh suggests nerve root irritation

Rib-Pelvis Distance
- Assesses height loss (due to vertebral compression fractures)
- Examiner's hands are inserted into the space between inferior margin of the ribs and superior surface of pelvis in the mid-axillary line while the patient is standing
- The rib-pelvis distance is determined in fingerbreadths to the closest whole value

EBM: Lumbar Vertebral Fractures

A rib-pelvis distance value <2 fingerbreadths has a good sensitivity (87%) and moderate specificity (47%).

Siminoski K, et al. 2003. *Am J Med* 115(3):233-236.

Screen the Hips
- Both osteoarthritis of the hip and a prolapsed intervertebral disc (at L2-L3 or L3-L4) are often confused with spinal stenosis

Peripheral Vascular System
- Crucial to obtain a thorough history to distinguish between claudication due to vascular insufficiency versus spinal stenosis
  - i.e. vascular claudication versus neurogenic claudication
- **Claudication due to Vascular Insufficiency:** constant pain, worse with walking, occurs after walking a very consistent distance; involves stocking type of sensory loss; peripheral pulses usually absent; is rapidly relieved by rest
- **Claudication due to Spinal Stenosis:** relieved by changes in posture (sitting, bending, flexing spine) and rest; slower to be relieved of pain than claudication due to vascular insufficiency

Common Clinical Scenarios

Sciatica
- Pain due to entrapment of sciatic nerve
- Patients complain of pain, burning, or aching in buttocks radiating down posterior thigh to the posterolateral aspect of calf
- Pain is worsened by sneezing, laughing or straining during bowel movement
- Use straight leg raise test to help in diagnosis (see **Figure 7**)

Cauda Equina Syndrome

- Most frequent cause is large central disc herniation (do not miss this diagnosis!)[12]
- Progressive neurological deficit presenting with:
  - Saddle anesthesia
  - Decreased anal tone and reflex
  - Fecal incontinence
  - Urinary retention (overflow incontinence)
  - Bilateral lower leg weakness
  - Surgical emergency! Will cause permanent urinary/bowel incontinence

Thoracic Outlet Syndrome

- Compression of the lower trunk of the brachial plexus and the subclavian artery
- May be due to fibrous bands or abnormalities in the scalene attachments at the root of the neck or by a Pancoast tumor
- May also be due to a cervical rib (rare)

Cervical Spondylosis

- Compression of cervical nerve roots or cord
- Cervical pain: chronic suboccipital headache
- Cervical radiculopathy (C7>C6>C5): sensory dysfunction (e.g. radicular pain) and/or motor dysfunction (e.g. weakness)
- Cervical myelopathy classified into five categories: transverse lesion syndrome, motor syndrome, central cord syndrome, Brown-Séquard syndrome, and brachialgia/cord syndrome

Whiplash

- Cervical strain resulting from soft tissue trauma
- Suboccipital headache is most common symptom
- Progressive onset of neck pain peaking around 12-72 h following trauma
- Decreased active and passive range of motion
- Less commonly reported symptoms include visual disturbances, tinnitus, dizziness, neurologic symptoms, concussion, disturbed concentration and memory, and difficulty sleeping due to pain
- Palpation may reveal rigidity in neck musculature
- Alterations in mood, weakness of upper and lower extremities, decreased reflexes, reduction in sensation, decreased coordination, and altered gait may be present

Scoliosis

- Etiology classified into three categories: neuromuscular, congenital, and idiopathic
- Scoliosis often observed when viewing patient from behind: a plumb line dropped from the spinous process of C7 should pass through the gluteal cleft if scoliosis is not present
- Adam's forward bend test should be performed: observe patient from behind while he/she bends forward at the waist until parallel with the ground (patient with scoliosis will have a thoracic or lumbar prominence unilaterally)

Kyphosis

- Abnormal development of vertebra or degeneration resulting in vertebrae becoming wedge-shaped
- Normal curve of thoracic spine up to 40° on lateral radiograph measured from T4-T12

Ankylosing Spondylitis

- A chronic systemic inflammatory disease: symptoms related to inflammatory back pain (primarily sacroiliac and axial skeleton), peripheral enthesitis and arthritis, constitutional symptoms, and organ-specific manifestations
- Insidious onset of low back pain (>3 mo) in patients <40 yr
- Symptoms worse in morning and improve with exercise
- Disease progression can lead to decreased range of motion associated with fusion of vertebral bodies (e.g. stooped forward-flexed position in neck)
- Common signs include tenderness in sacroiliac (SI) joints and enthesitis (especially Achilles)
- Extra-articular manifestations include: uveitis, cardiovascular, pulmonary, renal, neurologic, gastrointestinal, and bone involvement

Spina Bifida Occulta

- Incomplete closure of one or several vertebral arches posteriorly
- Can present as a dimple or small lipoma, and is mostly asymptomatic and discovered incidentally during evaluation of back pain

Prolapsed Intervertebral Disc (Herniated Disc)

- Usually occurs in middle age; more common in men
- Mostly occurs at L4-L5 or L5-S1 levels
- May be asymptomatic or cause back pain, abnormal posture, limitation of spine motion, focal sensory or reflex changes (motor findings occur less frequently)
- Symptoms and signs are usually unilateral

Spinal Stenosis

- Narrowing of spinal canal, most common in lumbar region
- Mostly occurs with aging, but also caused by osteoarthritis and osteophytes, rheumatoid arthritis, spinal tumors, Paget's disease of the bone, trauma, and previous surgery
- Mostly present as back or buttock pain that is induced by walking or standing, but relieved by sitting or flexed positions such as pushing a shopping cart
- Focal weakness, sensory or reflex changes may occur if associated with neural foraminal narrowing and radiculopathy

Spondylolisthesis

- One of the vertebrae slips out of position onto the vertebra below it, most often L4 on L5 or occasionally L5 on S1
- More common in female patients >40 yr
- May be asymptomatic or may cause low back pain and hamstring tightness, nerve root injury, symptomatic spinal stenosis, or cauda equina syndrome in severe cases

Neural Foraminal Narrowing and Radiculopathy

- Caused by one, or frequently a combination, of conditions including osteophytes, lateral disc protrusion, facet joint hypertrophy, uncovertebral joint hypertrophy, congenital shortened pedicles
- Unilateral nerve root symptoms and signs due to bony compression at the intervertebral foramen or lateral recess
- Symptoms are indistinguishable from those caused by disc-related radiculopathy by history and neurological exam; therefore, requires spinal neuroimaging (CT or MRI) to identify the underlying cause

3.6 Hip

Common Symptoms

- Pain
- Stiffness

Physical Exam

Inspection

- With Patient Standing
  - Inspect from the front and from behind for any pelvic tilting or rotational deformity
  - Note any abnormalities of bony or soft tissue contours (see **Figure 8**)
  - From the side, note presence of lumbar lordosis that may indicate a fixed flexion deformity
  - Observe the contour of the buttock for any abnormality (gluteus maximus atrophy or atonia)
- Examine Gait
  - Note antalgic gait (to avoid pain, time spent on injured limb during stance phase is minimized)
  - Note Trendelenburg gait (dropping of the pelvis on the unaffected side during the stance phase of the affected side)
- Trendelenburg Test
  - Ask the patient to stand on one leg
  - Pelvis on non-weight bearing side should not drop, indicating functioning abductors on the weight bearing leg
  - If the pelvis drops, it is a positive test
    - Can be caused by gluteal muscle weakness (mainly gluteus medius), inhibition from pain, or a hip deformity
- Measurement of Leg Length
  - True leg length: pelvis must first be set square and feet placed 15-20 cm apart; measure each leg from anterior superior iliac spine (ASIS) to the medial malleolus
  - Apparent leg length: apparent shortening (e.g. uncorrectable pelvic tilting) may also be assessed by comparing the distances between the umbilicus and each medial malleolus
  - Acceptable leg length discrepancy: ± 1 cm[13]

Palpation

- Anterior Aspect
  - Palpate the iliac crest, greater trochanter and trochanteric bursa, ASIS, inguinal ligament, femoral triangle, and symphysis pubis (see **Figure 8**)
  - Palpate the hip flexors, adductor and abductor muscles for signs of pathology
  - Palpate for crepitus by placing your fingers over the femoral head (which is just lateral to the femoral artery below the inguinal ligament)
  - Roll the relaxed leg medially and laterally to detect any crepitus
- Posterior Aspect
  - Palpate the iliac crest, posterior superior iliac spine (PSIS), ischial tuberosity, greater trochanter, sacroiliac, lumbosacral, and sacrococcygeal joints (see **Figure 8**)

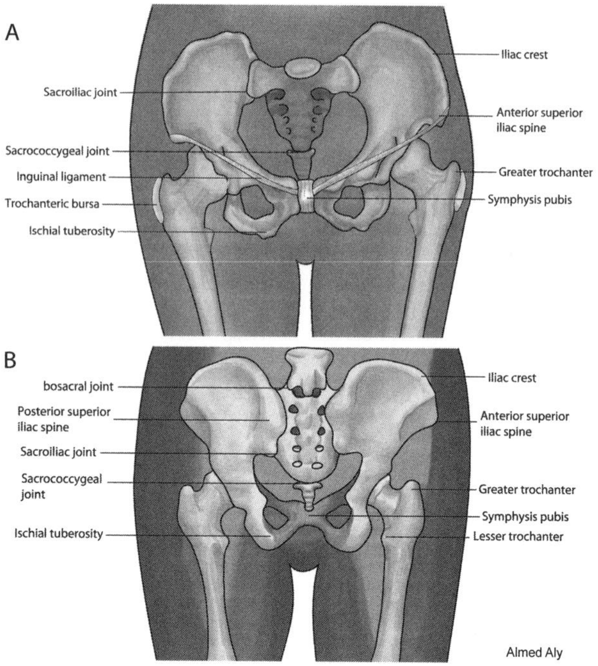

Figure 8. Anterior (A) and Posterior (B) Anatomy of the Pelvis and Hip

Range of Motion

- See **Table 17** for maneuvers and normal ROM

Table 17. Hip: Maneuvers and Normal Range of Motion

Maneuver	Range of Motion
Flexion: with patient lying supine, have patient pull knee to chest; knee is also flexed	120°
Extension: with patient lying on side, palpate the ASIS and PSIS and have patient fully extend the leg until pelvis shifts	30°
Abduction: place one hand on the contralateral ASIS and with the other hand, grasp the heel and abduct the patient's leg until the pelvis shifts	45°
Adduction: place one hand on the ipsilateral ASIS and with the other hand, grasp the heel and adduct the patient's leg until the pelvis shifts	30°
Rotation: flex knee and hip to 90°, grasp the lower leg and move medially (external rotation) and laterally (internal rotation) OR with patient lying supine with the leg fully extended, roll the leg medially and laterally	External Rotation in extension: 45° External Rotation at 90° flexion: 45° Internal Rotation in extension: 45° Internal Rotation at 90° flexion: 45°

ASIS = anterior superior iliac spine, PSIS = posterior superior iliac spine
Gross G, Fetto J, Rosen E. *Musculoskeletal Examination.* Malden: Blackwell; 2002.

Power Assessment/Isometric Movements

- Performed with patient in supine position (except for hip extension where patient is on his/her side), noting which movements cause pain or show weakness
- Since hip muscles are strong, instruction of "Don't let me move your leg" ensures that the movement is isometric
- All active movements performed should be tested isometrically

Special Tests

Patrick's Test (Fabere or Figure Four Test)

- Patient lies supine, with both knees flexed
- The foot of the test leg is placed on top of the knee of the opposite leg
- Gently press down on the knee of the test leg, lowering it toward the examining table
- Test is negative when test leg is at least parallel with the opposite leg
- Test is positive when the leg remains above the opposite leg
- Positive test indicates an affected hip or sacroiliac joint, or that iliopsoas spasms exist
- Pain indicates early osteoarthritic changes

Thomas Test

- Used to assess hip flexion contracture (fixed flexion deformity), the most common contracture of the hip
- With the patient supine, place your hand under the lumbar spine
- Reduce lumbar lordosis by passively flexing the hip by bringing the patient's knee to his/her abdomen (or ask the patient to hold his/her leg against his/her abdomen)
- Elevation of the opposite thigh suggests a loss of extension in that hip (tight hip flexors) and a fixed flexion deformity
- Useful observations to accompany this test:
  - o Note the degree of knee flexion in the free leg (knee flexion <90° suggests tight quadriceps)
  - o Note the degree of leg abduction in the free leg (abduction of the leg suggests tight abductors and/or tight iliotibial band)

Anterior Impingement Test

- Used to assess for femoroacetabular impingement syndrome[14]
- With patient supine, the hip and knee of affected limb are flexed to 90°
- The leg is adducted and internally rotated
- Sudden onset of pain, typically in the groin, is considered a positive test

EBM: Patrick's Test and Thomas Test

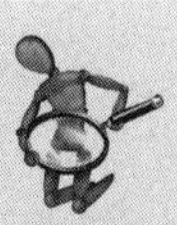

Patrick's Test
- Sensitivity of 77% and specificity of 100%*

Thomas Test
- Reliability of 91%†

*van der Wurff P, Meyne W, Hagmeijer RH. 2000. *Manual Therapy.* 5(2): 89-96.
†Vizniak N. *Physical Assessment.* Burnaby: Professional Health Systems; 2008.

Common Clinical Scenarios

Hip Fracture

- May be due to trauma or fragility fracture secondary to osteoporosis
- Injured leg is unable to bear weight, is shorter, and is classically externally rotated
- Patient experiences sharp pain in groin and down thigh

Avascular Necrosis
- Bone cell death due to decreased blood flow to the head of the femur
- Causes include hip fracture, prolonged steroid use, idiopathic, alcoholism, diving to depth

> **Clinical Pearl: Referred Pain**
> Pain referred to groin and thigh is HIP pain.
> Pain referred to buttocks is BACK pain.

3.7 Knee

Common Symptoms
- Pain
- Instability
- Swelling
- Locking

Physical Exam
Inspection
- SEADS
  - **S**welling: note any swelling in knees; specifically, look at the medial fossa and any bulging on the sides of the patellar ligament (indicative of small effusion)
  - **A**trophy: inspect quadriceps for muscle atrophy (vastus medialis)
  - **D**eformity: ask the patient to stand with his/her feet together; inspect for genu valgum (knock-knee), genu varum (bow-leg), genu recurvatum (hyperextended knee) or flexion contracture
- Gait
  - Patient will limit extension and flexion of a painful knee and minimize time spent on the injured knee while walking (antalgic gait)

Palpation
- Anterior palpation with knee extended
  - With the back of the hand, palpate the knee for temperature; compare both sides proximal to the joint, over the patella, and distal to the joint; normally, the patella is the coolest area of the knee
  - Palpate the anatomical structures noting tenderness, swelling or nodules; patellar tendon, tibial tuberosity, suprapatellar pouch (check for thickening or swelling of the suprapatellar pouch starting 10 cm proximal to the superior border of the patella), quadriceps muscles, medial collateral ligament
- Anterior palpation with knee flexed
  - Using thumbs, palpate the tibiofemoral joint line; noting the lateral aspect for swelling (meniscal cysts), tibial condyles, femoral condyles
- Posterior palpation with knee flexed
  - Palpate the popliteal fossa (for a Baker's cyst), hamstrings, and gastrocnemius muscles
- ROM: active movement (see **Table 18**)

Table 18. Knee: Normal Ranges of Motion

Maneuver	Range of Motion
Flexion	135°
Extension	0°

Gross G, Fetto J, Rosen E. *Musculoskeletal Examination.* Malden: Blackwell; 2002.

Range of Motion

- While patient is lying prone, have him/her actively flex and extend knee
- With the patient supine, passively flex and extend the patient's knee by placing one hand over the joint, and one hand on the lower leg
  - Note any crepitus, clicking, and end feel of the motion
- Passive, medial and lateral movement of patella is also tested for mobility, symmetry:
  - Normally, patella should move half of its width laterally and medially
  - Note whether patella tilts, rotates or stays parallel to femoral condyles

Special Tests: Tests for Effusion

Patellar Tap Test

- Place hand on the top of the femur, about 15 cm proximal to the patella, with index finger and thumb placed on either side
- Displace fluid from the suprapatellar pouch by sliding hand distally to just above the patella
- While maintaining pressure with the left hand, push down quickly on the patella with the tips of your thumb and 3 fingers of free hand
- In the presence of an effusion, a palpable tap (click) will be transmitted and felt by index finger and thumb on either side of the patella
- If the effusion is slight, the exam will be negative

Fluctuation/Ballotment Test

- Compress suprapatellar pouch back against the femur with your left hand as above
- With your right hand placed just below the patella, feel for fluid entering the patellar fossae, spaces next to the patella, with your right thumb and index finger
- If you feel fluid, confirm its presence by pushing the fluid between the medial and lateral fossae
  - ***Note:*** do not move the patella itself back and forth
  - Press the patella backward against the femur with your right hand and feel fluid returning to the suprapatellar pouch

Fluid Displacement/"Milk" Bulge Test (for detecting small effusions)

- Place hand on the top of the femur, about 15 cm proximal to the patella, with index finger and thumb placed on either side
- Displace fluid from the suprapatellar pouch by sliding hand distally to just above the patella
- With the back of the hand, stroke upward on the medial side of the knee to milk fluid into the lateral compartment
- Stroke downward on the lateral side of the knee and observe for fluid returning to the medial compartment, distending the medial fossa
- The wave of fluid may take up to 2 s to appear
- Normally, the knee contains 1-7 mL of synovial fluid
- This test shows as little as 4-8 mL of extra fluid in knee
- This test is positive if the effusion is small and negative if the effusion is large

Special Tests: Ligament Tests

Anterior Drawer Test for Anterior Cruciate Ligament (ACL) Tear

- With the patient supine, flex the hips to 45° and flex both knees to 90°
- Inspect the joint lines of both knees; a false positive can occur if the tibia was initially subluxed posteriorly due to a torn posterior cruciate ligament (PCL) (see **Posterior Sag Sign**, p.162)
- Sit close to the foot to steady it, grasp the leg just below the knee with both hands, ensure the hamstrings are relaxed, and pull the tibia forward (see **Figure 9**)

- Compare both knees, noting any abnormal forward displacement of the tibia
- Movement ≥1.5 cm is indicative of an ACL tear (sensitivity 62%)[10]

Lachman Test for ACL Tear
- Relax the knee in 15° of flexion
- Grasp the distal femur with one hand and the upper tibia with the other
- With the thumb of the tibial hand resting on the joint line to detect movement, simultaneously pull the tibia forward and push the femur back
- This exam is the most sensitive test (84%) for ACL insufficiency[10]
- A positive test shows anterior tibial movement and a spongy end point

Posterior Drawer Test for Posterior Cruciate Ligament (PCL) Tear
- Perform the same maneuver as the anterior drawer test, including inspection for subluxed tibia, but push the tibia backward instead (see **Figure 9**)
- Movement of >1.0 cm is indicative of a complete PCL tear (sensitivity 55%)[10]

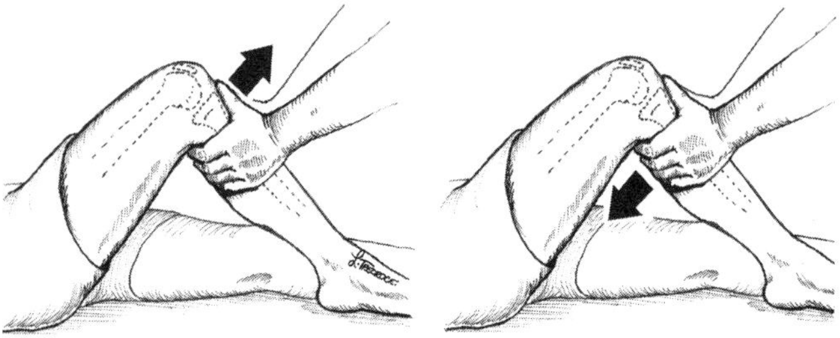

Anterior Drawer Test

Posterior Drawer Test

Lorraine Trecroce

Figure 9. Anterior and Posterior Drawer Tests for ACL and PCL Tears

Posterior Sag Sign
- Patient is supine with hips flexed to 45° and test knee flexed to 90°
- If the PCL is torn, the tibia drops back or sags on the femur; compare to the other knee
- A positive posterior sag sign can cause a false positive anterior drawer test

Medial Collateral Ligament (MCL)
- With knee extended, place one hand on the lateral aspect of the knee at the level of the joint
- Pull the lower leg laterally with the other hand, applying a valgus force
- This test opens up the MCL
- A positive test is indicated by pain on the inside of the knee

Lateral Collateral Ligament (LCL)
- Place one hand on the medial aspect of the knee at the level of the joint
- Push the lower leg medially with the other hand, applying a varus force
- This test opens up the LCL
- A positive test is indicated by pain on the outside of the knee

Special Tests: Menisci Tests

General Examination of the Meniscus

- Examine for joint line tenderness
- Discern if there is a springy block to full extension
- These two signs in association with quadriceps wasting are the most consistent and reliable signs of a meniscus tear

McMurray Maneuver for Medial Meniscus

- Fully flex the knee and place the thumb and index finger along the joint line with the palm of the hand resting on the patella
- Externally rotate the foot and extend the knee joint smoothly with the other hand
- A meniscal tear is suggested if the patient's pain is reproduced or if a click accompanies the pain
- Asymptomatic, nonpathological clicks may be caused by tendons or other soft tissues snapping over bony prominences

McMurray Maneuver for Lateral Meniscus

- Similar to the test above, but with the foot internally rotated

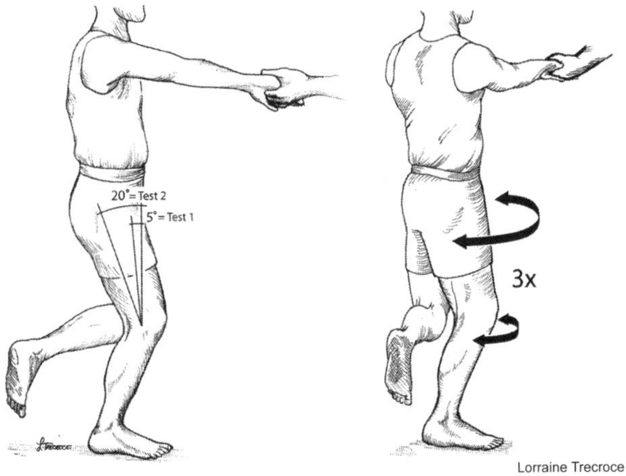

Lorraine Trecroce

Figure 10. Thessaly Test for Medial and Lateral Meniscus Tears

Thessaly Test for Medial or Lateral Meniscus

- This test is completed first on the normal (unaffected) leg and then on the injured leg
- The examiner supports the patient while he/she stands flatfooted on the normal leg
- The patient slightly flexes the knee (5°) and internally and externally rotates the knee and body three times
- The same process is completed with the knee flexed at 20°
- A meniscal tear is suggested if the patient experiences medial or lateral joint line discomfort[15]
- The patient may also experience the sensation of locking or catching of the knee joint (see **Figure 10**)

Common Clinical Scenarios

Patellofemoral Syndrome

- May be due to misalignment in the articulation between the femur and the patella

- Pain is a dull ache at the anterior surface of the knee
- Pain is normally worse when going downstairs, while squatting, or after getting up after sitting for prolonged periods[16]
- Examination may reveal atrophic quadriceps muscles and mild knee swelling

EBM: Torn Meniscus

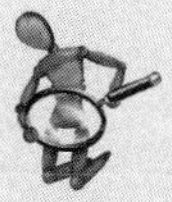

The gold standard for the diagnosis of a torn meniscus of the knee is arthroscopy.

Test	Sensitivity	Specificity
Joint Line Tenderness*	63%	71%
McMurray Maneuver*	71%	71%
Thessaly Test (5°)†	66% Med/81% Lat	96% Med/91% Lat
Thessaly Test (20°)†	89% Med/92% Lat	97% Med/96% Lat

*Hegedus EJ, et al. 2007. *J Orthop Sports Phys Ther* 37(9):541-550.
†Karachalios T, et al. 2005. *J Bone Surg Joint Am* 87(5):955-962.

Meniscal Injury
- Tear of the fibrocartilage cushioning the joint
- Knee may lock and/or click
- Tell-tale sign is tenderness of the joint line over the involved meniscus

Ligamentous Injury
- Tear of a ligament due to trauma
- Pain is acute and severe
- Examination will reveal effusion (possibly hemarthrosis if rapid in onset), instability, bruising, limited ROM due to muscle spasm
- ACL injuries are commonly accompanied with MCL and medial meniscus injuries (O'Donoghue's triad)

3.8 Ankle and Foot

Common Symptoms
- Pain
- Instability
- Swelling

Physical Exam
Inspection
- SEADS
  - Inspect the feet and ankles with and without weight bearing
  - Inspect bony and soft tissue prominences, noting any deformities or asymmetries, edema, scars, bruising, toe alignment, skin, or nail changes
  - Inspect the plantar surface of the foot for ulcerations, fungal infection, excess callous formation
- With the patient weight bearing
  - Inspect the posture of the ankle and foot anteriorly, posteriorly, and laterally, noting any splaying of the forefoot
  - With the patient standing, assess, from behind, for pronation (valgus) deformity of subtalar joint
  - Slip fingers under the arch to detect pes cavus (high arch) or pes planus (flatfoot)
  - Have patient stand on toes to differentiate between a flexible and fixed flatfoot

- Assess gait with and without shoes
  - Note the posture of the foot during walking (e.g. pronation of the ankle during the stance phase)

Palpation
- Palpate the feet and ankles
  - Palpate the bony prominences for tenderness and swelling
  - Note any temperature differences that exist between the feet
  - Place one hand over the anterior surface of the ankle and passively plantar flex and dorsiflex the ankle, noting any crepitus
  - Examine the pedal pulses and the more proximal pulses if required
  - Screen for tenderness of the metatarsophalangeal (MTP) joints by compressing the forefoot between thumb and fingers
  - To evaluate joints individually, firmly palpate the metatarsal heads and grooves between them with thumbs and index fingers

Range of Motion: Active Movements
- Ankle (Tibiotalar) Joint
  - Dorsiflex and plantar flex the foot
  - Invert and evert the foot; note that these motions involve the transverse tarsal and subtalar joints
- MTP joints
  - Ask the patient to flex and extend the toes
  - See **Table 19** for the complete list of active movements to be examined

Table 19. Ankle: Normal Ranges of Motion

Maneuver	Range of Motion
Plantar Flexion	50°
Dorsiflexion	20°
Inversion of Heel	35°
Eversion of Heel	15°
Supination of the Forefoot	35°
Pronation of the Forefoot	15°
Toe Extension	Lateral Toes: (MTP: 40°, PIP: 0°, DIP: 30°) Great Toe: (MTP: 70°, IP: 0°)
Toe Flexion	Lateral Toes: (MTP: 40°, PIP: 0°, DIP: 60°) Great Toe: (MTP: 45°, IP: 40°)

IP = interphalangeal, MTP = metatarsophalangeal
Gross G, Fetto J, Rosen E. *Musculoskeletal Examination*. Malden: Blackwell; 2002.

Range of Motion: Passive Movements
- Ankle (Tibiotalar) Joint
  - Test passive dorsiflexion and plantar flexion by grasping the foot proximal to the subtalar joint (or lock the subtalar joint in inversion) as subtalar dorsiflexion may be confused with ankle dorsiflexion
- Subtalar Joint
  - Stabilize the ankle with one hand, grasp the calcaneus with the other hand, and invert and evert the forefoot
  - This should be done with the ankle in dorsiflexion to lock the ankle joint
- MTP Joints
  - Steady the heel with one hand and flex and extend the MTP and interphalangeal (IP) joints of the great toe and lesser toes

Special Tests

Anterior Drawer for Ankle Stability

- With the knee at 90° and the foot flat on the table, stabilize the tibia and pull the foot forward to detect abnormal movement
- Alternatively, immobilize the foot and shift the tibia backward

Ligament Tests

- When testing the integrity of each ligament, it is important to stabilize the lower leg
- Each ligament is preferentially stressed passively as follows:
  - Anterior talofibular ligament (ATFL): plantar flexion and inversion
  - Calcaneofibular ligament (CFL): inversion at 90°
  - Posterior talofibular ligament (PTFL): dorsiflexion and inversion
  - Deltoid ligament: eversion

Ottawa Ankle Rules

- The purpose is to discern the need for X-ray
- Rules do not apply to patients <16 yr
- Palpation of bone, not the soft tissue
- An ankle X-ray is indicated if a patient suffers an inversion injury and has any one of the following[17]:
  - Tenderness at the tip of either malleolus or 6 cm proximal to malleolus
  - Tenderness at the base of the fifth metatarsal
  - Tenderness over the navicular
  - Inability to walk four steps
  - Age >50 yr
- An X-ray is indicated in the presence or absence of bone pain if the patient cannot walk
- During palpation, note the presence of isolated medial tenderness
  - Palpate the proximal fibula to rule out a Maisonneuve's fracture (fracture of the fibular head and disruption of the interosseous membrane secondary to an ankle fracture)
- Sensitivity is 100%, negative predictive value is 1 (i.e. by applying the rules, no significant ankle fractures are missed)[17]

Common Clinical Scenarios

Ankle Sprain

- Ligaments supporting ankle joint are torn due to trauma
- Pain is acute and localized, accompanied by swelling, hematoma, loss of ROM, and inability to bear weight
- Tenderness over the bony prominences should be examined more closely for fracture

Bunion (Hallux Valgus)

- Proximal phalanx of the great toe begins to drift producing a valgus deformity
- A protective bursa forms over the deformed MTP joint
- On examination, gross deformity associated with localized pain and stiffness is observed

Tibialis Posterior Dysfunction

- Tendinosis and resulting fibrosis of the tibialis posterior tendon leads to an acquired flatfoot deformity
- Prevalence increases with age, pes planus (flatfoot), HTN, DM, and steroid injections around tendon[18]
  - Early stages: swelling and tenderness behind and below medial malleolus and some weakness or pain with inversion of the foot

  - Late stages: less swelling and pain, flatfoot deformity acquired (valgus position of affected heel, flattening of medial longitudinal arch, and forefoot abduction)
- Too many toes sign: more than normal (1.5-2) toes are seen along lateral border of the foot when examining patient from behind
- Patients are unable to perform ipsilateral unsupported single heel rise (i.e. on affected foot)

4. COMMON CLINICAL SCENARIOS

4.1 Fracture

- Establish mechanism of injury, activity at the time of the injury, magnitude of the applied forces (e.g. fell from a height), point of impact, and the direction of the applied force (e.g. fall on an outstretched hand)
- Inspect injury for bony deformation, instability, hematoma, loss of function, localized edema, localized pain and severity
- Note any paresthesia, loss of pulse or decrease in capillary refill below the fracture
- Fracture Description
  - Open/closed
  - Involvement of joint (intra-/extra-articular)
  - Part of bone (epiphyseal, metaphyseal, diaphyseal – proximal, middle, distal)
  - Displacement
    - Angulation: distal fragment position relative to proximal fragment; orientation (degrees) of the distal bone fragment toward (valgus) or away (varus) from the midline
    - Translation: "sliding" (percentage) of distal bone fragment in relation to proximal fragment
    - Rotation: movement of distal fragment (longitudinal axis) in relation to proximal fragment
    - Impaction: bone ends are compressed together

4.2 Compartment Syndrome

- Increased tissue pressure decreases the perfusion and function of the tissues and nerves within the compartment
- Establish underlying mechanism: trauma, hemorrhage, previous fracture or surgical procedure, external compression (cast, wound closure)
- Perform motor and sensory exams, note 5 **P**'s:
  - **P**ain (early, increases with passive stretch)
  - **P**allor
  - **P**aresthesia
  - **P**aralysis (late)
  - **P**ulselessness (very late, tissue damage likely)

4.3 Osteoporosis

- In Canada, affects 1 in 3 women and 1 in 5 men >50 yr[19]
- Systemic disease characterized by low bone mass and micro-architectural deterioration of bone tissue
- Leads to increased risk of fragility fractures
- Areas of main concern are wrist, humerus, ribs, vertebral body, pelvis, and hip
- May present with height loss and a history of fragility fractures
- Osteoporosis related history:
  - Age (>65 yr)
  - History of low trauma fractures
  - Family history of osteoporotic fracture

- Height loss (4 cm historical or 2 cm prospective height loss)
- Systemic glucocorticoid therapy of >3 mo duration
- Early menopause (age <45 yr)
- Dietary calcium intake
- Weight <57 kg

4.4 Osteoarthritis

- Degeneration of cartilage within joints, damage to underlying bone, and new bone formation at joint margins
- Disease occurs most commonly in weight-bearing joints
- Patient complains of pain with movement and pain on palpation
- Decreasing joint ROM, grinding (crepitus), swelling and stiffness, bony enlargement of joint, fixed flexion deformity, limb shortening, referred hip pain to the knee, generally worse with activity, better with rest

4.5 Rheumatoid Arthritis

- Systemic inflammatory disorder characterized by destructive hypertrophic synovitis
- Symptoms include:
  - Symmetrical peripheral polyarthritis causing pain and stiffness that is most prominent in the morning and lasts >30 min
  - Insidious onset with involvement of an increasing number of joints including wrists, elbows, shoulders, ankles, knees, and hips
  - Systemic features such as malaise, weight loss, and low-grade fever
  - Soft tissue problems such as carpal tunnel syndrome and flexor tenosynovitis
- Physical signs include:
  - Soft tissue swelling, tenderness, stiffness, erythema, and increased temperature of affected synovial joints (often peripheral joints)
  - Synovial effusions
  - Raynaud's phenomenon, tenosynovitis, carpal tunnel syndrome
  - Swan-neck and boutonnière deformities of the fingers (see **Table 7**), volar and ulnar subluxation of the fingers at the MCP joints
- Diagnosis is made if ≥4 of the American College of Rheumatology 1987 Criteria are met: morning stiffness (>1 h, >6 wk), arthritis in at least three areas (>6 wk), arthritis of hands or wrists (>6 wk), symmetrical arthritis (>6 wk), rheumatoid nodules, positive rheumatoid factor, radiographic changes in wrists/hands[10]

REFERENCES

1. O'Brien SJ, Pagnani MJ, Fealy S, McGlynn SR, Wilson JB. 1998. The active compression test: A new and effective test for diagnosing labral tears and acromioclavicular joint abnormality. *Am J Sports Med.* 26(5):610-613.
2. Michener LA, Walsworth MK, Doukas WC, Murphy KP. 2009. Reliability and diagnostic accuracy of five physical examination tests and combination of tests for subacromial impingement. *Arch Phys Med Rehabil* 90(11):1898-1903.
3. Gerber C, Krushell RJ. 1991. Isolated rupture of the tendon of the subscapularis muscle. Clinical features in 16 cases. *J Bone Joint Surg Br* 73(3):389-394.
4. Bickley LS, Szilagyi PG, Bates B. *Bates' Guide to Physical Examination and History Taking,* 10th ed. Philadelphia: Lippincott Williams & Wilkins; 2009.
5. Swartz MH. *Textbook of Physical Diagnosis: History and Examination,* 6th ed. Philadelphia: Saunders Elsevier; 2010.
6. McRae R. *Clinical Orthopaedic Examination.* Edinburgh: Churchill Livingstone; 2004.
7. Foye PM, Stitik TP, Sinha D. Olecranon Bursitis. *Medscape Reference.* Available from: http://emedicine.medscape.com.
8. D'Arcy CA, McGee S. 2000. The rational clinical examination. Does this patient have carpal tunnel syndrome? *JAMA* 283(23):3110-3117.
9. Engstrom JW, Deyo RA. Back and Neck Pain. In: Longo DL, Fauci AS, Kasper DL, Hauser SL, Jameson JL, Loscalzo J (Editors), *Harrison's Principles of Internal Medicine,* 18th ed. New York: McGraw-Hill; 2011. Available from: http://www.accessmedicine.com.
10. Magee DJ. *Orthopedic Physical Assessment.* St Louis: Saunders Elsevier; 2008.
11. Vroomen PC, de Krom MC, Knottnerus JA. 1999. Diagnostic value of history and physical examination in patients suspected of sciatica due to disc herniation: A systematic review. *J Neurol* 246(10):899-906.
12. Storm PB, Chou D, Tamargo RJ. 2002. Lumbar spinal stenosis, cauda equina syndrome, and multiple lumbosacral radiculopathies. *Phys Med Rehabil Clin N Am* 13(3):713-733.
13. Harvey WF, Yang M, Cooke TD, Segal NA, Lane N, Lewis CE, et al. 2010. Associations of leg length inequality with prevalent, incident, and progressive knee osteoarthritis: A cohort study. *Ann Intern Med* 152(5):287-295.
14. Dooley PJ. Femoroacetabular impingement syndrome: Nonarthritic hip pain in young adults. *Can Fam Physician* 54(1):42-47.
15. Karachalios T, Hantes M, Zibis AH, Zachos V, Karantanas AH, Malizos KN. 2005. Diagnostic accuracy of a new clinical test (the Thessaly test) for early detection of meniscal tears. *J Bone Joint Surg Am* 87(5):955-962.
16. Juhn MS. 1999. Patellofemoral pain syndrome: A review and guidelines for treatment. *Am Fam Physician* 60(7):2012-2018.
17. Stiell IG, McKnight RD, Greenberg GH, McDowell I, Nair RC, Wells GA, et al. 1994. Implementation of the Ottawa Ankle Rules. *JAMA* 271(11):827-832.
18. Kohls-Gatzoulis J, Angel JC, Singh D, Haddad F, Livingstone J, Berry G. 2004. Tibialis posterior dysfunction: A common and treatable cause of adult acquired flatfoot. *BMJ* 329(7478):1328-1333.
19. Osteoporosis Canada. 2013. What is Osteoporosis? Available from: http://www.osteoporosis.ca/osteoporosis-and-you/what-is-osteoporosis/.
20. Dandy DJ, Edwards DJ. *Essential Orthopaedics and Trauma.* Edinburgh: Churchill Livingstone/Elsevier; 2009.

MUSCULOSKELETAL

The Neurological Exam

Editors:
Giorgia Tropini
Vahagn Karapetyan

Faculty Reviewers:
David Chan, MD, FRCP(C)
Liesly Lee, MD, FRCP(C)

TABLE OF CONTENTS

1. APPROACH TO THE NEUROLOGICAL HISTORY AND PHYSICAL EXAM

The following approach is generally used in neurology:

1. Where is the lesion? (anatomical diagnosis)
   - Cerebrum, basal ganglia, brainstem, cerebellum, spinal cord, motor neuron, peripheral nerve, neuromuscular junction, muscle (see **Table 1**)
   - The history and physical exam provide important clues
2. What is the lesion? (pathological diagnosis)
   - Vascular, infectious, congenital, traumatic, neoplastic, autoimmune/inflammatory, nutritional/toxic, metabolic, degenerative (see **Table 2**)
     - Is the disease process focal or diffuse?
     - Focal/asymmetrical (traumatic, neoplastic, vascular, degenerative)
     - Diffuse/symmetrical (infectious, autoimmune, nutritional/toxic, metabolic, degenerative)
     - Use of investigative tests

In addition to the general history, important aspects of the neurological history are:

- Neurological symptoms (see **Table 3**)
  - Onset, timing, distribution
- Focal vs. diffuse symptoms
- Precipitating events (e.g. trauma, medications)
- Past neurological history (e.g. TIA, stroke)

Table 1. Where is the lesion?

Level of Lesion	Signs and Symptoms
Cerebrum	Seizures, confusion, hemianopsia, aphasia, cortical findings, hemiparesis on contralateral side
Basal Ganglia	Tremor, rigidity, involuntary movements
Brainstem	Diplopia, vertigo, ipsilateral facial involvement with contralateral limb impairment (alternating hemiparesis)
Cerebellum	Ataxia, intention tremor, dysarthria, hypotonia Impairments ipsilateral to the lesion
Spinal Cord	Paraparesis, sensory level, incontinence Defects frequently bilateral, at and below level of lesion
Motor Neuron (anterior horn)	Diffuse weakness, fasciculations, atrophy
Peripheral Nerve	Glove/stocking paresthesia, areflexia
Neuromuscular Junction	Fatigable muscle weakness, ptosis, diplopia, dysarthria, dysphagia
Muscle	Proximal weakness

Table 2. What is the Lesion?

Type of Lesion	Signs and Symptoms, DDx
Vascular	Acute with focal deficits, HTN, fibrillation, bruit e.g. TIA, infarction, SAH, ICH
Infectious	Acute, diffuse, headache, fever, nuchal rigidity, back pain e.g. Meningitis, encephalitis, osteomyelitis, discitis
Congenital	Early onset, static, suggestive habitus e.g. Hydrocephalus, cerebral palsy
Traumatic	Focal, pain, tenderness e.g. SDH, vertebral fracture, sciatica
Neoplastic	Progressive, accelerating, focal, headache, back pain e.g. Primary or metastatic tumor
Autoimmune/ Inflammatory	Subacute, relapsing, multifocal/diffuse e.g. Polymyositis, myasthenia gravis, GBS, MS
Nutritional/Toxic	Acute/chronic, diffuse e.g. Medications, substance abuse, pernicious anemia
Metabolic	Acute/chronic, diffuse e.g. DM, electrolyte disturbances, uremia, cirrhosis, myxedema, sepsis
Degenerative	Chronic, diffuse, familial e.g. DMD, CMT, ALS, Parkinson's, Alzheimer's

ALS = amyotrophic lateral sclerosis, CMT = Charcot-Marie-Tooth disease, DMD = Duchenne muscular dystrophy, GBS = Guillain-Barré syndrome, ICH = intracerebral hemorrhage, SAH = subarachnoid hemorrhage, SDH = subdural hematoma

2. COMMON CHIEF COMPLAINTS (*see **Table 3**)

- Change in consciousness*
- "Dizziness" or vertigo*
- Frequent tripping or falls*
- Headache*
- Involuntary movements (e.g. tremors, seizures, restless leg syndrome)*
- Numbness or tingling (paresthesia)*
- Pain*
- Speech difficulties (dysphasia)*
- Visual loss
- Visual disturbances (e.g. transient scotoma, flashing lights)*
- Weakness*
- Sleeping difficulties
- Swallowing difficulty (dysphagia)
- Loss of coordination
- Loss of taste and/or smell
- Memory problems
- Paralysis
- Personality change

3. FOCUSED HISTORY

- See **General History and Physical Exam** for a detailed approach to history taking
- **OPQRSTUVW** questions regarding each complaint
- Complaint-specific questions (see **Table 3**)
- Associated risk factors for diseases (e.g. stroke: hypercholesterolemia, hyperlipidemia, HTN, family history of stroke, etc.)

Table 3. Chief Complaints and Specific Queries to Elicit History

Chief Complaint	Specific Queries, Signs and Symptoms
Headache	• Onset (e.g. thunderclap) • Pattern (e.g. worse in the morning = increased intracranial pressure [ICP]) • Preceding symptoms/aura • Associated symptoms (e.g. nausea and/or vomiting, neck stiffness, fever) • Differences from previous headaches • Systemic conditions (e.g. infections) • Current medications/addictions
Loss of Consciousness	• Syncope vs. seizure • Duration • Preceding symptoms (e.g. lightheadedness) • Associated symptoms (e.g. tongue-biting, body movements, incontinence) • Post-attack symptoms (e.g. confusion, drowsiness) • Previous diagnosis of systemic disorders (e.g. cardiovascular problems) • Current medications • Collateral/corollary information (e.g. bystanders)
Dizziness	• Vertigo vs. presyncope vs. ataxia • Associated symptoms: o Inner ear (N/V, nystagmus, tinnitus, hearing loss) o Brainstem/cerebellar (ataxia, diplopia, dysarthria) o Migraine aura o Changes in sensation between eyes open vs. closed, or with head positioning • Current medications
Visual Disturbances	• Duration • Diplopia (vertical, horizontal, or skew) • Associated symptoms (e.g. eye pain, headache) • Positive symptoms (e.g. flashing lights) • Negative symptoms (e.g. monocular vs. binocular scotoma)

Table 3. Chief Complaints and Specific Queries to Elicit History (continued)

Chief Complaint	Specific Queries, Signs and Symptoms
Numbness	• Paresthesia vs. dysesthesia • Distribution (hemibody vs. radicular vs. peripheral nerve) • Course (e.g. worse on exertion, worse in the morning)
Pain	• Onset, timing (acute/transient vs. chronic/permanent) • Distribution (dermatome vs. diffuse) • Associated symptoms • Previous trauma, surgery, family history
Weakness	• Nerve vs. neuromuscular junction vs. muscle • Associated activities (one activity vs. all activities) • Pattern: o Proximal vs. distal o Unilateral vs. bilateral o Hemiparesis vs. para/quadriplegia • Course, especially fatigability
Tremor	• Character (e.g. worse at rest, with posture, with movement) • Activity-specific vs. general • Associated symptoms (e.g. postural instability, bradykinesia) • Medications and food: o Alcohol, tea, coffee, chocolate, medication, drugs o Symptom-alleviating vs. symptom-enhancing effects
Speech Disturbance	• Onset • Dysphasia vs. dysarthria • Impaired naming, forming new nonsense words (paraphasia) • Reading problems vs. writing problems vs. comprehension problems
Gait	• Onset (e.g. on exertion) • Weakness vs. ataxia • Course • Associated symptoms (sensory impairment, muscle fatigability) • Associated signs: o Loss of position sense, postural instability o Weakness, fatigability, spasticity

4. FOCUSED PHYSICAL EXAM

4.1 Mental Status Examination (MSE)

The mental status exam can help identify neurological disease and help distinguish focal deficits from diffuse processes. Before making judgments about a patient's mental status, the examiner should ensure the patient is alert, cooperative, attentive, and has no language impairment.

- In general, testing proceeds from global functions to more specific and localized functions
  - Global brain function
  - Alertness (see **Table 4**)
  - Cooperation
  - Orientation
- Attention
- Language (speech production, repetition, naming, comprehension, reading, writing)
- Memory (working memory, short-term memory, long-term memory)
- Logic and abstraction

- Mood, Delusions, Hallucinations (see **Psychiatric Exam**, p.323)
  - Popular test batteries to assess mental status include:
    - Folstein MMSE to assess orientation, registration, attention, calculation, memory, and language (see **Psychiatric Exam**, p.322)
    - Montreal Cognitive Assessment (MoCA) to assess orientation, attention/concentration, executive function, memory, language, visuoconstructional skills, conceptual thinking, and calculation

> **Clinical Pearl: Limitations of the MMSE**
> The MMSE is affected by age, education, gender, and cultural background, giving it limited sensitivity and specificity. It will not detect mild cognitive impairment and should not be used as more than a screening instrument.

- Assessment of the following is not covered in this handbook but is included for completeness:
  - Left parietal dysfunction (Gerstmann's syndrome)
  - Right parietal dysfunction (neglect and extinction)
  - Frontal dysfunction (sequencing tasks, frontal release signs) (see **Motor and Reflexes Examination, Primitive Reflexes,** p.190)
  - Apraxia

Glasgow Coma Scale (GCS)

- Used to assess the patient's level of consciousness
- Scored as a total between 3 and 15, but it is best to report each of the three components separately (e.g. E3 V2 M4 instead of a total of 9)
- Coma is defined as (1) not opening eyes, (2) not obeying commands, and (3) not producing a verbal response
- As a general rule, 90% of patients with a score of ≤8 will be in a coma
- When testing response to pain, apply central pressure to the supraorbital region (deep pinching of the skin) or the sternum (firm twisting pressure applied with the examiner's knuckles) because spinal reflexes may occur with peripheral stimulation
- The GCS can reliably predict the outcome for head trauma, nontraumatic coma, ischemic stroke, subarachnoid and intracerebral hemorrhage, and meningitis[1,2]. However, it has some limitations:
  - An examiner cannot perform a full assessment in aphasic or aphonic patients, as well as those who have craniofacial trauma or are intubated and/or sedated; therefore, the GCS should be obtained on admission prior to sedation or intubation
  - The GCS does not directly assess brainstem function

Table 4. Glasgow Coma Scale

Best Eye Response (E)	Best Verbal Response (V)	Best Motor Response (M)
1. No eye opening	1. No verbal response	1. No motor response
2. Eye opening to pain	2. Incomprehensible sounds	2. Extension to pain
3. Eye opening to verbal command	3. Inappropriate words	3. Flexion to pain
4. Eyes open spontaneously	4. Confused	4. Withdraws from pain
	5. Oriented	5. Localizes pain
		6. Obeys commands

4.2 Cranial Nerve Examination

- Cranial nerves may have sensory function, motor function, or both (see **Table 5**)

Table 5. The Cranial Nerves

Nerve	Name	Function	S/M/B
CN I	Olfactory	• Smell	S
CN II	Optic	• Vision • Afferent limb of accommodation and pupillary light reflex	S
CN III	Oculomotor	• Innervates medial/superior/ inferior rectus, inferior oblique, and levator palpebrae superioris • Efferent limb of accommodation and pupillary light reflex	M
CN IV	Trochlear	• Innervates superior oblique	M
CN V	Trigeminal		
	V1 = ophthalmic	• Forehead and tip of nose • Afferent limb of corneal reflex	S
	V2 = maxillary	• Lower eyelid, cheek, and upper lip	S
	V3 = mandibular	• Sensory from chin, except angle of the jaw (C2-C3) • Innervates jaw muscles • Afferent and efferent limb of jaw jerk reflex	B
CN VI	Abducens	• Innervates lateral rectus	M
CN VII	Facial	• Innervates muscles of facial expression • Taste to anterior 2/3 of tongue • Sensory from skin posterior to ear, external acoustic meatus • Efferent limb of corneal reflex • Articulation • Lacrimation and salivation (except parotid gland)	B
CN VIII	Vestibulocochlear (Acoustic)	• Hearing and balance	S
CN IX	Glossopharyngeal	• Innervates stylopharyngeus (swallowing and articulation) • Afferent limb of gag reflex • Taste to posterior 1/3 of tongue • Salivation (parotid gland)	B
CN X	Vagus	• Swallowing • Phonation and articulation • Efferent limb of gag reflex • Sensory from skin posterior to ear, external acoustic meatus, dura in posterior cranial fossa	B
CN XI	Spinal Accessory	• Innervates sternocleidomastoid and trapezius	M
CN XII	Hypoglossal	• Innervates tongue muscles	M

S/M/B = Sensory/Motor/Both

CN I

- **Smell Test:** test each nostril separately using cloves, coffee, mint; patient closes eyes and occludes one nostril; note unilateral vs. bilateral loss
- **Pathology:** nasal disease, head trauma, smoking, aging, cocaine use, congenital

> **Clinical Pearl: CN I Dysfunction**
> The common cold is the most common cause of CN I dysfunction.

CN II

- **Visual Acuity** (tests central acuity)
  - Test each eye separately for best corrected vision using a Snellen chart or near card (use a pinhole card if patient's glasses are not available); patient covers other eye with palm of hand, avoiding pressure on the covered eye; estimate best corrected vision
  - Snellen chart: numerator = distance patient can read chart, denominator = distance normal eye can read chart (e.g. 20/200: what the normal eye can see at 200 ft, this patient reads at 20 ft) (see the **Eye Chart** at the back of the handbook)
- **Visual Fields by Confrontation:**
  - Face patient; patient closes left eye and looks into the examiner's left eye (examiner closes right eye)
  - Test using "counting" or "object" method in each of 4 quadrants (upper and lower temporal, upper and lower nasal)
    - Counting method: hold up 1 or 2 fingers in quadrant being tested and ask patient, "How many fingers?"
    - Object method: bring finger or a pen tip slowly toward the quadrant being tested; ask patient to "Tell me when you first notice the object"
  - Repeat for the other eye
  - Visual extinction: patient looks with both eyes uncovered into examiner's eyes; simultaneously hold up fingers to both sides of the visual field and ask "How many fingers?"
  - Neglect of visual field can suggest a parietal lesion (see **Ophthalmological Exam**, **Figure 3**, p.236)
- **Pupillary Light Reflex** (see **CN III/CN IV/CN VI**)
- **Color Test:** have patient read Ishihara plates
- **Fundoscopic Exam** (see **Ophthalmological Exam**, p.241)
- **Pathology:** optic neuropathy, papilledema

CN III/CN IV/CN VI

- **Inspect:** ptosis, pupil size/shape/asymmetry, eye position, resting nystagmus; defects may help localize lesions (see **Table 6**)
- **Eye Alignment:** hold penlight in front of patient; patient looks straight ahead into the distance; normal: location of light in center of both pupils
- **Ocular Movements:** test both eyes simultaneously
  - Smooth pursuit: patient tracks a target without moving his/her head; move the target through an "H" pattern, pausing at the ends to observe for endpoint nystagmus; normal if binocular diplopia and nystagmus are absent
  - Saccades: patient shifts gaze quickly between two closely placed targets (e.g. examiner's nose and index finger) in the horizontal then vertical directions; normal if eyes move together and find targets quickly

- Accommodation reflex: patient alternates between focusing on a distant object and an object held 10-15 cm from the nose; normal if eye convergence and pupil constriction observed at the near object

Table 6. Defects of CN III, IV, VI

Defect	Location of Lesion
Eye position down and out, ptosis, mydriasis	CN III palsy (complete)
Ptosis, miosis, anhydrosis (Horner's syndrome)	Sympathetic pathway
Difficulty looking down and in (e.g. walking down stairs)	CN IV palsy
Difficulty looking laterally	CN VI palsy
Impaired adduction of ipsilateral eye and nystagmus in abduction of contralateral eye	Medial longitudinal fasciculus (MLF) internuclear ophthalmoplegia (can suggest MS)

Note: Outer CN III fibers control pupillary constriction. Inner CN III fibers control ocular movements and upper eyelids.

- **Pupillary Light Reflex:** dim lights; as the patient looks into the distance, shine light obliquely into pupils; normal if direct and consensual responses present
- **Swinging Light Test**[3]**:**
  - Shine light in eye **A**, then swing light to eye **B**
  - If CN II of **B** is damaged, A and B will paradoxically dilate when light is swung to **B**
    - Neither **A** or **B** will constrict when light is at **B**, but both will constrict when light is at **A**
    - **B** will have more consensual response (when light is at **A**) than direct response (when light is at **B**)
    - This describes a relative afferent pupillary defect (RAPD) or a "Marcus Gunn pupil" in eye **B**
  - If CN III of **B** is damaged but CN II is intact, no pupillary constriction in **B** will be observed
    - Light at **B** will cause a consensual response in **A**
    - Light in **A** will cause a direct response in **A**

> **Clinical Pearl: RAPD and MS**
> RAPD is an important finding in optic neuritis, which is common in MS.

CN V

- **Inspect:** temporal wasting, jaw alignment with open mouth (jaw deviates toward side with lower motor neuron [LMN] lesion)
- **Motor:** ask patient to
  - "Clench your teeth": palpate masseter and temporalis muscles
  - "Open your mouth against resistance": lateral pterygoids
  - "Divert your jaw to the side against resistance": medial and lateral pterygoids
- **Sensory:**
  - Light touch: patient closes eyes; apply tip of cotton wool at single spot and have patient respond with "yes" when contact is made; compare both sides of forehead (V1), upper lip/cheeks (V2), and lower lip/chin (V3); avoid nose (V1) and angle of jaw (C2-S3) (see **Figure 1** for trigeminal dermatomes)

- Pain: patient closes eyes; vary application of end of broken tongue depressor vs. rounded end in same distribution as for light touch; have patient respond with "sharp" or "dull" when contact is made
- Temperature: use a cold tuning fork (if necessary run it under cold water) and apply it to the same distribution as for light touch and pain; have patient respond with "cold" when contact is made

- **Reflexes[4]:**
  - Corneal reflex: patient looks up and away as examiner approaches with a piece of cotton/tissue from side; touch cornea avoiding the eyelashes, conjunctiva or sclera; normal if direct and consensual blink response is observed
  - Jaw jerk reflex: patient opens mouth slightly; place finger over patient's chin and tap downward with reflex hammer; normal if elevation is minimal; increased reflex = pseudobulbar palsy

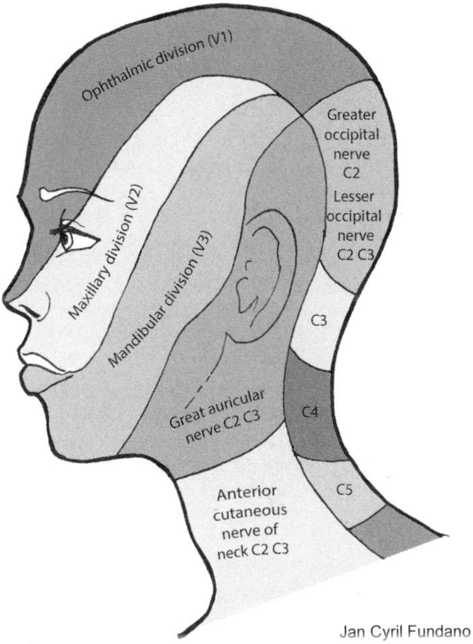

Figure 1. Trigeminal Dermatomes

NEUROLOGICAL

CN VII

- **Inspect:** nasolabial fold (e.g. flattened), palpebral fissure (e.g. eyelid retracted), mouth (e.g. drooping), involuntary facial movements
- **Motor:** ask patient to
  - "Raise your eyebrows": frontalis
  - "Close your eyes tight and don't let me open them": orbicularis oculi
  - "Show me your teeth": buccinator
  - "Puff your cheeks out and don't let me pop them": orbicularis oris
  - "Show me your bottom teeth only": platysma
  - Distribution of paralysis differs between LMN and upper motor neuron (UMN) lesions (see **Table 7**)
- **Sensory:** test taste; patient sticks out tongue; touch each side of tongue on anterior 2/3 (CN VII) and posterior 1/3 (CN IX) with 4 primary tastes (sweet = sugar, salty = salt, sour = vinegar, bitter = quinine); keeping tongue protruded, ask patient to point to taste perceived on card displaying taste options; provide sip of water between tests
- **Corneal Reflex** (see above)

Table 7. Defects of CN VII

Type of Lesion	Distribution of Paralysis
LMN Lesion (e.g. Bell's palsy)	Facial paralysis on same side as lesion, including forehead
UMN Lesion (e.g. cortex, corticobulbar tract)	Partial facial paralysis contralateral to lesion; forehead relatively spared

CN VIII

- **Hearing Tests[5]:** test each ear separately
  - **Whisper Test:** mask sounds entering one ear by rubbing tragus or snapping fingers; whisper numbers/letters into other ear and ask patient to repeat
  - **Rinne Test:** strike 512 Hz tuning fork and place on patient's mastoid process; ask patient to indicate when sound disappears; immediately place tines of fork in front of auditory canal without touching ear; normal if patient notes the reappearance of sound (air > bone conduction)
  - **Weber Test:** strike 512 Hz tuning fork and place on patient's forehead in midline; normal if there is an absence of sound lateralization (equal on both sides)
  - Rinne and Weber tests can be used to differentiate between conductive and sensorineural hearing loss (see **Table 8**)

> **Clinical Pearl: Conductive Deafness**
> Wax is the most common cause of conductive deafness.

- **Vestibular Function:** not usually tested in office setting except for
  - Romberg test (see **Sensory Examination**, p.191)
  - Positional nystagmus: induced with changes in head position
  - Gaze-evoked nystagmus: induced at extreme eccentricities of gaze (see **CN III/CN IV/CN VI,** p.177)

Table 8. Defects of CN VIII

Pathology	Rinne (affected ear)	Weber
Normal	Air > Bone Conduction	No lateralization
Conductive Loss	Bone > Air Conduction	Lateralization to affected ear
Sensorineural Loss	Air > Bone Conduction	Lateralization to unaffected ear

CN IX/CN X

- **Motor:**
  - **Palatal Elevation:** depress patient's tongue with tongue depressor; ask patient to "Say Ahh"; normal if elevation of soft palate and uvula is symmetrical (uvula deviates to unaffected side)
  - **Swallowing:** ask patient to swallow a sip of water; normal if there is no retrograde passage of water through nose after the nasopharynx is closed off
  - **Articulation:** ask patient to say "Pa Pa Pa" (labial), "La La La" (lingual), "Ka Ka Ka" (palatal), "Ga Ga Ga" (guttural)
    - Note that CN V, VII, IX, X, XII are all involved in articulation; CN IX and X are specifically involved in guttural and palatal articulation

- **Sensory** (Taste) (see **CN VII,** p.179)
- **Gag Reflex:** touch posterior wall of pharynx with tongue depressor; normal if palate moves up, pharyngeal muscles contract, uvula remains midline, and palatal arches do not droop
  - ***Note:*** CN IX is the afferent limb, CN X is the efferent limb of this reflex
  - The gag reflex is normally only tested in patients with suspected brainstem pathology, impaired consciousness, or impaired swallowing
    - ***Note:*** an absent gag reflex can be normal

> **Clinical Pearl: Deviations of Uvula and Tongue**
> Uvula deviates to the unaffected side; jaw and tongue deviate to the affected side.

CN XI
- **Inspect:** neck and shoulder; look for fasciculations, atrophy, asymmetry
- **Motor:** ask patient to
  - "Shrug your shoulders" (with and without resistance): trapezius
  - "Turn your head to the side" (with and without resistance): sternocleidomastoid
- **Pathology:**
  - Weak trapezius: shrugging of shoulders on the ipsilateral side is impaired
  - Weak sternocleidomastoid: turning head to the contralateral side is impaired

CN XII
- **Inspect:** tongue at rest in the floor of the mouth; look for fasciculations, atrophy, asymmetry
- **Motor:** ask patient to
  - "Stick your tongue out and move it side-to-side"; normal if protrusion of tongue is symmetrical (tongue deviates to affected side)
  - "Push your tongue into your cheek" (with and without resistance)

> **Clinical Pearl: Correcting for Facial Weakness**
> If there is facial weakness, support the upper lip on the side of weakness; otherwise, the tongue may erroneously appear to deviate. Once the facial weakness is corrected for, the tongue will no longer appear to deviate.

Table 9. Causes of Multiple CN Abnormalities

CN Combination	Likely Cause
Unilateral III, IV, V1, V2, VI	Cavernous sinus lesion
Unilateral V, VII, VIII	Cerebellopontine angle lesion
Unilateral IX, X, XI	Jugular foramen syndrome
Bilateral X, XI, XII	Bulbar palsy (LMN), pseudobulbar palsy (UMN)

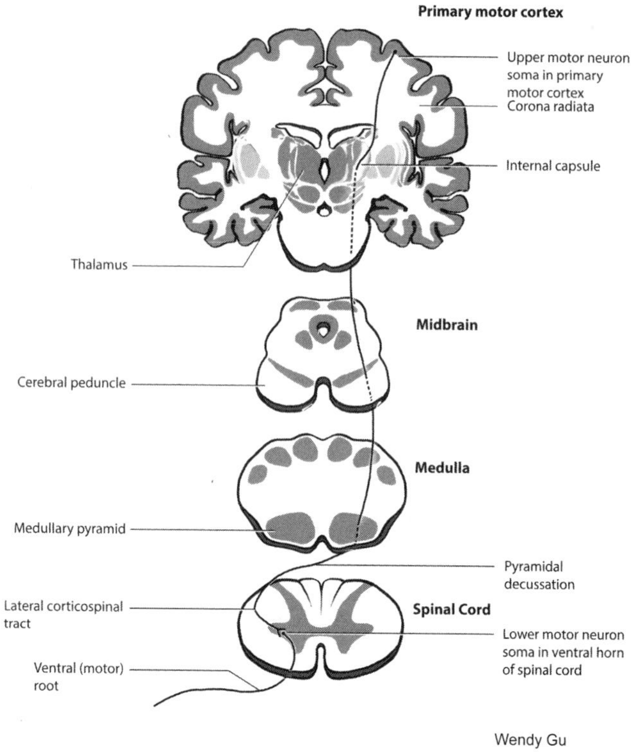

Figure 2. Motor Pathways: Corticospinal Tract

4.3 Motor and Reflexes Examination

- Considerations for pathology:
  - UMN vs. LMN pattern (see **Table 10**)
  - Pyramidal (corticospinal tract) vs. extrapyramidal tract lesion
  - Localization to specific root or peripheral nerve

NEUROLOGICAL

Table 10. Pattern of Upper and Lower Motor Neuron Lesions

	UMN Lesion	LMN Lesion
Appearance	Atrophy of disuse, arms flexed, legs extended	Atrophy, fasciculations
Power	Extensors < Flexors in upper extremities Extensors > Flexors in lower extremities	Weak/absent
Tone	Increased/spastic	Decreased
Coordination	Impaired due to weakness	Impaired due to weakness
Reflexes		
Superficial	Absent	Absent
Deep	Increased clonus	Decreased
Plantar	Upgoing (dorsiflexion of big toe)	Downgoing (plantar flexion of big toe)

Inspection

- Muscle bulk (atrophy, hypertrophy, abnormal bulging/depression); distribution of muscle wasting can suggest possible causes (see **Table 11**)
- Symmetry
- **Fasciculations:** quivering of the muscle under skin; typically benign, may be associated with LMN lesion (e.g. ALS)
- Abnormal movements and positioning (see **Table 12**)

Table 11. Distribution of Muscle Wasting or Weakness

Pattern	Possible Causes
Focal (one limb)	Nerve root or peripheral nerve pathology
Proximal (bilateral)	Myopathy (no sensory loss)
Distal (bilateral)	Peripheral neuropathy (distal sensory loss)

Table 12. Abnormal Movements and Positioning

Movement	Description	Possible Causes
Asterixis	Brief, jerky downward movements of the wrist when patient extends both arms with wrists dorsiflexed, palms forward and eyes closed	• Toxic/metabolic encephalopathies • Electrolyte disturbances • Wilson's disease
Tics	Involuntary contractions of single muscles or groups of muscles	• Tourette syndrome
Myoclonus	Sudden, rapid muscle jerk; may be focal, unilateral or bilateral	• Epilepsy • CNS injury/infection • Neurodegenerative disease
Athetosis	Repetitive, involuntary, slow, sinuous, writhing movements, especially severe in the hands	• Perinatal hypoxia • Kernicterus • Huntington's disease • Antipsychotics/antiemetics
Dystonia	Muscle contraction that is more sustained or prolonged than athetosis and results in spasms and distorted positions of limbs, trunk or face	• Basal ganglia disorders (Parkinson's/Huntington's/ Wilson's diseases) • Anoxic brain injury • Infections (TB/encephalitis)
Tremor	Rhythmic/semi-rhythmic oscillating movements; can be fast or slow; both agonist and antagonist muscles simultaneously activated (unlike in myoclonus or asterixis); classified as resting, postural, and intention (ataxic)	• Physiological tremor • Parkinson's disease (resting tremor) • Essential tremor (postural tremor) • Hyperthyroidism (postural tremor) • Cerebellar appendicular ataxia (intention tremor)
Chorea	"Dance" – fleeting random involuntary movements that affect multiple joints; may be fluid or jerky and varying in quality	• Huntington's disease • SLE/Sydenham's chorea • Chorea gravidarum • Tardive dyskinesia (levodopa/antipsychotics/ antiemetics)

Table 12. Abnormal Movements and Positioning (continued)

Movement	Description	Possible Causes
Hemiballismus	Violent flinging movement of half of the body	• Lesions of the subthalamic nucleus
Seizure Automatisms	Stereotyped semi-purposeful movements; repeated eye blinks, tonic or clonic motor activity	• Seizures

Yaman A, Akdeniz M, Yaman H. 2011. *J Fam Pract* 60(12):721-725.

Muscle Tone

- Slight residual tension in a normal muscle when it is relaxed voluntarily: test by flexion/extension, pronation/supination of joint through its ROM
- **Hypotonia (decreased tone)** is seen in LMN lesions, acute stroke, spinal shock, some cerebellar lesions
- **Hypertonia (increased tone)** may manifest as spasticity or rigidity
- Patterns of tone: the characteristic of abnormal tone suggests possible causes (see **Table 13**)
  - **Spasticity[6] (velocity-dependent):** limb moves, then catches, and then goes past catch (spastic, clasp-knife); best appreciated during rapid supination of forearm or flexion of knee; pyramidal lesion
  - **Rigidity[6] (velocity-independent):** increased tone through range of movement (cogwheeling, lead-pipe); best detected with circumduction of the wrist; extrapyramidal lesion

Table 13. Causes of Abnormal Tone

Characteristic	Possible Causes
Decreased Tone: Flaccidity	LMN lesion, cerebellar; rarely myopathies, "spinal shock" (e.g. early response after a spinal cord trauma)
Increased Tone: Spasticity ("clasp-knife", velocity-dependent)	UMN lesion: corticospinal tract (commonly late or chronic stage after a stroke)
Increased Tone: Rigidity ("lead-pipe", "cogwheeling")	Extrapyramidal tract lesion: parkinsonism, phenothiazines
Increased Tone: Paratonia (inconsistently increased tone of limb tested)	Inability for patient to relax

Power

- Measure active motion of the patient against resistance; compare both sides; grade power on a standard scale (see **Table 14**)
- Ensure all muscle groups are tested (see **Table 15**)

Table 14. MRC Scale for Grading Muscle Strength

Grade		Assessment
0	Absent	No contraction detected
1	Trace	Slight contraction detected but cannot move joint
2	Weak	Movement with gravity eliminated only
3	Fair	Movement against gravity only
4	Good	Movement against gravity with some resistance
5	Normal	Movement against gravity with full resistance

Note: Since this rating scale is skewed toward weakness, many clinicians further subclassify their finding by adding a (+) or a (-), e.g. 4- or 4+.

Table 15. Muscle Groups to Test (Myotomal Distribution)

Muscle	Movement	Nerve	Spinal Roots
Deltoid	Arm abduction	Axillary	**C5**, C6
Triceps	Forearm extension	Radial	C6, **C7**, C8
Biceps	Forearm flexion	Musculocutaneous	C5, C6
Wrist Extensors	Wrist extension	Radial	**C7**, C8
Wrist Flexors	Wrist flexion	Median	
Flexor carpi radialis			C6, C7
Palmaris longus			C7, **C8**, T1
Flexor Pollicis Longus	Thumb DIP flexion	Median (anterior interosseous branch)	C7, **C8**
Interossei of Hand	Fingers abduction/ adduction	Ulnar	C8, **T1**
Iliopsoas	Hip flexion	Femoral	
Iliacus			L1, L2, **L3**
Psoas			L2, **L3**, L4
Hip Adductors	Hip adduction	Obturator	**L2**, **L3**, L4
Hip Abductors	Hip abduction (and medial rotation)	Superior gluteal	**L4**, **L5**, S1
Quadriceps	Knee extension	Femoral	L2, **L3**, **L4**
Hamstrings	Knee flexion	Sciatic	L5, **S1**, S2
Tibialis Anterior	Foot dorsi-flexion and inversion	Deep peroneal (branch of sciatic)	L4, L5
Tibialis Posterior	Foot plantar flexion and inversion	Tibial (branch of sciatic)	L4, L5
Gastrocnemius, Soleus	Foot plantar flexion	Tibial (branch of sciatic)	S1, S2

Table 15. Muscle Groups to Test (Myotomal Distribution) (continued)

Muscle	Movement	Nerve	Spinal Roots
Peroneus (Fibularis) Longus and Brevis	Foot plantar flexion and eversion	Superficial peroneal (branch of sciatic)	L5, S1
Extensor Hallucis Longus	Great toe extension	Deep peroneal (branch of sciatic)	**L5**, S1

Blumenfeld H. *Neuroanatomy Through Clinical Cases*, 2nd ed. Sunderland: Sinauer Associates; 2010.

Pronator Drift

- Have the patient stand or sit with his/her eyes closed and arms held straight out from his/her body with hands supine
- Pronator drift is positive if patient cannot maintain position; may be due to:
  - Muscle weakness (may see pronation and outward drift of arm and hand)
  - UMN lesion (may see pronation and downward drift of arm and hand)

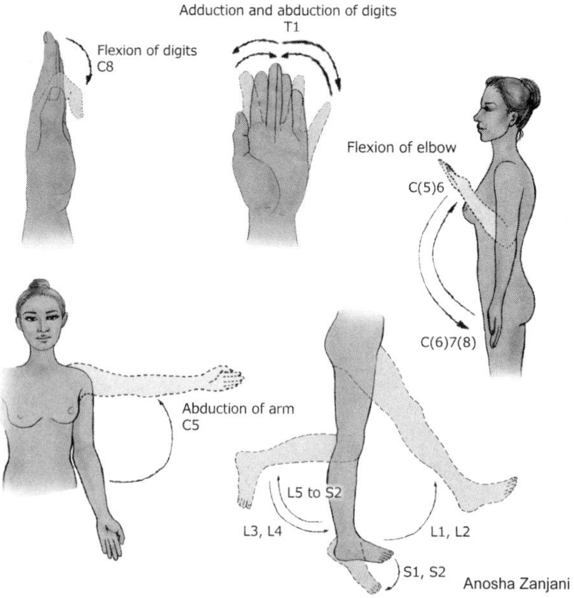

Figure 3. Myotomes of the Upper and Lower Limbs

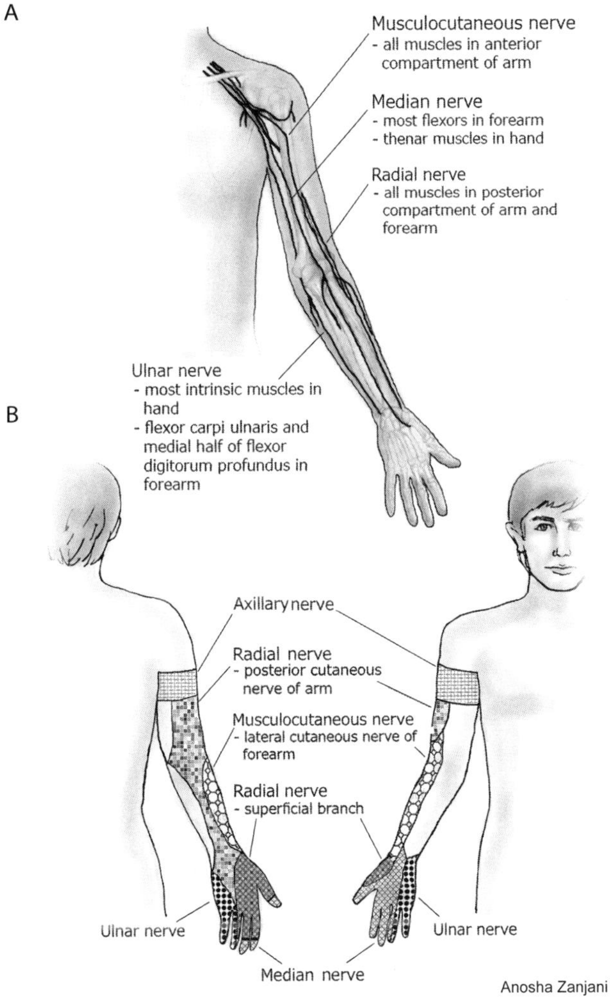

Figure 4. Motor (A) and Cutaneous (B) Distribution of Upper Limb Nerves

NEUROLOGICAL

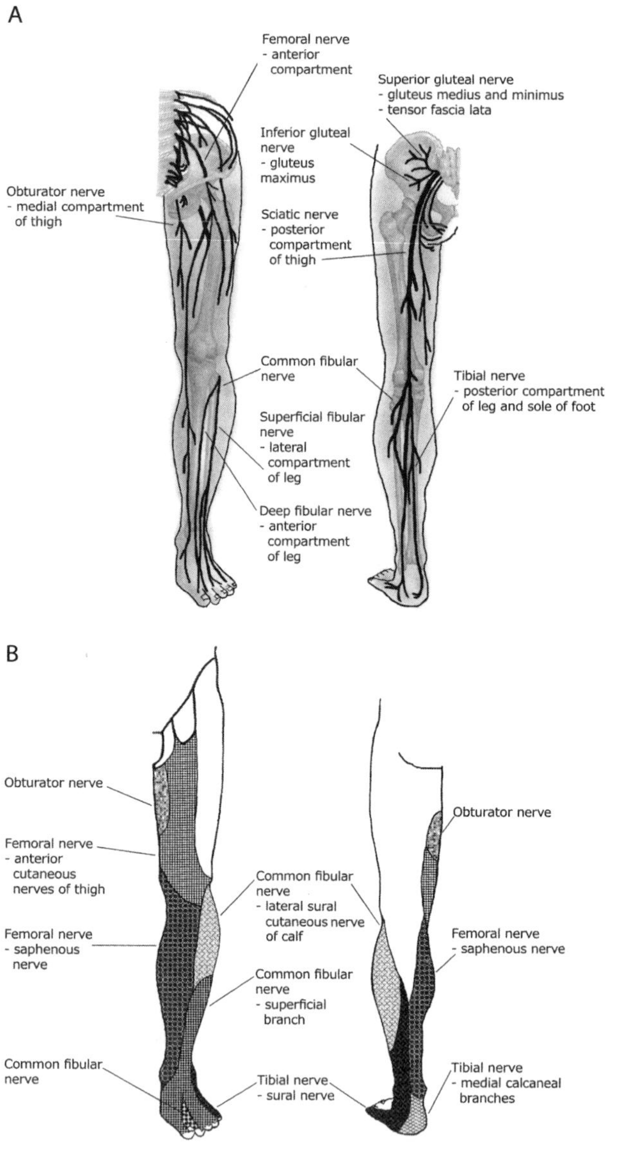

Anosha Zanjani

Figure 5. Motor (A) and Cutaneous (B) Distribution of Lower Limb Nerves

Deep Tendon Reflexes

- Monosynaptic spinal segmental reflexes
- Patient should be relaxed with muscle mildly stretched
- Strike tendon briskly and compare both sides
- Make sure that you watch or feel muscle for contraction
- If reflexes appear to be hyperactive, examine for clonus at the ankle and knee (patella)

- If reflexes are absent, have patient use reinforcement:
  - For upper body reflexes: clench teeth or push down on bed with thighs
  - For lower body reflexes: lock fingers and try to pull hands apart (Jendrassik maneuver)
- Graded on a standard scale (see **Table 16**)
- Characteristics of deep tendon reflex can suggest possible causes (see **Table 17**)

Table 16. Grading Reflexes

Grade	Response
0	Absent
1+	Hypoactive, or seen only with reinforcement
2+	Normal
3+	Brisk (no clonus)
4+	Hyperactive (associated with clonus; pathological)

- **Biceps Tendon Reflex** (C5, C6):
  - Have patient relax arm and pronate forearm midway between flexion and extension
  - Place your thumb on the tendon and strike the hammer on your thumb
  - Observe for contraction of the biceps followed by flexion at the elbow
- **Brachioradialis Tendon Reflex** (C5, C6):
  - Have patient rest forearm on the knee in semiflexed, semipronated position
  - Strike hammer on stylus process of radius about 2.5-5 cm above wrist
  - Observe for flexion at elbow and simultaneous supination of the forearm
- **Triceps Tendon Reflex** (C6, C7, C8):
  - Have patient partially flex his/her arm at the elbow and pull toward his/her chest
  - Alternatively, allow patient's arm to hang relaxed while supporting anterior arm
  - Strike hammer on tendon above insertion of the ulnar olecranon process (2.5-5 cm above the elbow)
  - Observe for contraction of triceps with extension at the elbow
- **Patellar Tendon Reflex** = knee jerk (L3, L4):
  - Bend the knee to relax the quadriceps muscle
  - With your hand on the quadriceps, strike the patellar tendon firmly
  - Observe for extension at the knee and contraction of the quadriceps
- **Achilles Tendon Reflex** = ankle jerk (S1, S2):
  - Place your hand under the foot to dorsiflex the ankle; strike the tendon
  - Observe for plantar flexion at the ankle and contraction of the calf muscle

Clonus

- **Ankle:** with knee flexed, quickly dorsiflex foot and maintain flexed position
- **Knee:** with knee extended, grasp quadriceps muscle just proximal to patella and exert sudden downward force
- Clonus is present if sudden movements elicit rhythmic involuntary muscle contractions; suggests UMN lesion

Table 17. Interpreting Deep Tendon Reflexes

Characteristic	Possible Causes
Increased Reflexes or Clonus	UMN lesion above root at that level
Absent Reflex	Generalized: peripheral neuropathy Isolated: peripheral nerve or root lesion
Reduced Reflex (insensitive)	Peripheral neuropathy Cerebellar syndrome (reflexes may also be absent in early phases of UMN lesion, e.g. "spinal shock")
Inverted (reflex tested is absent [e.g. biceps], but there is spread to lower or higher level [e.g. produces a triceps response])	LMN lesion at level of the absent reflex, with UMN below (spinal cord involvement at the level of the absent reflex)
Pendular (reflex continues to swing for several beats)	Cerebellar disease
"Hung" (slow to relax, especially at ankle)	Hypothyroidism

Primitive Reflexes

- Generally not present in adults: when present, they may signify diffuse cerebral damage, particularly of the frontal lobes (e.g. "frontal lobe release") (see **Pediatric Exam**, p.258 for further details)
  - **Glabellar:** tap forehead and watch if eyes blink. Abnormal if individual cannot overcome the reflex and continues blinking as long as the tapping continues[7]
  - **Snout and Pout:** tap filum (above upper lip) and watch for protrusion of lips[7]
  - **Palmo-Mental:** scrape palm over thenar muscles and watch for chin muscle contraction on the ipsilateral side[7]
  - **Grasp:** place fingers in palm to see if grasp reflex is elicited[7]

Superficial and Other Reflexes

- **Abdominal Reflex:** stroke abdomen toward umbilicus along the diagonals of the four abdominal quadrants
  - Normal: ipsilateral muscles contract, umbilicus deviates toward the stimulus
  - Above umbilicus tests T8-T10
  - Below umbilicus tests T10-T12
- **Cremasteric Reflex:** draw line along medial thigh
  - Normal: elevation of ipsilateral testis in the scrotum
  - Spinal roots involved are L1-L2
  - Abdominal and cremasteric reflexes may be absent on the side of a corticospinal tract lesion
- **Plantar Response**[8] (Babinski's sign, L5-S1): stroke the sole from the heel to the ball of the foot curving medially across the heads of the metatarsal bones
  - Normal (downgoing): plantar flexion of big toe, curling of the other toes
  - Abnormal (upgoing): dorsiflexion of the big toe, fanning of the other toes; associated with UMN lesion
    - Stroking the lateral aspect of the foot (Chaddock's sign) and downward pressure along the shin (Oppenheim's sign) can elicit the same reflex

NEUROLOGICAL

- **Anal Reflex** (anal wink): stroke perianal skin
  - Normal: contraction of the muscles around the rectal orifice
  - Loss of reflex signifies lesion in S2-S3-S4 reflex arc (e.g. cauda equina lesion)

4.4 Sensory Examination

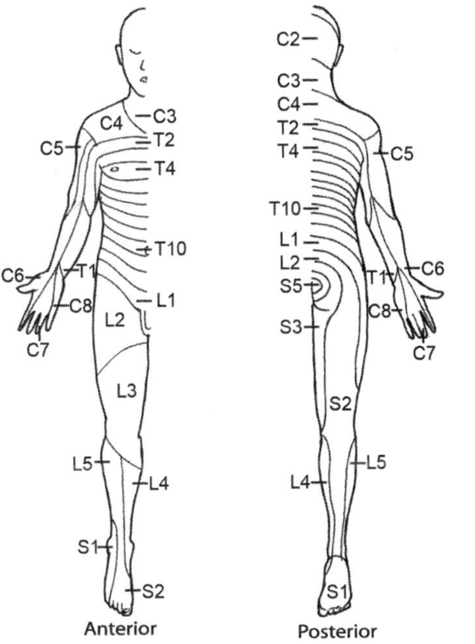

Figure 6. Map of Dermatomes

- Primary sensory exam: peripheral sensory nerve tests (light touch, pain, temperature, vibration, proprioception)
- Secondary sensory exam: test cortical functions regarding sensation (two-point discrimination, stereognosis, graphesthesia, extinction, point localization); test fails if spinal/peripheral nerves are severely impaired
- Always explain the test beforehand so that patients know exactly how to respond (i.e. run a sample test with the patient's eyes open, and ask him/her to say whether sensation is 'sharp', 'dull', etc.)
- Have the patient close his/her eyes before testing
- Test both sides of the body and ask the patient to compare sensation on each side
- Start each test distally with fingers and toes; if normal, proceed to next test; if abnormal, proceed proximally until the abnormality is mapped out
- Compare sensory function: right to left; distal to proximal; peripheral nerve to spinal nerve dermatomes (see **Figure 4**, **Figure 5**, and **Figure 6**)
- Note the location, magnitude, and quality of each sensory deficit found
- There is considerable overlap and variation in peripheral nerve distribution; therefore, a deficit in one area may be compensated for by another area
- Distribution of sensory loss can suggest location of lesion (see **Table 18**)

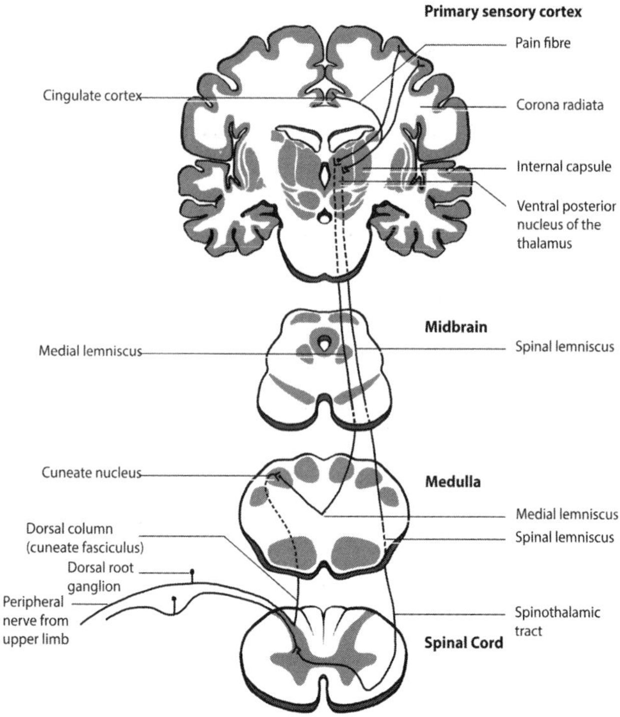

Figure 7. Sensory Pathways: Dorsal Columns/Medial Lemniscus & Spinothalamic Tract

NEUROLOGICAL

Primary Sensory Exam

- Aspects of touch sensation are carried by both the dorsal column pathway (fine, discriminative touch) and the spinothalamic pathway (crude touch/pain); touch sensation is not eliminated by isolated lesions to either pathway
- **Fine Touch[9]:** dorsal column pathway (see **Figure 7**)
  - Use cotton or tissue paper tip to touch skin; ask patient to say "yes" if touch is felt
- **Pain[9]:** spinothalamic pathway (see **Figure 7**)
  - Alternate between sharp and dull touches (and false touches to see if the patient is using other cues)
  - Ask the patient to identify sensation as sharp or dull
- **Temperature:** spinothalamic pathway (often not done if pain sensation is normal)
  - Run your tuning fork under cold water
  - Ask the patient to identify whether the tuning fork feels cold, and compare to the other side
- **Vibration:** dorsal column pathway
  - Place a 128 Hz tuning fork on joint (e.g. DIP) and ask the patient when the 'buzzing' stops and compare to control (i.e. examiner)
  - If the patient is unable to feel any vibrations, move proximally and repeat testing (e.g. from DIP to PIP to MCP joint, to wrist, to elbow, to shoulder) until a level with normal vibration relative to control is established

- **Proprioception** (position sense): dorsal column pathway
  - Hold the patient's joint (e.g. DIP) from the sides so he/she does not get cues from the pressure of your hand
  - Begin with the joint in the neutral position; raise or lower the digit and ask the patient to state the direction of movement ('up' or 'down'); increment 1-2 mm in upper limbs and 2-3 mm in lower limbs
  - Return the digit to the neutral position before moving it in another direction
- **Romberg Test[10]:** tests proprioception and vestibular sense in the absence of visual input
  - Have the patient stand in front of you with his/her feet together; be prepared to catch or support patient if he/she falls
  - Ask the patient to close both eyes and stand still for one minute
  - Positive Romberg sign if the patient falls in any direction without being aware of the fall
  - If the patient sways, ask him/her to stand perfectly still: this is NOT a positive Romberg sign
  - This test has low specificity because a positive test may be present in peripheral sensory denervation, vestibular dysfunction, or cerebellar disease
  - ***Note:*** if there is a more serious proprioceptive or vestibular lesion (or a midline cerebellar lesion causing truncal instability), the patient will be unable to maintain his/her position even with his/her eyes open

Table 18. Lesions Involving Sensory Modalities

Location of Lesion	Distribution of Sensory Loss	Examples
Single Nerve	Within distribution of single nerve; commonly median, ulnar, peroneal, lateral cutaneous nerve of the thigh	Entrapment, most commonly in carpal tunnel syndrome, rheumatoid arthritis, and hypothyroidism; mononeuritis multiplex
Root(s)	Confined to single root or roots in close proximity; commonly C5, C6, C7 in arm and L4, L5, S1 in leg	Compression by disc prolapse
Peripheral Nerves	Distal glove and stocking deficit	DM, alcohol-related, B12 deficiency, drugs
Spinal Cord	Depends on level of lesion and complete vs. partial lesion	Trauma, spinal cord compression by tumor, cervical spondylitis, MS
Brainstem	Loss of pain and temperature sensation in ipsilateral face and contralateral body	Demyelination (young) Brainstem stroke (older)
Thalamic Sensory Loss	All modalities; contralateral hemisensory loss (face, body) and pain – dysesthesia (e.g. burning feeling)	Stroke, cerebral tumor, MS, trauma
Cortical (parietal)	Able to recognize all primary modalities but localizes them poorly; loss of secondary modalities	Stroke, cerebral tumor, trauma

Secondary Sensory Exam

- Must first confirm that primary modalities are intact
- Inability to perform the following tests suggests a lesion in sensory cortex
- **Neglect and Extinction:** parietal lobe
  - Touch right hand, left hand, and then both hands
  - Patients with parietal lobe lesions can identify when each side is touched independently, but will neglect the side contralateral to the lesion when both sides are touched
  - Can also test extinction using visual and less commonly, auditory stimuli
  - For hemineglect, draw a line and ask the patient to bisect the line in the middle; patient with neglect will bisect the line away from the middle toward the affected side (usually right side)
- **Two-Point Discrimination:** parietal lobe
  - Ask patient if he/she feels two stimuli or one (use an untwisted paper clip)
  - Normal minimum values for discrimination are 2 mm on fingertips, 3-8 mm on toes, 8-12 mm on palms, 40-60 mm on back
- **Stereognosis[11]:** integration between parietal and occipital lobes
  - Place objects in the patient's hand one at a time and ask the patient to recognize them by feeling the object (e.g. a coin, pen, key, paperclip)
  - Patient must only use one hand to feel object
  - Tactile agnosia: inability to recognize objects by touch; suggests a parietal cortex lesion
- **Graphesthesia[11]:** parietal lobe
  - Use a blunt object to write numbers on a patient's hand in the correct orientation to the patient; patient tries to identify the numbers
- **Point Localization:** sensory cortex
  - Touch the patient and ask him/her to point to the area touched

4.5 Coordination and Gait Examination

- Assess speech, nystagmus, tremor, head titubation
- Inspect for erratic nonrhythmic movements; movements should normally be rapid, smooth, and accurate

Gross Motor Coordination

- **Finger-To-Nose Test:**
  - Ask the patient to alternate between touching his/her nose and your finger (held at an arm's length from the patient)
  - Make sure that your finger is far enough away from the patient in order to stress the system; keeping your finger too close makes the test too easy
  - Watch for:
    - "Past pointing" where patient persistently overshoots target
    - Tremor as the finger approaches the target
    - Inability to perform test (dysmetria) may indicate cerebellar disease
- **Heel-To-Shin Test:**
  - Have patient slide the heel of one foot down the opposite shin, starting at knee
  - Watch for wobbling of the heel from side-to-side
- **Rebound Test:**
  - Have the patient close his/her eyes, extend his/her arms and maintain that position; push the arms down and out of position; examine if there is asymmetry in the degree of compensation

Fine Motor Coordination

- **Rapid Alternating Movements (RAM):**
  - Dysdiadochokinesia: an abnormality in doing RAM (may be due to cerebellar lesion)
- Upper Extremities:
  - Pronate and supinate one hand on the other hand rapidly[11]
  - Touch the thumb to each finger as quickly as possible
- Lower Extremities:
  - Tap toes of foot and then heel of foot to floor in rapid alternation

Gait

- Ask patient to:
  - "Walk straight ahead"
  - "Stop and return to me, now on tiptoe" (also tests strength of plantar flexors)
  - "Walk away again but this time on your heels" (also tests strength of dorsiflexors)
  - "Stop, return by walking in tandem gait with one foot placed in front of the other (like walking on a tightrope)"
- Pathologic pattern of gait may suggest possible causes (see **Table 19**)

Table 19. Pathologic Patterns of Gait

Gait Pattern	Possible Causes
Hemiplegic	Unilateral UMN lesion due to stroke, MS
Parkinsonian (shuffling)	Parkinson's, extrapyramidal effects of antipsychotics, tranquilizers
Spastic or Scissor (legs held in adduction at the hip, thighs rub together, knees slide over each other)	Cerebral Palsy, MS
Cerebellar Ataxia (spreads legs wide apart to provide wider base of support – veers toward side of lesion)	Drugs (e.g. phenytoin), alcohol, MS, cerebrovascular disease
Foot Drop/Steppage (takes high steps as if climbing a flight of stairs)	Unilateral: common peroneal palsy, corticospinal tract lesion, L5 radiculopathy Bilateral: peripheral neuropathy
Sensory Ataxia	Joint position sense deficit (see Romberg test) due to peripheral neuropathy, dorsal column lesion

Viswanathan A, Sudarsky L. 2012. *Handb Clin Neurol* 103:623-634.

Balance

- Observe the patient while standing; look for swaying from side-to-side
  - ***Note:*** this is not the Romberg test; the Romberg test is part of the sensory examination to assess the dorsal columns, not cerebellar function
- **Pull Test:**
  - Stand behind the patient and give a sudden but gentle pull backward
  - Normally, the patient remains steady or takes one or a few steps back
  - A posturally unstable patient falls backward or festinates (takes multiple small rapid steps), e.g. in Parkinson's disease

5. COMMON INVESTIGATIONS

- See **Essentials of Medical Imaging**, p.512 for a detailed approach to neuroimaging
- **Lumbar Puncture:** laboratory assessment of cerebrospinal fluid (CSF) for biochemical, microbiological, and cytological (e.g. immunological/ hematological) analysis
- **CT:** utilizes computer-processed X-ray images to produce tomographic images of the body; useful to image blood vessels, bony details, hemorrhage (e.g. trauma), and neoplasms with injected contrast
- **MRI:** high resolution imaging that uses nuclear magnetic resonance properties to visualize nuclei of atoms within the human body; MRI is especially useful to image soft tissues; different types of MRI scans are available, and each allows differential visualization of tissues (see **Table 20**)
  - T1-weighted: useful to visualize anatomical details
  - T2-weighted: useful to identify pathology
  - FLAIR (fluid attenuated inversion recovery): useful to identify pathology, particularly if adjacent to fluid (fluid brightness is attenuated in FLAIR)
- **Functional MRI (fMRI):** functional imaging to map language, motor, and sensory areas (e.g. post-stroke)
- **X-ray:** useful to image bony deviations or fractures; imaging of calcified pineal glands can be used to determine midline deviation
- **Positron Emission Tomography (PET):** imaging of functionally activated brain regions using positron-emitting radionuclide tracers
- **Conventional Angiography:** uses imaging (CT or MRI) and contrast agents to visualize blood vessels; useful to visualize aneurysms, arterial thrombosis, arteriovenous (AV) malformations
- **CT Angiogram/MRI Angiogram:** useful to visualize intracranial vasculature; a noninvasive alternative to conventional angiography
- **Electroencephalography (EEG):** graphic record of the electrical activity of the brain over time: can reveal characteristic patterns in disease – useful especially for seizures/epilepsy
- **Electromyography (EMG) & Electrooculography (EOG):** graphic record of the electric currents associated with muscle (EMG) or eye (EOG) activity over time: useful especially for myasthenia gravis (EMG), eye movement disorders/saccades/nystagmus (EOG)
- EEG + EMG + EOG = sleep studies
- **Nerve Conduction Studies (NCS):** multiple electrodes placed along known course of a specific nerve: one electrode stimulates nerve and a second electrode picks up this stimulation → time between stimulation and recording determines nerve conduction velocity (compared to known standards) – useful especially for nerve entrapment syndromes (e.g. carpal tunnel syndrome)
- **Evoked Potentials:** an electrical test to examine the functional integrity of the central nervous system (usually looks at the optic nerve, brainstem auditory and spinal somatosensory pathways)

Table 20. Common MRI Scans and the Appearance of Tissues

Tissue Type	T1-Weighted	T2-Weighted	FLAIR
Gray Matter	Gray	Light gray	Light gray
White Matter	White	Dark gray	Gray
CSF or Water	Black	White	Dark gray
Fat	White	White*	White*
Air	Black	Black	Black
Bone or Calcification	Black	Black	Black
Edema	Gray	White	White
Demyelination or Glyosis	Gray	White	White
Ferritin Deposits	Dark gray	Black	Black
Proteinaceous Fluid	White	***Variable***	***Variable***

Note: While fat appears dark on T2 and FLAIR images using spin echo (SE) imaging, subcutaneous and epidural fat appears bright with the commonly used fast spin echo (FSE) imaging, unless fat saturation is applied.

Blumenfeld H. *Neuroanatomy Through Clinical Cases*, 2nd ed. Sunderland: Sinauer Associates; 2010.

6. COMMON DISORDERS

Disorders marked with (✓) are discussed in **Common Clinical Scenarios**

✓ Stroke
✓ Headache
✓ Brain tumors
✓ Diabetic neuropathy
✓ Alzheimer's disease (AD)
✓ Seizures
✓ Parkinson's disease (PD)
✓ Multiple sclerosis (MS)
✓ Herpes simplex encephalitis
✓ Lumbar disc prolapse
✓ Spinal cord disorders

- Huntington's disease
- Bell's (CN VII) palsy
- Guillain-Barré syndrome (GBS)
- Amyotrophic lateral sclerosis (ALS)

7. COMMON CLINICAL SCENARIOS

7.1 Stroke

- Classification
  - Ischemic (80%): thrombosis, embolism, and systemic hypoperfusion
  - Hemorrhagic (20%): intracerebral, subarachnoid, subdural/extradural bleeds
- History
  - Onset of the symptoms
  - Temporal progression of the symptoms: maximal at onset vs. progressive
  - Activity during the onset of the symptoms
  - Past history of strokes and TIAs
  - History of seizures, migraines, tumors, aneurysms, head trauma, MS
- Risk Factors
  - HTN
  - Hyperlipidemia
  - Age
  - Cardiac disease: angina, MI, palpitations, valvular heart disease, atrial fibrillation, CHF, patent foramen ovale, low ejection fraction
  - Peripheral vascular disease
  - Smoking

NEUROLOGICAL

- DM
- Positive family history
- Clotting disorders
- Medications, illicit drug use

EBM: Stroke

The presence of 3 specific clinical findings (acute facial paresis, arm drift, or abnormal speech) increases the likelihood of stroke (LR of ≥1 finding = 5.5; 95%CI: 3.3-9.1), while the absence of all 3 findings decreases the odds (LR of 0 findings = 0.39; 95%CI: 0.25-0.61). Furthermore, while clinical findings such as headache, vomiting, neck stiffness, severe hypertension (diastolic blood pressure >110 mmHg) and coma increase the probability of hemorrhagic stroke, no finding or combination of findings is ultimately diagnostic in all patients, and thus neuroimaging is required.

Goldstein LB, Simel DL. 2005. *JAMA* 293(19):2391-2402.
Runchey S, McGee S. 2010. *JAMA* 303(22):2280-2286.

- Physical Exam
  - Head and Neck
    - Signs of trauma
    - Retinal changes: hypertensive changes, cholesterol crystals, papilledema
  - PVS
    - Bruits over the carotid, common iliac, and femoral arteries
    - Decreased pulses
    - Signs of ischemic skin changes
  - CVS
    - Murmurs
  - Neurological findings can help localize location of occlusion (see **Table 21**)
- Imaging
  - CT: imaging of choice in acute stroke to determine if hemorrhagic
  - MRI: used to follow patient over time

Table 21. Common Stroke Syndromes

Type of Stroke	Clinical Findings
Anterior Cerebral Artery (ACA)	• Frontal lobe dysfunction (disinhibition, speech perseveration, presence of primitive reflexes, altered mental status, impaired judgment) • Contralateral weakness (greater in legs than arms) • Contralateral cortical sensory deficits • Gait apraxia • Urinary incontinence
Middle Cerebral Artery (MCA)	• Contralateral hemiparesis (greater in face and arms than legs) • Contralateral sensory loss • Contralateral hemianopsia • Gaze preference toward the side of the lesion • If stroke is in dominant hemisphere, also agnosia, receptive/expressive aphasia • If in nondominant hemisphere, neglect, inattention, and extinction
Internal Carotid Artery (ICA)	• Contralateral MCA and ACA signs • May also have ipsilateral transient monocular blindness (amaurosis fugax)

Table 21. Common Stroke Syndromes (continued)

Type of Stroke	Clinical Findings
Posterior Cerebral Artery (PCA)	• Contralateral homonymous hemianopsia • Cortical blindness • Visual agnosia • Altered mental status • Impaired memory
Vertebrobasilar Artery	• Posterior circulation strokes can present with ipsilateral CN deficits and contralateral motor deficits. Findings include: o Vertigo o Nystagmus o Diplopia o Visual field deficits o Dysphagia o Dysarthria o Facial hyperesthesia o Syncope o Ataxia
Lacunar	• Pure contralateral motor weakness • Pure sensory loss • Ataxic hemiparesis
Left-Sided	• Aphasia • Right hemiparesis or hemiplegia • Impaired memory
Right-Sided	• Left hemiparesis or hemiplegia • Neglect of left space • Motor impersistence • Apathy • Impulsivity • Impaired memory

Cruz-Flores S. *Ischemic Stroke*. New York: WebMD LLC. 2013. Available from: http://emedicine.medscape.com/article/1916852-overview.

7.2 Headache

- Different types of headaches have characteristic symptoms (see **Table 22**)
- Depending on the clinical context, neuroimaging may be required (see **Figure 8**)

NEUROLOGICAL

Table 22. Common Headache Syndromes

Type	Characteristics
Tension	• Lasts 30 min-7 d • Nonpulsating, mild-moderate in intensity, bilateral • Not aggravated by exertion, not associated with N/V or sensitivity to light, sound, or smell
Migraine	• Lasts 4-72 h • Throbbing, moderate to severe intensity, unilateral (not always same side) • Worse with exertion • Associated with photophobia, phonophobia, N/V • May be preceded by short prodromal period of depression, irritability, restlessness, or anorexia; 10-20% of occurrences associated with an aura: transient, reversible visual, somatosensory, motor, and/or language deficit – usually precedes headache by ≤1 h, can be concurrent

Table 22. Common Headache Syndromes (continued)

Type	Characteristics
Cluster	• Lasts 15-180 min, occurs up to 8 times/d • Severe, unilateral, located periorbitally and/or temporally associated with at least one of: tearing, red eye, stuffy nose, facial sweating, ptosis, miosis
Subarachnoid Hemorrhage	• Acute, severe, "thunderclap" • May have neurologic deficits or changes in level of consciousness

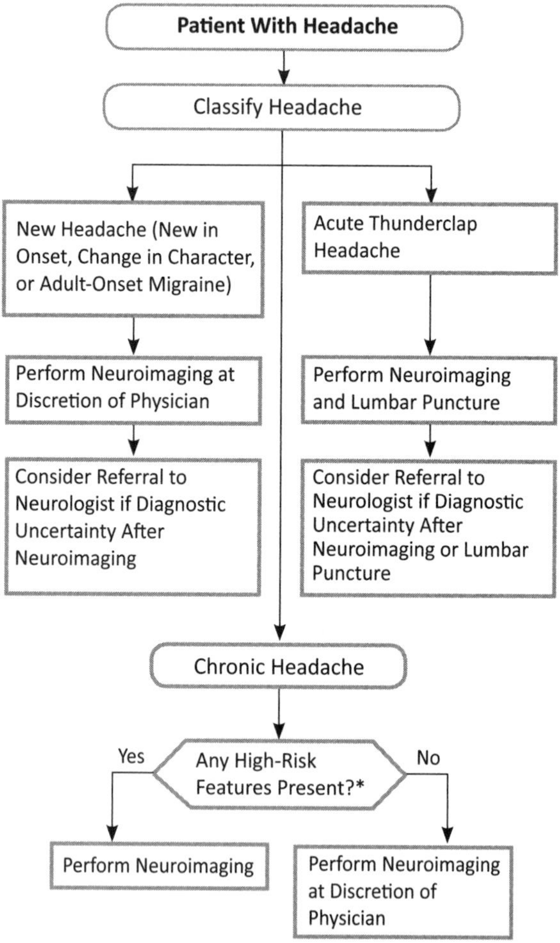

Figure 8. Headaches Requiring Neuroimaging
*Cluster-type headache, abnormal findings on neurologic examination, undefined headache (i.e, not cluster-, migraine-, or tension-type), headache with aura, headache aggravated by exertion or Valsalva-like maneuver, headache with vomiting.
Detsky ME, et al. 2006. *JAMA* 296(10):1274-1283.

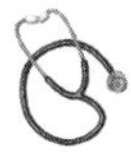

Clinical Pearl: Temporal Arteritis
The presence of symptoms such as scalp tenderness, jaw claudication, diplopia or other visual disturbances, and fever in a patient >50 yr should arouse suspicion of temporal arteritis (see **Essentials of Emergency Medicine**, p.436).

EBM: Who has a Migraine?

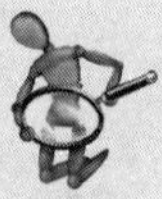

The presence of at least 4 out of 5 clinical criteria summarized by the mnemonic POUNDing (Pulsating, duration of 4-72 hOurs, Unilateral, Nausea, Disabling) is useful to diagnose migraine. The likelihood ratio for definite or possible migraine for 4 criteria is 24 (95%CI: 1.5-388); for 3 criteria, the LR is 3.5 (95%CI: 1.3-9.2), while for 2 criteria, the LR is 0.41 (95%CI: 0.32-0.52).

Detsky ME, et al. 2006. *JAMA* 296(10):1274-1283.

7.3 Brain Tumors

- Commonly present with:
  - Progressive focal neurological deficits
  - Headache: worse in the morning, improves during the day, worse when lying down or with Valsalva maneuver, may be associated with signs of increased intracranial pressure (N/V, blurring of vision, papilledema, transient visual obscuration)
  - Seizures
  - Cognitive deficits
- Most often metastases from other locations, spread hematogenously
- Benign tumors are still significant due to mass effect within fixed space

7.4 Diabetic Neuropathy

- Peripheral nerve damage from poor glucose control
- More common and more severe with increasing age
- Signs of diabetic neuropathy[12]:
  - Peripheral polyneuropathy
  - Autonomic neuropathy (e.g. orthostatic hypotension, gastroparesis)
  - Sensory ataxia (large fiber involvement)
  - Motor weakness (starts distally)
  - Pain/paresthesia/hyperesthesia (small fiber involvement)
  - Loss of deep tendon reflexes
  - Impotence
  - Pupil abnormalities

EBM: Large Fiber Peripheral Neuropathy (LFPN) in Diabetic Patients

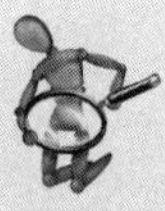

Peripheral neuropathy is a serious issue for diabetic patients, as it can increase the likelihood of developing foot ulcers and infections by 7-fold. LFPN is usually characterized by numbness and tingling in the feet, and its prevalence ranges from 23-79% of patients. However, the presence or absence of neuropathic symptoms is less useful in diagnosing LFPN than a clinical exam combining evaluation of the appearance of the feet, the presence of ulcers, and the testing of vibration perception and ankle reflexes. In particular, testing vibration perception with a 128 Hz tuning fork, and pressure sensation with a 5.07 Semmes-Weinstein monofilament are particularly useful in diagnosing LFPN.

Kanji JN, et al. 2010. *JAMA* 303(15):1526-1532.

7.5 Alzheimer's Disease (AD)

- Progressive neurodegenerative disorder characterized by cognitive decline that interferes with social and occupational functioning
- Characterized by anterograde amnesia (inability to form new memories), and one or more of:
  - Aphasia
  - Apraxia
  - Agnosia
  - Deficits in executive function
- Condition often worsens and symptoms become more prevalent as the disease progresses[13]
  - Anterograde amnesia
  - Speech becomes halting, with grasping for words
  - Slower comprehension
  - Errors in calculation
  - Defective visuospatial orientation
  - Disorientation
  - Amnesia
- In later stages[13]
  - Involuntary primitive reflexes
  - Significant cognitive impairment leading to a loss of ability to carry out self-care activities

7.6 Seizures

- Simple partial seizures
  - Motor, sensory, or psychomotor phenomena without loss of consciousness/awareness of surroundings
  - Seizures can begin in one part of the body and spread to other parts
- Complex partial seizures
  - May be preceded by an aura (sensory or psychic manifestations that represent seizure onset)
  - Staring, performing automatic purposeless movements, uttering unintelligible sounds, resisting aid
  - Motor, sensory, or psychomotor phenomena
  - Postictal confusion
- Tonic-clonic seizures (formerly known as grand mal)
  - Tonic phase: stiffening of limbs
  - Clonic phase: jerking of limbs
  - Respiration may decrease during tonic phase but usually returns during clonic phase, although it may be irregular
  - Incontinence may occur
  - Postictal confusion
- Atonic seizures
  - Brief, primarily generalized seizures in children
  - Complete loss of muscle tone, resulting in falling or pitching to the ground
  - Risk of serious trauma, particularly head injury
- Absence seizures (formerly known as petit mal)
  - Brief, primarily generalized attacks manifested by a 10-30 s loss of awareness of surroundings
  - Eyelid fluttering
  - No loss of axial muscle tone
  - No postictal symptoms
- Status epilepticus: a medical emergency!
  - Repeated seizures lasting >5-10 min with no intervening periods of normal neurologic function
  - Generalized convulsive status epilepticus may be fatal
  - With complex partial or absence seizures, an EEG may be needed to diagnose seizure activity

EBM: Status Epilepticus

While exact definitions vary, status epilecticus (SE) generally refers to a continuous seizure lasting more than 5-10 min, or two or more sequential seizures without full recovery of consciousness between episodes. Over 50% of patients with SE do not have a diagnosis of epilepsy, and the main acute causes of SE in adults are stroke, hypoxia, metabolic disturbances, and alcohol intoxication and withdrawal. In people with a diagnosis of epilepsy, SE can also be induced by anticonvulsant drug withdrawal or noncompliance.

Emergency treatment of SE involves close monitoring of respiratory and cardiovascular function, and first-line treatment with intravenous benzodiazepines, followed by phenytoin or fosphenytoin. If the first-line treatment fails, patients should be transferred to an intensive care unit and be administered an anesthetic agent (intravenous barbiturates, propofol or continuous midazolam infusion are commonly used).

Stecker MM. *Status Epilepticus in Adults.* Waltham: Wolters Kluwer Health. 2012. Available from: http://www.uptodate.com/contents/status-epilepticus-in-adults.
Walker M. 2005. *BMJ* 331(7518): 673-677.

7.7 Parkinson's Disease (PD)

- Extrapyramidal neurodegenerative disorder of unknown origin
- Neuronal loss in the substantia nigra (especially pars compacta) with Lewy bodies in the substantia nigra and other brainstem nuclei
- **TRAP** mnemonic:
  - **T**remor (resting tremor, pill-rolling)
  - **R**igidity (lead-pipe with cogwheeling due to tremor)
  - **A**kinesia/bradykinesia
  - **P**ostural instability
- Other findings
  - Fixed, immobile facial expression
  - Shuffling, festinating gait with decreased arm swing
  - Micrographia
  - Dysarthria
  - Hypophonia
  - Cognitive decline

EBM: Parkinson's Disease

Clinical features that suggest a diagnosis of Parkinson's disease (PD) include a history of rigidity and bradykinesia, micrographia, shuffling gait, and a history of loss of balance. In addition, difficulty turning in bed, opening jars, and rising from chairs can also aid the diagnosis of PD. The glabellar tap, heel-to-toe walking, and rigidity should also be examined.

Rao G, et al. 2003. *JAMA* 289(3):347-353.

7.8 Multiple Sclerosis (MS)

- A demyelinating disease characterized by focal disturbances of function and a relapsing and remitting course, later becoming progressive
- A minority of cases are primary progressive
- Women are affected more than men
- Most common presenting symptom is optic neuritis characterized by partial/total loss of vision and associated pain with eye movement
- Neurologic dysfunction in different parts of the nervous system at different times

- Diagnosis requires dissemination of neuronal dysfunction in both space and time (different parts of the body affected on at least two separate occasions)
- Other symptoms/signs include:
  - Brainstem: diplopia, internuclear ophthalmoplegia, trigeminal neuralgia (tic douloureux), Bell's palsy
  - Cerebellum: nystagmus, ataxia, intention tremor, gait disturbances
  - Spinal cord: weakness, spasticity, hyperreflexia/clonus, upgoing toe(s), bladder or bowel dysfunction/incontinence, sexual dysfunction, paraparesis, Lhermitte's sign (sensation of electric shock down the back and into the limbs with forward flexion of neck)
- Investigations:
  - MRI (shows hyperintense, demyelinating plaques on T2-weighted or FLAIR scans; active lesions enhance with gadolinium contrast)
  - CSF (shows oligoclonal IgG banding)
  - Evoked potentials (abnormal findings on visual, brainstem auditory, and somatosensory evoked potentials)

7.9 Herpes Simplex Encephalitis

- 1/3 cases due to primary HSV cases, 2/3 due to reactivation of latent HSV
- Rapidly progressive disease with profound neurologic derangement
- Mortality if untreated is 70%; 50% of treated individuals are left with significant morbidity[14]
- Infection commonly involves the temporal lobes; involvement of basal ganglia, cerebellum, and brainstem is uncommon
- Clinical findings include[14]:
  - Alteration of consciousness
  - Fever
  - Headache
  - Dysphasia
  - Psychiatric symptoms
  - Ataxia
  - Seizures
  - Vomiting
  - Focal weakness or hemiparesis
  - Cranial nerve defects
  - Memory loss
  - Visual field defects
  - Papilledema
  - Encephalopathy
  - Less common findings: photophobia, movement disorders
  - MRI shows temporal lobe involvement, active CSF

NEUROLOGICAL

7.10 Lumbar Disc Prolapse

- Disc prolapse (herniation) can occur without any recent history of traumatic injury, but can be caused or exacerbated by trauma (e.g. falling, lifting heavy weights)
- Due to the strength of the posterior longitudinal ligament in the midline, most herniated discs occur slightly off to one side and compress the nerve root exiting through the foramen below the affected level
- Findings:
  - Burning, tingling pain in the distribution of irritated/compressed root
  - Restricted spinal movement
  - Loss of reflexes (radicular distribution)
  - Decreased motor strength and sensation (radicular distribution)
    - ***Note:*** while sensation may be diminished, it is usually not absent because of overlap of adjacent dermatomes

- » Testing with pinprick is more sensitive than touch when assessing radicular sensory loss
  - » Reproduction of pain and paresthesias with straight leg raise test or crossed straight leg raise test (elevating the asymptomatic leg causes symptoms in the affected leg; this latter test has over 90% specificity for lumbosacral root compression)
- Motor, sensory, and reflex abnormalities can help localize level of disc prolapse; the majority of lumbosacral radiculopathies occur at the L4/L5 (40-45%) and L5/S1 (45-50%) disc levels (see **Table 23**)

Table 23. Lumbar Disc Prolapse Patterns and Physical Findings

Disc	Root	Motor Weakness	Sensory Loss	Reflex Affected
L3/L4	L4	Quadriceps Hip adductors	Medial leg/ foot	Patellar (knee jerk)
L4/L5	L5	Foot dorsiflexors, EDL, EHL, foot evertors/invertors Hip abductors	Lateral calf, dorsum of the foot, big toe	None
L5/S1	S1	Foot plantar flexors Hip extensors	Lateral foot, sole	Achilles tendon (ankle jerk)

EDL = extensor digitorum longus, EHL = extensor hallucis longus

7.11 Spinal Cord Disorders

- Paraplegia or quadriplegia due to complete or partial cord lesions
- Effect depends on level (e.g. C1-C3: death from respiratory paralysis)
- Two stages:
  - o Spinal shock
    - » Loss of all reflex activity below level of lesion
    - » Atonic bladder/bowel with overflow incontinence
    - » Gastric dilatation
    - » Loss of vasomotor control
  - o Heightened reflex activity
    - » Hyperactive tendon reflexes
    - » Frequency and urgency of urination, automatic emptying of bladder
    - » Hyperactive vasomotor and sweating reactions
- **Central Cord Syndrome**[15]**:**
  - o Occurs more often in older people or in patients with cervical spondylosis
  - o Weakened hands with impaired pain sensation (most prominent symptom)
  - o Relatively few long tract signs
- **Anterior Cord Syndrome**[15]**:**
  - o Caused by infarction in anterior spinal artery territory, tumor invasion or inflammatory myelitis in same region
  - o Paraplegia or quadriplegia
  - o Urinary retention
  - o Bilateral loss of pain and temperature sensation below the lesion
  - o Sparing of posterior column (joint position and vibration) sense
- **Conus Medullaris (CM) and Cauda Equina (CE) Syndromes**[15]**:**
  - o Pain localized to the low back with radiation to legs
  - o Bowel and bladder dysfunction (e.g. urinary retention, laxity of the anal sphincter)
  - o Erectile dysfunction
  - o Loss of sensation in sacral segments (saddle paresthesia)

- Leg weakness with upper and lower motor neuron signs
  - Weakness usually asymmetric in CE; atrophy more common in CE
  - Knee jerk reflexes preserved in CM but absent in CE; ankle jerk reflexes absent in both

REFERENCES

1. Stevens RD, Bhardwaj A. 2006. Approach to the comatose patient. *Crit Care Med* 34(1):31-41.
2. Young GB. *Stupor and Coma in Adults.* Waltham: Wolters Kluwer Health. 2012. Available from: http://www.uptodate.com/contents/stupor-and-coma-in-adults.
3. Wilhelm H. 1998. Neuro-ophthalmology of pupillary function--practical guidelines. *J Neurol* 245(9):573-583.
4. Smith JH, Cutrer FM. 2011. Numbness matters: A clinical review of trigeminal neuropathy. *Cephalalgia* 31(10):1131-1144.
5. Bagai A, Thavendiranathan P, Detsky AS. 2006. Does this patient have hearing impairment? *JAMA* 295(4):416-428.
6. Ivanhoe CB, Reistetter TA. 2004. Spasticity: The misunderstood part of the upper motor neuron syndrome. *Am J Phys Med Rehabil* 83(10 Suppl):S3-9.
7. Walterfang M, Velakoulis D. 2005. Cortical release signs in psychiatry. *Aust N Z J Psychiatry* 39(5):317-327.
8. Kumar SP, Ramasubramanian D. 2000. The Babinski sign--a reappraisal. *Neurol India* 48(4):314-318.
9. Walk D, Sehgal N, Moeller-Bertram T, Edwards RR, Wasan A, Wallace M, et al. 2009. Quantitative sensory testing and mapping: A review of nonautomated quantitative methods for examination of the patient with neuropathic pain. *Clin J Pain* 25(7):632-640.
10. Lanska DJ, Goetz CG. 2000. Romberg's sign: Development, adoption, and adaptation in the 19th century. *Neurology* 55(8):1201-1206.
11. Buchanan RW, Heinrichs DW. 1989. The Neurological Evaluation Scale (NES): A structured instrument for the assessment of neurological signs in schizophrenia. *Psychiatry Res* 27(3):335-350.
12. Tesfaye S, Boulton AJ, Dyck PJ, Freeman R, Horowitz M, Kempler P, et al. 2010. Diabetic neuropathies: Update on definitions, diagnostic criteria, estimation of severity, and treatments. *Diabetes Care* 33(10):2285-2293.
13. Bird TD, Miller BL. Alzheimer's Disease and Other Dementias In: Hauser S, Josephson S (Editors). *Harrison's Neurology in Clinical Medicine*, 2nd ed. New York: McGraw-Hill; 2010.
14. Steiner I. 2011. Herpes simplex virus encephalitis: New infection or reactivation? *Curr Opin Neurol* 24(3):268-274.
15. Levine AM. *Spine Trauma.* Philadelphia: Saunders; 1998.
16. Agur AMR, Dalley AF. *Grant's Atlas of Anatomy.* Philadelphia: Wolters Kluwer Health/Lippincott Williams & Wilkins; 2009.
17. Benarroch EE. *Medical Neurosciences: An Approach to Anatomy, Pathology, and Physiology by Systems and Levels.* Philadelphia: Lippincott Williams & Wilkins; 1999.
18. Bickley LS, Szilagyi PG, Bates B. *Bates' Guide to Physical Examination and History Taking,* 10th ed. Philadelphia: Lippincott Williams & Wilkins; 2009.
19. Blumenfeld H. *Neuroanatomy Through Clinical Cases*, 2nd ed. Sunderland: Sinauer Associates; 2010.
20. Campbell WW. *DeJong's the Neurological Examination*, 6th ed. Philadelphia: Lippincott Williams & Wilkins; 2005.
21. Carter LP, Spetzler RF, Hamilton MG. *Neurovascular Surgery.* New York: McGraw-Hill, Health Professions Division; 1994.
22. Greenberg MS. *Handbook of Neurosurgery.* New York: Thieme Medical Publishers; 2001.
23. Kandel ER, Schwartz JH, Jessell TM. *Principles of Neural Science.* New York: McGraw-Hill, Health Professions Division; 2000.
24. Ross RT. *How to Examine the Nervous System.* Totowa: Humana Press; 2006.
25. Snell RS. *Clinical Anatomy for Medical Students.* Philadelphia: Lippincott Williams & Wilkins; 2000.
26. Zigmond MJ. *Fundamental Neuroscience.* San Diego: Academic Press; 1999.

The Obstetric Exam

Editors:
Mary Ellen Gedye
Minji Kim
Alia Sunderji

Faculty Reviewers:
Rory Windrim, MD, FRCS(C)
Adrian Brown, MD, FRCS(C)

TABLE OF CONTENTS

1. ESSENTIAL ANATOMY

Refer to the **Gynecological Exam**, p.79 for diagrams of the external and internal genitalia.

2. COMMON CHIEF COMPLAINTS

Table 1. Common Chief Complaints

Complaint	Trimester	Possible Causes
Chief Complaints Secondary to Physiologic Changes		
Breast Tenderness/ Heaviness	1	Growth of breast tissue ↑ blood flow to breast
Fatigue	1	Unknown
N/V	1	↑ estrogen and β-hCG ↑ gastric motility
Weight Loss	1	Decreased appetite from N/V
Heartburn	1, 2, 3	Relaxation of lower esophageal sphincter allows reflux from stomach
Backache	1, 2, 3	Relaxation of joints and ligaments Growth of uterus Weight of fetus
Amenorrhea	1, 2, 3	↑ estrogen, progesterone, β-hCG
Constipation	1, 2, 3	Decreased peristalsis

OBSTETRIC

Table 1. Common Chief Complaints (continued)

Complaint	Trimester	Possible Causes
Chief Complaints Secondary to Physiologic Changes		
Urinary Frequency	1 2, 3 Term	↓ plasma osmolality ↑ vascularity, pressure of enlarged uterus Pressure of fetal head on bladder
Leukorrhea	1, 2, 3	Hormonal effects of pregnancy lead to increased blood flow to vagina
Chief Complaints Secondary to Potentially Pathological Processes		
Bleeding	1, 2	Spontaneous abortion Abnormal pregnancy (ectopic/molar) Trauma
	2, 3	Placenta previa Abruptio placentae
	3	Bloody show (= bloody mucus loosened free of the cervical mucus plug due to effacement of cervix prior to delivery)
Decreased Fetal Movements	2, 3	Fetal distress Fetal demise
Contractions	2, 3	Preterm labor Normal labor Braxton-Hicks contractions (nonpainful uterine activity)
Leaking of Fluid	3	Premature rupture of membranes Labor Yeast or other infection Normal secretions Urine

3. FOCUSED HISTORY, PHYSICAL EXAM, AND COMMON INVESTIGATIONS

3.1 Preconception Counseling

Table 2. Routine Objectives in Preconception Care

Goals of Care	
Risk Assessment	
Genetic Screening and Family History	Assess based on family history, ethnic background, and age
Nutritional Assessment	Assess anthropometric (BMI), biochemical (e.g. anemia), clinical, and dietary risks
Substance Abuse	Assess tobacco, alcohol, and drug use
Infections and Immunizations	Screen for periodontal, urogenital, and sexually transmitted infections as indicated Update immunization for hepatitis B, rubella, varicella, Tdap, HPV, and influenza as needed
Toxins and Teratogens	Review exposures at home, neighborhood, and work (e.g. chemical/radiation exposure)

OBSTETRIC

Table 2. Routine Objectives in Preconception Care (continued)

Goals of Care	
Risk Assessment	
Past Medical History	Assess for diseases that could affect future pregnancy (see **Gynecological Exam,** p.81)
Psychosocial Concerns	Screen for depression, anxiety, intimate partner violence, and major psychosocial stressors (see **EBM: ALPHA Form**, p.209)
Health Promotion	
Healthy Weight and Nutrition	Promote healthy pre-pregnancy weight through exercise and nutrition. Discuss nutrient intake including intake of a multivitamin with a minimum of 0.4 mg of folic acid (should begin after discontinuation of birth control and for 10-12 wk after last menstrual period)
Health Behaviors	Promote nutrition and exercise, and discourage risky behaviors such as smoking, alcohol consumption, and substance abuse
Medical and Psychosocial Intervention	
Medications	Review medications and avoid use of FDA category X and D drugs
Stress Resilience	Address ongoing stressors such as intimate partner violence; identify resources to help patient with positive mental health and stable living conditions

Liston R, et al. 2007. *J Obstet Gynaecol Can* 29(Suppl 4):S3-56.

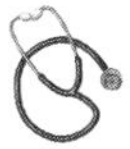

Clinical Pearl: Intimate Partner Abuse

Intimate partner violence is a serious and surprisingly common problem, affecting around 7% of pregnant women.[1] Physical abuse during pregnancy is associated with increased risk of antepartum hemorrhage, intrauterine growth restriction (IUGR), and perinatal death.[2] Routine screening questions addressing personal safety and violence should be included during the prenatal period.

EBM: ALPHA Form

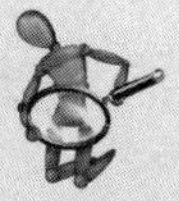

In a 2005 study, the use of the Antenatal Psychosocial Health Assessment (ALPHA) form was found to help healthcare providers detect psychosocial risk factors for poor postpartum outcomes. Specifically, the use of the form was associated with the increased detection of risk factors associated with family violence, an area previously shown to be problematic. As such, the incorporation of the ALPHA form into routine prenatal care may become a useful tool for assessing pregnant women's psychological health.

Blackmore ER, et al. 2006. *J Obstet Gynaecol Can* 28(10):873-878.

3.2 Diagnosis of Pregnancy

Table 3. Signs and Symptoms of Pregnancy

Diagnosis of a New Pregnancy	
History	Amenorrhea N/V Fatigue Breast tenderness Urinary frequency
Physical Exam	Signs on pelvic examination = **CHUG** **C** = Chadwick's sign: bluish discoloration of cervix and vagina (9-12 wk) **H** = Hegar's sign: softening of lower segment of uterus (6 wk) **U** = Uterine enlargement **G** = Goodell's sign: softening of cervix and vagina (8 wk)
Investigations	Serum β-hCG follow the Rule of 10's **10 IU** at time of missed menses (double every 1-2 d) **100,000 IU** at **10 wk** (peak) **10,000 IU** at term

Note: Confirmation of pregnancy with fetal heart rate can be heard via transvaginal ultrasound as early as 5 wk gestational age (GA).
Liston R, et al. 2007. *J Obstet Gynaecol Can* 29(Suppl 4):S3-56.

3.3 Initial Prenatal Assessment

Focused History

Patient Identification

- Age, occupation, and marital status

Fertility Summary

- Menstrual history (see **Gynecological Exam**, p.80)
  - Date of last menstrual period (LMP), last cycle frequency
  - Estimated date of birth (EDB)
    1. By date of LMP using Naegele's rule: 1st day of LMP + 7 d - 3 mo (if cycle is not 28 d, add number of additional days, i.e. add 4 if 32-day cycle)
    2. By ultrasound (most accurate in first trimester); once established by U/S, EDB does not change
- Contraception
  - Type, duration of use, last use
- History of current pregnancy
  - Physiologic symptoms (see **Table 1** and **Table 2**)
  - Potentially harmful exposures: smoking, alcohol, radiation, etc.
  - Nutritional assessment: diet, calcium, folate; avoid unpasteurized milk products, raw meats, and sushi
  - Red flags: bleeding (duration, amount, any clots), discharge/leaking fluid, cramping/contractions, abdominal pain
- **GTPALM** status
  - **G**ravida — # of pregnancies
  - **T**erm — # of deliveries at 37-42 wk gestation
  - **P**remature — # of deliveries <37 wk gestation
  - **A**bortion — # of abortions (spontaneous and therapeutic)
  - **L**ive — # of live deliveries
  - **M**ultiples — # of multiple pregnancies

OBSTETRIC

Obstetrical History of All Previous Pregnancies
- Year, place of birth
- Sex, gestational age, birth weight of baby
- Abortion (medical vs. surgical dilatation/curettage)
- Labor duration, type of delivery (vaginal, forceps, vacuum, Cesarean section [classical vs. lower segment])
- Pregnancy/delivery/perinatal/postpartum complications (e.g. pulmonary embolism, gestational DM, postpartum depression)
- Health status of previous children (alive, well, illnesses)

Medical History
- Including, but not limited to:
  - Infections (e.g. TORCH, HIV, STIs/HSV/bacterial vaginosis, varicella status, TB risk)
  - Psychiatric history
  - Transfusion history
  - Surgical history
  - Anesthesia complications
  - Allergies and medications

Other Discussion Topics
- Exercise: encourage regular low-moderate physical activity with a target HR of 3/4 of their non-pregnant target HR; discourage high impact activities (e.g. scuba diving, horseback riding)
- Coitus: safe during pregnancy (except placenta previa)
- Prenatal classes
- Avoiding cat litter boxes (risk of toxoplasmosis)
- Home pregnancy tests: accuracy depends on number of days since missed menstrual period and ease of use of test

Focused Physical Exam

Baseline Physical Assessment
- Height
- Pre-pregnancy weight and current weight
- BP
- Bimanual pelvic exam (uterine size and adnexa)

Systematic Assessment (see **Table 4** for description of expected changes)
- Thyroid (see **Head and Neck Exam**, p.114)
- Cardiovascular (see **Cardiovascular Exam**, p.52)
- Breasts (see **Breast Exam**, p.39)
- Abdominal (see **Abdominal Exam**, p.20): may be able to palpate the uterine fundus if pregnancy is 12 wk or further along

Table 4. Physiological Changes During Pregnancy

Parameter	Changes	Comments
General		
Weight	↑ 25%	0.5 kg/wk in second half of pregnancy
Energy Needs	↑ 15%	
Respiratory		
Arterial Blood Gases	pCO_2 98% (28-32 mmHg)	pCO_2 in maternal blood facilitates placental pCO_2 transfer
Tidal Volume	↑ 40%	

Table 4. Physiological Changes During Pregnancy (continued)

Parameter	Changes	Comments
Cardiovascular		
Cardiac Output	↑ 30-50% (6.0 L/min)	CO peaks at 24 wk due to ↑ stroke volume
Heart Rate	↑ 15-20 bpm	
Plasma Volume	↑ 45%	
Blood Pressure	Systolic: ↓ 5-10 mmHg Diastolic: ↑ 10-15 mmHg	BP lowest at 20-24 wk and then gradually increases
Hematologic		
Hemoglobin (Hb)	↓ 15-20 g/L	Hb starts ↓ by 12 wk, lowest at 30-34 wk
WBC	↑ 3.5 x 10^9/L	
Coagulation	↑ Factor VII to X ↑ venous stasis	1.8-fold ↑ risk of thromboembolism
Renal		
GFR	↑ 50%	No change in urine output due to tubular reabsorption

Common Investigations

Blood Work

- CBC (Hemoglobin [Hb], mean corpuscular volume [MCV])
- Blood group and type, Rh status
- Rubella titer
- Venereal disease research laboratory (VDRL) test
- Hepatitis B surface antigen
- HIV

Urinalysis

- Routine and microscopy
- Culture and sensitivity: for asymptomatic bacteriuria

Cervix

- Pap smear
- Culture for chlamydia and gonorrhea

3.4 Subsequent Prenatal Assessment

Recommended frequency of prenatal visits is outlined in **Table 5**

Table 5. Schedule for Uncomplicated Pregnancies

Gestational Age	Usual Frequency of Visit
Up to 32 wk	Monthly
32-36 wk	Every 2 wk
36 wk to Delivery	Every wk

Focused History

Note any changes from the initial assessment

- Ask about the **ABCDE**s
  - **A**ctivity (of the fetus)
  - **B**leeding
  - **C**ontractions
  - **D**ripping (discharge or fluid)
  - **E**stimated date of birth
- Other discussion topics:
  - Diet/nutrition, rest
  - Signs of labor, premature labor
  - Prenatal education classes
  - Review labor and delivery plans (e.g. supports, pain relief)
  - Breastfeeding

Focused Physical Exam

General Assessment

- Height
- Weight (see **Table 6**)
- BP
- Bimanual pelvic exam (see **Gynecology Exam**, p.84)

Table 6. Appropriate Weight Gain in Pregnancy

Expected Weight Gain	
BMI (kg/m²)	**Weight (kg)**
<19	12.7-18.2
19-25	11.3-15.9
>25	6.8-11.3
General Rule: 1-3 kg/wk during T1, then 0.45 kg/wk until delivery	

Society of Obstetricians and Gynecologists. *Healthy Beginnings: Guidelines for Care During Pregnancy and Childbirth.* SOGC Clinical Practice Guidelines, Policy Statement. Ottawa: SOGC; 1998.

Other Physical Assessments

- Abdominal Exam
  - Symphysis-fundal height (SFH) (see **Table 7** and **Figure 1**)
  - From 20-37 wk, SFH = GA ± 2 cm e.g. 30 weeks = 30 cm
- Fetal Heart Rate Assessment
  - Every visit beginning at 12 wk with doppler U/S or fetoscope

Table 7. Symphysis-Fundal Height

Symphysis-Fundal Height Reference Chart	
Weeks	**Top of Uterus**
12	Pubic symphysis
20	Umbilicus
36	Just below xiphoid
Term	No longer reliable due to engagement and descent

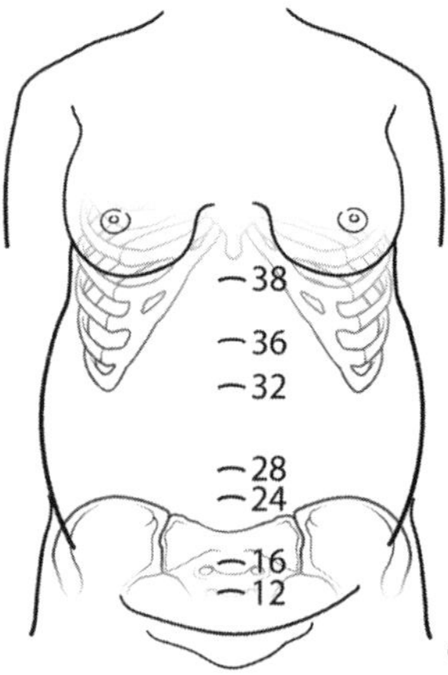

Figure 1. Expected Symphysis-Fundal Height by Gestational Age (weeks)

- Leopold Maneuvers (see **Figure 2**)[3]
  - Done in T3 to identify lie, presentation, and position of the fetus
  - First maneuver: determines which part of the fetus occupies the fundus
    - **How to perform:** face patient's head and palpate the fundal area
      - Buttocks at fundus/vertex: soft or irregular
      - Head at fundus/breech: round, hard, ballotable
  - Second maneuver: determines side on which fetal back lies
    - **How to perform:** place hands on lateral sides of the abdomen and palpate
      - Back: linear and firm
      - Extremities: multiple parts ("small parts")
  - Third maneuver: determines the presenting part
    - **How to perform:** place one hand just above the symphysis and grasp the presenting part between the thumb and third finger
      - Unengaged head/vertex: round, firm, and ballotable
      - Breech: irregular and nodular
  - Fourth maneuver: determines head flexion or extension
    - **How to perform:** face patient's feet and place hands on either side of lower abdomen just above inlet. Exert pressure in direction of inlet; one hand will usually descend further than the other
      - Head flexed: cephalic prominence prevents descent of one hand, which is on the same side as the small parts (suggests occiput presentation)
      - Head extended: occiput is felt prominently on the same side as the back (suggests face presentation)

OBSTETRIC

Common Investigations

Urine Dip

- Glucose and protein
  - Done at each visit

Genetic Screening Tests

- Offered to all pregnant women
- First Trimester Screening (FTS): 11-14 wk GA
  - Measures nuchal translucency (U/S), β-hCG, and pregnancy-associated plasma protein A (PAPP-A)
  - Estimates risk of Down syndrome (Trisomy 21)

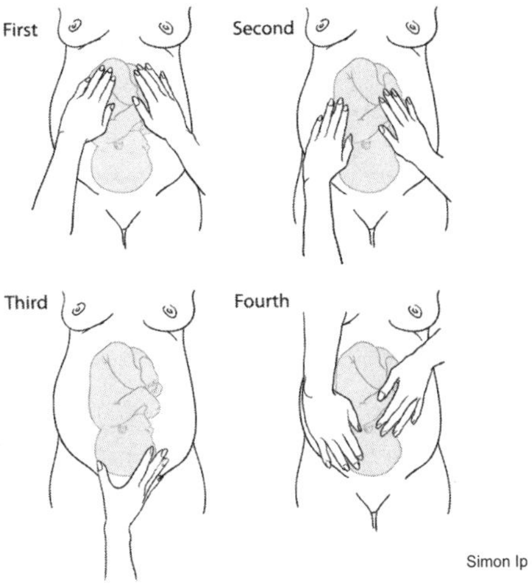

Figure 2. Leopold Maneuvers

- Maternal Serum Screen (MSS): 16 wk GA
  - Measures maternal serum α-fetoprotein (MSAFP), β-hCG, and estriol (μE3)
  - Estimates risk of trisomies 21 and 18, and neural tube defects (NTDs)
- Integrated Prenatal Screen (IPS)
  - Integrates part of FTS and MSS
  - Part 1 done at 11-14 wk: NT by U/S and PAPP-A
  - Part 2 done at 15-18 wk: MSS markers
  - More specific estimated risk of trisomies 21 and 18 and NTDs

Genetic Diagnostic Tests

Offered to women at higher risk as determined by genetic screening, family history or personal medical history

- Chorionic Villus Sampling: 10-13 wk GA
  - Placental biopsy (transabdominal or transcervical)
  - Additional miscarriage risk <1%
  - Indications: high risk population for chromosomal abnormalities:
    - Ashkenazi Jewish
    - Increased maternal age
    - FHx of abnormality
- Amniocentesis
  - Aspirate of amniotic fluid (U/S guided transabdominal)
  - Additional miscarriage risk <0.5%
  - Indications: high risk population for chromosomal abnormalities
- Ultrasound (U/S): 18 wk GA
  - Anatomic scan or when indicated (e.g. evidence of intrauterine growth restriction [IUGR], preeclampsia, or other abnormalities)
  - Transabdominal or transvaginal

Other Screening Tests (see **Table 8**)

- TB skin test, sickle cell/thalassemia screen
- Other genetic screens indicated by FHx/ethnicity
- Oral glucose challenge test for gestational DM
- Group B *Streptococcus* swab

OBSTETRIC

Antenatal Monitoring

- Non-Stress Test (NST):
  - Assess fetal heart rate patterns
  - Indications: suspected uteroplacental insufficiency or fetal distress
- Biophysical Profile (BPP)[4]:
  - U/S assessment of fetus
  - Indications: nonreassuring NST, fetal distress, postterm pregnancy
  - Goal: to detect fetal hypoxia early enough to allow for delivery
  - Scores:
    - » Amniotic fluid volume (most important parameter) /2
    - » Fetal tone /2
    - » Fetal movement /2
    - » Fetal breaths /2
    - » Fetal heart rate

Table 8. Gestational Age-Dependent Tests

Gestational Age (wk)	Tests
All Visits	Urine dip for proteinuria, glucosuria, ketones
12-14	CVS, U/S (nuchal translucency and dates), blood work
15-16	Amniocentesis
16	MSS
18-20	U/S (anatomical scan)
24-28	Oral glucose challenge test (50 g load)
26	Screen for Rh and give RhoGAM® at 28 wk to Rh negative women
28-32	Repeat CBC to determine need for iron supplementation
36-37	Group B *Streptococcus* culture (anovaginal)

CVS = chorionic villus sampling, MSS = maternal serum screen, Rh = Rhesus factor

3.5 Labor

Labor = regular uterine contractions leading to cervical dilatation and effacement and resulting in the expulsion of the products of conception (fetus, membranes, and placenta)

- Preterm labor: 20-37 wk GA
- Term labor: 37-42 wk GA
- Postterm labor: >42 wk GA

Braxton-Hicks contractions ("false labor") = irregular, occur throughout pregnancy and do not result in cervical dilatation, effacement or fetal descent (see **Table 9**)

History

Table 9. True vs. False Labor

	True Labor	False Labor
Contraction Intervals	Regular	Irregular
Duration of Time Between Contractions	Gradually shortens	Remains long
Intensity of Contractions	Gradually increases	Remains unchanged

OBSTETRIC

Table 9. True vs. False Labor (continued)

	True Labor	False Labor
Discomfort	Back and abdomen	Lower abdomen
Relief by Sedation	Not relieved by sedation	Often relieved by sedation
Cervix	Effacement and dilatation	No effacement and dilatation

Physical Exam and Investigations During Labor and Delivery

On Admission

- Vital signs and fluid status
- Abdominal examination
  - o Determine fetal lie, position, and station of presenting part
- Urine for protein, glucose, and ketone bodies
- If placenta previa known/suspected, do not attempt vaginal exam

Cervical Changes (see **Figure 3**)

- Effacement:
  - o Thinning of cervical walls caused by pressure of fetal head
  - o Expressed as % of total effacement
    - » 0%: none, 100%: complete thinning
  - o May result in release of mucus plug within cervical canal ("bloody show")
- Dilatation:
  - o Opening of cervical canal
  - o Expressed in cm:
    - » 0 cm: no dilatation, 10 cm: full dilatation

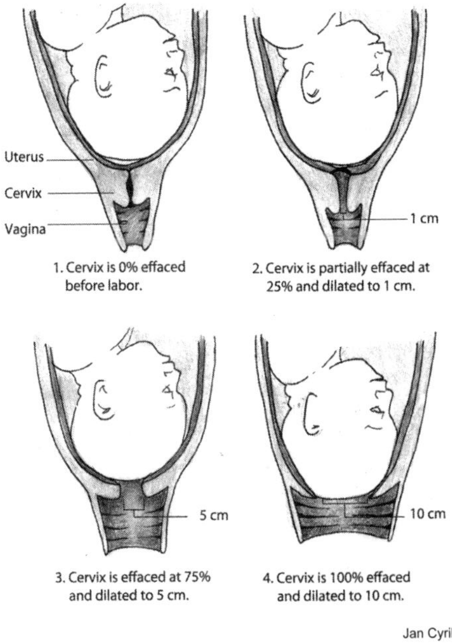
Uterus
Cervix
Vagina
1 cm
5 cm
10 cm
1. Cervix is 0% effaced before labor.
2. Cervix is partially effaced at 25% and dilated to 1 cm.
3. Cervix is effaced at 75% and dilated to 5 cm.
4. Cervix is 100% effaced and dilated to 10 cm.
Jan Cyril Fundano

Figure 3. Stages of Cervical Effacement and Dilatation

Stages of Labor

- First Stage: onset of true labor to full dilatation of the cervix[5]
  - Duration: 8-12 h in nulliparous women and 3-8 h in multiparous women
    - Latent phase: cervical effacement and dilatation (from 0-3 cm)
    - Active phase: rapid cervical dilatation (3-10 cm where 10 cm = full dilatation)
- Second Stage: full dilatation of cervix to delivery of baby
- Third Stage: delivery of placenta
- Fourth Stage: delivery of placenta until patient is stable (usually 1 h)

Table 10. Duration of Normal Labor

Stage	Nulliparous	Multiparous
First	6-18 h	2-10 h
Second	30 min-3 h	5-30 min
Third	5-30 min	5-30 min
Fourth	Until postpartum condition of patient has stabilized (usually 1 h)	

First Stage of Labor

- Vaginal examination: repeat every 2-3 h or as indicated
  - **How to perform:** separate vulva and labia with left hand and use right index and middle fingers to examine
    - Assess position of cervix: anterior vs. posterior
    - Assess degree of dilatation and effacement of cervix
    - Assess if membranes have ruptured
      - Pooling of fluid in speculum exam
      - ↑ pH of vaginal fluid
      - Ferning of fluid under light microscopy
      - ↓ amniotic fluid volume (AFV) on U/S

Table 11. Assessing Latent Phase of Labor: Bishop Score for Assessing Cervical Ripeness

	0	1	2	3
Cervical Length (cm)	1	1 or 2	<1	Fully taken up
Cervical Dilatation (cm)	0	1 or 2	3 or 4	≥5
Cervical Consistency	Firm	Medium	Soft	NA
Position of Cervix	Posterior	Central	Anterior	NA
Station of Presenting Part (cm above ischial spines)	3	2	1 or 0	Below spines

- After membranes have ruptured, examine the amniotic fluid, noting any meconium
- Assess position of the presenting part
  - **How to perform:** palpate suture lines and fontanelles in relation to pelvic diameters
- Assess the level of the presenting part in relation to the pelvic brim or ischial spines (**Figure 4** and **Table 11**)
  - 0 = level of ischial spines
  - **How to perform:** using index and middle fingers, palpate the ischial spines; locate most inferior aspect of presenting part, determine whether it is above, at or below level of ischial spines

- Estimate level in thirds or fifths above (+) or below (-) zero
- Electronic fetal heart rate (FHR) monitoring
  - Assess baseline FHR, variability, and periodicity (decelerations and accelerations)

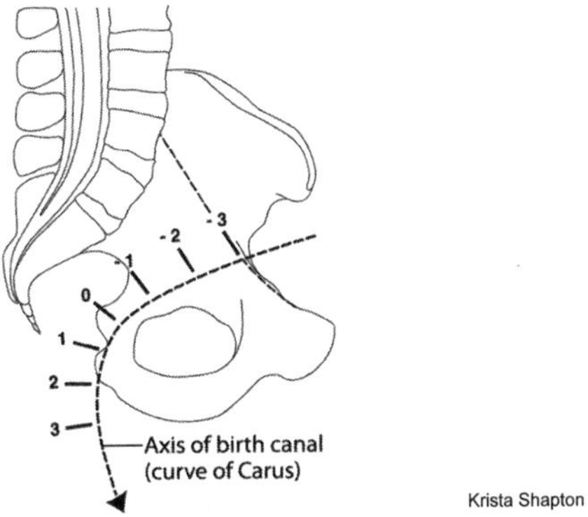

Figure 4. Level of Head in Thirds Above or Below Ischial Spines

Table 12. Intrapartum FHR Monitoring (see also **Figure 5**)

	Normal	Atypical	Abnormal
Baseline FHR (bpm)	• 110-160	• Slow 100-110 • Fast >160 for 30-80 min • Rising baseline	• Slow <100 • Fast >160 for >80 min • Erratic baseline
Variability (bpm)	• 6-25 • <5 for <40 min	• <5 for 40-80 min	• <5 for >80 min • >25 for >10 min • Sinusoidal
Decelerations	• None or occasional • Early or variable decels	• Repetitive (>3) variable decels • Occasional late decels • Single prolonged decel for 2-3 min	• Repetitive (>3) variable decels • Late decels >50% of contractions • Single prolonged decel for 3-10 min • Slow to return to baseline
Acceleration	• Spontaneous • Occurs with fetal scalp stimulation	• Absence of accel with fetal scalp stimulation	• Absent
Management	• Routine intrapartum monitoring	• Frequent reassessment and further management as indicated clinically	• Confirm fetal wellbeing • Fetal scalp blood sample • Consider operative delivery • Intrauterine resuscitation

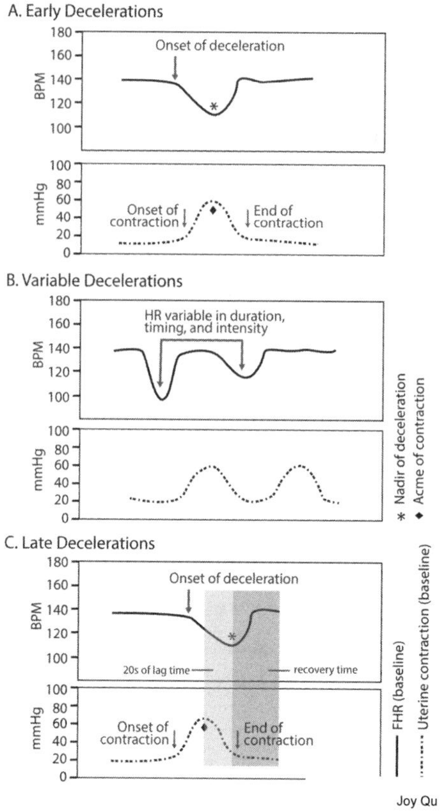

Figure 5. Fetal Heart Monitoring Strips

Second Stage of Labor

- Cardinal movements of fetus during delivery (see **Figure 6**)

1. Descent
   - Begins before onset of labor or during first stage
   - Continues until fetus is delivered
2. Flexion
   - Fetal head flexes chin to chest
   - Reduces diameter of presenting part
3. Internal Rotation
   - Fetal head rotates laterally during descent through the pelvis
4. Extension
   - Fetal neck extends to negotiate under the symphysis pubis
   - Crowning: largest diameter of fetal head is encircled by vulvar ring (station +3 or +5 if measuring station by thirds or fifths respectively)
5. Restitution/External Rotation
   - Fetal head returns to the position at the time of engagement
   - Fetal back and shoulders align
6. Expulsion
   - Delivery of anterior shoulder, posterior shoulder, then the rest of the body

OBSTETRIC

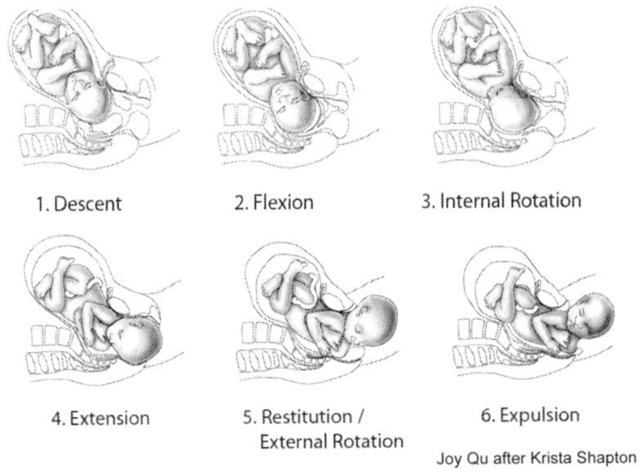

Figure 6. Cardinal Movements of the Fetus During Delivery

- Delivery of the fetus
  - Mother is positioned left lateral decubitus or supine
  - Episiotomy (incision in perineum) only if necessary
    - Midline: better healing but increased risk of deep tear
    - Mediolateral: reduced risk of extensive tear but poorer healing and more pain
  - Delivery of fetal head
    - Ritgen maneuver: exert forward pressure on the chin of the fetus through the perineum just in front of coccyx with left hand while exerting pressure superiorly against occiput with right hand
  - Check for nuchal cord
  - Consider clear fetal airway using suction bulb: oral cavity first, then nares
  - Delivery of anterior shoulder
    - Hold sides of the head with two hands and apply gentle downward pressure
  - Delivery of posterior shoulder
    - Gently elevate the head and apply upward pressure
  - Delivery of rest of body
  - Check fetal Apgar scores 1 and 5 min after birth (**Table 13**)

Table 13. Apgar Scores

Sign	0	1	2
Appearance	Blue, pale	Body pink, extremities blue	Completely pink
Pulse	Absent	<100 bpm	>100 bpm
Reflexes: stimulation with NG tube	No response	Grimace	Sneeze or cough
Activity: muscle tone	Flaccid	Some flexion of extremities	Good flexion
Respiratory Effort	Absent	Weak, irregular	Good, crying

EBM: Apgar Scores

In a 1988 study, the 5 min Apgar score was found to be a more powerful predictor of mortality than the 1 min Apgar score. Apgar scores are not useful predictors of later disability.

Specificity of Apgar score depression as a prognostic tool is far better than sensitivity. An infant with an Apgar score of 3 or less at 10 min has a 75% chance of either dying or developing major handicaps, while high scores do not rule out death or later developmental problems.

Schmidt B, et al. 1988. *J Clin Epidemiol* 41(9):843-850.

Third Stage of Labor

- Signs of placental separation:
  - Uterus becomes firm and globular
  - Gush of blood
  - Umbilical cord visibly lengthens
  - Uterine fundus rises in abdomen
- Patient is positioned supine
- Place left hand on abdomen over the uterine fundus
- Exert gentle pressure on uterine fundus while keeping the umbilical cord slightly taut with right hand
- Do NOT pull on umbilical cord!
- Monitor vital signs and ensure patient is stabilized
- Inspect placenta for completeness (i.e. no retained products) and blood vessels (2 arteries and 1 vein)
- Send cord blood gas samples of umbilical artery and umbilical vein cord to lab after every delivery
- Palpate to ensure uterine contraction and check for uterine bleeding
- Repair episiotomies or tears
- Administer oxytocic agent

Operative Delivery

- Use of forceps, vacuum extraction or surgery to deliver the fetus
- Common indications for Cesarean section (C/S)[6]:
  - **Maternal:**
    - Obstruction of birth canal
    - Active herpetic lesions on vulva
    - Underlying maternal illness (eclampsia, HELLP [hemolysis, elevated liver enzymes, low platelet count] syndrome)
    - Previous C/S
    - Elective
    - Poor obstetrical history
  - **Maternal-Fetal:**
    - Failure to progress
    - Cephalopelvic disproportion (CPD)
    - Multiple gestations
    - Placenta previa
    - Abruptio placentae
    - Prolapsed cord
  - **Fetus:**
    - Malpresentation: breech (3-4% of deliveries), transverse lie (0.3-0.4% of deliveries)
    - Malposition (e.g. occiput posterior)
    - Fetal distress, nonreassuring fetal heart rate (1-2% of cases)
    - Low-birth weight infant
    - Macrosomic infant (>4 kg)

- Maternal risks associated with C/S:
  - Uterine hemorrhage (due to atony, extension of incision, uterine rupture, presence of leiomyomata)
  - Deep vein thrombosis
  - Pulmonary embolism
  - Postoperative infection (determined by length of labor, rupture of membranes, number of vaginal examinations)
  - Risk of placenta previa or placenta accreta in future deliveries

Examination of the Newborn

- Full neonatal examination within 24 h of delivery (see **Pediatric Exam**, p.253)

3.6 Puerperium and Postpartum Period

- Postpartum period extends from 1 h after delivery of placenta to 6 wk period after pregnancy when pregnancy-related anatomic and physiologic changes are reversed

Physiologic Changes of the Uterus

- Uterus
  - Uterus decreases in size and cervix regains firmness
  - Uterus should involute 1 cm below umbilicus per day for first 4-5 d
  - Uterine spasms can cause pain 4-7 d postpartum
  - Returns to non-pregnant state in 4-6 wk
- Resumption of ovarian function
  - Ovulation resumes in 45 d in non-lactating patients, and 3-6 mo in lactating women
  - Breastfeeding is NOT a method of contraception: unless patient wishes to conceive, use a barrier method
- Lochia: normal vaginal discharge postpartum
  - Decreases and changes color from red (lochia rubra) to yellow (lochia serosa) to white (lochia alba)
- Breast changes
  - Engorgement in late pregnancy
  - Colostrum expression can occur in late pregnancy up to 72 h postpartum
  - Full milk production by 3-7 d
  - Mature milk by 15-45 d

Postpartum Disorders

Postpartum Hemorrhage (PPH)

- Loss of >500 mL of blood at time of vaginal delivery or >1000 mL in C/S
- Early (within 24 h of delivery) or delayed (24 h-6 wk post-delivery)
- Incidence 5-15%, significant cause of maternal mortality
- Causes: **4 T**'s
  - **T**one: uterine atony
  - **T**issue: retained products (e.g. retained placenta)
  - **T**rauma
  - **T**hrombosis: coagulopathy (e.g. DIC)

Endometritis

- Entry of normal GI or gynecological bacteria into the usually sterile uterus
- Incidence: 1-3% of vaginal deliveries
- High risk: C/S delivery, chorioamionitis, premature rupture of membranes (PROM)
- Suspect if foul smelling lochia

Urinary Incontinence
- Prevalence: 2.7-23.4% in the first year postpartum
- Higher risk in higher prepregnancy body mass index, parity, urinary incontinence during pregnancy, smoking, longer duration of breastfeeding, and vaginal delivery

Postpartum Depression
- Predictors: stressful life events, past history of depression, family history of mood disorders, poor marital relationship, and poor social support
- Screening: postpartum visits, well baby visits
- Postpartum "baby blues"
  - A physiologic phenomenon triggered by hormonal changes and augmented by sleep deprivation and nutritional deficiencies
  - Occurs in up to 70% of new mothers
  - Onset: first week postpartum and resolution by 10 d postpartum
  - Presentation: weeping, sadness, irritability, anxiety, confusion, extreme elation
- Postpartum depression (PPD)
  - Major depression occurring within 4 wk postpartum
  - Lasts about 7 mo if untreated
  - Incidence: 10-20%, 50% recurrence
  - Presentation: despondent mood, feelings of inadequacy as a parent, impaired concentration, changes in appetite and sleep, thoughts of harming the infant
  - Long-term adverse effects for mother and child if untreated
- Postpartum psychosis[7]
  - Acute psychotic episode or abrupt onset of depressive symptoms over 24-72 h within first postpartum month
  - Occurs in approximately 1-2 in 1000 women after delivery
  - Presentation: psychosis with delusions, hallucinations, or both, plus mood disorder
- Symptoms may appear to resolve then reoccur acutely and severely
- More likely to act on thoughts of harming their infants if untreated
- Mother is at increased risk of recurrence following future pregnancies and stressful life events
- Rapid referral to psychiatry is critical

4. COMMON DISORDERS

Disorders marked with (✓) are discussed in **Common Clinical Scenarios**

✓ Pregnancy-induced conditions
  - Hypertensive disorders
  - Gestational diabetes mellitus
  - Rhesus discrepancies
  - UTI
  - Anemia
  - Hyperemesis gravidarum

✓ Antenatal complications
  - Miscarriage
  - Ectopic pregnancy
  - Abruptio placentae
  - Placenta previa
  - Premature rupture of membranes (PROM)
  - Intrauterine growth restriction (IUGR)

✓ Labor and postpartum complications
  - Breech presentation
  - Postpartum depression

5. COMMON CLINICAL SCENARIOS

5.1 Pregnancy-Induced Conditions

Hypertensive Disorders:

- Gestational hypertension without proteinuria (pregnancy-induced hypertension)
  - HTN (>140/90 mmHg or an increase from baseline of 30 systolic or 15 diastolic BP) that develops during pregnancy and regresses postpartum (usually within 10 d)
- Gestational hypertension with proteinuria (preeclampsia)
  - Clinical triad of HTN, proteinuria, and edema (not always seen)
  - Classified as either mild or severe
- Eclampsia
  - Preeclampsia with seizures or coma
  - Signs and Symptoms:
    - History:
      - Swelling of face, hands, feet
      - Excessive weight gain
      - Headache
      - Visual disturbances
      - Seizures
      - Dyspnea
      - Right upper quadrant (RUQ) or epigastric abdominal pain
    - Physical Exam:
      - HEENT: facial edema, scotomas, loss of peripheral vision
      - Respiratory: crackles (pulmonary edema)
      - Cardiovascular: S3, S4, murmurs (CHF)
      - Abdominal: RUQ tenderness
      - Neurological: hyperreflexia, clonus
      - Fetal evaluation: abnormal FHR, NST, BPP

Gestational Diabetes Mellitus:

- Glucose intolerance present only in pregnancy
- Signs and Symptoms:
  - Asymptomatic, therefore must screen
- Investigations:
  - Screening (at 24-28 wk):
    - Oral glucose challenge test (OGCT): 50 g oral glucose
  - Confirmation (if OGCT abnormal)
    - Oral glucose tolerance test (OGTT): 75 g oral glucose including fasting, measure blood glucose 1 h and 2 h later
- Effects of diabetes on pregnancy
  - Increased perinatal loss
  - Increased incidence of fetal abnormalities
  - Macrosomia (large fetus size)
  - Delayed lung maturation
- Management:
  - Treated nutritionally: focus on complex vs. simple carbohydrates and limiting intake to 35-40% of diet, restricting calories in overweight and obese patients to 25 kcal/kg body weight
  - Addition of insulin or oral antidiabetic agents if maternal glucose levels and/or fetal size parameters indicate risk[8]

Other Conditions:

- Rhesus Discrepancies: 10% deliveries; with treatment only affects 0.5%
  - Sensitization of Rh negative mother to Rh positive blood from fetus
  - Prevention by blood typing and administering Rh immune globulin (RhIg) injection

- UTI: 4% pregnancies
- Anemia: 3/4 of cases due to iron deficiency; deficient RBC production due to increased iron and folate demands
- Hyperemesis gravidarum: intractable N/V in T1, T2; in 3.5 of 1000 pregnancies

5.2 Antenatal Complications

Miscarriage

- 40% caused by fetal abnormality (e.g. structural, chromosomal, genetic)
- Signs and Symptoms:
  - Crampy pelvic pain
  - Vaginal bleeding
  - Eventual expulsion of tissues
- Investigations:
  - Serum β-hCG (will be decreasing)
  - Ultrasound
- Management:
  - Follow-up ultrasound to confirm expulsion of all tissues
- Complications:
  - Retained products of conception resulting in infection which causes pain, fever, and potentially sepsis

Ectopic Pregnancy

- Most commonly occurs in fallopian tube, especially ampulla (80%)
- Signs and Symptoms:
  - Vague lower abdominal pain (95% of cases)
  - Minimal vaginal bleeding (50-80% of cases)
  - Catastrophic shock if ruptured
- Investigations:
  - Serum β-hCG
  - Pelvic ultrasound
  - Sometimes laparoscopy
- Management:
  - Surgical resection
  - Medical (methotrexate)

Abruptio Placentae (see **Table 14**):

- Premature separation of normally implanted placenta
- Hemorrhage from decidual spiral arteries
- Signs and Symptoms:
  - Dark red, painful vaginal bleeding in 80% of cases, internal/concealed (no visible vaginal bleeding) in 20% of cases

Placenta Previa (see **Table 14**):

- Occurs in 1 in 150-250 births in T3
- Abnormal location of placenta at or near the cervical os
  - Low-lying (NOT a previa)
  - Marginal
  - Partial
  - Total
- More than 90% resolve by T3
- Signs and Symptoms:
  - Bright red, painless bleeding at 30 wk
- Patient should be delivered by C/S
- Do not perform vaginal exams and counsel against coitus

OBSTETRIC

Table 14. Placenta Previa vs. Abruptio Placentae

Feature	Placenta Previa	Abruptio Placentae
Onset of Symptoms	Depends on degree of previa Mean: 30 wk GA 1/3 present before 30 wk GA	After 20 wk GA
Vaginal Bleeding	Painless and recurrent Bright red blood	Painful Dark, bright or clotted blood
Uterus	Soft, nontender	Tender, increased tone
Diagnosis	U/S	Clinical

Premature Rupture of Membranes (PROM)

- Rupture of fetal membranes prior to onset of labor
- Signs and Symptoms:
  - Pooling of fluid in vaginal vault
  - Valsalva fluid leakage from cervical os
- Investigations:
  - Nitrazine paper indicator: turns blue with amniotic fluid (also with blood, urine, and semen)
  - Ferning: allow fluid to evaporate on slide; if amniotic fluid, pattern visible on microscopy
    - Gold standard test
- Management:
  - Delivery

5.3 Labor and Postpartum

Breech Presentation

- Presentation of fetal buttocks or lower extremities into the maternal pelvis
- Occurs in about 3-4% of term pregnancies vs. 30% at 30 wk
- 3 types:
  - Complete (5-10%)
    - Thighs and knees flexed, feet above buttocks
  - Frank (50-75%)
    - Thighs flexed, knees extended
  - Footling (20%)
    - Single: one thigh extended; foot is presenting part
    - Double: both thighs extended
- Investigations:
  - Leopold maneuvers
  - U/S
- May be avoided with successful external cephalic version (attempted after 34 wk)
- Management:
  - Delivery: best done by C/S, but vaginal breech delivery is an option

Postpartum Depression (see **Postpartum Depression**, p.223)

REFERENCES

1. Janssen PA, Holt VL, Sugg NK, Emanuel I, Critchlow CM, Henderson AD. 2003. Intimate partner violence and adverse pregnancy outcomes: A population-based study. *Am J Obstet Gynecol* 188(5):1341-1347.
2. Daoud N, Urquia ML, O'Campo P, Heaman M, Janssen PA, Smylie J, et al. 2012. Prevalence of abuse and violence before, during, and after pregnancy in a national sample of Canadian women. *Am J Public Health* 102(10):1893-1901.
3. Liston R, Sawchuck D, Young D, Society of Obstetrics and Gynaecologists of Canada, British Columbia Perinatal Health Program. 2007. Fetal health surveillance: Antepartum and intrapartum consensus guideline. *J Obstet Gynaecol Can* 29(Suppl 4):S3-56.
4. Manning FA, Platt LD, Sipos L. 1980. Antepartum fetal evaluation development of a fetal biophysical profile. *Am J Obstet Gynecol* 136(5):787-795.
5. Steer P, Flint C. 1999. ABC of labour care: Physiology and management of normal labour. *BMJ* 318(7186):793-796.
6. Chamberlain G, Steer P. 1999. ABC of labour care: Operative delivery. *BMJ* 318(7193):1260-1264.
7. O'Hara MW, McCabe JE. 2013. Postpartum depression: Current status and future directions. *Annu Rev Clin Psychol* 9:379-407.
8. Buchanan TA, Xiang AH, Page KA. 2012. Gestational diabetes mellitus: Risks and management during and after pregnancy. *Nat Rev Endocrinol* 8(11):639-649.
9. Chalmers I, Erkin M, Keirse MJNC (Editors). *A Guide to Effective Care in Pregnancy and Childbirth*. Oxford: Oxford University Press; 2000.
10. Hacker NF, Gambone JC, Moore JG. *Essentials of Obstetrics and Gynecology*. Philadelphia: Saunders; 2009.

The Ophthalmological Exam

Editors:
Harleen Bedi
Yao Wang

Faculty Reviewers:
Alan Berger, MD, FRCS(C)
Kenneth Eng, MD, FRCS(C)
Nupura Bakshi, MD, FRCS(C)
Daniel Weisbrod, MD, FRCS(C)

TABLE OF CONTENTS

GLOSSARY

Common Abbreviations:

- OD (oculus dexter) = right eye
- OS (oculus sinister) = left eye
- OU (oculus uterque) = both eyes

Common Prefixes and Suffixes:

- *presby-* = old
- *core-* = pupil
- *blepharo-* = eyelid
- *kerato-* = cornea
- *dacryo-* = tear
- *-phakos/-phakic* = lens
- *-opsia* = vision

1. ESSENTIAL ANATOMY

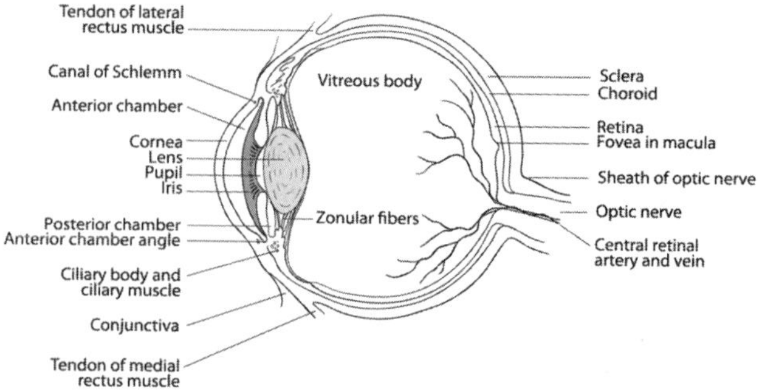

Figure 1. Anatomy of the Eye

2. DEFINITION OF REFRACTIVE ERROR

- Emmetropia: no refractive error
- Myopia: nearsightedness
  - **LMM** = **L**ong eyeball, **M**yopic (nearsighted), corrected with a **M**inus lens
- Hyperopia: farsightedness
  - Light rays focused beyond retina; correct with a plus lens or accommodation
- Presbyopia: decreased accommodation with aging (not a true refractive problem)
  - Correct with a positive lens for reading
- Astigmatism: nonspherical cornea or lens; light rays not refracted uniformly
  - Correct with a cylindrical lens

3. APPROACH TO THE OPHTHALMOLOGICAL HISTORY AND PHYSICAL EXAM

Overview of the History

In addition to general history taking, aspects of the ophthalmological history include:

- Ocular symptoms (see **Ocular Symptoms: Common Chief Complaints**)
- Past ocular history (e.g. corrective lens use, prior trauma, surgery, infections, eye diseases)
- Past medical history (for ocular effects of systemic diseases)
- Family history of eye disease
- Ocular and systemic medications

Overview of the Physical Exam

- Visual acuity (distance/near with correction)
- Visual fields (by confrontation)
- Pupillary examination (with hand-held light)
- External exam (orbit and **4 L**'s, see below)
- Extraocular muscle evaluation (motility, alignment)
- Slit lamp (front to back: sclera/conjunctiva to back of lens)
- Intraocular pressure (applanation or indentation)
- Fundoscopy (direct covered here, indirect more advanced)

4. FOCUSED HISTORY

Ocular Symptoms: Common Chief Complaints

- Pain
- Loss of vision: sudden vs. gradual, transient vs. prolonged, central vs. peripheral, binocular vs. monocular
- Drooping eyelid (ptosis)
- Redness
- Double vision (diplopia)
- Tearing
- Dryness (sicca)
- Foreign body sensation
- Itchy (pruritus)
- Discharge
- Eyelid crusting
- Eyelid swelling
- Floaters
- Flashes (photopsia)
- Halos
- Sensitivity to light (photophobia)
- Headache

Pain

Associated with:

- Blinking (e.g. corneal abrasions, foreign bodies, keratitis)
- Eye movement (e.g. optic neuritis)
- Headache and nausea (e.g. acute angle-closure glaucoma)
- Brow or temporal pain (e.g. may indicate temporal arteritis)
- Photophobia (e.g. iritis, corneal irritation)
- Irritation or "gritty sensation" (e.g. blepharitis, conjunctivitis, corneal abrasion)

Table 1. Common Differential Diagnoses for Pain and Possible Interpretation

	Acute Conjunctivitis	Acute Iritis	Acute Angle-Closure Glaucoma	Corneal Abrasion
History	Sudden onset	Fairly sudden onset, often recurrent	Rapid onset, possible previous attack	Trauma, pain
Vision	Normal, discharge may mildly obscure	Impaired if untreated	Impaired and permanently lost if untreated	Can be affected if central
Pain	Gritty feeling	Photophobia, tenderness	Severe	Sharp
Bilateral	Frequent	Occasional	Rarely	Not usually
Vomiting	Absent	Absent	Common	Absent
Cornea	Clear	Variable	Cloudy/ edematous	Irregular light reflex
Pupil	Normal, reactive	Sluggishly reactive, may be irregular shape, usually miotic	Partially dilated, nonreactive, oval	Normal, reactive
Iris	Normal	Nonreactive due to synechiae	Hard to see due to corneal edema	Defect shadow often detected on iris
Ocular Discharge	Watery and mucopurulent	Watery	Watery	Watery or mucopurulent
Prognosis	Self-limited	Poor (untreated)	Poor (untreated)	Good

Red Eye

Causes for a red eye can be divided into traumatic and nontraumatic:

Table 2. Traumatic vs. Nontraumatic Causes of Red Eye

Traumatic Red Eye	Nontraumatic Red Eye
Corneal abrasion*	Blepharitis
Corneal foreign body*	Conjunctivitis*
Foreign body under eyelid*	Subconjunctival hemorrhage*
Hyphema*	Iritis*
UV keratitis	Orbital or periorbital cellulitis*
Chemical injury	Herpes simplex keratitis*
Intraocular foreign body	Acute angle-closure glaucoma
Corneal laceration	Episcleritis
	Scleritis

*Common

Further questions to ask:
- Associated eye pain or discharge?
- Contact with anyone with a red eye?

Diplopia (Double Vision)
- Due to misalignment of the eyes (compensatory head postures may be used)
- Can be with both eyes open (binocular) or noted only in one eye or with one eye open (monocular)
- Occurs in one or multiple fields of gaze when cranial nerves are affected

Table 3. Causes of Diplopia

Classification	Example
Ocular Motor Palsies	Cranial nerves III, IV, VI
Trauma	Blowout fracture
Thyroid Abnormalities	Graves' disease
Autoimmune Disease	Myasthenia gravis
Inflammatory	MS
Endocrine	DM (pupil-sparing)
Other	Brainstem lesions, Circle of Willis aneurysms, neoplasm

- Common causes of binocular diplopia are CN palsies, strabismus, and dysthyroid orbitopathy; common cause of monocular diplopia is a cataract

Loss of Vision

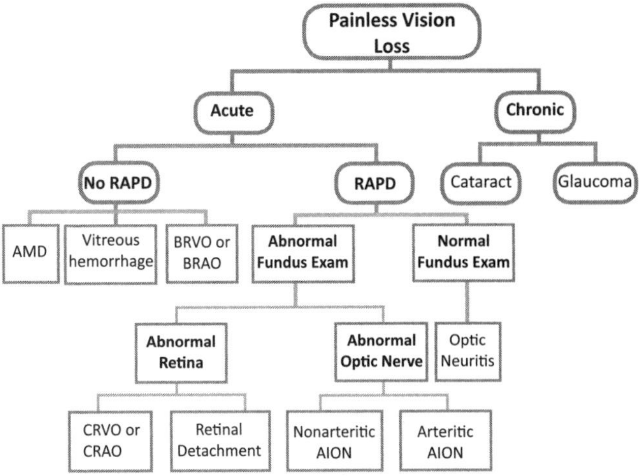

Figure 2. Common Causes of Painless Vision Loss
AION = anterior ischemic optic neuropathy, AMD = age-related macular degeneration, BRVO/BRAO = branch retinal vein/artery occlusion, CRVO/CRAO = central retinal vein/artery occlusion, RAPD = relative afferent pupillary defect

- 3 common causes of acute painful vision loss: acute angle-closure glaucoma, acute iritis, optic neuritis (may or may not be painful)
- ***Note:*** chronic vision loss can still present as sudden or unrecognized by patient and can result from any of the acute causes

Table 4. Other Common Visual Eye Symptoms and Disease States

Visual Symptom	Possible Causes
Colored Halos Around Light	Acute angle-closure glaucoma, opacities in lens or cornea
Color Vision Changes	Cataracts (rarely noticed by patient), drugs (e.g. digitalis increases yellow vision, Viagra® can cause a blue hue)
Difficulty Seeing in Dim Light	Myopia, vitamin A deficiency, retinal degeneration, cataract, diabetic retinopathy
Distortion of Vision	Wet age-related macular degeneration, macular pucker, central serous retinopathy, diabetic macular edema, macular hole
Flashes (photopsias) and Floaters	Migraine, retinal tear/detachment, posterior vitreous detachment, vitritis, vitreous hemorrhage, choroiditis
Glare, Photophobia	Iritis, cataracts
Loss of Visual Field or Presence of Shadow or Curtain	Retinal detachment or hemorrhage, branch retinal vein or arterial occlusion, NAION or AION, chronic glaucoma, stroke

(N)AION = (non) anterior ischemic optic neuropathy

Table 5. Common Nonvisual Ocular Symptoms with Possible Causes

Nonvisual Symptom	Possible Causes
Discharge	Watery: allergy/viral infection Mucoid (yellow): allergy/viral infection Purulent (creamy white/yellow): bacterial infection
Dryness	Decreased secretion due to aging, corneal abrasion, damage to lacrimal apparatus, dry-eye syndrome, Graves' disease, Bell's palsy, Sjögren's syndrome, anticholinergic drugs
Eyelid Swelling	Chalazion, stye, conjunctivitis, cellulitis, dermatitis, systemic edema, dacryocystitis
Protrusion of Eyes	Graves' proptosis, aging changes in the lid, retrobulbar tumor
Itching	Dry eyes, eye fatigue, allergies
Sandiness, Grittiness	Conjunctivitis
Tearing	Hypersecretion of tears, blockage of drainage, cholinergic drugs, ocular inflammation, abnormal lid positions, corneal abrasion/keratitis, normal emotion

Past Ocular History

- Use of eyeglasses and/or contact lenses: duration, frequency, cleaning practice
- Previous eye surgery, laser treatment, infections, trauma, foreign body presence (e.g. metal workers)
- Presence of chronic eye disease such as amblyopia, glaucoma, cataracts, macular degeneration, diabetic retinopathy

Past Medical History

- Systemic diseases: many have ocular sequelae (e.g. DM, HTN, thyroid, autoimmune, systemic infections such as HIV, MS, connective tissue disorders)
- Lung disease and kidney stones are possible contraindications for the prescription of topical β-blockers and carbonic anhydrase inhibitors, respectively
- Allergies: rhinoconjunctivitis (hay fever)

Family History

- Corneal disease, glaucoma, cataracts, retinal disease, strabismus, amblyopia
- Family history of systemic diseases that can affect eyes (see **Past Medical History**, above)

Medications

- Ocular medications, current and prior use
- Common topical ocular medications include the following:
  - Anti-infectives (antibacterial, antivirals)
  - Anti-inflammatories (anti-allergy, NSAIDs, steroids)
  - Glaucoma drops:
    - Carbonic anhydrase inhibitors
    - Adrenergic agonists
    - Prostaglandin analogues
    - Mitotic agents
    - β-blockers

- Many systemic medications have ocular side effects (e.g. corticosteroids can cause glaucoma, cataracts, and central serous retinopathy)

5. FOCUSED PHYSICAL EXAM

5.1 Visual Acuity (VA)

- Tests the integrity of the macula, optic nerve, optic tract, and visual cortex
- Test distance and near vision for best corrected visual acuity (BCVA, i.e. with glasses/contacts); one eye at a time (right eye first) with the other eye occluded
- A pinhole occluder improves vision in an eye with uncorrected refractive error but NOT neural lesion or media opacity (e.g. pinhole can help with cataract sometimes if the cataract has caused a shift in refractive error)
- Legal blindness = 20/200 best corrected visual acuity (BCVA) in better eye or <20° of binocular visual field
- Canadian Ophthalmological Society recommends 20/50 BCVA with both eyes open, and a continuous visual field of 120° horizontally plus 15° both above and below fixation for driving in Canada

Distance Visual Acuity Testing

- Snellen chart: test at 20 ft (6 m)
- Recorded as a ratio: the numerator is the testing distance for the patient; the denominator is the distance at which a normal eye can read the line of letters
  - e.g. 20/100 = the patient can read at 20 feet what a "normal" eye can read at 100 feet
- If the patient cannot see the largest letters, then test VA from a closer distance and record a new numerator as the new distance (e.g. 5/70)
- If unable to read letters at closer distance, then do the following from patient's best distance:
  1. **Count Fingers** (CF): (e.g. CF 1 ft)
  2. **Hand Motion** (HM): (e.g. HM 2 ft)
  3. **Light Perception** (LP) with a penlight: (e.g. LP or NLP)

$\overline{\text{SC}}$

V 20/70+1 → 20/60 PH
HM 1 FT

VA of R eye is recorded first
CC = corrected acuity (i.e. with glasses); **SC** = uncorrected acuity

- **20/70+1** = all of 20/70 plus one letter of 20/50
- **20/60 PH** = improved VA with pinhole occluder
- **CF 3 ft** = counting fingers at 3 ft; **HM 1 ft** = hand motion at 1 ft; **LP (with projection)** = light perception (with projection); **NLP** = no light perception

Near Visual Acuity Testing

- Test if near vision complaint or if distance testing is difficult (e.g. no vision chart available)
- Use pocket vision chart with or without correction (e.g. Rosenbaum Pocket Vision Screener **found on the inside back cover**)
- Test at 14 in (30 cm) and record as Jaeger values (e.g. J2 at 14 in), which can be converted to distance equivalent (e.g. 20/30)

Testing of Patients Who Cannot Read
- Use tumbling "E" chart or Landolt "C" chart with the patient describing/motioning the direction of the "E" or "C"
- Picture chart and the Sheridan-Gardiner matching test are often used for children between 2-4 yr and adults with expressive aphasia

5.2 Color Vision
- Ishihara pseudoisochromatic plates
- Assess macula/optic nerve function; often in pediatrics to screen for color blindness

5.3 Confrontation Visual Field Testing
- Approximates large field defects in the four quadrants of each eye
- Testing the patient's right eye:
  - Sit ~3 feet directly in front of the patient and close your right eye
  - Tell patient to cover left eye and focus right eye on your open left eye
  - Hold up 1 or 2 fingers in each quadrant (one quadrant at a time) and ask the patient to count fingers while looking at your nose or open eye
- Repeat for the patient's left eye by covering the patient's right eye
- Note any areas of field loss and record as below:

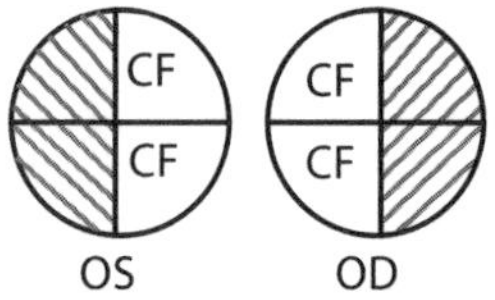

- Normal monocular visual field: 100° temporally, 60° nasally, 60° superiorly, and 75° inferiorly
- Blind spot: 15° temporal to fixation, below the horizontal meridian
- Amsler grid: tests central or paracentral scotomas
- Formal perimetry: Goldmann, Humphrey

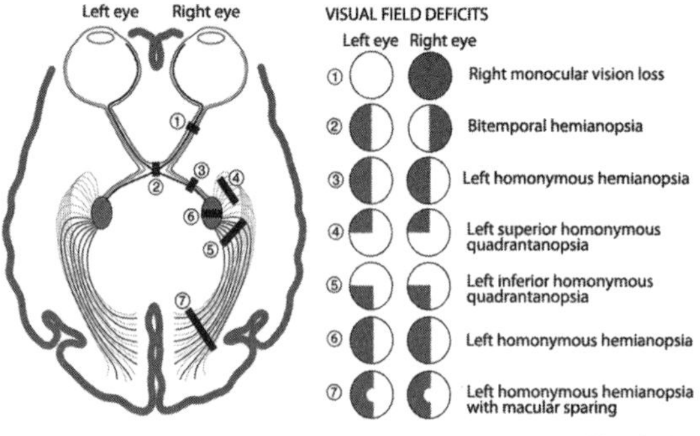

Marta Scythes

Figure 3. Brain Lesions and the Resulting Visual Field Defects

5.4 Pupil Examination (see **Neurological Exam**, p.177)
- Ask patient to fixate on distant target in dimly-lit room room
- Shine a penlight obliquely to both pupils; assess pupil size, shape, and symmetry (measure using the pupil gauge found on the near vision card)
- Common causes of anisocoria (asymmetrical pupils): physiologic, CN III palsy, Horner's syndrome, ocular trauma or inflammation, mydriatic eyedrops, recreational drugs, ocular surgery

Pupillary Light Reflex

- Shine penlight directly into the right eye and observe symmetric pupillary constriction in the right eye (direct response) and the left eye (consensual response)
- 3+ to 4+ = pupil constricts rapidly and completely; 1+ to 2+ = slowly and incompletely; 0 = does not constrict

Table 6. Differential Diagnosis of Constricted and Dilated Pupils

Constricted Pupil	Dilated Pupil
Horner's syndrome	CN III palsy
Iritis	Acute glaucoma
Drug-induced*	Drug-induced†; Adie's pupil (mostly considered normal variant); post-trauma

*Parasympathetic activation and/or sympathetic block
†Sympathetic activation and/or parasympathetic block

Swinging Light Test (see **Neurological Exam**, p.178)

- Swing light from one pupil to the other to assess relative afferent pupillary defect (RAPD)/Marcus Gunn pupil
- Pupil dilation in either eye as the light is shone on it indicates a RAPD, a sign of an optic nerve or retinal lesion
- Common causes of RAPD: optic neuritis, ischemic optic neuropathy, central retinal artery or vein occlusion, retinal detachment

Accommodation Reflex

- Ask patient to look into the distance and then at an object (e.g. your finger) positioned 10 cm from the patient's nose
- Observe normal pupil constriction and eye convergence

Clinical Pearl: Recording a Normal Pupil Exam
Record normal pupil examination as "PERRLA": Pupils Equal, Round, Reactive to Light and Accommodation.

5.5 External Ocular Examination

- Inspect the orbits looking for exophthalmos (protruding eye) and enophthalmos (sunken eye)
- Inspect the **4 L**'s (see **Figure 4**):
  - **Lymph Nodes:** preauricular, submandibular nodes
  - **Lids:**
    - Ptosis, swelling (allergy), crusting, xanthelasma (lipid deposits), smooth opening and closure, entropion/ectropion (inversion/eversion)
    - Chalazion: chronic inflammation of meibomian gland; localized painless swelling
    - Hordeolum/stye: acute inflammation of meibomian gland
    - Blepharitis: chronic inflammation of lid
  - **Lashes:**
    - Direction and condition
    - Trichiasis: inward turned lashes
  - **Lacrimal Apparatus:**
    - Tearing, obstruction, discharge, swelling
    - Dacryocystitis: infection of lacrimal sac
    - Keratoconjunctivitis sicca: dry eye syndrome
    - Epiphora: excessive tearing

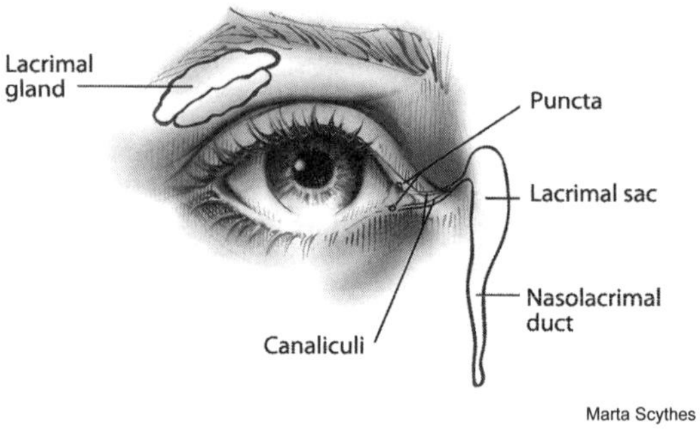

Figure 4. Lacrimal Apparatus

5.6 Upper Lid Eversion

- To look for foreign bodies or other conjunctival lesions
- May require topical anesthetic
- As patient looks down, grasp eyelashes and upper lid between thumb and index finger; with other hand, place cotton tip applicator gently on the skin at the lid fold (8 mm above lid margin), and press down as the lid margin is pulled up by the lashes

5.7 Extraocular Muscle Evaluation (see **Neurological Exam,** p.177)

Motility

- Smooth pursuit: instruct patient to follow an object (e.g. tip of pen) in six cardinal positions of gaze; look for nystagmus (horizontal, vertical, or rotator) and ask patient to report diplopia (double vision) in any position of gaze
- Saccadic movement: instruct patient to shift gaze rapidly from your index finger (positioned in the periphery) to your nose

Alignment

- Strabismus: any type of ocular misalignment. Use the following tests:
  - **Hirschberg Corneal Reflex Test:** ask patient to fixate on a distant object. Shine penlight into both eyes from ~14 in (30 cm) away. Aligned eyes show symmetric light reflection near the center of both corneas. Misaligned eyes show displacement of corneal reflection in one eye
  - **Cover Test:** ask patient to fixate on a distant object. Cover the patient's right eye with a hand or an occluder, and observe for positional shift in the left eye. Rapidly change the cover to the patient's left eye, and observe for shift in the right eye. Positional shift in the non-covered eye indicates presence of a tropia (a manifest or apparent deviation)
  - **Cover-Uncover Test:** ask patient to fixate on a distant object. Cover the patient's right eye and then uncover it. Repeat for the left eye. Positional shift in the testing eye upon uncovering indicates presence of a phoria (a latent deviation not apparent when both eyes are fixating)

Table 7. Possible Outcomes of Eye Alignment Tests

	Eye Movement*			
	Outward	**Inward**	**Up**	**Down**
Tropia	Esotropic	Exotropic	Hypotropic	Hypertropic
Phoria	Esophoric	Exophoric	Hypophoric	Hyperphoric

*Tropia (constant misalignment) vs. phoria (latent deviation); eso/exo/hypo/hyper describe movement of eye during the application of the cover in each test

Common Causes of Motility/Alignment Defects
- Congenital and late-onset strabismus, cranial nerve palsies, Graves' disease, myasthenia gravis, stroke, brain tumor, and orbital trauma

5.8 Slit Lamp Examination
- Provides binocular, stereoscopic, and magnified views of all structures of the anterior segment of each eye, including eyelid, sclera, conjunctiva, cornea, iris, anterior chamber, and lens
- Stereoscopic view of the fundus and vitreous can be obtained with special lenses (78 or 90 diopter)
- Using a cobalt blue filter, corneal abrasions can be visualized upon staining with fluorescein dye

Pupillary Dilation (Mydriasis)
- Mydriatics provide significantly better viewing of the lens, vitreous, and retina
- Contraindications: narrow angles, acute angle-closure glaucoma
- Usually with tropicamide 1% and phenylephrine hydrochloride 2.5%
- Wait 15-20 min after instilling mydriatic to allow dilation to occur
- To instill eye drop:
  - Seat patient, tilt head back, have patient look up, pull down on lower eyelid
  - Instill drop into sac made by lower eyelid and globe
  - Instruct patient to close eyes for a few seconds, provide a clean tissue

Anterior Segment
- Examine the following structures of the anterior segment:
  - Lids and lashes (with lids everted if necessary)
  - Conjunctiva
    - Blood vessel dilatation, pigment, pallor, hemorrhage, redness (note pattern), swelling, nodules
    - Pinguecula: areas of benign elastotic degeneration of the conjunctiva near the nasal or temporal limbus
    - Pterygium: growth of fibrovascular tissue of the conjunctiva onto cornea
  - Sclera
    - Nodules, redness, discoloration (jaundice)
    - Episcleritis: self-limiting inflammation of the episclera, asymptomatic or with mild pain
    - Scleritis: bilateral, severely painful red eye with photophobia and decreased vision
  - Cornea
    - Abrasion, foreign body, clarity/opacity, scarring, ulceration
    - Keratitis: inflammation of cornea with pain, redness, and tearing with blinking
    - Corneal edema: cornea with irregular reflection and haze

- » Arcus senilis: white ring of lipid deposits in peripheral cornea related to atherosclerosis
  - » Kayser-Fleischer ring: Wilson's disease
  - » AFTER examining corneal clarity, use fluorescein dye and cobalt blue filter to visualize corneal abrasions, ulcers, and foreign bodies; Rose Bengal dye for devitalized corneal epithelium
- o Anterior chamber
  - » Examine for blood (hyphema), pus (hypopyon), cells (graded 1+ to 4+)
  - » Depth measurement:
    - Slit lamp: direct narrow beam onto peripheral cornea at an oblique angle of 60°; chamber is shallow if distance between corneal endothelium and iris surface ≤1/4 of corneal thickness
    - Penlight: shine light at an oblique angle from the temporal side of the head; chamber is shallow if ≥2/3 of nasal iris is covered by the shadow

> **Clinical Pearl: Ulcers vs. Abrasions**
> To differentiate corneal ulcers from abrasions, view the cornea before staining with fluorescein. Ulcers have an opaque base, whereas abrasions have a clear base.

- o Iris
  - » Cysts, nodules, color differences between eyes (congenital Horner's), neovascularization, synechiae (adhesions to cornea or lens)
  - » Iritis/anterior uveitis: unilateral, usually accompanied by concurrent inflammation of ciliary body, iridocyclitis
- o Lens
  - » Opacities (cataracts), dislocation, intraocular lens implant

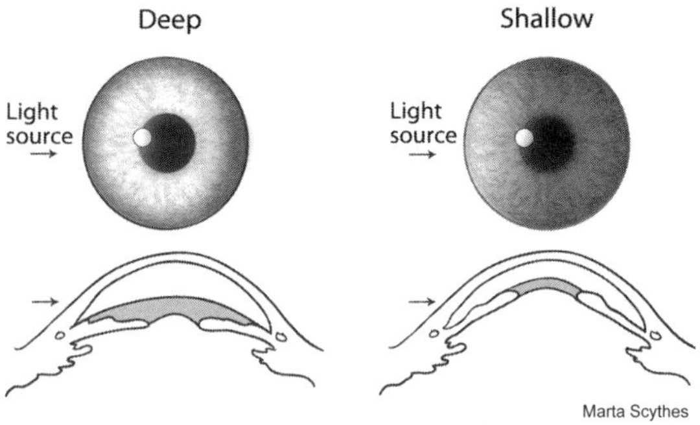

Figure 5. Anterior Chamber Depth Assessment

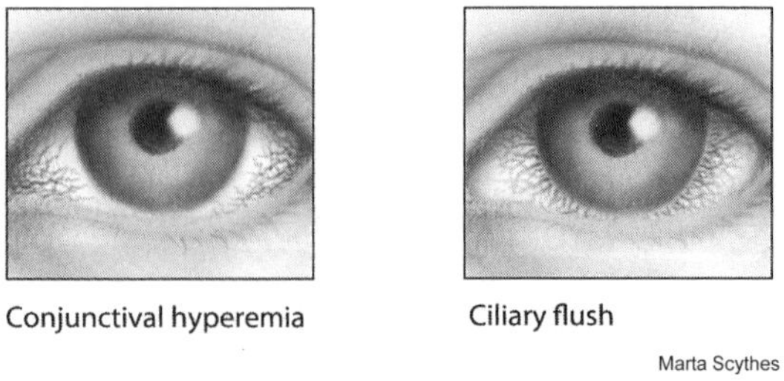

Figure 6. Conjunctival Hyperemia vs. Ciliary Flush

OPHTHALMOLOGICAL

Intraocular Pressure (IOP) Measurement

- Normal = 10-21 mmHg, mean = 16 mmHg
- Elevated IOP a risk factor for glaucoma
- Measured by:
  - Applanation: Goldmann applanation tonometry (GAT) using slit lamp, gold standard
    - Tono-pen is widely utilized as a handheld, portable instrument that provides IOP readings that correlate closely with GAT
  - Indentation: Tono-pen or Schiotz; topical anesthetic with patient supine
  - Noncontact applanation: air-puff tonometry

5.9 Direct Ophthalmoscopy/Fundoscopy

- Filters: red-free (visualize blood vessels and hemorrhages); polarizing (reduce corneal reflection); cobalt blue (corneal abrasions upon fluorescein stain)
- Red numbers = minus lenses for myopic eye; green numbers = plus lenses for hyperopic eye
- Technique:
  - Hold the ophthalmoscope in your R hand and use your R eye to examine the patient's R eye
  - Use large aperture for dilated pupil, small aperture for undilated pupil. Use low light intensity!
  - Set the focusing wheel at +5 and begin to look at the R eye at 1 foot away to detect the red reflex
  - Slowly come closer to the patient at 15° temporally until <2 inches from the eye (as close as possible!). Turn the focusing wheel in the negative direction until patient's retina comes into focus
  - Follow a retinal vessel until it widens into the optic disc (nasal to the macula). Examine the following landmarks in order:
    - Optic disc: size, shape, color, margin (normal = sharp), symmetry, hemorrhages, elevation, cup-to-disc ratio (normal <0.5)
    - Retinal vessels: arteries are thinner and have a brighter reflex than veins. Follow arteries from the disc and veins back to the disc in each quadrant, noting arteriovenous (A/V) crossing patterns
    - Retinal background: color (normal red-orange), pigmentation, lesions (diffuse flecks, flame-shaped, cotton wool spots)
    - Macula: ask patient to look directly into the light; usually appears darker than surrounding retina and produces the foveolar reflex
  - Repeat for the L eye (use L hand and L eye to examine patient's L eye)

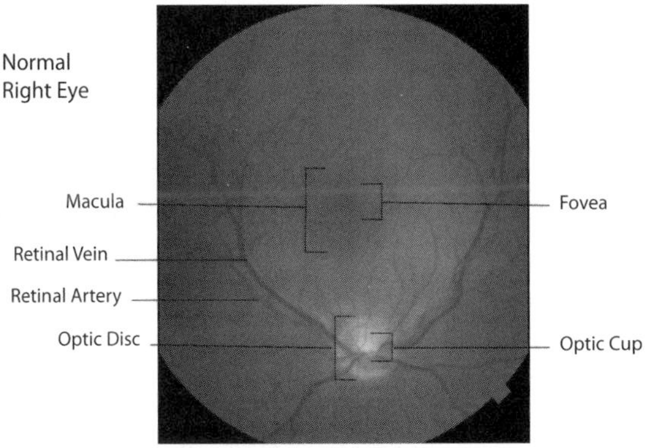

Figure 7. Fundoscopy Examination View
Dr. Kenneth Eng, 2013.

OPHTHALMOLOGICAL

Red Reflex

- Shine ophthalmoscope light into the pupils from ~30 cm away and look through the viewer
- Observe for evenness of color, presence of shadows/opacities
- An eye with clear ocular media (cornea, anterior chamber, lens, and vitreous) gives off bilaterally even red reflexes
- Common causes of abnormal red reflex (absent or dull): corneal scar, hyphema (blood in aqueous humor), cataract, vitreous hemorrhage, vitritis (infectious/noninfectious), large refractive error, ocular misalignment

> **Clinical Pearl: Pupillary Reflexes and Dark Irises**
> When checking pupillary reflexes in patients with dark irises, use the ophthalmoscope to focus on the red reflex to get a better view than using a penlight.

Table 8. Findings on Ophthalmoscopy

Retinal Disease	Findings on Ophthalmoscopy
Diabetic Retinopathy	
Nonproliferative	Retinal hemorrhages, microaneurysms, cotton wool spots, exudates
Proliferative	Neovascularization, vitreous hemorrhage
Central Retinal Artery Occlusion (CRAO)	Whitened retina, cherry red spot in macula ± plaque
Central Retinal Vein Occlusion (CRVO)	Dilated, tortuous veins, flame-shaped hemorrhages, cotton wool spots, optic disc hyperemia/edema
Hypertensive Retinopathy	Arteriolar narrowing, and straightening with areas of silver-wire appearance, changes in arteriovenous crossings, cotton wool spots, flame-shaped hemorrhages, disc edema
Papilledema	Optic disc edema, blurred elevated disc margins, ± flame-shaped hemorrhages
Glaucomatous Optic Neuropathy	Increased cup-to-disc ratio, asymmetric cup size between eyes, cup approaching disc margin, notching, optic nerve pallor, vessel displacement in disc
Retinal Detachment	Elevated retinal folds
Age-Related Macular Degeneration	Drusen (yellow deposits), retinal pigment epithelium atrophy (depigmentation in macula), subretinal fluid, subretinal hemorrhage or lipid

5.10 Application of an Eye Patch

- Can be used for corneal abrasions
- Contraindicated if suspicion of infection present or contact lens wearer
- Instill antibiotic drops if necessary
- With eye closed, apply two patches on the eye, tape patches to eye with moderate pressure using four strips of tape

6. COMMON DISORDERS

Disorders marked with (✓) are discussed in **Common Clinical Scenarios**

Acute Diseases

• Acute conjunctivitis	Inflammation of the conjunctiva (bacterial, viral or allergic)
• Acute iritis	Inflammation of the iris
• Uveitis	Inflammation of the iris, ciliary body, and/ or choroid
• Blepharitis	Inflammation of the eyelid
• Corneal abrasion	Self-limited loss of the corneal epithelium
• Corneal ulcer	Infection of the cornea: deeper than corneal abrasion (i.e. into stroma), with less defined contours
• Anterior ischemic optic neuropathy (AION)	Acute small-vessel infarct of optic nerve head
• Optic neuritis (ON)	Inflammation of the optic nerve (often associated with MS)
• Papilledema	Bilateral optic disc swelling secondary to elevated intracranial pressure
• Retinal vascular occlusion (venous or arterial)	Common cause of sudden unilateral visual loss; due to a blockage/obstruction of the retinal vascular lumen by an embolus or thrombus, or inflammatory/ traumatic vessel wall damage or spasm

✓ Acute angle-closure glaucoma (ACG)

✓ Retinal detachment (RD)

Note: amaurosis fugax is the transient loss of unilateral vision due to an arterial occlusion; an important sign of carotid atheroma

Chronic Diseases

- Strabismus
  - Ocular misalignment
- Amblyopia
  - A neurodevelopmental visual acuity due to inadequate stimulation of the eye(s) during early childhood and cannot be corrected by optical means

✓ Diabetic retinopathy

✓ Age-related macular degeneration (ARMD)

✓ Glaucoma

✓ Cataract

7. COMMON CLINICAL SCENARIOS

7.1 Retinal Detachment (RD)

- Neurosensory retina separates from the underlying retinal pigment epithelium
- Classification:
  - **Rhegmatogenous:** most common type; happens in the setting of a retinal tear, often due to detachment of the vitreous humor from the retina (posterior vitreous detachment), and subsequent retinal tear
  - **Tractional:** occurs via mechanical forces on the retina; usually mediated by fibrotic tissue resulting from diabetic retinopathy, injury, surgery, infection, inflammation or sickle cell
  - **Exudative (or serous):** results from accumulation of serous and/or hemorrhagic fluid in subretinal space due to hydrostatic factors (e.g. severe acute hypertension), inflammation or neoplastic effusions
- Signs and Symptoms:
  - Retinal tears may occur without symptoms, but often photopsia (light flashes in vision) and/or floaters are noted; if untreated, retinal tears can progress to retinal detachment
  - Acute floaters and acute vision loss; altered red reflex
  - Visual field loss usually in the periphery that progresses toward the central visual axis over hours to weeks
- Risk Factors: aging, cataract surgery, myopia, family history, history of RD in the other eye, trauma, congenital, and diabetic retinopathy
- Treatment:
  - Retinal detachment **is a true ophthalmic emergency**
  - Prevention is best achieved by treating retinal breaks by laser before they progress to retinal detachment
  - Surgical correction usually required for repair
    - Pneumatic Retinopexy: injection of a gas bubble into the vitreous cavity, done if there are few and localized retinal breaks within the superior 8 clock hours (8 to 4 o'clock) of retina
    - Scleral Buckling: affix a silicone band on outside surface of sclera
    - Vitrectomy (more difficult cases): vitreous gel is removed and replaced with a large gas bubble (can be combined with scleral buckling)

7.2 Glaucoma

- Progressive optic neuropathy often associated with elevated intraocular pressure (IOP)
- Categorized into open- and closed-angle forms; as well as primary and secondary forms
- Complication of many other disorders that affect the eye

Table 9. Characteristics of Major Types of Glaucoma

	Congenital Glaucoma	Primary Open-Angle Glaucoma (POAG)	Normal-Tension Glaucoma (NTG)	Acute Angle-Closure Glaucoma
Definition/ Etiology	**Primary Infantile:** abnormal development of anterior chamber **Secondary Infantile:** linked with various ocular and systemic syndromes and surgical aphakia (removal of lens)	Progressive loss of optic nerve without occlusion of outflow tract	A variety of POAG with normal IOP	Iris apposition or adhesion to the trabecular meshwork, causing a decrease in outflow and an increase in IOP and optic nerve damage
Epidemiology	Arises in children <2 yr; seen in 1:10000 to 1:15000 live births in U.S.	2% of general population; 55% of all glaucoma cases; leading cause of irreversible world blindness	A significant proportion of POAG cases	0.1% of general population; older individuals, especially those with hyperopia
Signs	Corneal edema/ clouding, epiphoria and/or red eye, corneal enlargement	Elevated IOP >21, optic nerve cupping, visual field loss especially in the periphery	IOP within normal range, optic nerve cupping ± hemorrhage, peripheral vasospasm, visual field changes	Corneal edema resulting in blurring of red reflex, conjuctival injection, mid-dilated, nonreactive, vertically oval pupil, IOP elevated often due to shallow anterior chamber, flare, and cells in anterior chamber
Risk Factors	Lensectomy, small cornea	IOP >25 mmHg, enlarged optic nerve cup (>0.5 cup-to-disc ratio), age >40 yr, black race, family history, myopia, vascular diseases	Similar to POAG	Family history, age >40 yr, female, family history of angle-closure symptoms, hyperopia, pseudoexfoliation race (Inuit > Asian > Caucasian = African)
Management	Surgical (not medical)	Directed at lowering IOP: medications, laser trabeculoplasty/ trabeculectomy	Directed at lowering IOP: correction of circulatory deficiencies at optic nerve head (theoretical)	Directed at lowering IOP: laser iridotomy or trabeculectomy

IOP = intraocular pressure

EBM: Glaucoma

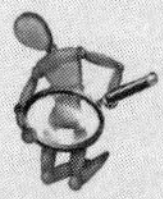

The essential clinical exam for glaucoma should include visual acuity, assessment for relative afferent pupillary defect, IOP (as well as method and time of measurement), central corneal thickness (CCT), gonioscopy, dilated optic disc and fundus evaluation, and VF testing[*].

There is a beneficial effect of immediate therapy to lower the IOP versus late or no treatment on the progression of newly detected open-angle glaucoma, as measured by increasing visual field loss and/or optic disc changes[†].

Topical ocular hypertensive medication is effective in delaying or preventing onset of glaucomatous visual field loss and/or optic disc damage in ocular hypertensive individuals at moderate or high risk for developing primary open-angle glaucoma[‡].

*Canadian Ophthalmological Society Glaucoma Clinical Practice Guideline Expert Committee. 2009. *Can J Ophthalmol* 44(Suppl 1):S1-S93.
†Leske MC, et al. 1999. *Ophthalmology* 106(11):2144-2153.
‡Kass MA, et al. 2002. *Arch Ophthalmol* 120(6):701-713.

7.3 Cataracts

- Clouding and opacification of the crystalline lens of the eye
- Opacity may occur in the cortex, nucleus of the lens, or posterior subcapsular region, but it is usually in a combination of areas
- Epidemiology: highest cause of treatable blindness; peak incidence is >40 yr (senile cataract) and in early life
- Etiology: most are age-related but may be related to heredity, trauma, corticosteroid use (causes posterior subcapsular cataract), radiation, inflammation, DM, and other systemic/congenital illnesses
- Signs and Symptoms: blurred vision, decreased acuity and glare around lights at night; cloudiness and opacification of lens, and altered red reflex on physical exam
- Treatment: surgery to remove the lens and replace with intraocular lens implant

7.4 Age-Related Macular Degeneration (AMD or ARMD)

- A common, chronic degenerative disorder that affects older individuals; severe central visual loss as a result of geographic atrophy, serous detachment of the retinal pigment epithelium (RPE) and choroidal neovascularization (CNV)
- Drusen (small yellowish deposits in the retina) are generally accepted to be precursor lesions when they are soft or indistinct
- Epidemiology: average age at onset of visual loss is about 75 yr
- Risk Factors: female, family history, smoking, age, sunlight exposure, obesity, elevated cholesterol level, HTN
- Classification:
  - **Non-Neovascular (Dry):** 90% of cases; hallmark are multiple drusen; advanced cases develop geographic atrophy (depigmentation or hypopigmentation of RPE), which causes approximately 21% of all cases of legal blindness in North America
  - **Neovascular (Wet):** hallmark is ingrowth of CNV from choriocapillaries under the macular region; less prevalent but responsible for nearly 80% of significant visual disability associated with AMD; more rapid progression of visual loss compared to non-neovascular AMD
- Signs and Symptoms:
  - Subacute onset except in some cases of neovascular AMD, where abrupt visual loss is noted

- Blurred vision or distortion (metamorphopsia) usually bilateral but often asymmetric, may be asymptomatic
  - Decreased reading ability, especially in dim light
  - Clinical exam findings may include drusen, pigmentary changes, subretinal fluid, macular edema, hemorrhage, yellow-green discrete discoloration and/or RPE detachment
- Treatment:
  - **Dry AMD:** vitamin A, C, E and zinc supplementation in patients with moderate to severe dry AMD decreases risk of progression to wet form (Age-Related Eye Disease Study [AREDS] supplement)[1]
  - **Wet AMD with CNV:** intravitreal injections of anti-VEGF; consider referral to the Canadian National Institute for the Blind (CNIB) and low vision aids for those with legal blindness or low vision

7.5 Eye Complications in Diabetes Mellitus

- Diabetic Retinopathy (DR)
  - Progressive dysfunction of the retinal vasculature caused by chronic hyperglycemia
  - Nonproliferative DR: microaneurysms, retinal hemorrhages, retinal lipid exudates, cotton wool spots, capillary nonperfusion, macular edema
  - Proliferative DR: retinal neovascularization
  - Successful management via a combination of glucose control, laser therapy, anti-VEGF drugs, and vitrectomy reduces the risk of severe visual loss
  - Best predictor for the disease is duration of DM (71–90% with DM type 1 for 10 yr have diabetic retinopathy; incidence is slightly lower for type 2)
- Cataracts
- Cornea
- Glaucoma
- Optic Neuropathy

EBM: Diabetic Retinopathy (DR)

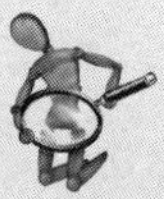

A screening evaluation for DR (within 5 yr of onset for type 1 and 1 yr of onset for type 2) should include measurement of visual acuity, intraocular pressure, and an evaluation to look for the presence of neovascularization of the iris and angle. Pupils should be dilated for the fundus examination, except where non-mydriatic photography is used*.

Early panretinal photocoagulation is recommended for high-risk proliferative DR†.

*Hooper P, et al. 2012. *Can J Ophthalmol* 47(Suppl 1):1-30.
†Early Treatment Diabetic Retinopathy Study Research Group. 1985. *Arch Ophthalmol* 103(12):1796-1806.

Sample Ophthalmology Note[2]

ID: Mrs. A is a retired 50-yr-old African American female.

CC: Patient complains of sudden onset of right eye pain, severe headache, blurred vision, N/V.

HPI: These symptoms began 2 h ago without any inciting event. The patient was watching television when the symptoms began. The patient also reports seeing rainbow colored halos around lights. There is no history of trauma, flashing lights, curtains, metamorphopsia or diplopia.

Vcc: 20/70 / 20/20

P: Mildly dilated, sluggishly responsive to light / Normal
± RAPD

Tap: 52 / 11

Extraocular muscles intact

SLE:
L/L: Normal OU
C/S: Injected conjunctiva OD, normal OS
K: OD demonstrates corneal edema, normal OS
A/C: Shallow anterior chamber OD, normal depth OS
Iris: Appears pushed forward OD, normal OS
Lens: Normal OU
Anterior Vit: Normal OU
Gonioscopy: Closed-angle OD, demonstrating iris bombé; normal angle, but no apparent obstruction of trabecular meshwork OS

DFE:

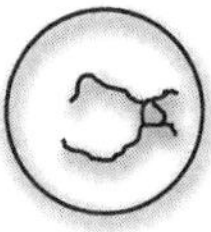

Hazy view through edematous cornea
Macula: normal with no signs of retinal breaks or detachments
Vessels: no AV nicking
Periphery: normal
Disc: cup-to-disc ratio 0.3 OU

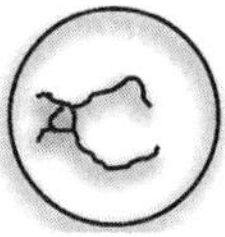

PMH:
Osteoarthritis (knees)

POH:
Mild myopia
No surgeries, laser, injection or other treatment

FH:
Mother: Chronic primary angle-closure glaucoma
No history of macular degeneration, retinal detachment, blindness or autoimmune disorders

Social History:
20 pack yr smoking history
Drinks alcohol on occasion
No illicit drug use

Meds:
Daily Multivitamin
Tylenol 3 PM (uses it about 1 day/month when knee pain worsens

Allergies:
NKDA

Assessment Plan:
- Acute angle-closure glaucoma
- Acetazolamide 500mg IV x 1 to reduce IOP
- Prednisolone acetate 1% to suppress inflammation
- Laser peripheral iridotomy for definitive treatment
- Follow-up with gonioscopy to assess the extent of peripheral anterior synechiae (PAS), and consider fundus exam as clinically indicated

ID (identifying data), **CC** (chief complaint), **HPI** (history of present illness), **Vcc** (vision with glasses), **POH** (past ocular history), **FH** (family history), **SLE** (slit lamp exam), **Ext** (external), L/L (lids and lacrimation), **C/S** (conjunctiva and sclera), **K** (cornea), **A/C** (anterior chamber), **Vit** (vitreous chamber), **NKDA** (no known drug allergies), **DFE** (dilated fundus exam), **OD** (right eye), **OS** (left eye), **OU** (both eyes)

REFERENCES

1. Age-Related Eye Disease Study Research Group. 2001. A randomized, placebo-controlled, clinical trial of high-dose supplementation with vitamins C and E, beta carotene, and zinc for age-related macular degeneration and vision loss: AREDS report no. 8. *Arch Ophthalmol* 119(10):1417-1436.
2. Medical College of Wisconsin. *Department of Ophthalmology Case Studies*. Milwaukee: Medical College of Wisconsin. 2013. Available from: http://www.mcw.edu/ophthalmology/education/ophthcstudies.htm#.UDRCxe1Qh8s.

PEDIATRIC

The Pediatric Exam

Editors:
Thomas McLaughlin
Suparna Sharma

Faculty Reviewers:
Sheila Jacobson, MBBCh, FRCP(C)
Shawna Silver, MD, FAAP, PEng, FRCP(C)

TABLE OF CONTENTS

1. APPROACH TO THE PEDIATRIC EXAM

- Overview
  - Often given by third party: identify relationship with child
  - Observe parent-child interaction for nonverbal cues and family dynamics
  - Allow parent to discuss his/her feelings and acknowledge his/her concerns
  - Ask parents about specific concerns (for hidden or unexpressed fears/agendas)

PEDIATRIC

1.1 Chief Complaint
- There may be more than one CC (e.g. cough, runny nose, and earache)
- Elicit duration and temporal sequence of complaints
- Child's CC may not be the main issue and child may not in fact be the real patient

1.2 History of Presenting Illness
- Use the **OPQRSTUVW** approach:
  - **O**: Onset of symptoms: "When was child last well?" In infants, "When was child last feeding or sleeping well?"
  - **P**: Palliating/Provoking factors: "What makes it better?", "What makes it worse?"
  - **Q**: Quality of symptoms (e.g. for pain, "burning", "sharp" vs. "dull")
  - **R**: Radiation (of pain)
  - **S**: Severity of symptoms
  - **T**: Timing: continuous vs. episodic symptoms, duration, progression over time
  - **U**: How is the illness affecting "U" (i.e. functioning at school, play, activities)
  - **V**: Déjà vu: "Has this ever happened before?"
  - **W**: "What do you think is causing this?"
- Associated Symptoms (e.g. if child presents with a cough, ask about sore throat, runny nose, fever, etc.)
- Risk Factors
  - Similar problems in relatives/daycare contacts?
  - Recent travel
  - Family history of similar problems
  - Related problems (e.g. eczema and asthma)
- Care/interventions prior to this encounter

1.3 Past Medical History
- Prenatal (see **Approach to the Neonate**, p.252)
- Labor and Delivery (see **Approach to the Neonate**, p.253)
- Feeding History (see **Approach to the Neonate**, p.253)
- Growth and Development (see **Table 22** in **Appendix**, p.291)
- Immunizations
  - Which and when? (see **Table 23** in **Appendix**, p.292)
  - Adverse reactions: local, systemic, or allergic
- Allergies
  - Environment, food, and medication: reaction experienced, action taken, time to resolution of symptoms, presence of a viral illness, exercise, heat, cold
  - Family history of atopy (hypersensitivity to environmental allergens)
- Medications, including vitamins and supplements
  - Any recent changes to medications
  - Compliance
  - Recent antibiotic use
- Previous illnesses, hospitalizations, or surgeries
- Other healthcare providers/services involved

1.4 Family History
- Genogram may be helpful
- Ask about consanguinity
- Broader family: congenital abnormalities, allergies, recurrent illnesses, early deaths, frequent miscarriages

1.5 Social History

- Family
  - Extended/reconstituted family, birth parents, custody and access
  - Household: space, pets, occupants, frequency of moves
  - Family dynamics: who cares for child?
  - Support systems, stress/discord/violence
  - Recreation history: "What does the family do as a group?"
  - Major life events (deaths, accidents, separations, divorce)
- Parents
  - Occupational history (prolonged absences, exposures to toxins or infection)
  - Approach to discipline
  - Financial issues/problems (including any social assistance)
  - Substance abuse
- Child
  - Interests and activities
  - School performance
  - Screen time

1.6 Review of Systems

- See age-appropriate sections (**Neonate**, p.252; **Infant and Child**, p.258; **Adolescent**, p.270)

1.7 The Physical Exam

- No history is complete without a physical exam; a full physical exam should be done for every pediatric exam, except in emergency or walk-in situations where a more focused exam may be more appropriate[1]
- Knowledge of adult exam is assumed for pediatric exam. See the following "**Approach to...**" sections for more details on age-specific physical examinations for each organ system

Vital Signs

Temperature

- In children up to 2 yr:
  - For definitive temperature, take rectal temperature:
    - Use disposable slipcovers
    - Lubricate the thermometer prior to insertion. Spread the buttocks and insert a rectal thermometer slowly through the anal sphincter to 1-3 cm; read after 1 min
    - Reading >38°C constitutes fever[2]
- For screening low-risk children, take axillary temperature:
  - Reading >37.3°C constitutes fever

Clinical Pearl: Temperature[3]

Normal rectal temperature > oral temperature > axillary temperature

Method	Normal Temperature
Rectal	36.6-38°C
Tympanic	35.8-38°C
Oral	35.5-37.5°C
Axillary	34.7-37.3°C

Respiratory Rate

- Count breaths for at least 30 s
- Measure RR while baby/child is calm, prior to intrusive procedures

- Place your hand just below the child's xiphoid process or listen to breath sounds through the stethoscope to get an accurate RR
- For each 1°C rise in temperature, the RR increases by ~3 breaths/min

Pulse
- Auscultate or palpate for 15-30 s (sinus arrhythmia is normal)
- For each 1°C rise in temperature, the pulse increases by ~10 beats/min

Blood Pressure
- Measurement is not indicated for those under 3 yr, unless hospitalized or specific indication
- Systolic = 60-70 mmHg
  - Lower limit for children up to 10 yr: 70 + 2(age) mmHg
  - Lower limit for children >10 yr: >90 mmHg
- Diastolic ~2/3 systolic
- In the neonatal period, mean arterial pressure (MAP) should be at least the gestational age

Oxygen Saturation
- For pediatric patients in a hospital setting (or as an outpatient if available), the oxygen saturation is a valuable piece of information
- Can be measured by attaching the probe to any well-perfused body part (e.g. finger, toe, or earlobe)

Table 1. Average Ranges for Pediatric Vital Signs

Age	Respiratory Rate	Heart Rate	Systolic Blood Pressure	Weight (kg)
Infant	30-50	120-160	>60	3-4
6 mo-1 yr	30-40	120-150	70-80	8-10
2-4 yr	20-30	110-140	70-80	12-16
5-8 yr	14-20	90-120	90-100	18-26
8-12 yr	12-20	80-110	100-110	26-50
>12 yr	12-16	60-100	100-120	>50

Schafermeyer R. 1993. *Emerg Med Clin North Am* 11(1):187-205.

2. APPROACH TO THE NEONATE

2.1 Neonatal History
- Follow the outline in **Approach to the Pediatric Exam** p.249, including the following sections:
  - CC, HPI, PMHx, FHx, SHx, ROS
- Inquire about the family's adaptation to the newborn, mother's emotional state (postpartum blues/depression), and supports for the parents
- Ask about future follow-up visits: baby's pediatrician or family doctor
- Common problems: jaundice, poor feeding, weight gain, sleeping, difficulty breathing, cyanosis

Prenatal
- Mother's obstetrical history: previous pregnancies, miscarriages, abortions
- Pregnancy: planned or not, number of weeks, single or multiple pregnancies, complications

- Mother's health during pregnancy: age, hospitalizations, medications, bleeding, illnesses, accidents, vitamins, supplements, herbals, HTN, DM
- Tests: U/S, Amniocentesis/CVS (when and why), Group B *Streptococcus* (GBS)
- Both parents: alcohol, smoking, drug exposure

Labor and Delivery

- Spontaneous labor or induced? If induced, why?
- Premature or prolonged rupture of membranes?
- Labor duration and problems (maternal fever, nonreassuring fetal heart rate [FHR], meconium)
- Vaginal, forceps, vacuum or Cesarean delivery
- Gestational age at birth, birth weight, Apgar scores (see **Obstetric Exam**, p.221)
- Did the baby require neonatal intensive care unit (e.g. for ventilation) or antibiotics after birth? Was the baby kept in hospital for any reason?
- Postnatal period: jaundice, cyanosis, hypoglycemia, breathing or feeding problems, seizures

Feeding

- Breastfeeding or formula?
  - Breastfed: frequency, duration
    - Vitamin D 400 IU/d
  - Formula: type, dilution, any formula changes, feeding frequency, and amount
- Associated problems: difficulty latching on breast, vomiting
- Supplements: including vitamins and natural products
- Regurgitation: amount, frequency, bilious/non-bilious
- Outputs: urine/stool (number of diapers/d)

Review of Systems

- Head: any swelling of the head post-delivery, has it decreased?
- Eyes: conjunctivitis, scleral icterus
- Mouth/throat: cleft lip/palate, neck masses
- Cardiovascular: fatigue/sweating during feedings, cyanosis
- Respiratory: congenital stridor
- GI: appetite, weight gain, height, growth, vomiting
  - Bowel movements: timing of first meconium, frequency, consistency, color, blood, mucus, diarrhea or constipation, hernia
- GU: number of wet diapers
- Dermatological: jaundice (distribution, worsening or improving), birthmarks, rash

2.2 Neonatal Exam

- Opportunistic exam, with baby undressed
- To optimize the exam, keep the baby quiet by placing the tip of your gloved finger in a crying baby's mouth, or ask parent to do so
- As much as possible, keep the baby warm

General Survey and Vitals

- Appearance: Well or septic? Any signs of respiratory distress (i.e. intercostal or sternal indrawing, nasal flaring, stridor, etc.), color change, or abnormal vital signs?
  - Vital signs: measure the RR, pulse, temperature, blood pressure, and oxygen saturation
  - Assuming the patient is stable, note alertness, activity, facial features/expressions

PEDIATRIC

- Assess Dehydration and Volume Depletion
  - Detailed signs of dehydration/volume status (see **Common Clinical Scenarios**, p.277)
  - Weight loss is the gold standard; capillary refill time, mucous membranes, skin turgor, fontanelles, urine output, blood pressure, heart rate
  - Approximate child's level of dehydration (as this affects management) correlate with % lost from birth weight
    - Mild dehydration: ~5% body weight lost
    - Moderate dehydration: ~10% body weight lost
    - Severe dehydration: ≥15% body weight lost
- **Height:** supine length
- **Weight:** loss of up to 10% of birth weight in first few days of life is normal (see **Table 2**)
  - Classify birth weight on an intrauterine growth curve
  - Small for gestational age (SGA) is <10th percentile
  - Asymmetric SGA: weight <10th percentile with head circumference and length >10th percentile
    - Implication: brain growth may be relatively spared
  - Symmetric SGA: weight, head circumference, and length all <10th percentile
    - Implication: brain growth restricted
  - Appropriate for gestational age (AGA) is 10-90th percentile
  - Large for gestational age (LGA) is >90th percentile
  - See **Common Clinical Scenarios**, p.287 for associated disorders
- **Head Circumference:** measure the greatest circumference around the occipital, parietal, and frontal prominences above the brows and ears
  - Average circumference at term is ~35 cm
- To assess growth, plot height, weight, and head circumference on growth chart and determine percentiles. In the neonatal period, goal is 20-25 g/d of weight growth. Birth weight should be regained by 10-14 d of age

Table 2. Gestational Age and Birth Weight

Birth Weight Classification	Weight
Extremely Low Birth Weight	<1000 g
Very Low Birth Weight	<1500 g
Low Birth Weight	<2500 g
Normal Birth Weight	≥2500 g
Gestational Age Classification	**Gestational Age**
Preterm	<37 wk
Term	37-42 wk
Postterm	≥42 wk

H.E.E.N.T.

Head

- Size, shape (macrocephaly, microcephaly, dolicocephaly, brachiocephaly), and symmetry of head
- After vaginal vertex delivery/prolonged labor:
  - Occipitally elongated head (for ~1 wk)
  - Harmless scalp swelling
  - Caput succedaneum: subcutaneous edema in occipitoparietal region that resolves 1-2 d postpartum; does not respect suture lines

- Cephalohematoma: subperiosteal hemorrhage that resolves in weeks to months; respects suture lines
- Sutures and fontanelles
  - Sutures feel like ridges and usually flatten by 6 mo; persistent ridging suggests craniosynostosis
  - Fontanelles feel like soft concavities: anterior fontanelle is 4-6 cm, and usually closes in 4-24 mo, posterior fontanelle is 1-2 cm, and usually closes by 2 mo
- Palpebral fissures

Eye
- Newborns respond best to human faces, so place your face directly in front of theirs
- Observe position of eyes, eyelids (ptosis), conjunctivae (for purulent conjunctivitis, hemorrhage), sclerae (for scleral icterus), irises, pupils
- Observe palpebral fissure: angle from line drawn from inner and outer canthus (e.g. up slanting may indicate Down's syndrome, down slanting may indicate Noonan's syndrome, short may indicate fetal alcohol syndrome [FAS])
- Fundoscopy
- Always observe for the red reflex (fundus): absence due to opacification suggests glaucoma, cataract or retinoblastoma
- Examine the optic disc (lighter in color than adults, foveal light reflection may not be visible) (see **Table 8** in **Common Clinical Scenarios**, p.277)

Ear
- A neonate's ears are flat against the head
- The tympanic membrane is obscured with accumulated vernix caseosa (white cheesy substance that covers baby's skin at time of birth) for the first few days of life
- Position, shape, and features of ears
- If an imaginary line is drawn from outer canthi of eyes, it should cross pinna or auricle
- Low-set ears present if pinna is below this line; may indicate chromosomal anomaly

Nose
- Test for patency of nasal passages by gently occluding each nostril alternately while holding the baby's mouth closed

Mouth
- Look at lips, gingival, and buccal mucosa for hydration and cyanosis
- Check hard and soft palate and uvula for cleft palate with tongue depressor and otoscope
  - Palpate the upper hard palate to make sure it is intact
- Notching of the posterior margin of the hard palate or a bifid uvula are clues of a submucosal cleft palate
- Epstein's pearls: tiny white or yellow rounded mucus retention cysts along the posterior midline of the hard palate
  - Disappear within month
- A prominent protruding tongue may signal congenital hypothyroidism or Down's syndrome

Neck
- Webbing or extra neck folds may indicate Turner syndrome or Down's syndrome
- Midline or lateral congenital neck mass (e.g. thyroglossal duct cyst)
- Feel for enlarged nodes/glands, and the thyroid

- Palpable thyroid in newborns is always abnormal
- Congenital torticollis: "wry neck", bleeding into the sternocleidomastoid leaving a firm fibrous mass (fibromatosis coli) during the stretching process of birth; disappears over months
- Clavicles, to look for evidence of fracture (i.e. tenderness or a lump)

Respiratory

- Use the bell of an adult stethoscope, or a pediatric stethoscope diaphragm; always compare both sides
- Signs of respiratory distress: tachypnea, tracheal tug, indrawing, retractions, nasal flaring, cyanosis
  - Infants display more abdominal breathing
- AP diameter is round in neonates
- Chest wall deformities (pectus excavatum)
- Respiration phases, depth, and rhythm
  - Rhythm irregularities may signify abnormalities such as apnea
  - Periodic breathing (up to 10 s of apnea) can be normal, especially in premature infants

> **Clinical Pearl: Percussion**
> Percussion is of little clinical benefit in young children and should be avoided, especially in low birth-weight or preterm infants, as it may cause injury or bruising.

Cardiovascular

- Cyanosis, pallor, perfusion, respiratory distress
- Noncardiac findings that may indicate cardiac disease (e.g. poor feeding may be due to tachypnea)
- Heaves, thrills
- Capillary refill time
- Peripheral pulses help assess major branches of the aorta: note strength/quality of femoral pulses
  - Normal pulse has sharp rise, is firm, and well localized
  - Patent ductus arteriosus is indicated by bounding pulses
  - Coarctation of the aorta is indicated by absence of femoral pulse, or its diminution relative to the brachial pulse
- Note rate, rhythm, S1 and S2, murmurs (see **Common Clinical Scenarios**, p.280)
  - Soft precordial systolic murmur common in first few days after birth
  - May be patent ductus arteriosus if persists and is heard over back
- Listen to the back, neck, and axillae as murmurs can radiate there
- Listen over both sides of the skull for an intracranial arteriovenous malformation
- Sinus arrhythmia is a normal finding in children, with heart rate increasing on inspiration and decreasing on expiration

Gastrointestinal

Inspection

- Protuberant abdomen expected in neonates; distended abdomen may indicate obstruction (see **Common Clinical Scenarios**, p.282)
- Scaphoid abdomen together with respiratory distress may suggest congenital diaphragmatic hernia in a neonate
- Umbilicus
  - Check for umbilical hernia
  - Check umbilical cord for 2 umbilical arteries and 1 umbilical vein
  - Examine cord for discharge or signs of infection
  - Presence of a single umbilical artery is correlated with a variety of congenital anomalies (e.g. renal anomalies)

- Abdominal wall
  - Omphalocele: incomplete closure of anterior abdominal wall; herniated, overlying sac, typically associated with other anomalies
  - Gastroschisis: defect in anterior abdominal wall just lateral to umbilicus; herniated intestine with no covering sac; no associated abnormalities
- Signs of jaundice, especially in neonates
- Anus
  - Examine perianal skin for redness, rash
  - Check for imperforation and prolapse
  - Look for passage of meconium in newborns; ask if meconium passage was delayed in a neonate or infant with constipation

Auscultation
- Listen for bowel sounds over each quadrant
  - Bowel sounds normally present every 10-30 s, but must listen for several minutes before determining that sounds are absent

Percussion
- Rarely done in a neonate
- Should be tympanic except over the liver, fecal masses, or full bladder

Palpation
- Make sure your hand is warm
- Liver edge (1-2 cm below costal margin) and kidneys are often palpable in the normal infant
- Palpate for an umbilical, epigastric, or inguinal hernia

Liver Size and Position
- Palpate liver lower margin; if margin indefinite, use percussion
- Normal liver margin is palpated no more than 1-2 cm below costal margin
- Can use 'scratch test' to delineate liver size by auscultating for change in quality of sound when scratching over top and bottom edge of liver

Genitourinary
- Male
  - Ensure testes are descended, further work-up required if bilateral undescended testes
  - Check for hernia, hydrocele, hypospadias
- Female
  - Patent vagina, swollen labia, bloody or white vaginal discharge from maternal estrogen withdrawal
  - In some newborns the genitalia may appear ambiguous as to gender, indicating either a chromosomal or endocrine abnormality

Musculoskeletal
- With patient supine, test for developmental dysplasia of the hip with Barlow and Ortolani maneuvers; check each hip individually
- Barlow (mnemonic: *back*): flex knees, flex and slightly adduct hips, apply posterior pressure
  - POSITIVE if able to dislocate unstable hip
- Ortolani (mnemonic: *out*): flex knees and hips, abduct hips and apply anterior pressure
  - POSITIVE if audible and palpable clunk, able to reduce dislocated hip
- Club foot: plantar flexion of foot, heel inversion, medial forefoot deviation (such fixed deformity is pathological)
- Birth injury: clavicle fracture, brachial plexus injury (e.g. Erb's palsy)

- Full-term newborns exhibit 20-30° hip and knee relative flexion 'contractures' that will disappear by 4-6 mo

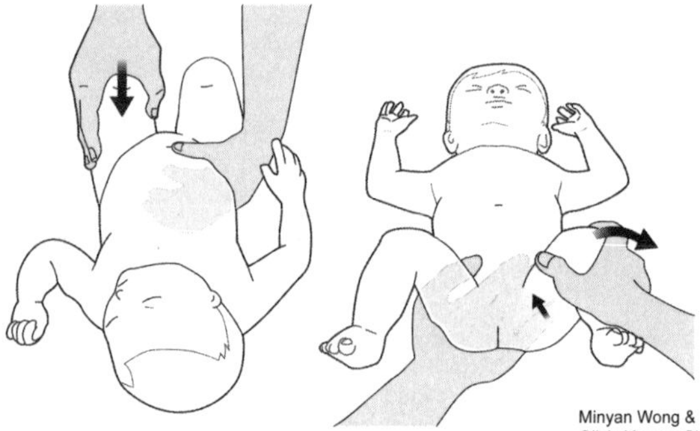

Figure 1. Barlow's and Ortolani's Tests for Hip Dislocation

Neurological

Findings are greatly affected by internal factors: alertness, timing from last feeding, sleeping

- Moving all limbs symmetrically? Bilaterally?
- Tone: normal or low?
- Positive Babinski is normal until 2 yr
- Deep tendon reflexes are variable in newborns since corticospinal pathways are not yet developed, so little diagnostic significance unless response is extreme or different from previous
- Primitive reflexes: galant, placing, rooting, palmar/plantar grasp, moro, parachute, asymmetric tonic neck reflex
- Neural tube defects
  - Spine/back: sacral dimple/hair tuft (spina bifida occulta), midline skin lesions

Dermatological

- Jaundice, pallor, mottling, diaper dermatitis, rashes, birthmarks, hemangiomas
- Skin temperature should be assessed as well
- If lesions are present, describe their distribution, configuration, thickness, primary/secondary changes present, and color
- Be certain to distinguish physiological lesions and those from child abuse

3. APPROACH TO THE INFANT/CHILD

3.1 Infant/Child History

- If the infant/child is presenting for a regular "well-baby" check-up, document history, physical, immunizations, and patient education on the Rourke Baby Record
- Ask about and arrange future follow-up visits with pediatrician or family doctor
- Common problems: pharyngitis, earache, cough, asthma, dehydration, vomiting/diarrhea, urinary problems, limping/pain, headache, rashes, school or behavior problems (see **Common Clinical Scenarios**, p.277)
- Follow the outline in **Approach to the Pediatric Exam** p.249, including the following sections:
  - CC, HPI, PMHx, FHx, SHx, ROS

3.2 Infant/Child Physical Exam

- For infants, do an opportunistic "head-to-toe" exam with child undressed and lying down
- Tips for examining children[1]:
  1. Use parent as a helper to soothe child: with younger children/infants, do most of exam with infant sitting/lying in the caregiver's lap. Ensure cranky infants are well-fed
  2. Begin by observation: much of the neurologic exam can be done by observing the child play, move, and respond to outside stimuli
  3. Introduce yourself and your tools: let child see, and safely touch tools you will be using during the exam. You can also use toys as distractions
  4. Be flexible: perform distressing maneuvers toward the end of the exam. Give the child as much choice as possible (e.g. which body part to examine first?)
  5. Make a game out of the exam:
     - **Head and Neck (H&N):** often best saved for the end, as many children dislike having their ears and throat examined. "Let me see how big your tongue is!"
     - **Cardiac:** if the child is afraid of the stethoscope ask Mom or Dad if it would be OK to listen to their chest first. Make a show of listening to the heart go "ba-boom!"
     - **Respiratory:** to get the child to take a deep breath in and out, hold up your finger and tell them to practice blowing out the candle
     - **Abdomen:** have them put their hands on top of yours while you palpate the abdomen: this may make them less ticklish
     - **MSK/Neurological:** to test upper body strength, have the child "show you how strong they are". For lower body strength, use descriptors, such as "push on the gas". For the cranial nerve exam, "Simon Says" is a favorite

General Survey and Vitals

- Appearance: Well or septic? Any signs of respiratory distress (intercostal or sternal indrawing, nasal flaring, stridor, etc.) or color change?
- Assuming the patient is stable, note alertness, activity, facial features/expressions
- Assess dehydration and volume depletion
  - See **Table 7** in **Common Clinical Scenarios**, p.277 for detailed signs
- Body weight loss is gold standard of dehydration[4]
  - Mild dehydration: ~3% body weight lost
  - Moderate dehydration: ~6% body weight lost
  - Severe dehydration: ≥9% body weight lost

Growth and Development

- **Height:** supine length up to 2 yr, then standing >2 yr
- Weight
- **Head Circumference:** measure the greatest circumference around the occipital, parietal, and frontal prominences above the brows and ears
- To assess growth, plot height, weight, and head circumference on growth chart and determine percentiles
  - Growth charts are available from the World Health Organization (WHO) and the Centers for Disease Control and Prevention (CDC) (both available online): WHO charts are now the Canadian standard and include only breastfed children (50% of the CDC sample) and are based on a multi-ethnic population. They also include different percentile range cut-offs

  - Focus on trend of growth longitudinally rather than individual values
  - Pay attention to crossing of percentile ranges
- **Failure to Thrive (FTT):** when a child's weight for age falls below the 5th percentile of the standard CDC growth chart or if it crosses two major percentile curves. With the WHO charts, investigations for FTT should occur BEFORE the child crosses 2 percentile lines
- **BMI:** can be used in children aged ≥2 yr; growth chart available
- Find out parents' sizes and appearance, and their child's age before judging apparent abnormalities. Calculate mid-parental height (MPH) to determine expected height of child when full-grown

> **Clinical Pearl: Weight and Height**[5]
> **Weight Estimate (kg): (2 x age) + 8**
> - Weight should be doubled at 4-6 mo, tripled at 1 yr, and quadrupled at 2 yr
> - Height should grow by half at 1 yr, and doubled from birth height at 4 yr
> - Head circumference grows by 12 cm in the first 12 mo
>
> **Calculating Mid-Parental Height (MPH)**
> This formula can be used to estimate child's future adult height (in cm):
> MPH for girl = (father's height + mother's height - 12.5) / 2
> MPH for boy = (father's height + mother's height + 12.5) / 2

- **Development:** always assess developmental milestones in infants/children, noting results on the Rourke Baby Record or chart
  - If infant was born premature (<37 wk GA), use the "adjusted age": the age based on the child's due date
  - e.g. if an 8 mo old baby was born 2 mo premature, use the 6 mo milestones

H.E.E.N.T.

Head

- See **Approach to the Neonate**, p.254
- Asymmetry of the cranial vault (plagiocephaly) may result from consistently placing the child supine; ask about child's sleeping or playing positions
- Bulging, tense fontanelle when infant upright, suggests increased intracranial pressure and is seen when baby cries, vomits, or has underlying pathology (CNS infection, neoplasm, hydrocephalus, injury)
- An enlarged posterior fontanelle may be seen in congenital hypothyroidism

Eye

- Observe position of eyes, eyelids (ptosis), conjunctivae (for purulent conjunctivitis, hemorrhage), irises, pupils
- Observe palpebral fissure (see **Approach to the Neonate**, p.255)
- Assess fixation of eyes, if any strabismus found refer to ophthalmology
- **Cover-Uncover Test:** assess fixation by alternately covering one eye and observing for strabismus (present if covered eye moves toward object after being uncovered)
- **Corneal Light Reflex:** assess fixation by shining a bright light (e.g. penlight) in child's eyes. If the position of the reflected light on the child's pupil is different between the left and right eye, it may indicate a less-obvious constant strabismus
- Pseudostrabismus: false appearance of eye misalignment. Commonly found in infants of East Asian and Aboriginal origin, where the medial epicanthal folds are especially apparent and the nasal bridge is widened. Unlike strabismus, the corneal light reflex will be normal in pseudostrabismus

PEDIATRIC

- **Visual Acuity**
  1. <3 yr old:
     - » Use Tumbling E's or LEA Symbols eye chart
     - » LEA Symbols eye chart: child holds chart with several shapes on it, points to matching shape held on a separate chart by the doctor
     - » Visual acuity may not be possible if patient cannot identify pictures on eye chart
     - » Optic blink reflex: for preverbal infants: blinking in response to bright light, or quick movement of object toward eyes
  2. >3 yr old:
     - » Use Snellen eye chart; average acuity is not 20/20 until 2-4 yr
- **Visual Fields**
  - o Bring toy in from periphery; child's eyes should conjugately deviate toward object when it is seen
- **Fundoscopy**
  - o Examine the red retinal (fundus) reflex and optic disc (lighter in color than adults, foveal light reflection may not be visible), looking for retinal hemorrhages, cataracts, corneal opacities (see **Table 8** in **Common Clinical Scenarios**, p.277)

Ear

- Inspection
  - o Position, shape, and features of ears
  - o If an imaginary line is drawn from outer canthi of eyes, it should cross pinna or auricle
  - o Low-set ears occur if pinna is below this line; may indicate chromosomal anomaly, FAS, or other syndromes
  - o Look for discharge (rupture of tympanic membrane) and blood (foreign body irritation or scratching)
  1. Infant
     - » Pull auricle gently downward rather than upward for best view, since ear canal will be directed downward from the outside
     - » Once tympanic membrane is visible, the light reflex may be diffuse and may not become cone-shaped for several months
     - » Use smallest otoscope tip available to better visualize tympanic membrane
  2. Child
     - » Young children may sit in the parent's lap or may need to be restrained while lying down by parents to examine ears
     - » To restrain a child, have the parent hold the child's elbows firmly by the side of the child's head while you lean over the child's body
     - » Pull the auricle upward, outward, and backward for best view
- Hearing
  - o Grossly test for hearing by whispering a command or question 2.5 m away and not in the line of the child's vision
  - o Children >4 yr should have a full-scale acoustic screening test
  - o An infant or child of any age can be referred for formal audiometric testing: if children fail screening maneuvers or you are doubtful in any way, have them tested!

Nose

- Nasolabial folds: asymmetry indicates facial nerve impairment or Bell's palsy
- With otoscope, inspect nasal mucous membranes, noting color and condition
- Look for nasal septal deviation and polyps

Table 3. Neonate and Infant Signs of Hearing

Age	Sign of Hearing
3 mo	• Turns eyes and/or head to follow voice • Responds to environmental sound
6 mo	• Turns eyes and/or head to localize source of sound/voice • Vocalizes with variety
9 mo	• Babbling • Able to take turns when vocalizing with adult • Able to associate a sound with its source

Mouth and Pharynx

- Inspection
  - Look at lips, gingival and buccal mucosa for hydration and cyanosis
  - Check hard and soft palate, uvula, and tonsils for exudates or infection
  - Assess breath
    - Odor indicates oropharyngeal/gingival infection, dehydration, constipation, or poor oral hygiene
- Inspecting a child
  - Teeth: examine for timing and sequence of eruption, number, character, condition and position; all of these characteristics are very variable between children (see **Figure 2**)
    - First teeth erupt at around 6 mo; permanent teeth erupt at 6 yr
    - Significant delay may be a sign of delayed skeletal development
    - Malformed teeth may indicate systemic insult
    - Look for maxillary protrusion (overbite) and mandibular protrusion (underbite) by asking child to bite down hard and part the lips
  - Inspect tongue:
    - Common abnormalities include coated tongue from viral infection, and strawberry tongue found in scarlet fever, streptococcal pharyngitis, or Kawasaki disease
  - Tonsils: note size, position, symmetry, and appearance
  - Size of tonsils is assessed from 1+ (easy visibility of gap between tonsils) to 4+ (tonsils which touch in the midline with the mouth wide open)

Neck

- Inspection
  - Look for enlarged nodes/glands and the thyroid size, masses, and texture
- Palpation
  1. Infant
     - Best palpated while patient is supine since the neck is short
  2. Child
     - Best examined while sitting
     - Neck mobility, either passive or active, depending on child's age
     - Ensure the neck is supple and mobile in all directions
     - Nuchal rigidity: for suspected meningitis, ask child to touch chin to chest and note pain/restriction
     - Lymph nodes and presence of any additional masses (congenital cysts)
     - The majority of enlarged lymph nodes in children are due to infection, not malignant disease
     - Malignancy is more likely if node is >2 cm, hard, fixed, and accompanied by systemic signs such as weight loss

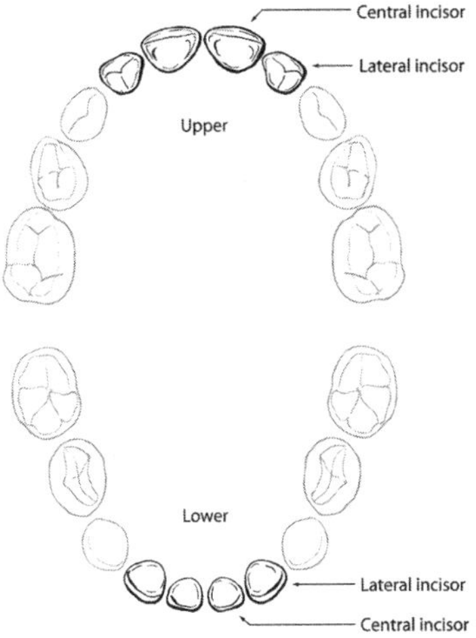

Figure 2. Dentition in Children 5-12 Months Old

Respiratory

- The pediatric respiratory exam should be completed using the same criteria as in the adult exam (see **Respiratory Exam**, p.351)
- Infants and young children should have the respiratory exam done while sitting on a parent's lap: if they become agitated by the examiner's presence, they may need to be observed from a distance to better assess their respiratory status at rest

Inspection

- AP diameter
  - In infants, the chest is rounder than in older children
  - Increased AP diameter is seen in cystic fibrosis, chronic asthma or chronic diffuse small airway obstruction
- Chest wall deformities
  - Pectus excavatum may be an isolated finding or may be associated with a chronic cardiorespiratory problem
  - Other chest wall deformities may be congenital or due to surgery
  - Spinal configuration
  - Kyphoscoliosis can affect shape of thoracic cage and pulmonary function
- Signs of respiratory distress
  - Retractions (suprasternal, intercostal, subcostal)
  - Nasal flaring is nonspecific, but is an important distress sign
- Respiration phases, depth, and rhythm
  - Infants display more abdominal breathing, with a shift to chest excursion as they get older (thoracic breathing at ~6 yr)
- Rhythm irregularities beyond the neonatal period may signify abnormalities such as apnea
  - Periodic breathing (up to 10 s of apnea) can be normal, especially in infants
- Finger clubbing: may indicate chronic disease such as cystic fibrosis, respiratory, cardiac, and GI disorders
- Cyanosis: central cyanosis (indicates cardiorespiratory disease) vs. peripheral cyanosis

EBM: Pneumonia in Infants

The respiratory rate should be determined by observing the chest of a quiet infant over two 30 s intervals, or over a full min. When examining infants, auscultation is relatively unreliable.

To rule out pneumonia, the best individual finding is the absence of tachypnea. Signs that can be helpful for ruling in pneumonia include abnormal auscultatory findings, chest indrawing, and other signs suggesting increased work of breathing (e.g. nasal flaring). In developed countries, multiple findings are needed to increase the likelihood of pneumonia.

If all clinical signs (i.e. respiratory rate, auscultation, and work of breathing) are negative, a CXR is less likely to be positive.

Margolis P, Gadomski A. 1998. *JAMA* 279(4):308-313.

Palpation

- Use one or two fingers (based on size) to assess tracheal position
- Chest expansion and tactile fremitus have little use in young children

Percussion

- Diaphragmatic excursion is usually only performed on older child
- Can be used to assess for consolidation/atelectasis

Auscultation

- The bell of an adult stethoscope, or a pediatric stethoscope diaphragm, should be used in young children
- The examiner should ask about and listen for respiratory sounds (see **Respiratory Exam**, p.348)
- As in the adult exam, always compare both sides

Cardiovascular

Inspection

- See **Cardiovascular Exam**, p.52
- General signs of health: nutritional status, responsiveness; failure to thrive is one presentation of heart failure
- Nail clubbing may be associated with cyanotic congenital heart disease

Clinical Pearl: Tachypnea
Tachypnea paired with increased respiratory effort is usually pulmonary in origin, while "effortless tachypnea" is usually of cardiac or metabolic origin.

Palpation

- Chest wall to assess volume change in heart and thrills
- Peripheral pulses help assess major branches of the aorta: palpate brachial artery pulse (antecubital fossa), temporal arteries in front of the ear, and femoral pulses
- Normal pulse has sharp rise, is firm, and well localized
- Point of maximal impulse is found in the 4th intercostal space before age 7, 5th space after age 7
- Patent ductus arteriosus is indicated by bounding pulses
- Coarctation of the aorta is indicated by absence of femoral pulse (or its diminution relative to brachial pulse), or much greater upper limb BP than lower limb BP

Auscultation

- Note rate, rhythm, S1 and S2, murmurs
  - Murmurs are a common finding: up to 80% of children have murmurs, but only 0.35% have confirmed organic heart disease (see "Murmurs" under **Common Clinical Scenarios**, p.280)
- Listen to the back, neck, and axillae as murmurs can radiate there
- Sinus arrhythmia is a normal finding in children, with heart rate increasing on inspiration and decreasing on expiration

Gastrointestinal

- It is important when inspecting the abdomen to relax the child
- Useful tips include flexing the child's knees, talking and playing with the child, and putting your hand flat on the abdomen
- Make sure your hand is warm
- Distract older children by asking simple questions

Inspection

- Protuberant abdomen
  - Expected in infants; feature disappears as early as 4 yr
  - Distended abdomen may indicate obstruction
  - A large abdomen, with thin limbs and wasted buttocks, suggests severe malnutrition; seen in celiac disease or cystic fibrosis
- Umbilicus
  - Check for umbilical hernia
- Abdominal wall
- Signs of jaundice, especially in neonates and young infants
- Ask if meconium passage was delayed in a neonate or infant with constipation
- Anus
  - Examine perianal skin for redness
  - Check for imperforation and prolapse
  - Redness and rash may indicate inadequate cleaning, diaper rash, or irritation from diarrhea

Auscultation

- See **Approach to the Neonate**, p.257

Percussion

- Systematically percuss all areas of the abdomen
- Should be tympanic except over the liver, fecal masses, or full bladder

Palpation

- Observe child's face carefully for pain while lightly palpating for tenderness and deeply palpating for abnormal masses
- Localized tenderness with guarding and rebound tenderness is a sign of peritoneal irritation
- Palpate for an umbilical or inguinal hernia
- Liver size and position
- Palpate liver's lower margin; if margin indefinite, use percussion
- Pyloric stenosis: in later stages, described as an "olive", palpable just to the right of the midline in the epigastric area (usually in the first few months of life), associated with vomiting
- Rectal exam should be done only if abdominal or pelvic disease suspected
- Prostate gland is not palpable in the young male

Table 4. Differential Diagnosis of Abdominal Pain

Area of Pain	Differential Diagnosis
Right Upper Quadrant	Hepatitis, enlarged liver
Right Lower Quadrant or Around the Umbilicus	Appendicitis
Lower Quadrants	Feces, gastroenteritis*, pelvic infection, tumor
Left Upper Quadrant	Intussusception†, splenic enlargement

*Infants/children under age 5 experience gastroenteritis 1-2 times/yr (episodes usually resolve in 3-7 d; causes: bacterial or viral; signs/symptoms: N/V, fever, pain)
†Intussusception: most common cause of bowel obstruction under 5 yr (signs/symptoms: "currant jelly" stools and colicky pain)

Clinical Pearl: DRE
While the DRE is only performed if required for diagnosis or treatment, physicians should not forget its utility. DRE can help differentiate functional constipation from constipation due to organic causes. Functional fecal retention is the most common cause of childhood constipation.

Genitourinary: Male

Inspection

1. Infant
   - Penis
     - Foreskin completely covers the glans penis and is not retractable until months to years after birth
     - Shaft of penis: ensure penis appears straight, and note any ventral surface abnormalities. Fixed downward bowing of the penis is a chordee, and may accompany a hypospadias
     - Look for fibrous ring around meatus of foreskin (phimosis)
     - A small amount of white, cheesy material under the foreskin around the glans (smegma) is normal
   - Scrotum: poorly developed scrotum may indicate cryptorchidism (undescended testes)
   - Note rugae and presence or absence of testes in sac
2. Child
   - In precocious puberty, the penis and testes are enlarged due to conditions of excess androgens, including pituitary and adrenal tumors
   - As with adult men, swelling in the inguinal canal, especially after a Valsalva maneuver may indicate inguinal hernia

Palpation

1. Infant
   - Palpate the testes in the scrotum and then palpate up the spermatic cord to the external inguinal ring
   - If testis is palpated in the inguinal canal, gentle pressure can ease them down
   - Testes should be ~10 mm in width and ~15 mm in length
   - Differentiate any swelling found in the scrotum from the testes
   - Hydroceles and inguinal hernias are two common scrotal masses
     - Hydroceles transilluminate

PEDIATRIC

2. Child
   - An extremely active cremasteric reflex may cause testis to retract upward and appear undescended
   - To minimize retraction, examine when child is relaxed, use warm hands, and palpate from the lower abdomen, along inguinal canal toward scrotum
   - Cremasteric reflex test: scratch the medial aspect of the thigh, ipsilateral testis moves upward
   - Common causes of painful testicle are infection, trauma, torsion of the testicle, and torsion of the appendix testis

Genitourinary: Female

Inspection

- Examine child in supine position; in younger children, child can sit in parent's lap with parent holding knees outstretched
- Inspect labia majora, labia minora, size of clitoris, presence of rashes, bruises or other lesions
- To examine more internal structures, separate the labia majora at midpoint to inspect urethral orifice and labia minora
- Internal examination of genitalia in female child not typically performed unless specific complaint
- Infant: use the thumbs of each hand
- Older children: grasp labia between thumb and index finger of each hand
- Note condition of labia minora, urethra, hymen, and proximal vagina
- Child:
  - Labia majora and minora flatten out after infancy
  - Check for any rashes, bruises or external lesions
  - Examine labia minora, urethra, hymen, and proximal vagina by inspection only
  - Hymen becomes thin, translucent, and vascular, often with easily identifiable edges
  - Pubic hair before age 7 yr indicates premature adrenarche and potential precocious puberty
  - Labial adhesions (fusion of the labia minora) posteriorly may be noted in prepubertal girls

Musculoskeletal

- Inspection, palpation, and range of motion with the greatest number of findings involving the spine and lower extremities
- Become familiar with normal MSK changes during development to recognize abnormalities and conditions that spontaneously regress
- Range of motion is greatest in the infant and then decreases with age

Infant

- Feet
  - Toeing-in:
    - 6-18 mo: commonly caused by internal tibial torsion
    - Rotate knees so patella faces forward, feet should face inward (usually disappears at 2 yr)
  - Flat feet are normal in children <2-3 yr
- Knee Alignment
  - Mild bow-legged (genu varum) pattern is normal until age 2 yr
  - Mild knock-knee (genu valgum) pattern is normal from 2-8 yr
- Hips
  - Barlow's and Ortolani's tests are useful in the first 6 wk of life; after this time the radiological exam provides a more accurate diagnosis

PEDIATRIC

- See **Approach to the Neonate**, p.257
- Asymmetry of buttocks and thigh folds suggests congenital hip dysplasia
- Spine
  - Look for vertebral deformities and pigmented spots, hairy patches, sacral dimple, or overlying skin in lumbosacral region (spina bifida)

Child

- As child gets older, MSK exam is generally the same as an adult exam (see **Musculoskeletal Exam**, p.134)
- Feet: In-toeing >12 yr: commonly caused by femoral anteversion
  - Rotate knees so patella faces forward, feet should now face forward
- Hips: check for hip pain or instability using Trendelenburg test
- Spine: check for scoliosis
  - Ask child to lean forward
  - Inspect curvature of spinous processes, rib humps (prominence of ribs due to convexity of spinal curvature), and look for asymmetry in hips and scapulae

Common Injuries

- Ankle sprains are one of most common childhood MSK injuries
  - Signs and symptoms: pain, bruising, swelling
  - Ottawa Ankle Rules to determine presence of fracture do not apply for children

Neurological

- Findings are greatly affected by internal factors: alertness, timing from last feeding, sleeping, and external factors: fear and anxiety, presence of parents
- Neurologic and developmental exams are often combined since neurologic abnormalities can present in young children as developmental abnormalities

Infant

- Mental status
  - Observe activities during alert periods
- Motor exam
  - Watch position at rest and as the infant moves spontaneously
  - Test resistance to passive movement noting any spasticity or flaccidity, increased or decreased tone
  - Can place infant on abdomen to observe movements, head position
- Deep tendon reflexes
  - Can substitute index or middle finger for reflex hammer
  - Triceps, brachioradialis, and abdominal reflexes are hard to elicit before 6 mo
  - Anal reflex is present at birth and should be elicited if spinal cord lesion is suspected
  - Ankle reflex elicited by grasping infant's malleoli with one hand and abruptly dorsiflexing child's foot
  - Normal downgoing plantar response is seen in 90% of infants, but a normal infant can manifest an upgoing plantar (Babinski) response until 2 yr
  - Progressive increase in deep tendon reflexes in first year coupled with increased tone may indicate CNS disease such as cerebral palsy
- Sensory function
  - Pain sensation: touch or flick infant's palm or sole with your finger and observe for withdrawal, arousal, and change in facial expression

Child

- Motor Exam
  - Observe child's gait while walking and running, noting any asymmetry, tripping, or clumsiness
  - Heel-to-toe walking, hopping, jumping (if developmentally appropriate)
  - Use toy to test for coordination, strength of upper extremities
  - If concerned about strength, test by having child lie on the floor and then stand up
  - In certain forms of muscular dystrophy, children rise by rolling over prone and pushing off the floor with their arms while legs stay extended, then achieve upright position using arms to walk up legs (Gower's sign)
  - Hand preference in a child <18 mo-2 yr suggests weakness: must rule out hemiplegia
- Deep tendon reflexes
  - As assessed for adults (see **Neurological Exam**, p.188)
- Sensory exam
  - Test with cotton ball with child's eyes closed; do not use pinprick with young child
- Cerebellar exam
  - Finger-to-nose test with rapid alternating movements: make this a game!
  - Look for nystagmus and gait disturbances

> **Clinical Pearl: Pediatric Brain Tumors**
> Most pediatric brain tumors are located in posterior fossa (e.g. medulloblastomas, brainstem gliomas, astrocytomas), which present with cerebellar signs.

Dermatological

- Done almost entirely on history and inspection, with a good source of light
- Inspection should begin with general observation of skin, hair, and nail color, pigmentation, and texture
- Skin temperature should be assessed as well
- If lesions are present, describe their distribution, configuration, thickness, primary/secondary changes present, and color
- Be certain to distinguish physiological lesions and those from child abuse
- Dermatological findings vary with age
- Contact dermatitis
  - Vesicular, erythematous, well-defined lesions
- Atopic dermatitis (eczema)
  - Itchy, dry, slightly elevated papular lesions that form plaques
  - Face, neck, hands, and flexor surfaces of joints
- Café-au-lait spots: consider neurofibromatosis type 1 if six or more café-au-lait spots greater than 5 mm in diameter before puberty, or greater than 15 mm in diameter after puberty
- Ash leaf spots (hypomelanic macules): consider tuberous sclerosis complex (Ash leaf spots may be the only visual sign in infancy)

4. APPROACH TO THE ADOLESCENT

- Adolescence is a time of tremendous physical and psychosocial change
- History and Physical Exam should focus on the following:
  - Puberty: signs of normal vs. abnormal maturation
  - Screening: for safety and risk-taking behaviors

4.1 Adolescent History

- With the adolescent's permission, at least part of the history should be obtained without parent in the room
  - Discuss confidentiality: inform adolescent that you will have to disclose to other people if they are suicidal, homicidal, or if they are being abused or taken advantage of by a person of power
- ID: name, age, school grade, siblings, cohabitants in home
- CC: note that a teenager's initial CC may not represent his/her actual reason for seeking medical attention
- HPI (see **Approach to the Pediatric Exam**, p.250)
- PMHx: previous illnesses, surgeries, medications, allergies (medications and environmental), immunization history
- FHx: recurrent illnesses, early deaths, genetic diseases, cancer, psychiatric conditions, suicide, alcohol/substance abuse
- ROS: including menstrual patterns, urinary symptoms

Psychosocial History

The "HE^2ADS^3" Assessment

- **H**ome
  - Living arrangements, relationship with parents and siblings, other occupants
  - Attempts at running away, family issues, recent changes at home, feeling safe within the home
- **E**ducation
  - Name of school, current grade, academic performance, school attendance, behavior at school, plans for further education/vocation
- **E**ating
  - Diet: typical foods, types and frequency of skipped meals, vomiting, nutritional supplements, vitamin use, calcium/vitamin D intake
  - Body image: recent weight gain or loss, dieting, use of weight loss drugs
  - Compensatory behaviors: including vomiting, laxatives, exercise, diuretics, stimulants
  - Eating Disorder Screen: "SCOFF"[6]
    - Do you make yourself **Sick** because you feel uncomfortably full?
    - Do you worry that you have lost **Control** over how much you eat?
    - In 3 mo have you lost **Over** 15 lbs?
    - Do you think you are **Fat** when others think you are thin?
    - Does **Food** dominate your life?
- **A**ctivities
  - After school or work; exercise, sports, hobbies, parties/clubs
  - Part-time work, income for activities
- **D**rugs
  - Do you have any friends who drink, smoke or use drugs?
  - Have you ever tried smoking or drinking alcohol? What did you think? What about other drugs?
  - Have you ever gotten in trouble because of using these substances?
- **S**ex/**S**exuality
  - Current/past sexual activity, sexual identity, history of pregnancy
  - STI's
    - Contraception: what method(s)? Is it used every time and used properly?

PEDIATRIC

- **S**uicide/Mood
  - Screen for depression MSIGECAPS (see **Psychiatric Exam**, p.330)
  - Suicide assessment: past attempts, protective factors, current plan/means
- **S**afety
  - From physical and sexual abuse at home, school, in relationships
  - Recent injuries: motor vehicle accidents, sports injuries, concussions
  - Risk-taking behavior (e.g. driving while intoxicated or being a passenger with an intoxicated driver)
  - Internet and social media safety, sexting

4.2 Overview of the Adolescent Physical Exam

- Knowledge of adult exam is assumed for adolescent exam
- As per adult exam except:
  - **Growth:** height, mass, BMI: should be plotted on curve to monitor growth
  - **H&N:** thyroid examination, screen for visual acuity and hearing
  - **GU:**
    - » Male: external genitalia (Tanner staging), secondary sexual characteristics (body hair, pubic hair)
    - » Female: external genitalia/breast/pubic hair (Tanner staging), if indicated speculum (vagina and cervix) and bimanual examination
  - **MSK:** scoliosis
  - **Dermatological:** skin (acne, petechiae, pallor, pigmentation), hair (amount, distribution, hirsutism), breasts (development in females, gynecomastia in males)

4.3 Detailed Adolescent Physical Exam

General Survey and Vitals

- General Survey should consist of (1) General Inspection, (2) Growth Measurements
  1. General Inspection: does this adolescent look "sick"?
     - » Respiratory distress, level of alertness, general affect, nutritional status
  2. Growth Measurements: measure height, weight, calculate BMI
     - » Plot on growth chart and note trend and percentiles of growth
     - » Height: growth spurt occurs during puberty, which accounts for 20-25% of final adult height; onset and duration of growth spurt is highly variable
       - Females: onset 9.5-14.5 yr
       - Males: onset 10.5-16 yr
       - Growth spurt lasts about 2 yr longer in males (into 3rd decade)
     - » Weight: pubertal weight gain accounts for 50% of final adult body weight
       - Percentage body fat increases in females and decreases in male
     - » BMI = mass (kg) / height^2 (m^2)

Vital Signs

- As per adult
- Ensure teenager is comfortable and not anxious before measuring vitals
- Hypertension in children is often due to a secondary cause whereas adolescent hypertension is usually essential hypertension

H.E.E.N.T.

1. **Cranial Nerves** (see **Neurological Exam**, p.176)
2. **Oral Cavity and Pharynx** (see **Head and Neck Exam**, p.108)
   - Of particular note in adolescents:
     - Teeth: check for poor dental hygiene, enamel erosion from vomiting or tooth grinding (bruxism)
     - Tonsils
       - Infectious mononucleosis: can appear grayish
       - Viral pharyngitis: diffuse redness across tonsils and pharynx (without tonsillar exudate)
       - Streptococcal infection (strep throat): erythema, edema, exudates
       - Peritonsillar abscess ("quinsy"): asymmetric enlargement of tonsils (with lateral displacement of uvula toward unaffected tonsil)
3. **Nose and Paranasal Sinuses** (see **Head and Neck Exam,** p.106)
4. **Thyroid** (see **Head and Neck Exam**, p.114)
   - In adolescence, Hashimoto's thyroiditis > asymptomatic goiter > Graves' disease
   - Hypothyroidism: mostly caused by Hashimoto's thyroiditis in adolescence
     - Growth and pubertal delay, menstrual dysfunction
     - Abnormally high weight gain, cold and dry skin
   - Hyperthyroidism: almost always caused by Graves' disease in adolescence
     - Emotional lability and sleep disturbance, change in school performance
     - Skin changes: eczema, erythema, excoriations, or smooth skin
5. **Neck** (see **Head and Neck Exam**, p.114)
   - Lymph nodes
   - Palpate the occipital, posterior auricular, preauricular, anterior cervical, submandibular, submental, and supraclavicular nodes
   - Infection (vast majority): red, <2 cm, mobile, anterior (often strep throat) vs. posterior (mononucleosis) location
   - Malignancy (rare): hard, fixed, >2 cm, with constitutional symptoms
     - Supraclavicular lymphadenopathy (metastasis)
   - Neck stiffness: suggestive of meningitis
6. **Eyes** (see **Ophthalmological Exam**, p.235)
   - Adolescents should have visual acuity screened q2-3 yr
   - Use standard Snellen chart, with one eye covered
7. **Ears** (see **Head and Neck Exam**, p.101)

Clinical Pearl: Meningismus[4]
Neck stiffness is suggestive of meningitis and can be discerned with the following two clinical signs (both while the patient is supine):
1) **Brudzinski's Sign**: flexion of the neck causes involuntary flexion of the knee and hip
2) **Kernig's Sign**: extension of the knee while the hip is flexed 90° is limited by knee extensor spasm and hamstring pain

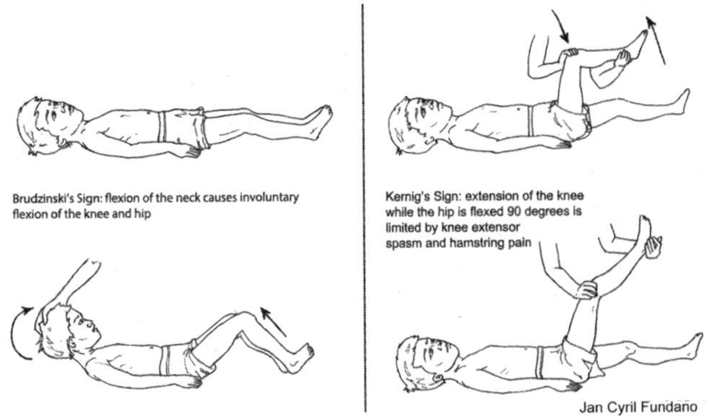
Brudzinski's Sign: flexion of the neck causes involuntary flexion of the knee and hip
Kernig's Sign: extension of the knee while the hip is flexed 90 degrees is limited by knee extensor spasm and hamstring pain
Jan Cyril Fundaño

Figure 3. Kernig's and Brudzinski's Signs

Respiratory

- Similar to the adult exam (see **Respiratory Exam**, p.351)
- In adolescents, should be particularly aware of the following:
  - Asthma: wheezing, variable coughing (can be dry or wet), worsening with certain triggers (exercise, cold weather, environmental allergens)
  - Bronchitis: cough that is loose and "rattling", bronchial breath sounds

Cardiovascular

- Similar to the adult exam (see **Cardiovascular Exam**, p.52 and **Peripheral Vascular Exam**, p.297)
- Specific sign in adolescents:
  - Bradycardia, orthostatic vitals (hypotension and tachycardia with standing): associated with anorexia nervosa

Gastrointestinal

- Similar to the adult exam (see **Abdominal Exam**, p.20)

Inspection

- Central adiposity vs. malnourishment/cachexia
- Lanugo (baby-like) hair: associated with anorexia nervosa

Auscultation and Percussion

- Bowel sounds
- Percuss all four quadrants, liver, and spleen
- Splenomegaly in infectious mononucleosis, leukemia/lymphoma, hemolytic diseases

Palpation

- Light and deep palpation (tenderness, masses, peritoneal signs)
- Liver and spleen
- Kidney
- Special tests: appendicitis (see **Abdominal Exam**, p.31)
- Appendicitis is the most common indication for emergency abdominal surgery in childhood; its frequency peaks between ages 15-30 yr

Genitourinary and Reproductive System

- Often the genitourinary/reproductive examination is left until the end, as teenagers can be embarrassed or sensitive about this area
- There should always be a chaperone for the GU and breast exams
- Onset of puberty is often variable, in general, onset is 8-13 yr in females, 9-14 yr in males
- Usual sequence of pubertal sexual maturation:
  - Females: thelarche (breast budding) → adrenarche (pubic hair) → growth spurt → menarche (onset of menstruation)
  - Males: testes enlargement → penile enlargement → adrenarche + axillary hair → growth spurt

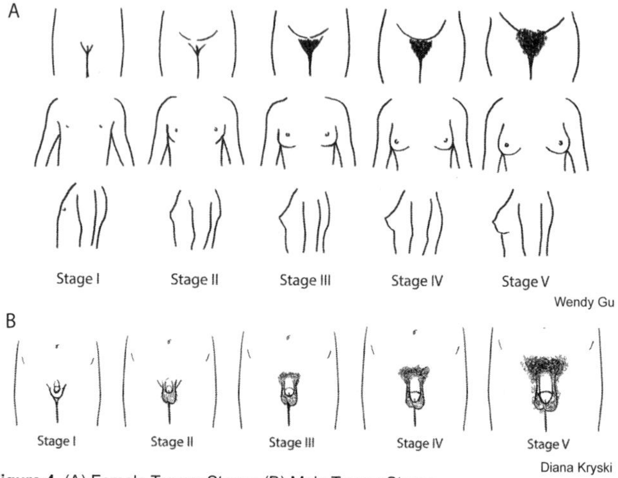

Figure 4. (A) Female Tanner Stages (B) Male Tanner Stages

Breast (see **Breast Exam**, p.39)

- Thelarche (budding of breast at onset of puberty) occurs at roughly 11 yr; is one of earliest signs of puberty
- Age of onset variable among different ethnicities; earlier in teenagers of African descent
- Inspect for development of chest hair (characteristic of increased androgens)
- Amount of chest hair highly variable
- If chest hair present in females, suspect excess androgen
- Inspection of breasts: **4 S**'s
  - **S**ize, **S**hape, **S**ymmetry, **S**kin changes
  - Normal to have asymmetry because one breast may develop more rapidly
- Inspection of nipples: **6 S**'s
  - **S**ize, **S**hape, **S**ymmetry, **S**kin changes, **S**pontaneous nipple discharge, **S**upernumerary nipples
- Sexual maturation: can assign Tanner Stage (see **Figure 4**)
  - Stage 1: preadolescent breast, with elevated papilla
  - Stage 2: breast bud stage; small elevation of breast and papilla; areola diameter enlarges
  - Stage 3: further enlargement of breast and areola, but their contours are not separated
  - Stage 4: projection of areola and papilla to form secondary mound
  - Stage 5: mature breast; areola recess to general contour of breast

- In males: inspect for gynecomastia
  - Usually benign, self-limited; seen in up to 50-60% of adolescent boys
  - Etiology: idiopathic, 1° or 2° hypogonadism, hyperthyroidism, antiandrogen drugs, cancer chemotherapy
  - Typical appearance: 1-3 cm, round, freely mobile, often tender, firm mass beneath areola
  - Further investigation if: large, hard, fixed enlargement or mass/nodules
- Palpation (see **Breast Exam**, p.41)

Table 5. Causes of Palpable Breast Masses in Children and Adolescents

Causes	
Classic or Juvenile Fibroadenoma	Intraductal Papilloma
Fibrocystic Changes	Fat Necrosis/Lipoma
Breast Cyst	Abscess/Mastitis
Neoplasm (carcinoma <1%)	Adenomatous Hyperplasia

Marcdante KJ, Kliegman RM, Jenson HB, Behrman RE (Editors). *Nelson Essentials of Pediatrics*, 6th ed. Philadelphia: Elsevier Saunders; 2011.

Genitourinary

Female

- See **Gynecological Exam**, p.82 for detailed description
- Important points with respect to the adolescent female:
- Indications for pelvic examination (otherwise not necessary until 21 yr of age or after 3 yr of being sexually active):
  - Abnormal vaginal discharge, pelvic pain, history of unprotected sexual intercourse, menstrual irregularities, suspicion of anatomic abnormalities, patient request
  - Rarely performed by pediatricians
- **Inspection**
  - External genitalia
  - Pubic hair: assign Tanner staging based on amount and quality
    - Stage 1: prepubertal
    - Stage 2: sparse hair at labia/base of penis
    - Stage 3: hair over pubis
    - Stage 4: coarse adult hair
    - Stage 5: hair extends to medial thigh
  - Internal genitalia (speculum examination)
  - Cervix, vagina
- **Palpation**
  - External genitalia (labia, clitoris, vagina), internal genitalia (cervix, uterus), adnexae as in adult

EBM: HPV Vaccine

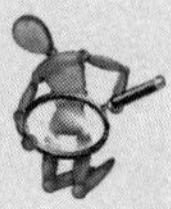

In a 2007 systematic review of 9 RCTs, prophylactic HPV vaccination was found to be highly efficacious in the prevention of HPV infection, high- and low-grade precancerous lesions, and genital warts among women aged 15-25 yr.

Rambout L, et al. 2007. *CMAJ* 177(5):469-479.

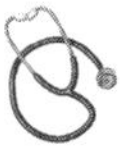

Clinical Pearl: The Ectopic Triad
Not to be missed: Triad of tender adnexal mass, vaginal bleeding, and abdominal/pelvic pain = ectopic pregnancy until proven otherwise.

Male

- See **Urological Exam**, p.367 for detailed description
- **Inspection**
  - Assign Tanner stages of pubertal maturation (see **Figure 4** and **Table 6**)
  - Pubic hair: assign Tanner staging
  - Not to be missed: red, tender, swollen testicle = torsion until proven otherwise (emergency)
    - DDx: testicular torsion, torsion of appendix testes or epididymitis
- **Palpation**
  - Penis, scrotum, inguinal hernias, inguinal lymph nodes
  - DDx of painless scrotal mass in adolescent male: testicular cancer, hydrocele, spermatocele, varicocele, indirect inguinal hernia, abscess

Table 6. Tanner Stages: Male Genitalia

Stage	Description
1	Testes: volume <1.5 mL Phallus: childlike
2	Testes: volume 1.6-6 mL Phallus: no change Scrotum: reddened, thinner, larger
3	Testes: volume 6-12 mL Phallus: increased length Scrotum: greater enlargement
4	Testes: volume 12-20 mL Phallus: increased length, circumference Scrotum: further enlargement, darkening
5	Testes: volume >20 mL Phallus: adult Scrotum: adult

Neinstein LS. *Adolescent Healthcare: A Practical Guide.* Philadelphia: Wolters Kluwer/ Lippincott Williams & Wilkins; 2008.

- **Common Investigations**
  - Gonorrheal and chlamydial swabs
  - STI testing
  - Pap smear (rarely performed on females <21 yr)
  - See **Gynecological Exam**, p.83 and **Infectious Diseases Exam**, p.494

Musculoskeletal (see **Musculoskeletal Exam**, p.134)

Neurological (see **Neurological Exam**, p.174)

Dermatological

- Pubertal changes
- Acne (comedonal, papular or pustular inflammatory, nodulocystic); seen in 85% of adolescents
- Pigmentation of areolae, external genitalia
- Development of pubic and axillary hair
- Tinea pedis (athlete's foot): fungal infection
  - Scaling, fissuring, erythema at soles of feet and toe webs
- Psoriasis: 25% of cases have onset in adolescent years
  - Erythematous, circumscribed plaques with silvery scaly appearance
- Pitting and ridging nail changes: associated with anorexia nervosa

5. COMMON CLINICAL SCENARIOS

5.1 General: Dehydration

Table 7. Signs of Dehydration/Volume Status

Sign/Symptom	Mild Dehydration (Children: <3% body wt lost; Infants: <5% body wt lost)	Moderate Dehydration Children: 3- 9% body wt lost; Infants: 5-15% body wt lost)	Severe Dehydration (Children: >9% body wt lost; Infants: >15% body wt lost)
Mental Status	Alert	Fatigued/irritable	Lethargic/ obtunded
Thirst	Drinks well	Thirsty, eager to drink	Drinks poorly/ unable to drink
Fontanelles/Eyes	Normal	Depressed	Sunken
Mucous Membranes	Moist	Dry	Parched
Heart Rate	Normal	Slightly tachycardic	Tachycardia → bradycardia
Blood Pressure	Normal	Normal/orthostatic change	Decreased
Respiratory Rate	Normal	Normal/tachypneic	Tachypneic
Capillary Refill	Normal	>2 s	>4 s
Skin Turgor	Warm, normal turgor	Cool, recoil <2 s	Cold, mottled, recoil >2 s
Peripheral Pulses	Normal	Normal to decreased	Weak, tready or impalpable
Urine Output	Normal to decreased	Decreased	Minimal

Lalani A, Schneeweiss S (Editors). *Handbook of Pediatric Emergency Medicine.* Mississauga: Jones and Bartlett Publishers; 2008.

5.2 H.E.E.N.T.

Eye

Table 8. Differential Diagnosis of Findings on Observation of Eyes

Finding	Differential Diagnosis
Absence of red reflex	Glaucoma, cataracts, retinoblastoma
Fixed eyes staring in one direction (doll's eye reflex), **intermittent alternating convergent strabismus** (crossed eyes), **or intermittent alternating divergent strabismus** (intermittent laterally deviated eyes)	Normal in newborns due to dysconjugate gaze Abnormal after 6 mo
Pendular nystagmus or roving eye movements	Highly suspicious for blindness after 6 wk
Hypertelorism, Brushfield's spots	Down's syndrome
Inner epicanthal folds	Normally found in Asian children, Down's syndrome

Table 8. Differential Diagnosis of Findings on Observation of Eyes (continued)

Finding	Differential Diagnosis
Appearance of sclera between upper lid and iris	Hydrocephalus, Graves' disease
Drooping eyelid	Paralysis of oculomotor cranial nerve
Painful, red, swollen eyelid	Stye
Nodular, nontender area	Cyst
Sunken area around eyelids	Dehydrated
Subconjunctival hemorrhages	Normal in newborn
Red conjunctivae	Bacterial or viral infection, allergy, irritation
Pale conjunctivae	Anemia
Yellow sclerae	Jaundice
Bluish sclerae	Premature baby, osteogenesis imperfecta, glaucoma, hyperbilirubinemia
Absence of color in iris	Albinism
Notch of outer edge of iris	Visual field defect
Constriction of pupils (miosis)	Iritis, drug-induced (morphine)
Fixed unilateral dilation of a pupil	Local eye injury or head injury
Dilaton of pupils (mydriasis)	Acute glaucoma, drug-induced, trauma, circulatory anesthesia, emotionally-induced
White pupils (leukocoria)	Coloboma (failure of retinal development), intraocular tumor (retinoblastoma), cataract, retinopathy of prematurity, congenital infection (toxoplasmosis)

Ear

- **Acute Otitis Media**
  - CC: ear pain, fever, irritability, pulling at ears, persistent crying
  - Signs: bulging, immobile, erythematous tympanic membrane, and painful ear
  - Diagnosis requires all three of: acute onset of symptoms; middle ear effusion (otorrhea, fixed tympanic membrane, visible air fluid levels); and middle ear inflammation (discoloration of tympanic membrane: opaque, hemorrhagic, red/yellow)
  - Causes: *S. pneumoniae*, *H. influenzae*, *M. catarrhalis* most common

EBM: Acute Otitis Media (AOM)

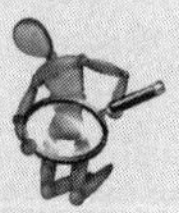

The most useful signs for detecting AOM are cloudiness, bulging, and distinct immobility of the tympanic membrane (adjusted LR+ = 34 [95%CI: 28-42], 51 [95%CI: 36-73], and 31 [95%CI: 26-37], respectively). Normal, as opposed to red color, makes AOM less likely (adjusted LR+ = 0.2 [95%CI: 0.19-0.21]).

Rothman R, Owens T, Simel DL. 2003. *JAMA* 290(12):1633-1640.

PEDIATRIC

Mouth

- **Oral Candidal Thrush**
  - Common up to 12 mo; investigate for underlying condition/ immunodeficiency in older child
  - Signs: cracking at mouth corners and whitish patches on buccal mucosa
  - Milk can be scraped off with a tongue depressor, while thrush cannot
- **Pharyngitis/Tonsillitis**
  - CC: sore throat, fever, stridor, shortness of breath, hoarseness, dysphagia, neck mass/swollen neck

Table 9. Common and Serious Causes of Pharyngitis/URTI

Illness	Clinical Characteristics
Viral Pharyngitis*	Gradual onset; low grade fever; rhinorrhea/cough; conjunctivitis; hoarseness
Group A Strep	Mclsaac Criteria: fever; age 3-14 yr; anterior cervical lymphadenopathy; no cough; tonsillar erythema/exudate
Mononucleosis (EBV)	Fever, severely exudative, erythematous, hypertrophic tonsils; posterior cervical adenopathy; hepatosplenomegaly
Vincent's Angina/ Trench Mouth	High fever; halitosis; adenopathy; bleeding, engorged, exudative tonsils with gray pseudomembrane
Quinsy/Peritonsillar Abscess	Asymmetric hypertrophied, erythematous, exudative, ulcerated tonsil(s); uvula deviated away from affected side
Oral HSV (primary infection)	Gradual onset; high fever; acute gingivostomatitis; ulcerating vesicles throughout anterior mouth including lips, with sparing of posterior pharynx, pain with oral fluids
Epiglottitis	Sudden onset; high fever; drooling; dysphagia; dysphonia (hot potato voice); significant respiratory distress; tripod sit; irritability/lethargy; thumb print sign on neck AP X-ray
Croup	Sudden onset; fever; barking cough, nonproductive cough; worse at night; stridor; hoarse voice; steeple sign CXR
Bacterial Tracheitis	Similar to croup, then rapid deterioration, high fever and lack of response to treatment for croup

*Most common cause (80% of pharyngitis cases)

5.3 Respiratory

Asthma

- CC:
  - Shortness of breath from: viral illnesses (most common trigger in younger children), physical activity, environmental allergens (animal dander, dust, house dust mites, pollen), food (eggs, seafood, peanut butter), smoke, weather changes, exposure to cold, and stress[7]
  - Dry, tight, occasionally wheezy cough especially at night
  - Eczema in atopic child, especially in flexural surfaces
- Signs: expiratory phase longer than inspiratory phase, with high-pitched wheezes throughout most of expiration[7]

EBM: Asthma

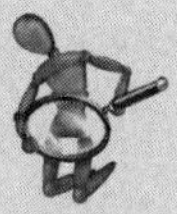

Asthma is considered well-controlled if daytime symptoms are <4 d/wk, nighttime symptoms are <1 night/wk, there is normal physical activity, infrequent exacerbations, no absence from school, and the need for a β2-agonist is <4 doses/wk.

Becker A, et al. 2007. *CMAJ* 173(6 Suppl):S12-S14.

Cough

- CC: productive or nonproductive, worse at night/day

Table 10. Qualities of Cough Associated with Common Respiratory Illnesses

Illness	Character of Cough
Asthma	Dry, "tight", occasionally wheezy; wet asthma cough can mimic cystic fibrosis cough; spasmodic asthma cough can mimic pertussis (without whoop)
Bacterial Tracheitis	Brassy cough that does not respond to standard croup therapies; inspiratory and/or expiratory stridor; rapid decompensation
Bronchiolitis	Initially dry; may become "loose and rattling"
Croup	Sounds like a seal's bark; sudden hoarse voice and inspiratory stridor at night
Cystic Fibrosis	Productive or purulent
Pertussis	During coughing spasm, sudden crowing inspiration (whoop) in between coughs, often followed by vomiting
Pneumonia	Paroxysmal, dry, and staccato (short inspiration between coughs)
Psychogenic	Uncommon, cough sounds like a loud goose "honk"; never occurs during sleep
Pulmonary Aspiration	Dry or loose; often associated with lower airway obstruction; can be similar to cough of asthma or bronchitis
Tracheomalacia	Loud, brassy or vibratory; can be associated with a coarse inspiratory and expiratory stridor/wheeze

Goldbloom RB. *Pediatric Clinical Skills.* Philadelphia: Saunders; 2003.

5.4 Cardiovascular

Murmurs in Infants and Children

- Soft precordial systolic murmur common in first few days after birth
- May indicate patent ductus arteriosus if it persists and is heard over the back

Innocent Murmurs (vibratory murmurs, venous hum, carotid bruits)

- All diastolic murmurs, or systolic that are coarse or >grade 3
- Heard best with bell of stethoscope and may change with patient position

Organic (non-innocent) Murmurs

- Systolic or diastolic, coarse, >grade 3
- <3 yr: congenital heart disease
- >3 yr: acquired heart disease (e.g. rheumatic carditis)

Table 11. Benign Heart Murmurs in Children

Murmur (age of presentation)	Location	Timing	Intensity, Quality, and Pitch
Closing Ductus (neonate to 1 yr)	Upper left sternal border	Transient	Soft
Peripheral Pulmonary Flow Murmur (neonate to 1 yr)	Left of upper left sternal border, and in lung fields and axillae	Systole	Soft, slightly ejectile
Still's Murmur (preschool to early school age)	Mid/lower left sternal border and over carotid arteries	Early and mid-systole	Grade I-II/VI Musical, vibratory, multiple overtones
Venous Hum (preschool to early school age)	Under clavicle	Continuous	Soft, hollow, louder in diastole, can be eliminated by maneuvers that affect venous return, or by contralateral neck rotation

Bickley LS, Szilagyi PG, *Bates B. Bates' Guide to Physical Examination and History Taking*, 10th ed. Philadelphia: Lippincott Williams & Wilkins; 2009.

Table 12. Pathologic Heart Murmurs in Children

Defect	Location	Timing	Intensity	Pitch	Quality
Atrial Septal Defect (acyanotic)	Second left interspace	Wide, fixed split S2, peaks in mid-systole	Soft	Medium	Nonmusical
Ventricular Septal Defect (acyanotic)	Left sternal border, third and fourth interspaces	Between S1 and S2	Very loud	High	Blowing
Patent Ductus Arteriosus	Second left interspace; may radiate to left clavicle/ sternum	Continuous; louder in late systole (just before S2); obscures S2; softer in diastole	Loud	Medium	Harsh
Tetralogy of Fallot (cyanotic)	Second and third left interspaces	Between S1 and S2	Not well transmitted		No distinct characteristics

Engel J. *Pocket Guide to Pediatric Assessment.* St. Louis: Mosby; 1989.

EBM: Murmurs in Children

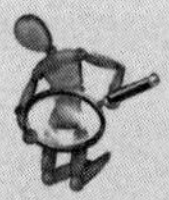

In a study of 30 office-based pediatricians, the average sensitivity was 82% and average specificity was 72% for differentiating innocent murmurs from pathological ones by auscultation, as compared to the gold standard of complete echocardiographic assessment.

Haney I, et al. 1998. *Arch Dis Childhood* 81(5):409-412.

PEDIATRIC

Heart Failure

- CC: shortness of breath, exercise intolerance, presyncope or syncopal episodes; diaphoresis and tiring with feeds in infants
- Signs: peripheral edema, failure to thrive, cyanosis, clubbing, heart murmur, hepatomegaly
- Investigations: CXR, ECG, 4 limb BPs, consider echocardiogram

Table 13. Timing of Heart Failure

Timing of Heart Failure	Significance
At Birth	Rare (e.g. hemolysis, fetal-maternal transfusion, neonatal lupus)
First Week of Life	Obstructive lesion or persistent pulmonary hypertension (this can present later in Trisomy 21 cases, as their lungs are more compliant to start with)
4-6 Weeks	Left-to-right shunting
After 3 Months	Myocarditis, cardiomyopathy or paroxysmal tachycardia

5.5 Gastrointestinal

- In neonates, common problems include congenital abnormalities (e.g. atresia, obstruction, Hirschsprung's disease)

Jaundice

- Common in the first wk of life
- Visible at serum bilirubin levels of 85-120 μM[8]
- Etiology (see **Table 14**)
- Clinical characteristics
  - Yellowed skin, scleral icterus
  - Acute bilirubin encephalopathy: lethargic, slight hypotonia, poor sucking, high pitched cry → no feeding, increased tone, coma
- Physical examination for hyperbilirubinemia can be unreliable; it is best to have a low threshold for bilirubin testing via heel prick

Table 14. Differential Diagnosis of Jaundice in the Neonatal Period

Time of Appearance	Possible Etiology
<24 h of Birth	***ALWAYS PATHOLOGIC*** • Hemolysis: Rh/ABO incompatibility • Sepsis: GBS/TORCH infection
24-72 h	• Physiologic • Breastfeeding/dehydration • Hemolytic: G6PD/PKU deficiency, thalassemia, spherocytosis • Nonhemolytic: hematoma, polycythemia, hypothyroidism, sepsis
72-96 h	• Physiologic • Breastfeeding • Sepsis
>1 wk	• Breast milk jaundice • Inborn errors of metabolism: galactosemia • Neonatal hepatitis • Idiopathic: total parenteral nutrition (TPN) • Biliary atresia

Maisels MJ. 2006. *Pediatr Rev* 27(12):443-454.

5.6 Genitourinary

Enuresis/Incontinence

- May be nocturnal (nighttime only), diurnal (day and night)
- Classification:
    - Primary: child has never achieved dryness; associated with family history of delayed bladder control; maturational
    - Secondary: child had achieved dryness for at least 6 mo before new onset of "accidents"
- DDx: psychosocial stressors, constipation, UTI, behavior, DM, abuse, neurodevelopmental condition, cauda equina syndrome

Urinary Tract Infection (UTI)

- CC: primarily age dependent, may present with fever, irritability, and smelly/cloudy urine at any age
- Signs:
    - Infant and young child (<2 yr)
        - Asymptomatic, or GI symptoms such as fever without a focus, vomiting, poor feeding, diarrhea or abdominal pain
    - Child (>2 yr)
        - Cystitis: dysuria, frequency, urgency, hematuria, urinary retention, suprapubic pain, pruritus, incontinence, enuresis, foul-smelling urine
    - Pyelonephritis: fever, chills, costovertebral pain and tenderness
- Causes: *E. coli*, *Klebsiella*, coagulase negative *Staphylococci spp.* most common

5.7 MSK

Limp

- CC: painful or painless limp
- Signs: antalgic gait, swelling/erythema of hip or knee joint, leg length discrepancy, unusual/fixed positioning of leg at rest, fever
- Differential Diagnosis: painless vs. painful
    - Painless limp: weakness secondary to hip dysplasia, cerebral palsy, leg-length discrepancy
    - Painful limp (see **Table 15**)

Common MSK Injuries

- Knee
    - Patellofemoral dysfunction: deep, aching anterior knee pain worsened by prolonged sitting, knee instability (common in female athletes)
    - Anterior cruciate ligament (ACL) tear: after "cutting" movement in sports
    - O'Donoghue's unhappy triad/skier's knee: (ACL, medial collateral ligament, medial/lateral meniscus): after valgus knee injury
- Ankle: most common acute injury in adolescent athletes
    - Inversion: 85% acute ankle injuries
    - Eversion: often more serious because higher risk of fracture or injury to tibio-fibular syndesmosis
- Uncommon, but not to be missed:
    - Legg-Calvé-Perthes disease: osteonecrosis of capital femoral epiphysis which can disrupt the growth plate
    - Most common in boys <12 yr
    - Common presentation: hip or groin pain, often minor; limp
    - Slipped capital femoral epiphysis (SCFE): displacement of proximal femoral epiphysis (usually posteromedially) due to disruption of growth plate
        - Most common in obese adolescent males

» Common presentation: acute, severe pain with limp
» Key signs: limited internal rotation of hip and obligate external rotation on hip flexion (Whitman's sign)

Table 15. Differential Diagnosis of Painful Limp

Differential Diagnosis	Peak Age (yr)	Features
Septic Arthritis	All ages	Fever, antalgic gait, refusal to weight bear, severely limited internal rotation, and adduction of hip
Osteomyelitis	All ages	Point tenderness, local edema, erythema, restricted movement/pseudoparalysis, ± fever
Transient Synovitis*	3-10	Antalgic gait, hip fixed in flexion/external rotation
Legg-Calvé-Perthes	4-10	Mild, intermittent hip pain, referred to thigh/knee, limited internal rotation and abduction of hip
Osgood-Schlatter	11-18	Pain with activity, relieved by rest, insidious onset over months, tenderness over tibial tuberosity ± erythema
Slipped Capital Femoral Epiphysis (SCFE)	8-17	Obese child, tenderness over hip joint capsule, restricted internal rotation and abduction; acute, painful limp
Malignancy		All: weight loss, constitutional symptoms
Leukemia	2-10	Night pain, pallor, petechiae, infections, bruising
Neuroblastoma	1-5	Abdominal mass, night pain
Osteosarcoma	5-20	Palpable mass, pathologic fracture
Juvenile Idiopathic Arthritis (JIA) (several types)	Varies	Persistent arthritis in children <16 yr; classified by affected joints; may have constitutional symptoms, fever, extra-articular signs, nail, and eye abnormalities
Henoch-Schönlein Purpura (HSP)	3-7	Following respiratory illness, purpuric rash over buttocks and legs, arthralgia, angioedema, abdominal pain
Growing Pains	3-10	Crampy night pain in calves and thighs, occasionally wakes child from sleep, bilateral; exam unremarkable

*Most common cause of hip pain/limp in children

5.8 Neurological

Table 16. Neonatal Primitive Reflexes

Reflex	How to Elicit	Reaction	Time Period
Galant	Stroke back about 1 cm from midline with baby held prone	Trunk curves toward stroked side	Birth to 4-6 mo
Placing	Baby upright, touch top of foot to table edge	Child mimics walking onto table	Birth to 4-6 mo
Rooting	Stroke cheek	Head turns to same side	Birth to 4 mo

Table 16. Neonatal Primitive Reflexes (continued)

Reflex	How to Elicit	Reaction	Time Period
Palmar/Plantar Grasp	Place finger into palm or sole of foot	Fingers and toes grasp together	Birth to 4-6 mo
Moro	Startle baby with loud noise or suddenly lower supine baby	Arms extend, abduct with hands open; then arms come together	Birth to 2 mo
Asymmetric Tonic Neck	Turn head to one side	Arm/leg on same side extend, flex on opposite side (fencing position)	Birth to 3-4 mo
Parachute Reflex	Tilting the infant to side while in sitting position	Ipsilateral arm extension	6-8 mo

Febrile Seizures

- CC:
  - Commonly in infants and young children 6 mo-5 yr with febrile illness
  - Associated with fever but without evidence of: 1) intracranial infection, 2) metabolic disturbance, or 3) history of previous afebrile seizures
- Features of simple febrile seizures
  - <15 min, generalized seizure occurring once in 24 h period
  - No focal neurological findings
- Features of complex febrile seizures
  - Prolonged (>15 min), focal, multiple in a 24 h period

5. 9 Dermatological

- Diaper dermatitis

Table 17. Differential Diagnosis of Diaper Dermatitis

Disease	Primary Lesion	Secondary Lesion	Flexural Involvement	Other Sites
Contact Irritant Dermatitis	Shiny, red macules/patches	Ulcerations, superficial erosions	Absent	None
Seborrheic Dermatitis	Yellow, greasy papules/ plaques on an erythematous base	Scales	Present	Scalp, axillae, trunk
Candidal Dermatitis	Bright red patches with peripheral scale, 'satellite lesions'	None	Present	Oral thrush
Psoriasis	Sharply well demarcated areas of papules/ plaques with thin scale	None	Present	Trunk, extremities, nails, scalp
Bullous Impetigo	Bullae on an erythematous base	Superficial erosions, crusts	Present	Axillae or other areas

5.10 Genetic Disorders

Table 18. Common Genetic Disorders: Autosomal

Condition	Cause	Signs
Down's Syndrome (Trisomy 21) 1/650-1/1,000 live births	Chromosomal abnormality, extra chromosome 21 Associated with ↑ maternal age	• Hypotonia and microcephaly • Epicanthal folds • Upward slanting palpebral fissures • Stenotic Eustachian tubes • Single palmar creases • Congenital heart and abdominal defects • Mild to moderate mental retardation • Frequent respiratory infections
Edwards Syndrome (Trisomy 18) 1/5,000 births <5% infants survive past 1 yr	Chromosomal abnormality, extra chromosome 18 Associated with ↑ maternal age	• Growth retardation • Simple, low-set ears • Prominent occiput • Micrognathia • Overlapping fingers • Rocker bottom feet • Congenital heart, genital, and CNS defects • Hypertonia

Table 19. Common Genetic Disorders: Sex Chromosome

Condition	Cause	Signs
Klinefelter Syndrome 1/1,000 live male births	Aneuploidy of sex chromosomes, XXY in 80% of cases Associated with ↑ maternal age	• Long arms and legs, slim build • Small testes 1-2 cm • Gynecomastia • Delays in language and emotional development • Cognitive deficits variable; average IQ ~90 • Often not diagnosed until adolescence
Turner Syndrome 1/2,000-1/5,000 live female births	Aneuploidy of sex chromosomes, usually XO	• Short stature • Streak gonads • Webbed neck • Lymphedema • Coarctation of aorta • Hypoplastic nails • Learning disabilities

5.11 Psychiatric and Behavioral Problems

Anxiety Disorders (see **Psychiatric Exam**, p.333)

- Note that transient development of age appropriate fears are common in childhood; therefore must evaluate degree of life disruption
- Watch for frequent repeat occurrences of anxiety related behaviors

Attention Deficit/Hyperactivity Disorder

- Triad of inattentiveness, impulsivity, and hyperactivity such that behavior interferes with functional ability (social and academic)
- Hyperactivity can be associated with this disorder; not always present
- Signs: distractible, tendency to fidget, tendency to interrupt, low attention span

Autism Spectrum Disorders

- Spectrum of developmental disorders characterized by impairment in:
  - Social interaction: nonverbal behavior, peer relationships, and social/emotional reciprocity, sharing of enjoyment/interests
  - Communication: delayed spoken language, difficulty conversing, repetitive use of language, lack of imaginative/make-believe play
  - Stereotyped behaviors: preoccupation with narrow interests or parts of objects, inflexible adherence to routines, motor mannerisms
- Checklist for Autism in Toddlers (CHAT screening tool) is available and has a good specificity; PPV = 83%, but a low sensitivity of 18%

Depression

- Persistent depressed or irritable mood present for most of nearly every day, or anhedonia (markedly diminished interest/pleasurable activities)
- Signs and Symptoms:
  - Changes in sleeping patterns and appetite, inability to concentrate, feelings of worthlessness, fatigue, suicidal ideations and behaviors
  - Atypical presentations in adolescents include anger, oppositional behaviors
- Highly associated with other psychiatric issues: anxiety, somatic complaints, relationship problems, academic concerns, drug usage
- Take suicide threats seriously; 80% of suicidal teens seek help beforehand

Eating Disorders (Anorexia Nervosa and Bulimia Nervosa)

- Risk Factors: family history, low self-esteem, immaturity, poor family dynamics
- Expresses fears of obesity associated with alteration in perception of body image, and preoccupation with becoming or staying thin
- Disordered eating (especially anorexia) can be found as part of the "Female Athletic Triad": disordered eating, osteoporosis, and amenorrhea
- See comparison in **Table 20**

PEDIATRIC

Table 20. Anorexia Nervosa and Bulimia Nervosa

	Anorexia Nervosa	Bulimia Nervosa
Key Feature	Refusal to maintain body weight at or above 85% expected	Recurrent binge eating with inappropriate compensatory behaviors (self-induced vomiting, laxatives, diuretics)
Amenorrhea	Yes	No
Epidemiology	0.5% adolescent females 0.05% adolescent males Peak incidence 15-19 yr	1-5% adolescent females Peak incidence early 20s
Subtypes	1. Restricting (no compensatory behaviors) 2. Binge eating/purging	1. Purging (vomiting, laxatives, diuretics) 2. Non-purging (compensatory behaviors: fasting, excessive exercise)
Physical Signs	Emaciation, muscle wasting, lanugo, hypothermia, starvation edema, bradycardia, arrhythmias, carotenemia (from excess carrot ingestion)	Muscle weakness, tooth decay, parotid gland enlargement, Russell's sign (knuckle calluses from self-induced vomiting), bloodshot eyes
Body Weight	BMI <18 kg/m^2	Normal or higher than average

Aggressive Behaviors

- **Oppositional Defiant Disorder**
  - Negativistic, hostile, and defiant behavior
  - Features: losing temper, arguing with parents, refusal to comply with rules, blames others for mistakes, angry/resentful
  - Must cause clinically significant impairment in social, academic, or occupational functioning
  - May progress to conduct disorder; usually onset before 8 yr
- **Conduct Disorder**
  - Repetitive, persistent pattern of behavior in which basic rights of others and age-appropriate social norms/rules are violated
  - Features
    - Aggression: bullying, initiating fights, cruelty to animals or people
    - Property destruction: setting fires, destroying others' property
    - Deceitfulness or theft: lying to obtain goods, breaking and entering
    - Serious violation of rules: staying out, running away from home, truancy

5.12 Child Abuse

- Definition: violence, mistreatment, or neglect of a child while in the care of a parent, sibling, relative, caregiver, or guardian

Physician's Role

- Mandatory Reporting Requirement: physicians are responsible to report any "reasonable grounds to suspect" child abuse; not reporting to Children's Aid Society is an offence (in Ontario)
- Physician's duty to report overrides provisions of confidentiality

History

- If possible, defer to expert
- Listen and believe reports with nonjudgmental and caring attitude
- Any statements made by a child about abuse should be recorded as direct
- Questions about what, who, when, how often, threats, bribes must be open-ended
- Observe behaviors of child and caretaker
- Are caretaker responses appropriate and consistent?
- Does the child have exaggerated aggressiveness or passivity, or suggest sexualized overtones?

Physical Exam

- Always do a complete physical exam (pictorializing on a diagram when ever possible), but especially noting the following:
  - **General:** height, weight, head circumference percentile
  - **H&N:** retina, eardrums, and oral cavity for signs of occult trauma
  - **GU:** genitalia, rectum
  - **MSK:** bone and joint tenderness, fractures (new or healed), ROM
  - **Dermatological:** bruises, bites, cuts, scars, puncture wounds; unusual number, shape, and location warrant further investigation
- Red Flags: lack of reasonable explanation, changing/vague history, history inconsistent with injury, or inappropriate level of concern by caretaker

> **Clinical Pearl: Consider Abuse**
> Rib fractures in children are highly predictive of nonaccidental injury. Bruises in a nonambulatory child are a concern of nonaccidental injury ("No cruising, no bruising").

Common Disorders Related to Abuse

- Malnutrition; developmental delay
- Emotional difficulty: anxiety, depression, self-harm, suicide attempts, post traumatic stress disorder (PTSD)
- Head injury: leading cause of death from child abuse
- Physical and mental health problems as adults and high-risk lifestyle choices

Table 21. Indicators of Child Abuse

Types of Abuse	Signs and Symptoms	
	Behavioral Indicators	**Physical Indictors**
Neglect: Failing to provide basic needs	• Frequent absence from school • Poor hygiene • Delinquent acts, alcohol/drug abuse	• Pale, listless, unkempt • Poor hygiene • Failure to thrive without identifiable organic disease • Indiscriminately seeks affection
Physical Abuse: Deliberately using force against child	• Cringe/flinch if touched unexpectedly • Infants may have a vacant stare • Extremely aggressive or withdrawn • Extremely compliant and/or eager to please • Delay in seeking medical attention • Fear, anxiety, depression, low self-esteem, social withdrawal, poor school performance, self-harm	• Posterior rib fractures • Distinct marks: cigarette burns, loop marks, belt buckles • Untreated fractures • Presence of several injuries over a period of time and/or in various stages of healing
Sexual Abuse: Includes fondling, sexual touching, intercourse, rape, sodomy, exhibitionism or child pornography	• Age inappropriate play with toys, self or others displaying explicit sexual acts • Age inappropriate sexually explicit drawing/description • Bizarre, sophisticated or unusual sexual knowledge • Prostitution and seductive behaviors	• Unusual or excessive itching in genital or anal area • Torn, stained or bloody underwear • Pregnancy; bruising, swelling or infection in genital or anal area, venereal disease, STIs
Shaken Baby Syndrome: Forceful shaking of infant or young child	• Acute: spectrum from vomiting to irritability to LOC or death • Long-term: Developmental disability, speech/ learning disability	• Minimal to no evidence of external trauma • Severe closed head injury, diffuse brain injury and swelling, subdural/subarachnoid and retinal hemorrhages • Fractures, especially posterior ribs • Paralysis, hearing loss, seizure, death

6. APPENDIX

Table 22a. Major Developmental Milestones (2-12 mo)

	2 mo	4 mo	6 mo	9 mo	12 mo
Gross Motor	Prone: lifts chin	Head Control Prone: raises head and chest Rolls from front to back	Tripod sitting	Pull to stand Crawling (optional)	First steps
Fine Motor	Pulls at clothes	Holds objects in midline Reaches	Transfers across midline	Finger-thumb grasp	Pincer grasp
Speech and Language	Coos	Responds to voice	Babbles Responds to name		First word
Adaptive and Social Skills	Follows moving person with eyes	Laughs	Raises arms for up Stranger anxiety	Pat-a-cake Waves bye-bye Peek-a-boo Separation anxiety	Drinks from a cup

Table 22b. Major Developmental Milestones (18 mo-5 yr)

	18 mo	2 yr	3 yr	4 yr	5 yr
Gross Motor	Runs stiffly	Runs well Climbs stairs 1 at a time	Rides a tricycle	Hops on one foot	Skips Rides bicycle
Fine Motor	Draws a line and scribbles Stacks 2 cubes	Stacks 6 cubes Runs Kicks ball	Pulls on shoes	Copies squares	Copies triangles
Speech and Language	20+ words Follows simple commands with cues	2 words together 50-100 words	3-4 word sentences Colors	Nursery rhymes Alphabet	Future tense in speech
Adaptive and Social Skills	Uses spoon Points to body parts	Temper tantrum Parallel play	Counts to 10 Dresses (except buttons) Toilet training	Cooperative play Buttons clothes	Knows 4 colors

Table 23. Publicly Funded Immunization Schedules (Ontario, 2011)

Age at Vaccination	DTaP-IPV	Hib	PCV13	Rot-1	Men-C-C	MMR	VZV	MMRV	Men-C-ACYW	HepB	HPV-4 (Girls)	Tdap	Flu
2 mo	X	X	X	X									
4 mo	X	X	X	X									
6 mo	X	X											
12 mo			X		X	X							
15 mo							X						
18 mo	X	X											
4-6 yr	X							X					
12 yr (Gr. 7)									X	X			
13 yr (Gr. 8)											X		
14-16 yr												X	
Every yr (in autumn)													X

Ministry of Health and Long-Term Care. *Publicly Funded Immunization Schedules for Ontario*. Toronto: MOHLTC. 2011. Available from: http://www.health.gov.on.ca/en/public/programs/immunization/docs/schedule.pdf.

DTaP	Diphtheria, tetanus, acellular pertussis
IPV	Inactivated poliovirus
Hib	Haemophilus influenzae type b
PCV13	Pneumococcal conjugate 13-valent
Rot-1	Rotavirus ORAL
MenC-C	Meningococcal conjugate C
MMR	Measles, mumps, rubella
VZV	Varicella zoster virus
MMRV	Measles, mumps, rubella, varicella
Men-C-ACYW	Meningococcal conjugate ACYW-135
HepB	Hepatitis B
HPV4	Human papillomavirus quadrivalent
Tdap	Tetanus, diphtheria, acellular pertussis
Flu	Influenza

REFERENCES

1. Goldbloom RB. *Pediatric Clinical Skills.* Philadelphia: Saunders; 2003.
2. Leduc D, Woods S. *Temperature Measurement in Paediatrics*. Ottawa: Canadian Paediatric Society. 2013. Available from: http://www.cps.ca/en/documents/position/temperature-measurement.
3. Neinstein LS. *Adolescent Healthcare: A Practical Guide.* Philadelphia: Wolters Kluwer/Lippincott Williams & Wilkins; 2008.
4. Lalani A, Schneeweiss S (Editors). *Handbook of Pediatric Emergency Medicine*. Mississauga: Jones and Bartlett Publishers; 2008.
5. Marcdante KJ, Kliegman RM, Jenson HB, Behrman RE (Editors). *Nelson Essentials of Pediatrics*, 6th ed. Philadelphia: Elsevier Saunders; 2011.
6. Anstine D, Grinenko D. 2000. Rapid screening for disordered eating in college-aged females in the primary care setting. *J Adolesc Health* 26(5):338-342.
7. Lougheed MD, Lemière C, Dell SD, Ducharme DM, Fitzgerald JM, Leigh R, et al. 2010. Canadian Thoracic Society Asthma Management Continuum - 2010 Consensus Summary for children six years of age and over, and adults. *Can Respir J* 17(1):15-24.
8. Lauer BJ, Spector ND. 2011. Hyperbilirubinemia in the newborn. *Pediatr Rev* 32(8):341-349.
9. Bickley LS, Szilagyi PG, Bates B. *Bates' Guide to Physical Examination and History Taking*, 10th ed. Philadelphia: Lippincott Williams & Wilkins; 2009.
10. Engel J. *Mosby's Pocket Guide to Pediatric Assessment.* St. Louis: Mosby; 2006.

The Peripheral Vascular Exam

Editors:
Lior Flor
Jieun Kim

Faculty Reviewers:
George Oreopoulos, MD, MSc, FRCS(C)
Tony Moloney, MD, MB, HDip, FRCS(C)

TABLE OF CONTENTS

1. COMMON CHIEF COMPLAINTS

- Chest, abdominal, or back pain (in the setting of acute aortic emergency)
- Pain in calf (especially with exercise)
- Skin ulceration
- Swelling
- Changes in skin temperature and color
- Transient ischemic attack (TIA, in setting of carotid artery disease)
- Varicose veins (in setting of cosmesis and/or symptomatic venous disease)

2. FOCUSED HISTORY

2.1 Risk Factors

- Atherosclerosis
  - Smoking
  - HTN
  - DM
  - Family history
  - Lifestyle (e.g. exercise, diet)
  - Elevated cholesterol
- Thromboembolic event
  - Atrial fibrillation, post-myocardial infarction <3 mo, valvular disease, prosthetic valves, endocarditis, cardiomyopathy, myxoma

PERIPHERAL VASCULAR

2.2 Previous Medical History

- Myocardial infarction (MI) or coronary artery disease (CAD)
  - Signs and symptoms of MI or CAD (see **Cardiovascular Exam**, p.58)
  - Peripheral vascular disease (PVD) often considered a "CAD equivalent"
  - Course of disease, hospitalization, medical and surgical treatment
- Congestive heart failure (CHF)
  - Peripheral edema, pulmonary congestion, exercise intolerance
- Stroke/TIA
  - Cerebrovascular occlusive disease
  - Signs and symptoms of stroke (see **Neurological Exam**, p.197) including: unilateral or bilateral weakness/paralysis of limbs, sensory deficits, speech difficulties, diplopia or amaurosis fugax, and facial droop
  - Neurological symptoms (e.g. dizziness, presyncope, and syncope)
  - Hemispheric symptoms
- Precipitants of venous thrombosis
  - Recent prolonged immobilization (deep vein thrombosis [DVT])
  - Postoperatively (especially orthopedic, thoracic, GI, GU)
    - Trauma (fractures of femur, pelvis, spine, tibia, etc.)
    - Post-MI, CHF
    - Long travel
  - Hormone-related: pregnancy, oral contraceptive pill use, hormone replacement therapy, selective estrogen receptor modulators (SERMs)
  - Inheritable hypercoagulability states:
    - APLA syndrome, Factor V Leiden, Prothrombin G20210A, etc.
  - Underlying malignancy or blood dyscrasias
- Vasculitis
  - Skin changes, mucosal ulcerations
  - Joint pain
  - Changes in vision and/or eye pain

2.3 Symptoms of Ischemia

6 P's

- **P**olar (cold): typically first notable symptom
- **P**ain: absent in 20% of cases due to prompt onset of anesthesia and paralysis
- **P**allor: replaced by mottled (network-like appearance) cyanosis within a few hours
- **P**aresthesia*: light touch lost first (small fibers) followed by other sensory modalities (larger fibers)
- **P**aralysis*/Power loss: further progression of ischemia, indicative of severity
- **P**ulselessness
- *Paresthesia and paralysis suggest critical ischemia
- Do NOT expect all of the **6 P**'s to be present and do NOT rely on pulses

Critical Ischemia

- Acute
  - **6 P**'s
  - Neuromotor dysfunction
- Chronic
  - Night pain
  - Pain at rest (pain at all times and not relieved by dependency)
  - Tissue loss (ulceration/gangrene)

PERIPHERAL VASCULAR

Pain

- **OPQRSTUVW** with emphasis on:
  - Onset (if acute, associated with paresthesia)
  - Location (temple, muscles, abdomen)
  - Pain in lower extremities during exercise (e.g. pain in calves, thighs, hips, buttocks)
  - Dependent upon exertion (e.g. amount of walking, rate of walking, degree of incline)
  - Reproducible pain with similar exertion (consistent pattern)

Skin

- Changes in color, temperature, appearance
- Ulceration
  - Classification (traumatic, ischemic, neoplastic, venous, mixed, malignant)
  - Time and rate of development
  - If resulting from minor trauma (e.g. toes, heel), may indicate chronic ischemia
- Gangrene: wet (infectious) vs. dry (noninfectious)

3. FOCUSED PHYSICAL EXAM

3.1 General

- Ensure the patient is adequately exposed with draping in between the legs
- Remember to compare sides
- Vitals: bilateral and orthostatic blood pressures (see **General History and Physical Exam**, p.12)

3.2 Inspection

- Specific locations
  - Upper extremities (from the finger tips to the shoulder)
  - Lower extremities (from the groin and buttocks to the toes)
  - Inspect for:
    - Masses, scars, lesions
    - Symmetry: muscle bulk (atrophy/hypertrophy)
    - Size: swelling, thickening
    - Skin: shiny, hair loss, erythema/discoloration, gangrene
    - Ulcers: arterial: between toes and heel; venous: medial malleolus
    - Nails: note color and texture
- Arterial insufficiency
  - Cyanosis: central (frenulum and buccal mucosa) and peripheral (nails)
  - Skin: cool, pale extremities, increased pigmentation, swelling, heaviness and aching in legs (usually medial lower third of legs)
  - Ulcers: ischemic ulceration due to trauma of the toes and heel, develops rapidly, painful, and has discretely visible edges
- Venous stasis
  - Skin: warm, thickening and erythema over the ankle and lower leg (dependent areas), thickened (woody) fibrosis/lipodermatosclerosis
  - Ulcers: stasis ulceration of ankle or above medial malleolus, develops slowly, painless, diffuses with no distinct borders
  - Veins: engorgement, varicosities
    - Prominent veins in edematous limb may be venous obstruction
    - Pemberton's sign: facial flushing, distension of neck veins, elevation of JVP, and stridor when patient raises arms above head (sign of vena cava obstruction)

- Chronic venous insufficiency: warm, erythematous, thickened skin, increased pigmentation, ± brown ulcers around ankles
- Superficial phlebitis: warm, painful, erythema secondary to inflammation around vein, superficial changes, swelling of distal part of extremity

> **Clinical Pearl: Deep Vein Thrombosis**
> Swelling in the affected limb is a common symptom of DVT, which is a risk factor for PE.

- **Vasculitis**
  - Skin:
    - Livedo reticularis rash (bluish-red discoloration, network pattern)
    - Malar or discoid rash on face in SLE
    - Raynaud's phenomenon: episodes of sharply demarcated pallor and/or cyanosis, then erythema of the digits (see **Common Clinical Scenarios**, p.314)
    - Purpura
  - Mucosa: oral or nasal ulcers (SLE, Wegener's, Behçet's)
  - Joints: look for "active" swollen joints
  - Eyes: episcleritis, scleritis, anterior uveitis (iritis)
  - Venous and arterial thrombosis/ulcers, gangrene as above

3.3 Palpation and Auscultation

Arterial

- Skin temperature: feel with back of hand: warm vs. cool
- Capillary refill: compress nailbeds and determine the duration for return of circulation: normal = 2-3 s
- **Pulses**
  - Rate: tachycardia >100 bpm, bradycardia <60 bpm
  - Rhythm: regular, regularly irregular (consistent pattern), irregularly irregular
  - Amplitude:

Amplitude of Pulses	
0	Absent
1	Diminished
2	Normal
3	Increased
4	Aneurysmal (often exaggerated, widened pulse)

  - Always compare both sides for presence and symmetry

Characteristic Pulse Patterns

- **Hyperkinetic Pulse**
  - Strong, bounding pulse
  - Increased stroke volume in heart block
  - Hyperdynamic circulation and increased stoke volume in fever, anemia, exercise, anxiety
  - Reduced peripheral resistance in patent ductus arteriosus, AV fistula
- **Pulsus Tardus**
  - Small, slowly rising pulse that is delayed with respect to heart sounds
  - Seen in aortic stenosis
- **Pulsus Parvus (Hypokinetic)**
  - Small, weak pulse due to diminished left ventricular (LV) stroke volume

- Seen in hypovolemia, LV failure, MI, restrictive pericardial disease, shock, arrhythmia

Table 1. Description of Characteristic Wave Forms

Waveform	Description	Representative Diagram	Associated with/ Etiology
Pulsus Parvus et Tardus (anacrotic)	Small, slow rising pulse with drop or notch in ascending portion	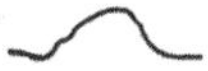	Aortic stenosis
Collapsing	Quick rise, quick fall	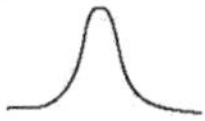	Increased CO_2
Water-Hammer	Sudden rapid pulse with full expansion followed by sudden collapse	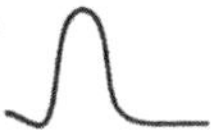	Aortic regurgitation or arterial obstruction
Bisferiens	Double-peaked pulse with mid-systolic dip	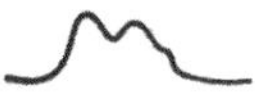	Aortic regurgitation, ± aortic stenosis, hypertrophic cardiomyopathy
Alternans	Alternating amplitude of pulses	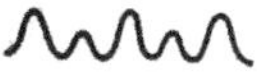	CHF, more easily detected in conjunction with BP measurement

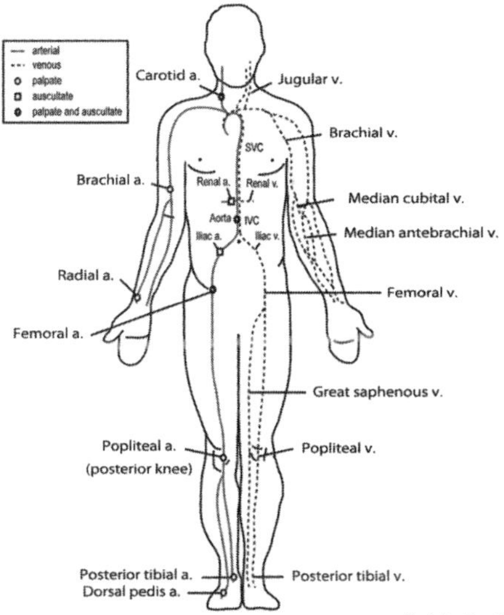

Varinder Randhawa

Figure 1. Location of Pulses

- Examine the following pulses (see **Figure 1**):
- **Carotid**
  - Auscultate for bruits (absent, mild/soft, harsh/loud)
  - If no bruits, palpate one carotid artery at a time
- **Brachial**
  - May use thumb to palpate

- **Radial**
  - Use the pads/tips of three fingers
  - Significant delay of the radial pulse after the brachial pulse may suggest aortic stenosis
- **Abdominal Aorta**
  - Normal width of abdominal aorta is about 2 cm
  - Palpate deeply for pulsations (lay patient flat, ensure abdomen is relaxed)
  - Auscultate for abdominal bruits
  - Midline pulsatile abdominal mass may be an abdominal aortic aneurysm (AAA)
  - Midline abdominal bruit suggests atherosclerotic disease of the aorta or renal vessels
- **Renal Arteries**
  - Auscultate for bruits at positions 5 cm above the umbilicus and 3-5 cm to either side of the midline or from the back
- **Femoral**
  - Palpate at midpoint of the inguinal ligament
  - Auscultate for bruits
  - Compare timing of femoral pulse with radial pulse to rule out radio-femoral delay
  - Significant delay of the femoral pulse after the radial pulse suggests coarctation of the upstream aorta (most commonly thoracic, however abdominal coarctation is also possible)
- **Popliteal**
  - Flex the knee approximately 10-20°
  - Using two hands, place thumbs on the tibial tuberosity and palpate deeply in the popliteal fossa with 3-4 fingers from each hand (allow knee to relax/fall into both hands)
  - A decreased or absent pulse indicates partial or complete arterial occlusion proximally; all pulses distal to occlusion are typically affected
  - Prominent pulse may predict popliteal aneurysm
- **Posterior Tibial**
  - Palpate behind and slightly below the medial malleolus
  - Chronic arterial occlusion of the legs causes intermittent claudication, postural color changes and skin alterations
- **Dorsalis Pedis**
  - Palpate on dorsum of the foot, lateral to extensor tendon of the big toe

> **Clinical Pearl: Dorsalis Pedis**
> Dorsalis pedis is absent in 15% of normal populations.

Venous

Edema

- Check for pitting (venous) or nonpitting (lymphatic) edema
  - Press firmly with thumb over bony prominences for >5 s
    - Over the dorsum of each foot
    - Behind each medial malleolus
    - Over the shins
    - If nonambulatory, check for sacral edema
  - Pitting: depression caused by the pressure from your thumb
    - Pitting suggests orthostasis, chronic venous insufficiency or CHF
    - Firm, nonpitting edema (lymphedema) suggests lymphatic obstruction (see **Lymphatic System and Lymph Node Exam**, p.130)
  - Note height of leg edema and if swelling is unilateral or bilateral
  - Unilateral edema may suggest DVT

- When following patients with chronic edema (venous or lymphatic), it may be useful to document calf circumference at serial visits
  - A difference between the two sides suggests edema
  - >1 cm at the ankles and 2 cm at the calf
  - Muscular atrophy can also cause differences in leg circumference
- Note unusually prominent veins
- Chronic venous insufficiency can lead to dependent edema ('heaviness in the legs')
- With DVT, extent of edema may suggest location of occlusion:
  - A calf DVT when the lower leg or ankle is swollen
  - An iliofemoral DVT when the entire leg is swollen

Special Tests

Arterial: Arterial Insufficiency

- Allen Test
  - Purpose: test for good collateral flow through the ulnar artery before proceeding with puncture of the radial artery for arterial blood gases
  - Method
    - Using your thumbs, occlude the patient's radial and ulnar arteries at the wrist
    - Ask patient to open his/her hand with the palm up: palm should be blanched
    - Then release pressure on the ulnar artery only, watch palm for "blushing"
  - Normal Result: color returns to the hand in 5-10 s
  - **Abnormal Result:** if color does not return within 10 s, DO NOT perform arterial puncture at this site, as this may indicate incomplete palmar arch or insufficient collateral flow
- Straight Leg Raise Test (Pallor on Elevation)
  - Raise the leg 45-60° for 30 s, or until pallor of the feet develops
  - Normal Result: mild pallor on elevation
  - **Abnormal Result:** marked pallor on elevation may suggest arterial insufficiency
- Rubor on Dependency
  - After performing the straight leg raise test, ask the patient to sit up and dangle both legs over the side of the bed
  - Normal Result: return of color within 10 s, filling of the superficial veins of the foot within 15 s
  - **Abnormal Result:** persistent pallor of the feet for >10 s followed by rubor (marked redness) on dependency (after 1-2 min) may be seen in patients with critical ischemia; the marked redness is due to arterial dilation following the tissue hypoxia induced by elevation of a leg with arterial insufficiency

Venous: Incompetent Saphenous Vein

- Test for Incompetent Saphenous Vein
  - Instruct patient to stand (dilated varicose vein will become obvious: note the location and distribution)
  - Compress the vein proximally with one hand and place other hand 15-20 cm distally on the vein
  - Briskly decompress/compress the distal site
  - Normal Result: the hand on the proximal site should feel no impulse
  - **Abnormal Result:** any impulse transmitted to the proximal site indicates incompetent saphenous valves between the two sites
- Brodie-Trendelenburg Maneuver
  - Ask the patient to lie supine and raise his/her legs 90° for 15 s to empty the veins
  - Place a tourniquet around the patient's upper thigh after the veins have drained (do not occlude arterial pulse)

- Instruct the patient to stand
- Watch for venous filling with the tourniquet on for 60 s
- Normal Result: superficial saphenous system should fill slowly from below the tourniquet within 35 s
- **Abnormal Result:**
  - Fast filling: indicates incompetence of the deep and perforator veins
  - Slow filling: remove the tourniquet and observe the superficial venous system
  - Retrograde flow: suggests superficial venous incompetence
- Tourniquet can be used above and below knee to differentiate between long and short saphenous incompetence

4. COMMON INVESTIGATIONS

Blood Work

- Hypercoagulability work-up:
  - CBC with peripheral smear
  - aPTT, PT/INR, fibrinogen, factor assay
  - Creatinine, albumin, lipid profile
  - Deficiency of antithrombin III, protein C or S
  - Lupus anticoagulant, anticardiolipin antibody
  - C-anti-neutrophil cytoplasmic antibody (C-ANCA), P-ANCA
  - D-dimers: useful to rule out venous thromboembolism (VTE) if negative and low clinical suspicion

Ankle-Brachial Index (ABI)

- ABI = ankle systolic pressure/brachial systolic pressure
- ABI diagnoses the presence (sensitivity = 95%, specificity = 100%) and severity of peripheral artery disease (PAD)
- A Doppler U/S probe is placed over the artery (ankle and antecubital fossa). Proximal to this, the cuff is inflated until the pulse ceases. The cuff is then deflated until the Doppler probe detects the peripheral pulse again, allowing for the detection of systolic pressure
- ABI >0.90 is normal, ABI >1.3 suggests calcification, 0.5-0.8 is claudication range, <0.4 suggests possible critical ischemia[1]

Duplex Ultrasonography

- Detects the direction, velocity, and turbulence of blood flow with an accurate anatomical view
- Can assess location and degree of stenosis as well as patency of bypass grafts; in detecting >50% stenosis in iliac arteries, generally has a sensitivity of 90% and a specificity of 95%
- Normal arteries produce biphasic or triphasic waveform signals, while monophasic signals are associated with an upstream stenosis; a significant increase in arterial flow velocity also suggests stenosis

CT Angiogram (CTA)

- Very helpful in assessing underlying atherosclerosis, aneurysm, and dissection
- Requires IV contrast, but is associated with less radiation than conventional angiogram
- In detecting >50% stenosis in iliac arteries, has a sensitivity from 89-100%, and a specificity from 92-100%
- MR angiography (MRA) using gadolinium is an emerging modality useful in delineating anatomy

Conventional Cathether-Based Angiography

- Inject IV contrast and image using X-ray based techniques; is often intraoperative to facilitate thrombolytic or endovascular therapy
- Detects narrowing of vessels and vessel anatomy
- Gold standard technique, but is invasive and uses high doses of radiation

5. COMMON DISORDERS

Disorders marked with (✓) are discussed in **Common Clinical Scenarios**

Arterial

- ✓ Acute occlusion (embolus/ thrombus)
- ✓ Chronic occlusion (claudication, critical ischemia)
- ✓ Mesenteric ischemia (acute/ chronic)
- ✓ Aortic dissection
- ✓ Abdominal aortic aneurysm (AAA)
- ✓ Cerebrovascular disease (carotid stenosis)
- ✓ Vasculitides

Venous

- ✓ Deep vein thrombosis
- ✓ Deep venous insufficiency
- ✓ Superficial thrombophlebitis
- ✓ Varicose veins

Lymphatic (see **Lymphatic System and Lymph Node Exam**)

- Lymphangitis
- Lymphedema

6. COMMON CLINICAL SCENARIOS

6.1 Arterial

Acute Arterial Occlusion/Insufficiency

- Patient has 6 h before irreversible muscle injury (in the setting of complete ischemia). This is a vascular emergency!

Etiology

- Important to differentiate embolism from thrombosis because the treatment for the two varies
- **Embolus**
  - Cardiogenic embolus: (80-90%)
  - Atrial fibrillation (most common)
    - MI <3 mo (anterior MI most common)
    - Valvular disease (e.g. endocarditis)
    - Cardiomyopathy with severe LV dysfunction
    - Atrial myxoma (very rare)
  - Arterial embolus:
    - Atheroembolism (e.g. ulcerated plaque)
    - Aneurysms (e.g. popliteal)
  - Paradoxical embolism
    - History of venous embolus passing through intracardiac shunt
    - May have history of oral contraceptive pill (OCP) use, VTE, PE, TIA, or stroke
- ***In situ* Thrombosis**
  - Atherosclerotic artery with underlying severe disease
  - Bypass graft occlusion (most common example)
  - Increased risk associated with hypercoagulable state (e.g. malignancy) and stasis (e.g. CHF)
- **Trauma**
  - Iatrogenic (e.g. arterial catheterization)
- **Idiopathic**

> **Clinical Pearl: Acute Arterial Occlusion**
> If there is neuromuscular compromise (i.e. paralysis and/or absent sensation) emergent revascularization is indicated.

Signs and Symptoms
- Depend on the etiology (see **Table 2**)
- Compartment syndrome:
  - Characterized by elevated interstitial pressure due to reperfusion injury and edema in the ridged compartments of the lower limb
  - Treatment is fasciotomy

Table 2. Embolus vs. *In situ* Thrombosis in Acute Arterial Occlusion

Feature	Embolus	*In situ* Thrombus
Onset of Pain	Sudden	Acute-on-chronic or gradual
Neuromuscular Status	Severe loss of function	Less severe loss (due to collaterals)
History of Claudication	Unlikely	Maybe
Contralateral Pulses	Usually normal	Diminished or absent
Chronic Skin Changes	No	Maybe
Possible Associated Symptoms	Focal neurological deficits (stroke), abdominal pain (splenic, mesenteric, renal), shortness of breath, blue toe syndrome	Usually local process

Physical Exam
- Vitals
- Inspect limbs for pallor, chronic skin changes, and signs of critical ischemia (e.g. ulcerations, gangrene)
- Palpate limbs for cool temperature, sluggish capillary refill, and arterial pulses
- Assess neuromuscular status of limbs
- Neurological, cardiorespiratory, and abdominal exams

Investigations
- If physical exam findings are severe, may have to immediately treat without the delay of investigations
- CBC, aPTT, PT/INR, troponin (consider: Cr, LFTs, lactate)
- ECG (rule out atrial fibrillation or MI)
- Echocardiogram (identify valvular disease, intracardiac thrombus, or aortic dissection)
- Bedside ABI with Doppler (consider duplex ultrasonography)
- Computed tomography angiography (CTA)
- Conventional angiography (usually intraoperatively)

Treatment
- Medical: immediate heparinization, consider long-term antiplatelet and/or anticoagulation depending on underlying etiology
- Surgical/endovascular: intraarterial thrombolysis, embolectomy, thrombectomy ± bypass graft ± endovascular therapy, primary amputation
- Treat underlying cause

Chronic Arterial Occlusion/Insufficiency

Etiology

- Atherosclerosis (most common)
- Rare causes include (vasculitis, see **Common Clinical Scenarios**, p.314): giant cell arteritis, Takayasu disease, Buerger's disease, polyarteritis nodosa

Signs and Symptoms

- Chronic atrophic changes of the skin and muscles
- Intermittent claudication: pain or discomfort in calves or thighs with exertion that is relieved rapidly with rest. Classically reproducible in same location with same distance
- Critical ischemia
  - Rest pain, night pain, and/or tissue loss
- Leriche's syndrome: if male patient complains of buttock or thigh pain while walking, inquire about impotence (intermittent claudication and impotence are features caused by chronic aortoiliac obstruction)
- Chronic mesenteric ischemia: classically describe history of weight loss, and "food fear" due to postprandial pain

Table 3. Vascular Claudication vs. Neurogenic Claudication vs. Musculoskeletal Pain

Feature	Vascular	Neurogenic	MSK
Onset of Pain	Dependent on discrete, reproducible amount of exercise	Sudden discomfort with locomotion	Sudden discomfort with locomotion or movement
Location of Pain	Can be unilateral - involves muscles of lower extremities (calf, thigh or buttock)	Usually bilateral - involves whole leg and can be associated with numbness and tingling	Localized to affected joints or muscles
Resolution of Pain	Rest (usually <5 min)	Rest (>5 min)	Rest (>5 min)
Alleviating and Provoking Factors	No change with position	Flexion of spine relieves pain	Pain is often insidious and gradually progresses over years, with flare-ups and remissions
Pulses	Diminished or absent	Present	Present
Skin	Atrophic changes	No changes	No changes

Physical Exam

- Inspect for signs of chronic poor perfusion: hair loss and/or shiny skin, pallor, arterial ulcers, hypertrophic nails, muscle atrophy
- Palpate for cool temperature and sluggish capillary refill
- Assess for decreased or absent pulses
- Auscultate for significant bruits, which may be heard if 50% occlusion (if severe stenosis present, bruits may be absent)
- Pallor on elevation/rubor on dependency
- Allen Test (upper extremity disease)

Investigations
- Routine blood work, fasting metabolic profile
- ABI
- Duplex ultrasonography
- CTA
- Consider conventional angiogram at time of procedure

Treatment
- Conservative:
  - Exercise rehabilitation, risk factor modification (smoking, HTN, dyslipidemia, type 2 DM [DM2])
- Medical:
  - Antiplatelet therapy (e.g. ASA, clopidogrel)
- Surgical/endovascular revascularization:
  - Endovascular angioplasty/stenting
  - Endarterectomy
  - Bypass graft
- Primary amputation

Aortic Dissection
- Disruption of aortic intima causing blood to flow into the media: considered acute if <14 d
- Classification[1]:
  - Stanford:
    - Type A: involves ascending aorta ± arch and/or descending aorta
    - Type B: does not involve ascending aorta (usually distal to left subclavian artery)
  - DeBakey:
    - Type I: involves ascending and variable amounts of descending aorta (50%)
    - Type II: involves only ascending aorta (35%)
    - Type III: involves aorta distal to left subclavian artery and confined to thoracic aorta (IIIA) or extends into abdomen (IIIB) (15%)
- Risk Factors: smoking, HTN, male, >70 yr, family history, history of vascular disease (CAD, cerebrovascular disease [CVD], PVD)

Etiology
- Atherosclerotic degeneration (most common)
- Other Factors: collagen vascular disease (Marfan's, Ehlers-Danlos), arteritis, bicuspid aortic valve, infection (e.g. syphilis), iatrogenic, trauma
- DDx: MI, massive PE, esophageal rupture, cardiac tamponade, aortic aneurysm

Signs and Symptoms
- Classically present with acute onset tearing chest/interscapular pain
- Dissection is painless in ~10% of cases[1]
- Signs and symptoms vary according to aortic branches involved: coronary (MI), carotids (syncope, Horner's, neurological deficits), mesenteric, renal, iliac (ischemic limb)
- Respiratory symptoms if dissection ruptures into pleura
- Heart failure if dissection ruptures into pericardium causing tamponade
- Hypovolemic shock if dissection ruptures into peritoneum

Physical Exam
- Vitals
  - Hypotension (Type A), HTN (Type B), asymmetrical pulse or BP (>20-30 mmHg suggests dissection)

- Abdominal exam
- Cardiorespiratory exam: aortic regurgitation (AR) murmur, heart failure, tamponade
- Peripheral vascular exam: limb ischemia, signs of heart failure
- Neurological exam: focal deficits

Investigations
- Blood work: CBC, creatinine, LFTs, troponin, lactate, type and cross
- ECG: may show LVH or ST changes
- CXR: may show widened mediastinum
- CTA (84-94% sensitive, 87-100% specific): allows rapid and accurate assessment of anatomy to diagnose and facilitate planning for surgical repair[1]
- Echocardiogram (transesophageal echocardiogram more sensitive and specific than transthoracic echocardiogram): can confirm dissection and assess aortic valve competence
- Consider conventional aortogram at time of procedure

EBM: Thoracic Aortic Dissection

Thoracic aortic dissections are life threatening, but can be difficult to diagnose with history, physical, and plain radiography. Most patients will have sudden severe pain (sensitivity 84-90%), thus the absence of sudden pain lowers the likelihood of dissection (LR- = 0.3). On physical exam, diastolic murmur does not significantly alter the pretest probability (LR+ = 1.4). However, asymmetrical pulses (LR+ = 5.7) and focal neurological deficits (LR+ = 6.6-33) significantly increase the likelihood of dissection in the appropriate setting. Chest radiographs are usually abnormal (sensitivity 90%), thus a normal radiograph decreases the likelihood of dissection (LR- = 0.3). A combination of sudden pain, asymmetric pulse, and abnormal radiograph is specific and can rule in a dissection (LR+ = 66). However, the author warns that due to the morbidity and mortality associated with a false-negative diagnosis, clinical examination alone is insufficient to rule out thoracic aortic dissection. CT scans with contrast have become the most commonly used diagnostic tool.

Klompas M. 2002. *JAMA* 287(17):2262-2272.

Treatment
- Hemodynamically unstable: aggressive resuscitation
- Medical: β-blockers, analgesia, vasodilators (target systolic BP: 100-120 mmHg)
- Surgical/endovascular repair:
  - Type A: open surgery is only definitive therapy
  - Type B:
    - Uncomplicated (i.e. no malperfusion syndrome or rupture): no surgery required
    - Complicated: open or endovascular repair (emerging technique)

Abdominal Aortic Aneurysm (AAA)
- Localized dilatation of an artery that is 2 times normal diameter
- True Aneurysm: wall is made of all 3 layers of the artery (intima, media, adventitia)
- False Aneurysm: wall is made of fibrous tissue or graft (e.g. complication postcatheterization)
- Classification: infrarenal (~90%), juxtarenal, suprarenal, thoraco-abdominal
- Risk Factors: smoking, cocaine, HTN, men who have sex with men (4 times the incidence), >70 yr, family history, history of vascular disease (CAD, CVD, PVD)

Etiology
- Atherosclerotic degeneration
- Other Factors: collagen vascular disease (Marfan's, Ehlers-Danlos), arteritis, infection (e.g. syphilis), trauma

Signs and Symptoms
- Aneurysms are generally asymptomatic until they rupture, and are often incidentally found on physical exam or imaging
- Ruptured AAA
  - Other symptoms include syncope and shock (pale skin, hypotension, shallow, fast respirations, decreased LOC)
  - Surgical emergency
  - Classic presentation is most often misdiagnosed as renal colic

> **Clinical Pearl: Ruptured AAA**
> Classic triad: abdominal pain radiating to back, pulsatile mass, hypotension.

Physical Exam (see **EBM: Abdominal Aortic Aneurysm (AAA)**, p.309)
- Do not delay treatment if highly suspicious history
- Vitals
- Inspect for flank ecchymosis (retroperitoneal hemorrhage)
- Abdominal exam: palpate for pulsatile mass
- Cardiorespiratory, peripheral vascular, and neurological exams
- Typical signs in classic triad may not be present
  - Expansile mass may be hard to feel if person is obese or aneurysm is well tamponaded
  - Hypotension may be absent in person who is normally hypertensive

Investigations
- Screening with abdominal U/S is recommended among men aged >50 yr with risk factors, all men >65 yr, and women >65 yr with risk factors
- Blood work: CBC, electrolytes, creatinine, aPTT, PT/INR, ESR, blood culture, type and cross (10 units pRBCs)
- Abdominal U/S (nearly 100% sensitive and specific for diagnosis)
- CT abdomen
  - Done to assess extent of aneurysms
  - Usually abdomen and pelvis, however include chest if thorax involved
  - Also identifies anatomic abnormalities: retroaortic vein, left sided vena cava, dilatation of ureters, enhancing rim of aorta seen with inflammatory aneurysm
- Conventional aortography
  - Only done when using endovascular aneurysm repair (EVAR)
  - Risk of false aneurysm, hematoma, or atheroembolism is 1-2%

Treatment
- Ruptured AAA:
  - Proximal aortic control by surgical or endovascular means (small-volume resuscitation can reduce the risk of further bleeding)
  - No investigations are necessary if patient is hemodynamically unstable
- Asymptomatic:
  - Conservative: exercise rehabilitation, risk factor modification, surveillance every 6 mo-3 yr with abdominal U/S
  - Surgical repair or EVAR

Clinical Pearl: AAA
Repair is recommended for aneurysms exceeding 5.5 cm (in men) and 5.0 cm (in women).

EBM: Abdominal Aortic Aneurysm (AAA)

The only physical exam maneuver of demonstrated value for diagnosis of an AAA is abdominal palpation to detect a widened aorta.

Width of Aorta by Palpation	Sensitivity (%)	LR+	LR-
≥3.0 cm (all)	39	12.0	0.72
3.0-3.9 cm	29		
≥4.0 cm		15.6	0.51
4.0-4.9 cm	50		
≥5.0 cm	76		

Reference standard: abdominal U/S
- Positive findings on abdominal palpation greatly increase likelihood of large AAA
- Abdominal palpation is useful in detecting AAA large enough to require surgery, but cannot be relied on to exclude the diagnosis
- Sensitivity is diminished by abdominal obesity and by routine abdominal exam not specifically targeted at measuring aortic width

Lederle FA, Simel DL. 1999. *JAMA* 281(1):77-82.

The long-term follow-up in the United Kingdom Small Aneurysm Trial (diameter 4.0 to 5.5 cm) indicated that, "there was no long-term survival benefit of early elective open repair of small abdominal aortic aneurysms. Even after successful aneurysm repair, the mortality among these patients was higher than in the general population."

Powell JT, et al. 2007. *Br J Surg* 94(6):702-708.

Physical Sign	Sensitivity (%)	Specificity (%)
Definite Pulsatile Mass	28	97
Definite or Suggestive Pulsatile Mass	50	91
Abdominal Bruit	11	95
Femoral Bruit	17	87
Femoral Pulse Deficit	22	91

Swartz MH. *Textbook of Physical Diagnosis: History and Examination*, 6th ed. Philadelphia: Saunders Elsevier; 2010.

Carotid Artery Disease

- Stenosis of the internal carotid artery, usually near the bifurcation of the common carotid artery
- Stenosis can be origin of thrombemboli to distal sites, leading to symptoms (e.g. TIA, amaurosis fugax, stroke)
- Risk Factors: age, smoking, HTN, DM2, dyslipidemia, family history, history of CAD, PVD, and AAA

Etiology

- Atherosclerotic degeneration (~90%)
- Other: dissection, aneurysm, arteritis, fibromuscular dysplasia
- DDx: cardioembolic (e.g. atrial fibrillation), *in situ* thrombosis of intracranial artery, vertebral artery disease, idiopathic (~32%)[2]

PERIPHERAL VASCULAR

Signs and Symptoms

- May be asymptomatic: incidental finding
- TIA: lateralizing neurologic deficit (usually middle cerebral artery [MCA] territory), lasting less than 24 h (usually 1 h), and that completely reverses (CT normal)
  - MCA territory: contralateral hemiplegia and hemianesthesia, aphasia
- Amaurosis fugax: transient blindness (total or sectorial) due to ipsilateral retinal insufficiency (Takayasu syndrome is associated with retinal findings)
- Stroke: similar to a TIA but lasting more than 24 h, and usually associated with CT findings (carotid stenosis is underlying etiology in 30% of ischemic strokes)[2]

Physical Exam

- Inspect retina by fundoscopy: look for "Hollenhorst plaques", emboli that are visible as small bright flecks at arterial bifurcations in the retina
- Auscultate for carotid bruits: bruits do not correlate with severity of stenosis, and absence of bruits does not rule out severe disease

> **Clinical Pearl: Carotid Artery Disease**
> If patient has known carotid artery atherosclerosis (especially symptomatic and/or bruits), do not palpate the carotid pulse due to theoretical risk of atheroembolism and ischemic stroke.

- Neurological exam: assess for lateralizing neurological deficits and cerebellar abnormalities
- Precordial and peripheral vascular exams: assess for arrhythmias, cardiomegaly, murmurs, extra heart sounds, and signs of arterial insufficiency in lower limbs

Investigations

- Blood work: CBC, creatinine, aPTT, PT/INR, metabolic profile
- Duplex ultrasonography: indicates presence of disease (for >50% stenosis, 98% sensitivity and 88% specificity) and severity of stenosis (mild/moderate/severe)[3]
- CT abdomen (88% sensitivity, 100% specificity)[3]
- MRA (95% sensitivity, 90% specificity): can concurrently evaluate cerebral circulation[3]
- Catheter-based angiography (gold standard): usually performed with angioplasty and stenting (not diagnostic test), and carries a 1/200 risk of stroke

Treatment

- Risk factor modification (smoking, HTN, DM2, dyslipidemia)
- Antiplatelet therapy (e.g. ASA ± clopidogrel)
- Asymptomatic disease[4]
  - >60-70% stenosis benefit from carotid endarterectomy (CEA): controversial
- Symptomatic disease[5]
  - >50% stenosis benefit from CEA (70-99% stenosis see greater benefit than 50-69%)
- Carotid angioplasty/stenting can be considered in poor surgical candidates with severe disease: controversial[6]

EBM: Carotid Artery Stenosis

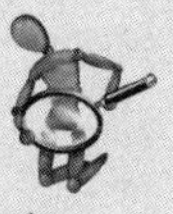

In the Northern Manhattan Study, the sensitivity and specificity of auscultation for the detection of clinically significant carotid stenosis was 56% and 98%, respectively. "The high false-negative rate suggests that auscultation is not sufficient to exclude carotid stenosis. An ultrasonography may be considered in high-risk asymptomatic patients, irrespective of findings on auscultation."

Ratchford EV, et al. 2009. *Neurol Res* 31(7):748-752.

6.2 Venous

Venous Thromboembolism (VTE)

- Blood clot formation, and subsequent inflammation, in one of the major deep veins in the leg, thigh, or pelvis

Etiology

- Virchow's triad: hypercoagulability, stasis, endothelial damage (see **Table 4**)
- Increasing age and family history are risk factors

Signs and Symptoms

- Establish index of suspicion according to risk factors (see **Table 4**)
- Classically presents as sudden unilateral pain, swelling, erythema, and warmth that is relieved with elevation

Table 4. Virchow's Triad

Hypercoagulability	Stasis	Endothelial Damage
Surgery/trauma	Obesity	Trauma
Neoplasms	Recent travel	Previous VTEs
Estrogen related (e.g. OCP, pregnancy, HRT)	Postoperative bed rest	Venulitis
Blood dyscrasias or hyperviscosity (e.g. polycythemia and sickle cell disease respectively)	Trauma and subsequent immobilization	
Antiphospholipid antibody syndrome	Right heart failure	
Nephrotic syndrome		
Inherited thrombophilias (e.g. protein C & S deficiency, antithrombin deficiency)		

HRT = hormone replacement therapy, OCP = oral contraceptive pill, VTE = venous thromboembolism

Physical Exam

- Absence of physical findings does not rule out VTE
- Examine the patient both upright and supine, venous distension is exacerbated in the upright position
- Vitals
- Inspect for erythema, collateral vein distension, and leg swelling (>3 cm difference in calf circumference is significant)
- Palpate for temperature difference, pitting edema, and indurated tender venous cord
- Attempt to elicit calf pain on dorsiflexion (Homans' sign)
- Cardiorespiratory exam

Investigations

- Blood work: CBC, aPTT, PT/INR, creatinine, LFTs
- D-dimer (if low index of suspicion: sensitive but nonspecific)[8,9]
- Consider hypercoagulability work-up
- ECG, CXR
- Doppler ultrasonography (highly sensitive and specific)
- CT abdomen/pelvis with contrast (if proximal veins suspected)
- Venography (definitive but rarely used)
- If suspicious of PE, consider: ventilation-perfusion (V/Q) scan or multi-detector CT (MDCT)

Treatment

- Prophylaxis
  - Conservative: early ambulation, compression stockings
  - Moderate to high risk: consider unfractionated heparin (UFH) or low molecular weight heparin (LMWH)
- Initial Therapy
  - UFH, LMWH, or fondaparinux
  - In select patients, catheter-directed thrombolytics or thrombectomy may be considered
- Long-Term Therapy
  - Anticoagulation (e.g. warfarin, dabigatran)
  - If anticoagulation is contraindicated (e.g. active bleeding), consider IVC filter
  - Duration ranges from 3-12 mo or indefinite therapy depending on risk factors
- Pulmonary Embolism (PE)
  - Admission for observation
  - Treatment for mild-moderate PE is similar to VTE
  - Massive PE: aggressive resuscitation, thrombolysis (systemic or catheter-directed) or thrombectomy ± IVC filter (with contraindication to anticoagulation)

EBM: Deep Vein Thrombosis

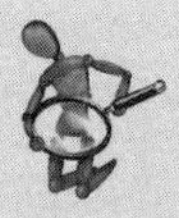

The use of a predictive tool (e.g. Wells *et al.*) to determine a pretest probability of DVT increases the utility of subsequent D-dimer testing.

Clinical Variable	Score
Active Malignancy	1
Immobilization of Lower Extremity	1
Bed Rest/Recent Surgery	1
Localized Tenderness along Deep Venous System	1
Entire Leg Swelling	1
Calf Swelling (>3cm difference)	1
Pitting Edema in Symptomatic Leg	1
Collateral Veins	1
Previous DVT	1
Alternate Diagnosis at Least as Likely as DVT	-2

≥3 is high probability, 1-2 is moderate probability, ≤0 is low probability
Wells PS, et al. 2006. *JAMA* 295(2):199-207.

In patients with low clinical probablity of DVT (prevalence <5%), a negative D-dimer test effectively rules out DVT. In patients with high clinical probablity of DVT, a D-dimer result should not be involved in clinical decision making.

Clinical Pearl: Pulmonary Embolism
About 10% of cases of VTE are associated with pulmonary embolism. Clinically significant symptoms and signs include: shortness of breath, tachypnea (RR >16), tachycardia (>100 bpm), cough, hemoptysis, chest pain, fever, and anxiety.

Superficial Venous Thrombosis (SVT)

Etiology
- 20% associated with occult VTE
- SVTs may be caused by varicose veins, trauma (e.g. recent sclerotherapy), intravenous indwelling catheters, autoimmune disease (e.g. Buerger's), malignancy, or hypercoagulable state
- Most commonly in greater saphenous vein
- Migratory SVT often associated with malignancy (Trousseau's disease)
- Can be misdiagnosed as cellulitis

Signs and Symptoms
- Often history of previous SVTs
- Tenderness, warmth, induration, redness, and localized swelling along course of vein
- Typically no generalized swelling of the limb

Physical Exam
- Inspect the area for redness, swelling, and varicose veins
- Palpate the affected vein and determine if it is hard and cord-like

Investigations
- Tests are not necessary for diagnosis of SVT, but should be done to rule out VTE
- Doppler ultrasonography

Treatment
- Conservative: warm compress, ambulation, NSAIDs
- Medical: depending on risk factors, consider antiplatelet or heparinization
- Surgical excision if conservative and medical measures fail

Varicose Veins
- Distended tortuous superficial veins due to venous insufficiency from incompetent valves in the lower extremities

Etiology
- Previous VTE
- Hereditary incompetence of venous valves
- Increasing age, female gender
- Situation of increased pressure (pregnancy, prolonged standing, ascites, tricuspid regurgitation)

Signs and Symptoms
- Dull aching, burning, or cramping provoked by prolonged standing or menstruation
- Edema which resolves overnight
- In some cases, chronic venous insufficiency (CVI) leads to skin damage
  - Pruritus, hyperpigmentation (hemosiderin deposits), stasis dermatitis, lipodermatosclerosis, bleeding, or ulceration

PERIPHERAL VASCULAR

Physical Exam

- Inspect for evidence of varicose veins, skin damage, swelling, or ulceration
- Palpate for tenderness or edema
- Test for incompetent saphenous vein with Brodie-Trendelenburg maneuver (see **Special Tests**, p.301)
- Peripheral vascular exam

Investigations

- Duplex ultrasonography: assess for reversed flow

Treatment

- Usually a cosmetic problem
- Conservative
  - Elastic/compression stockings
  - Leg elevation
- Surgical: indicated with symptomatic varices, prominent tissue changes, or failure of conservative measures
  - Sclerotherapy: injection of sclerosant drug by U/S-guidance into vein to cause vein shrinkage
  - Stripping, removal of all or part of saphenous vein trunk
  - Endovenous laser therapy (EVLT)

6.3 Vasculitis

Etiology

- Inflammation of any blood vessel, including arteries, arterioles, capillaries, venules, and veins
- Clinical presentation is diverse depending on the type of blood vessel involved and their location
- Can involve any organ system, but some may present with symptoms of peripheral vascular disease

Disease-specific Findings

- Behçet's Disease
  - Multisystem leukocytoclastic vasculitis
  - Ocular involvement
  - Recurrent oral and vaginal ulcers
  - SVT
  - Skin and joint inflammation
- Buerger's Disease
  - Thromboangiitis obliterans (TAO)
  - Inflammation secondary to clotting of small- and medium-sized vessels
  - Most common in Asian males
  - Strong association with cigarette smoking
  - May lead to distal claudication and gangrene
- Giant Cell (Temporal) Arteritis
  - Inflammation of aorta and its branches
  - New headache, jaw claudication
  - Scalp tenderness, may have pulseless or "ropy"/thickened temporal artery
  - Female > Male, >50 yr, elevated ESR
  - May present with sudden, painless loss of vision ± diplopia
  - Aortic arch syndrome: involvement of subclavian and brachial arteries
    - Pulseless disease, aortic aneurysm ± rupture
- Polyarteritis Nodosa
  - Necrotizing vasculitis of small- to medium-sized vessels
  - May lead to thrombosis, aneurysm or dilatation at any lesion site

- Associated with hepatitis B surface antigen positivity
  - Livedo reticularis of the skin
  - Diastolic BP >90 mmHg
  - Renal failure
  - Neuropathy
- Takayasu's Arteritis
  - "Pulseless" disease
  - Chronic inflammation of aorta and its branches
  - Usually in young Asian females
  - Constitutional symptoms
- Raynaud's Phenomenon
  - Pain and tingling in the digits due to vasospasm
  - Episodes of sharply demarcated pallor and/or cyanosis followed by erythema
  - Normal pulses present
  - Triggered by cold or emotional stress
  - May be primary or secondary; associated with SLE, scleroderma, rheumatoid arthritis (RA), cryoglobulinemia
- Antiphospholipid Antibody Syndrome
  - Multisystem vasculopathy often associated with SLE
  - Recurrent thromboembolic events (arterial and venous)
  - Recurrent spontaneous abortions
  - Skin changes (e.g. livedo reticularis, purpura, leg ulcers, gangrene)

Investigations
- Routine blood work
- Autoimmune work-up: ESR, CRP, ANCA, RF, C3, C4, antinuclear antibody (ANA), ferritin, anticardiolipin, and lupus anticoagulant antibodies
- Urinalysis (active sediment, proteinuria), BUN, creatinine
- Consider synovial fluid analysis if joint involvement
- Fundoscopy ± slit lamp examination
- CT scan
- Angiography
- Biopsy of affected organ, skin, or suspected blood vessel

Treatment
- Often dependent on condition
- Mainstay of treatment is immunosuppressive agents, most often with corticosteroids and/or cyclophosphamide
- Consider anticoagulation if thromboembolism involved
- NSAIDs for pain control with joints, eye and/or skin involvement

6.4 Lymphatics
- See **Lymphatic System and Lymph Node Exam**, p.130

PERIPHERAL VASCULAR

REFERENCES

1. Hagan PG, Nienaber CA, Isselbacher EM, Bruckman D, Karavite DJ, Russman PL, et al. 2000. The International Registry of Acute Aortic Dissection (IRAD): New insights into an old disease. *JAMA* 283(7):897-903.
2. Barnett HJ, Gunton RW, Eliasziw M, Fleming L, Sharpe B, Gates P, et al. 2000. Causes and severity of ischemic stroke in patients with internal carotid artery stenosis. *JAMA* 283(11):1429-1436.
3. Chappell FM, Wardlaw JM, Young GR, Gillard JH, Roditi GH, Yip B, et al. 2009. Carotid artery stenosis: Accuracy of noninvasive tests - Individual patient data meta-analysis. *Radiology* 251(2):493-502.
4. Halliday A, Mansfield A, Marro J, Peto C, Peto R, Potter J, et al. 2004. Prevention of disabling and fatal strokes by successful carotid endarterectomy in patients without recent neurological symptoms: Randomised controlled trial. *Lancet* 363(9420):1491-1502. Erratum in: *Lancet* 2004;364(9432):416.
5. North American Symptomatic Carotid Endarterectomy Trial Collaborators. 1991. Beneficial effect of carotid endarterectomy in symptomatic patients with high-grade carotid stenosis. *New Engl J Med* 325(7):445-453.
6. Brott TG, Hobson RW 2nd, Howard G, Roubin GS, Clark WM, Brooks W, et al. 2010. Stenting versus endarterectomy for treatment of carotid-artery stenosis. *New Engl J Med* 363(1):11-23. Erratum in: *New Engl J Med* 2010;363(5):498, and *New Engl J Med* 2010;363(2):198.
7. Wells PS, Owen C, Doucette S, Fergusson D, Tran H. 2006. Does this patient have deep vein thrombosis? *JAMA* 295(2):199-207.
8. Kearon C, Ginsberg JS, Douketis J, Crowther M, Brill-Edwards P, Weitz JI, et al. 2001. Management of suspected deep venous thrombosis in outpatients by using clinical assessment and D-dimer testing. *Ann Intern Med* 135(2):108-111.
9. Bickley LS, Szilagyi PG, Bates B. *Bates' Guide to Physical Examination and History Taking*, 10th ed. Philadelphia: Lippincott Williams & Wilkins; 2009.
10. Orient JM, Sapira JD. *Sapira's Art and Science of Bedside Diagnosis*, 4th ed. Philadelphia: Lippincott Williams & Wilkins; 2010.

The Psychiatric Exam

Editors:
Evan Lilly
Chris Tang

Faculty Reviewers:
Raed Hawa, MD, MSc, DABSM, FRCP(C)
Jodi Lofchy, MD, FRCP(C)
Mark J. Rapoport, MD, FRCP(C)

PSYCHIATRIC

TABLE OF CONTENTS

1. APPROACH TO THE PSYCHIATRIC INTERVIEW/HISTORY

General Approach

- Resembles traditional medical history, but with more emphasis on psychosocial factors (see **Focused Psychiatric History**, p.319)
- A Mental Status Examination (MSE) should be performed for all patients at every visit (see **Mental Status Examination**, p.322)
- With patient's permission (except in emergency situations), collateral source(s) for history (spouse, parent, adult child, friend, teacher, coworker) is/are almost always helpful
- Of particular importance in the psychiatric interview are the privacy and confidentiality of the patient
- If the patient has a history of violence against others, make arrangements to have security present

Initial Stages

- Try to ease initial concerns (anxiety, indignation, shame, etc.)
- Some general advice to make patients as comfortable as possible[1]:
  - Try to find a private room with a wall clock that allows you to check the time without consulting a wristwatch
  - Have a box of facial tissues ready
  - Meet patients at their eye level
  - Avoid desks between the patient and physician, if possible

    - Convey respect for the patient
- A succinct outline of the interview may be useful

Eliciting Information

- Different types of patients respond better to different interview approaches (see **Table 1**)

Table 1. Approach to Psychiatric Patients

Type of Patient	Strategies
Agitated	• Brief • Focus on most relevant/important symptoms • Keep your voice calm • Avoid gestures that may suggest an imminent attack/defence (e.g. hands behind back, hands raised in defence) • Resist the urge to touch the patient to help calm him/her down, and give him/her more space than usual
Shutdown	• Try to engage patient in an area of conversation that is of interest to him/her (music, sports, politics, etc.) • Avoid sensitive topics • Avoid long pauses • Increase ratio of open-ended to closed-ended questions, often with several consecutive open-ended questions
Rationalizing	• Collateral sources of information may be extremely valuable • Be nonjudgmental
Wandering	• Try to avoid gestures and sounds (note-taking included) that "feed the wanderer"[2] • Increase ratio of closed-ended to open-ended questions • Attempt to interject and focus the patient, gently at first, but gradually more directly • Avoid structuring the patient too early: during the open-ended phase of the CC/HPI, let the patient wander
Tearful	• Give patient some uninterrupted time to talk/cry • Interject sensitively: patients may experience this as containing and organizing • Monitor nonverbal cues, language, tone • Say something comforting ("It's all right to cry") • The moment immediately after crying subsides is a good opportunity to learn more about the patient's pain

Goldbloom DS (Editor). *Psychiatric Clinical Skills.* Philadelphia: Mosby Elsevier; 2006.
Shea S. *Psychiatric Interviewing: The Art of Understanding.* Philadelphia: W.B. Saunders Company; 1988.

- After setting the stage, begin with an open-ended question or statement (e.g. "Tell me about what brought you here.")
    - Let the patient talk relatively freely, making note of areas of interest that you wish to revisit
    - Use facilitative phrases and gestures: "Go on", "Uh-huh", head nodding
    - Avoid being too "directive" at this stage[1]
- When expanding any area of the history, avoid asking questions in a "laundry list" manner at this early stage, and attempt to let the questions flow naturally from what the patient says
- Leave adequate time to close the interview without being rushed. The following aspects are particularly important to convey:[1]
    - Why you think the patient has the problem
    - How common his/her problem is (to help normalize)
    - How often people with his/her problem improve (to provide hope)

- How treatment makes a difference (to provide psychoeducation and involve patients in their own care)

2. COMMON CHIEF COMPLAINTS OR REASONS FOR REFERRAL

- Hearing voices (auditory hallucinations)
- Mood changes (depression, mania)
- Thoughts of suicide (suicidal ideation [SI])
- Anxiety
- Delusions
- Confusion
- Medication side effects
- Agitation

3. FOCUSED PSYCHIATRIC HISTORY

Identifying Data

- Age
- Employment (or most recent job). If patient is unemployed, what is his/her source of income?
- Relationship status (be sure to ask about past relationships and any children from past relationships if single)
- Living arrangements, including dependents
- Ethnic, cultural, and racial heritage
- Source(s) of information and their reliability
- May include circumstances/setting of interview
- ***Note:*** should be kept brief to allow smooth transition to the open-ended phase of the CC/HPI

Reason for Referral (RFR)

- Who is referring this patient?
- What is the reason for referral?

Chief Complaint

- In patient's own words
- Include collateral versions of the patient's complaint if applicable

History of Present Illness

- Onset, frequency, progression of symptoms
- Possible precipitating factors (e.g. stressful life event, substance abuse): consider 3 domains of "love, work, and play"[2]
- Effects on functioning (work, social, family, daily activities)
- Current medications and adherence (including oral contraceptive pills)
- Suicidal and homicidal ideation (see **Suicide Risk Assessment**, p.327)

Psychiatric Review of Systems/Functional Inquiry

- Begin by normalizing the questions: "I want to ask you about some experiences that people can have when they feel this way"[3]
- **Mood:** depression, mania (see **Mood Disorders**, p.329)
  - "Have you been feeling down, depressed, or blue? How is it different from usual feelings of sadness for you?"
  - "Have you had little interest or pleasure in doing things that you usually enjoy doing?"
  - "Have you been feeling more irritable than usual?"
- **Psychosis:** hallucinations, delusions (see **Mental Status Examination**, p.322 for definitions)

PSYCHIATRIC

- **Substance Use**
  - Alcohol (type of alcohol and weekly consumption)
  - Recreational drugs, smoking, caffeine
  - OTC medications, alternative medicines
  - Phrase questions with an assumption of use[2] (e.g. "How much alcohol do you drink in a d/wk?")
- If alcohol abuse is suspected, the **CAGE** questionnaire is a valid screening tool (average sensitivity = 0.71, specificity = 0.90 in psychiatric inpatients[4])
  - **C** = "Have you ever felt the need to **Cut down** on your drinking?"
  - **A** = "Have people **Annoyed** you by criticizing your drinking?"
  - **G** = "Have you ever felt **Guilty** about your drinking?"
  - **E** = "Have you needed a drink in the morning to steady your nerves or get rid of a hangover (an '**Eye Opener**')?"
  - ≥2 affirmative responses is recommended as a cutoff for alcohol abuse or dependence[3]
  - Limitations of the CAGE questionnaire: does not perform as well in primary care settings, with women, or for detecting less severe forms of drinking
  - CAGE does not replace a full inquiry including symptoms of intoxication, withdrawal, dependence, and abuse (see **Substance-Related Disorders**, p.336)
- **Anxiety:** panic, agoraphobia, obsessions, compulsions
  - "Do you ever feel anxious or on edge?"
  - "Do you find yourself worrying about a lot of different things?"
  - "Do you have worries or fears that you know are not rational but are unable to suppress?"
- **Disordered Eating**
  - "Do you feel fat?" (for anorexia nervosa only)
  - "Do you find yourself constantly thinking about your weight? Food?"
  - "Do you purge?"
- **Cognitive:** memory, concentration, dementia
  - "Have you had trouble concentrating or remembering things lately?"
  - If yes: "Is this worse than prior to X? Worse than peers your age?"
- **Somatic Symptoms**
  - Anorexia, weight loss/gain, insomnia/hypersomnia and pattern (trouble falling/staying asleep, early morning awakening), lethargy, agitation, decreased sexual energy or interest
  - Neurological symptoms (seizures, recent head injury)
  - Somatic problems with no known physical basis (psychosomatic)

Past Psychiatric/Medical History

- Includes episodes for which the patient did not see a mental health professional
- Past psychiatric, psychosomatic, medical, or neurological history
  - Age of first symptoms and first contact with psychiatry
  - Allergies
  - Hospitalizations: number, diagnosis, treatment, outcome, date of last discharge
  - Surgeries: number, date(s), reason, outcome
  - Outpatient contacts: type, medications
  - Past psychotherapy or electroconvulsive therapy (ECT)
- Pregnancy (for women)
  - If patient has been pregnant, screen for current and/or previous postpartum psychiatric issues such as depression, mania, or psychosis
- Suicide attempts: lethality, medical attention, date of last attempt (see **Suicide Risk Assessment**, p.327)

- Common medical problems, as appropriate to patient age and health status (e.g. head injury, seizures, endocrine or renal disease, infections, malignancies, vascular fisk factors and disease)
- Medications: adherence, response, maximum dose, duration, side effects, allergies

Family History of Psychiatric Illness

- Determine if any of the patient's biological relatives have:
  - Major psychiatric illness (symptoms, diagnosis, duration, treatment, response, hospitalization)
  - Contact with a mental health professional
  - Attempted or completed suicide
  - Substance abuse
  - Legal history
- Begin by assuming there is relevant family history[2]. Questions that begin with "Who else in your family…?" elicit more information than those that begin with "Does anyone else in your family…?"
- May be useful to determine the roles of parents during the patient's childhood[2]: "How would you describe your parents to someone who has never met them?"

PSYCHIATRIC

Past Personal/Developmental History

- Adjust detail depending on age of patient, CC, and HPI
- A summary of the patient's life from infancy to present, with emphasis on relationships with family and major life events (e.g. illness, divorce, deaths, etc.)
- Goal is to look for two themes[2]
  1. Recurring patterns of behavior
  2. Evolving sense of identity in "love, work, and play"
- Can be divided into 5 phases[3]
  1. Prenatal and perinatal: maternal substance use; pregnancy/delivery complications
  2. Early childhood (to age 3 yr): developmental milestones (only whether, to the patient's knowledge, he/she reached major milestones at a roughly usual age); temperament/childhood personality; attachment figures; separations; earliest memories; breastfeeding; toilet training
  3. Middle/late childhood (ages 3-11 yr): development of gender identity; punishment; school performance; socialization, ability to make friends, etc.
  4. Puberty and adolescence: early intimate relationships, sexual and nonsexual (if there are/were many, try to figure out why they usually ended, and what attracts the patient to others); school performance; extracurricular activities; friends; psychosexual development; experimentation with drugs and alcohol; onset of puberty and how it affected social relationships
  5. Adulthood: education; occupational history; marital and relationship history; sexual history; religion(s); social activities; diet and exercise; current social support system; legal history; military history (if applicable); retirement (if applicable)
- Ask about the patient's strengths, competencies, and interests as well. Patients who are not willing participants in psychiatric interviews may appreciate these questions[1,2]

4. MENTAL STATUS EXAMINATION

Note: Should reflect the patient's current mental condition. Much of the evaluation can be gleaned from your observations during the interview, but some information may need to be actively sought. It should be done for every patient at every visit.

PSYCHIATRIC

Mnemonic for elements of the MSE[5]
Man, **A**ll **B**orderline **S**ubjects **A**re **P**retty **T**ough, **T**roubled **C**haracters

- **M**otor activity
- **A**ppearance
- **B**ehavior
- **S**peech
- **A**ffect and mood
- **P**erception
- **T**hought content
- **T**hought process/form
- **C**ognition: consciousness/alertness, orientation, attention and concentration, memory, insight, and judgment

Motor Activity

- Gait: festinating, ataxic
- Posture: slumped, stiffened
- Facial expression and eye contact: tearful, fearful/anxious
- Mannerisms
- Presence of nail biting, arms hugging the body, and echopraxia
- Agitated behavior (e.g. hair pulling, hand wringing)
- Presence of repetitive or involuntary movements (e.g. tics, chorea, tremor)
- Presence of tremor, jitteriness, lip-smacking, or tongue rolling that may indicate tardive dyskinesia (TD), akathisia, or medication-induced parkinsonism[3]
- ***Note:*** any abnormalities in motor activity should be further investigated with a neurological examination[6]

Appearance

- Apparent vs. chronological age
- Dress
- Grooming/hygiene
- Distinguishing physical features (including scars, tattoos)
- Facial expression
- Physical build
- Apparent physical health and presence of any physical limitations
- Get a sense of what the appearance says about the patient's self-esteem, and his/her interests, activities, attitudes, etc.[4]

Behavior

- Does the patient exhibit acute distress?
- Patient's attitude toward examiner: cooperative, disinterested, agitated, guarded, seductive
- Appropriateness of attitude to context (e.g. whether patient sought help voluntarily or against his/her will)

Speech

Mnemonic: **FLAVoR**

- **F**luency
  - o Gross fluency of English language
  - o Subtler issues such as stuttering, word finding difficulties, nonfluent aphasias, etc.

- **L**atency of response: there should normally be a short pause
- **A**mount: normal, increased, decreased
- **Vo**lume, tone: loud, soft, timid, angry, irritable, anxious, juvenile, insulting, etc.
- **R**ate: slowed, pressured/rapid

Affect and Mood

- Affect: patient's mood as observed by you (OBJECTIVE)
  - Quality: euthymic, depressed, elevated, anxious
  - Range: full, constricted, flat (an extreme form of constricted affect)
  - Intensity/Quantity: mild, moderate, severe
  - Stability: continuum from stable to labile
  - Appropriateness to thought content
- Mood: patient's mood as described by the patient (SUBJECTIVE)

PSYCHIATRIC

Perception

Note the presence or absence of the following, as appropriate:

- Hallucinations: sensory perception in the absence of external stimuli[3]
  - Most frequently auditory, but can occur in all five modalities
  - Describe how patient feels and what he/she subjectively experiences during hallucinations, when they occur, and how often they occur
  - For auditory hallucinations, describe whether patient hears words, commands, or conversations
- Illusions: misperception of a real external stimulus[3]
- Depersonalization: a sense that one feels unreal, or has been detached from one's body[3]
- Derealization: a sense that one's surroundings have become unreal[3]

Thought Content

Definition: ideas/themes the patient communicates (WHAT the patient is thinking about)

- Obsessions: recurrent, often anxiety-provoking thoughts that the patient cannot suppress[3] (e.g. fear of contamination, obsession with order)
- Delusions: fixed, false beliefs that the patient maintains despite contradictory evidence, and which cannot be accounted for by the beliefs of a religious, cultural, or subcultural group.[3] They can be classified into bizarre and non-bizarre delusions (see **Psychosis**, p.334 for types of delusions)
  - Bizarre: content has no basis in reality (e.g. having a GPS tracking device inside one's body)
  - Non-bizarre: content is not true, but is within the realm of possibility (e.g. being followed/investigated by the government)
  - Determine the degree to which the patient challenges the delusion(s), how preoccupied the patient becomes, how consistent the delusion is, and the bizarreness of the delusion
- Preoccupations, phobias, somatic concerns
- Suicidal and homicidal ideation

Listed are some questions that can be useful when broaching the often sensitive issues of perceptual and thought content disturbances (see **Table 2**).

Table 2. Questions for Perceptual and Thought Content Disturbances

MSE Subsection	Suggested Questions	Inquiring about...
Perception	"Have you ever felt as if the world around you suddenly changed or disappeared?"	Derealization
	"Have you ever felt as if you were outside your body and could watch yourself?"	Depersonalization
	"Have you ever heard/seen/felt/smelled/ tasted anything that others could not?"	Hallucinations*
	"Have you noticed that you hear the voices of people speaking to you or about you when you are alone?"	Hallucinations (auditory)
Thought Content	"Do you have experiences that you think might be hard for others to understand?"	Delusions
	"Do you ever feel like you are being followed, watched, or spied on?"	Delusions (non-bizarre)
	"Do you ever feel like someone else is controlling your mind or body?"	Delusions (bizarre)
	"Do you ever feel like the television or radio was addressing you personally?"	Delusions of reference
	"Do you have thoughts that you can't seem to get out of your head, no matter what you do?"	Obsessions

*Ask about only one modality at a time
Shader RI (Editor). *Manual of Psychiatric Therapeutics*, 3rd ed. Philadelphia: Lippincott Williams & Wilkins; 2003.

PSYCHIATRIC

Thought Process/Form

Definition: the way that a patient comes to a conclusion (HOW the patient thinks)

- Components
  - Rate and flow of ideas
  - Coherence/logic
  - Presence/absence of goal-directed thinking
- Normal thought process is linear, organized, and goal-directed[3]
- Abnormalities of thought process
  - Blocking: patient cannot complete a thought, leading to cessation of speech
  - Perseveration: patient cannot seem to switch topics, and will continually return to the same topic despite attempts to change the subject
  - Circumstantiality: patient is indirect and includes irrelevant details, but eventually answers the question
  - Tangentiality: patient digresses from initial topic, and never returns to original point
  - Flight of ideas: patient rapidly "jumps" from one topic to another, but all topics are logically connected
  - Loosening of associations: patient moves between topics that are not logically connected
  - Word salad: jumble of words/phrases that is often repetitious and has no coherent meaning
  - Neologism: a fabricated/made-up word that is often incomprehensible
  - Clang association: a sequence of thoughts that is driven by the sounds of preceding words, often leading to rhyming or punning

Cognition

- Asking patient to state age and date of birth as part of ID at the beginning of the assessment can be used as a quick cognitive screen
- Many cognitive screening tools are available, each with advantages and disadvantages (see **Cognitive Screening Tools**, p.326)
- Consciousness/alertness: hyperalert, alert, drowsy, confused, stuporous, unconscious
- Orientation: to time, person (others), place, and self
  - If patient has arrived on time to the appointment (by him/herself), orientation may not have to be assessed formally
  - For time and place, ask questions from easiest to hardest: "What year is it? Month? Day of the week? Date?" or "What country are we in? Province? City? Road? Address?"
- Attention and concentration
  - Digit span test (forward and backward)
  - Spelling the name of a city (forward and backward)
  - Serial 7's subtraction test (or serial 3's)
  - Aside from formal tests, observing how the patient interacts in the interview will give a good sense of his/her attention and concentration
- Memory[5,6]
  - Immediate recall: name 3-5 unrelated objects, and have patient repeat them back
  - Delayed recall: ask patient to repeat the same 3-5 objects after roughly 5 min
    - If the patient has trouble, offer a hint (category hint first, then multiple choice)
  - Long-delayed recall: ask patient to repeat the same 3-5 objects after roughly 30 min
    - More commonly tested by neuropsychologists, less commonly by physicians
  - Recall of remote personal memory
    - Names and dates from patient's past
    - Birthdays and anniversaries (spouse, parents, etc.)
  - Recall of general cultural knowledge
    - "Who was Christopher Columbus?"
    - "What happened on September 11th, 2001?"
    - "Name as many colors/animals/fruits/towns as you can"
- Abstraction
  - Take into consideration patient's education, IQ, native language, and culture
  - Proverb interpretation: "How would you explain the meaning of 'Don't judge a book by its cover'?"
  - Similarities test: "What do a baseball and an orange have in common?"
- Insight: the patient's degree of awareness and understanding of his/her illness and the potential causes
  - "What do you think is going on with you now?"
  - Insight can be good, partial, or poor
- Judgment: the patient's ability to make sound decisions and to act accordingly
  - "What do you think would be helpful for you right now?"
  - "What do you think would happen if…?"
  - Best determined by examining the decisions that the patient has made during the course of his/her illness rather than using hypothetical situations[3,6]

5. COGNITIVE SCREENING TOOLS

- Some patients may become agitated by the nature of the questions. Use introductory comments such as: "How would you describe your memory? I have a few questions that will help me see how your memory and concentration are functioning".
- Avoid using the word 'test' when introducing the questions

PSYCHIATRIC

Table 3. Common Cognitive Screening Tools

Comparison of Cognitive Screening Tools		
MMSE	Advantages	• Fast and easy to administer • Long history of clinical use • Focuses on short-term memory loss and recognition problems
	Limitations	• Not sensitive to early/mild changes in cognitive functioning • Does not test executive functioning • Emphasis on verbal ability • Fee for usage (copyrighted) • Affected by education levels • Developed for English speaking patients
MoCA	Advantages	• Free • More sensitive to mild or early cognitive changes (MMSE ≥24-26) • Useful when patients have cognitive complaints but no functional impairment • Better measures of apraxia, visuospatial function, and executive function vs. MMSE
	Limitations	• Slightly longer than MMSE (but not by much) • Affected by education levels
Mini-Cog	Advantages	• Not limited by education levels or language • Similar sensitivity and specificity for dementia compared to MMSE • Short testing time and easy to administer (three-item recall and clock drawing)[7]
	Limitations	• Relatively new • Limited cognitive dimensions are tested
Clock-Drawing	Advantages	• Score correlates with MMSE (high sensitivity, specificity, and inter-rater reliability) • Fast and easy to administer (less than 1 min to conduct and score)[8] • Widely used in clinical settings • Tests executive functioning • May be less affected by language and education
	Limitations	• Not a sensitive test for mild dementia • Not a direct test of memory

MMSE = Mini-Mental State Examination, MoCA = Montreal Cognitive Assessment

6. COMMON INVESTIGATIONS IN PSYCHIATRY

1. Laboratory Tests: TSH, vitamin B12, folate, ferritin, CBC, electrolytes, calcium profile, blood glucose, blood culture, serum and urine toxicology screen, BUN, creatinine, liver enzymes and liver function tests, serum medication levels
2. Imaging: CT head (e.g. first episode psychosis), MRI head
3. Weight and BMI
4. ECG
5. Cognitive assessments (see **Table 3**)
6. CT imaging guidelines (according to 2006 CCCD recommendations)[9]: A cranial CT scan is recommended if 1 or more of the following criteria are present:
   - Age <60 yr
   - Rapid (e.g. over 1-2 mo) unexplained decline in cognition or function
   - "Short" duration of dementia (less than 2 yr)
   - Recent and significant head trauma
   - Unexplained neurologic symptoms (e.g. new onset of severe headache or seizures)
   - History of cancer (especially in sites and types that metastasize to the brain)
   - Use of anticoagulants or history of a bleeding disorder
   - History of urinary incontinence and gait disorder early in the course of dementia (as may be found in normal pressure hydrocephalus)
   - Any new localizing sign (e.g. hemiparesis or a Babinski reflex)
   - Unusual or atypical cognitive symptoms or presentation (e.g. progressive aphasia)
   - Gait disturbance

7. SUICIDE RISK ASSESSMENT

Risk Factor Assessment

- Risk factors for suicide: **SAD PERSONS** scale[5,6,10]
  - **S**ex: male
  - **A**ge >60 yr
    - In males, increased suicide risk also occurs in late adolescence[4]
  - **D**epression
  - **P**revious attempts (including aborted attempts and acts of self-harm)
  - **E**thanol abuse
  - **R**ational thinking loss (psychosis, helplessness, hopelessness)
  - **S**uicide in family
  - **O**rganized plan
  - **N**o spouse/no support systems
  - **S**erious illness, intractable pain

Clinical Pearl: SAD PERSONS Scale and Suicide Risk
Do not rely solely on the SAD PERSONS scale to assess suicide risk, as it has been found to have low sensitivity and positive predictive value when predicting future suicide attempts.[11]

- Of particular concern are 3 elements that comprise Shea's "triad of lethality"[1]
  1. Recent suicide attempt
  2. Acute psychosis suggesting lethality
  3. Elements from history that strongly suggest that the patient intends to harm him/herself

PSYCHIATRIC

- 3 psychotic processes should be actively and carefully explored if they arise during history[1]:
  1. **Command Hallucinations:** hearing voices that tell the patient to perform an act
  2. **Sense of Alien/Outside Control:** the sensation that one's body is being controlled externally
  3. **Religious Preoccupation:** performing suicidal (or homicidal) acts to please a higher power; preoccupation with certain verses from religious texts suggesting violence
- 3 personality traits that may place patients at increased risk when stressed[12]:
  1. **Controlling:** may feel lack of control if living with a severely limiting illness
  2. **Dependent-Dissatisfied:** if all potential caregivers are alienated, patient is left without social support
  3. **Strongly Dependent Relationship:** if strong support dies or abandons the patient, he/she may be at increased risk
- If possible, interview collateral sources (friends, family, etc.) about presence of SI
- Determine the quality of the social environment to which the patient would be returning to if discharged: Are the family/friends supportive? Does the patient have unresolved interpersonal conflicts?
- Look for any rapid change in medical condition (positive or negative), as this may indicate increased risk[1]
- Assess patient to determine if he/she has a "framework for meaning"[4] (e.g. religion, cultural heritage, social obligations, children) that may deter him/her from suicide: "What has kept you from committing suicide?"

SI and Lethality Assessment

- Initially, try to create an atmosphere in which patient is more likely to disclose SI
  - Ambiguous questions may spontaneously elicit SI: "Have you ever thought of a way of ending your pain?"
  - Explore areas such as depression, psychosis, stressful life events, or abrupt social changes, from which disclosure of SI may naturally arise
  - May inquire here about passive ideation: "Have you ever thought life was not worth living?"
- Next, ask about SI directly: "Have you had thoughts of killing yourself/ taking your life/committing suicide?"
  - Minimize patient anxiety by normalizing: "Sometimes people who feel like you have been thinking about committing suicide. Do you ever feel that way?"
  - Be aware of your own reactions/attitudes toward suicide and suicidal patients. Monitor these feelings when discussing SI with patients to ensure that they do not discourage disclosure
  - If a patient spontaneously brings up a particular method of suicide, he/she has likely considered that method[4]
  - Patients may give nonverbal cues of deception or anxiety when discussing SI; note-taking may hinder observation of such cues
  - If patient initially denies active SI, ask again later
- Finally, determine the lethality of current SI
  - Frequency
  - Duration
  - Pervasiveness (fleeting, sustained)
  - Impulsivity of the patient
  - Extent and details of any suicide plans: lethality of method; availability of method; likelihood of rescue; motive
  - Extent and details of any action taken

- A commonly used framework used to elicit SI is the Chronological Assessment of Suicidal Events (CASE) approach[13]
    1. Assess present SI or suicide event
    2. Assess any SI over the preceding 2 mo
    3. Assess past SI
    4. Assess any immediate SI
- When using this framework, inquire about all pertinent characteristics of SI noted above

> **Clinical Pearl: Suicide**
> Discussing suicidal thoughts and plans does not put ideas into a patient's head.[4] It is important to screen every patient for suicidal tendencies.

Management Approaches

- Patients with active SI should be assessed on an emergency basis
    - Go to an emergency department to be referred for a psychiatric consultation
    - If patient does not or cannot agree to this plan, he/she may be issued a Form 1 (see **Mental Health Act Forms**, p.344); note that this form only applies in Ontario
- Hospitalization may be necessary (voluntary or involuntary)
- Recommendations for management of patients with active SI[14]
    - Treatment must be initiated immediately
    - Two phases of treatment:
        - Acute (8-12 wk): symptom remission
        - Maintenance (at least 6 mo): prevent symptom relapse/recurrence
    - Ensure patient safety by removing dangerous objects and monitoring patients more frequently
    - Optimize pharmacotherapy and address psychosocial issues, which may require formal psychotherapy (see **Depression, Management Approaches**, p.330)
    - Reassess patient for suicidal risk at every visit
- The utility of having a patient "contract for their safety" is highly controversial and should NEVER replace/supersede a clinical assessment

8. COMMON CLINICAL SCENARIOS/FEATURES

Note: The following sections are meant to assist in optimizing the interview process and setting for patients who present with psychiatric symptoms. For specific diagnostic criteria, classification, epidemiology, and differential diagnosis of psychiatric disorders, please refer to the DSM-IV or an equivalent manual. Clinical practice guidelines from the American Psychiatric Association (APA) are also available at http://psychiatryonline.org/guidelines.aspx.

Physicians must be diligent in monitoring for any drug-drug interactions with psychotropic medications. For more information, see English et al., 2012.[15]

8.1 Mood Disorders

- Always consider whether a patient has a mood disorder due to a general medical condition or substance (e.g. hypothyroidism masquerading as a mood disorder)

8.1.1 Depression

- Characterized by a combination of depressed mood, inability to experience pleasure, and neurovegetative symptoms, which suggest that "basic regulatory physiology has been disturbed"[4]

PSYCHIATRIC

Interview Techniques

- Be warm when appropriate, but do not neglect gathering clinical information for the sake of empathy
- Use broader vocabulary when asking about mood to uncover more cases of depression[1,2]: sad, low, blue, gloomy, down in the dumps, loss of interest
  - ***Note:*** depressed patients may also present with irritable/angry mood, or somatic pain[1]
- Try to use a single "anchoring episode"[2] when screening for depressive symptoms (worst, first, most recent, best recalled, longest)
- Introduce inquiry about every symptom with a "catch phrase" that acknowledges the time of the episode
  - "During that 2 mo period last winter, did you notice any changes in your appetite?"
  - "Throughout the summer of 2013, how was your sleeping?"
  - "For the first 4 mo after your baby was born, did you find it hard to focus and concentrate on your daily activities?"
- **Mnemonic for depressive symptoms: SIGMECAPS** (* indicates a neurovegetative symptom)
  - **S**leep*: ↑/↓
  - **I**nterest or pleasure*: ↓(anhedonia)
    - Including sexual interest/libido
  - **G**uilt or worthlessness
  - **M**ood: ↓
  - **E**nergy*: ↓
  - **C**oncentration*: ↓
  - **A**ppetite or weight*: ↑/↓
  - **P**sychomotor activity*: ↑(agitation)/↓(retardation)
  - **SI** (see **Suicide Risk Assessment**, p.327)
- For each symptom, ask about duration, frequency, and intensity
  - Patients often underestimate the duration of symptoms[1]
- Ask about only one symptom at a time, and avoid asking about them as a "laundry list"
- When inquiring about anhedonia, first explore what kinds of activities the patient enjoys normally[1]
- Use a level tone of voice when asking about libido to decrease the likelihood that patients will feel uncomfortable
- Explore personal history for life events (psychological) or medical conditions (physiological) that could account for symptoms
- Always ask directly about manic symptoms to avoid missing a diagnosis of bipolar disorder (see **Bipolar Disorder**, p.332)
- Must inquire about alcohol and substance history
- Mental status exam (MSE) signs[2]
  - **Appearance/Behavior:** signs of personal neglect; fidgety, tense, restless or slow movements; effort put into interview
  - **Speech:** quantity; volume; speed
  - **Mood/Affect:** sad; tearful; despondent; irritable/bored (more commonly in adolescents)
  - **Thought Process:** preoccupation; rumination; perseveration
  - **Thought Content:** guilt; worthlessness; helplessness; delusions (commonly somatic, nihilistic, or guilt); thoughts of self harm; SI
  - **Perception:** hallucinations; derealization; depersonalization

Management Approach

Nonpharmacological (see **Table 4**)

- **Cognitive Behavioral Therapy (CBT):** a formalized brief therapy aimed at changing the patient's automatic style of thinking, and engaging the patient in more pleasurable activities to experience more positive reinforcement

- **Interpersonal Therapy (IPT):** a formalized brief therapy that examines changes in the patient's interpersonal environment and how he/she relates to mood disorders
- **Psychodynamic Therapy/Brief Dynamic Psychotherapy (BDP):** a form of therapy that examines unresolved developmental conflicts to bring these conflicts into conscious awareness and foster acceptance
- **Motivational Interviewing (MI):** a brief therapy that uses a stages-of-change model to help move patients toward behavior modification
- **Cognitive-Behavioral Analysis System of Psychotherapy (CBASP):** a brief therapy that helps the patient recognize how negative thinking patterns and behaviors interact to produce negative outcomes
- **Behavioral Activation Therapy (BA):** a form of therapy that tries to increase patient activity and exposure to positive reinforcement
- **Emotion-Focused Therapy (EFT):** a form of therapy that helps the patient express emotions more readily
- **Bibliotherapy:** a form of therapy in which the patient reads self-help materials
- **Acceptance and Commitment Therapy (ACT):** a form of therapy that increases patient awareness and acceptance of subjective experiences

Table 4. Nonpharmacological Treatment of Depression

1st line	2nd line	3rd line
CBT IPT	Bibliotherapy BA CBASP	ACT BDP MI EFT

ACT = acceptance and commitment therapy, BA = behavioral activation therapy, BDP = brief dynamic psychotherapy, CBASP = cognitive-behavioral analysis system of psychotherapy, CBT = cognitive behavioral therapy, EFT = emotion-focused therapy, IPT = interpersonal therapy, MI = motivational interviewing
Parikh SV, et al. 2009. *J Affect Disord* 117(Suppl 1):S15-25.

Pharmacological (see **Table 5**)
- Choice of antidepressant should depend on factors such as patient age, tolerability, affordability, and preference[16]

Table 5. Pharmacological Treatment of Depression

1st line	2nd line	3rd line
SSRIs; SNRIs; bupropion; escitalopram; mirtazapine; moclobemide; mianserin; reboxetine; tianeptine	TCAs; quetiapine; trazodone; selegiline transdermal	Irreversible MAOIs (tranylcypromine, phenelzine)

SNRIs = serotonin norepinephrine reuptake inhibitors, SSRIs = selective serotonin reuptake inhibitors, TCAs = tricyclic antidepressants
Lam RW, et al. 2009. *J Affect Disord* 117(Suppl 1):S26-43.

- For patients who do not respond to other therapies, electroconvulsive therapy (ECT) should be considered; special circumstances may indicate ECT as first-line treatment[17]

Electroconvulsive Therapy
- A small electrical current is delivered to induce a therapeutic seizure in patients
- More commonly used for acute episodes, but can be used as maintenance therapy
- Most effective treatment for major depression, with efficacy estimated between 70-80%[3,18]

- Situations in which ECT may be a first-line therapy: psychotic depression; patients at high risk for suicidal behavior; rapidly deteriorating patients; patients with prior history of good response to ECT and/or poor response to pharmacotherapy; patient with preference for ECT over pharmacotherapy
- Other indications: medically refractive catatonia; schizophrenia; schizoaffective disorder; mania; intractable seizures; Parkinson's disease
- Adverse effects: cognitive disturbances (retrograde and/or anterograde amnesia); cardiac arrhythmias and, rarely, arrest

PSYCHIATRIC

8.1.2 Bipolar Disorder (BD)

- BD is defined by extreme, atypical fluctuations in mood. Mania and hypomania are periods of elevated mood, while depression is a period of decreased mood. Various subtypes of BD have been defined (see **DSM-IV** for specific criteria)

Interview Techniques

- Try to keep interview short
- Be flexible in your style of questioning
- Remain calm and objective in the presence of euphoria or disinhibition
- Do not engage in personal or intimate conversations[2]
- Inquire about all depressive symptoms (see **Depression**, p.329)
- ***Note:*** avoid using the terms "manic" and "hypomanic" with patients
- When considering behavior, need to understand what a patient is normally like (collateral informants are valuable)
- **Mnemonic for manic symptoms: I PAID GST**
  - **I**ncreased/elevated mood
  - **P**leasurable activities performed to excess (e.g. spending, sex, substance abuse) with potentially harmful consequences
  - **A**ctivity, increase in impulsive or disinhibited behavior
    - Avoid asking direct questions, as patients often have poor insight[2]
    - Collateral sources often valuable
  - **I**deas, flight of (racing thoughts)
    - Keep questions short, simple, and closed-ended
  - **D**istractible by irrelevant environmental stimuli
  - **G**randiosity (inflated self-esteem): "How would you describe your mood over the last…?"
  - **S**leep, decreased need: "What's the least amount of sleep you've been able to get away with in the last…?"
    - One of the "most useful and reliable" criteria for mania[2]
  - **T**alkative, more than usual or feels pressured to talk
- MSE signs for mania/hypomania[2]
  - **Behavior:** impulsive, disinhibited
  - **Cognition/Perception:** racing thoughts
  - **Speech:** incoherent

Management Approach

Nonpharmacological

- All patients should first receive psychoeducation[18]
- CBT, IPT, and family interventions are associated with positive clinical outcomes[18]

Pharmacological (see **Table 6**)

Table 6. Pharmacological Treatment of Bipolar Disorder

	1st line	2nd line
Acute Bipolar Mania*	Monotherapy: lithium; valproic acid; olanzapine; risperidone; quetiapine; aripiprazole; ziprasidone Combination: lithium/valproic acid + risperidone/quetiapine/olanzapine/aripiprazole	Monotherapy: carbamazepine; ECT; asenapine; paliperidone Combination: lithium + valproic acid; lithium/valproic acid + asenapine

*Please refer to references for treatment recommendations for bipolar depression and maintenance therapy
ECT = electroconvulsive therapy
Yatham LN, et al. 2005. *Bipolar Disord* 7(Suppl 3):5-69.
Yatham LN, et al. 2007. *Bipolar Disord* 8(6):721-39.

PSYCHIATRIC

8.2 Anxiety

- A spectrum from normal physiological response to severe functional impairment[19]
- See **DSM-IV** for specific criteria for disorders such as panic disorder, agoraphobia, generalized anxiety disorder, post-traumatic stress disorder, obsessive-compulsive disorder, specific anxiety, and social anxiety disorder

General Approach

- Become familiar with the referral prior to formal assessment
- Anticipate the possibility that anxiety might create difficulties for the patient to get to and from the clinic/hospital
- Rule out medical disorders and substance abuse that may trigger anxiety
- Screen for mood and psychotic disorders due to high prevalence and comorbidity in these patients
- Ensure the environment is comfortable for the patient and anticipate any anxiety provoking triggers that may be present during the assessment (e.g. leave the door slightly open for claustrophobic patients)

Interview Techniques

- Tools of assessment: structured clinical interview for DSM-IV axis I disorders (SCID-I) and anxiety disorder interview schedule (ADIS-IV)
- **Mnemonic for symptoms of acute anxiety: STUDENTS FEAR the 3 C's**[20]
  - **S**weating
  - **T**rembling or shaking
  - **U**nsteadiness or dizziness
  - **D**erealization or depersonalization
  - **E**xcessive heart rate, palpitations
  - **N**ausea or abdominal distress
  - **T**ingling and numbness (paresthesia)
  - **S**hortness of breath or smothering sensation
  - **F**ear of loss of control, going crazy, or dying
  - **C**hest pain or discomfort
  - **C**hoking sensation
  - **C**hills or hot flushes

- History and quantity of substance use, including alcohol or other substances that patients may be using to alleviate their symptoms (e.g. "self-medication")
- Medical history: patients who experience episodes of panic with chest pain should be screened for symptoms of heart disease
- Medications: cocaine, amphetamines, caffeine
- Past and family psychiatric history (be specific, e.g. obsessions, compulsions)

PSYCHIATRIC

Management Approach

Nonpharmacological: CBT

Pharmacological (see **Table 7**)

Table 7. Pharmacological Treatment of Anxiety

Disorder	Medications Indicated (approved by Health Canada)	
Anxiety*	SSRIs	Fluoxetine, Fluvoxamine, Paroxetine, Sertraline
	SNRIs	Venlafaxine
	Buspirone	
	BZDs	Useful as adjunct in early treatment (e.g. SSRI/SNRI + BZD). Consider short-term BZDs in severe anxiety, agitation or acute functional impairment. Be cautious in usage if comorbid substance abuse, elderly or pregnant.

*See reference below for specific indications according to DSM-IV criteria
BZDs = benzodiazepines, SNRIs = serotonin norepinephrine reuptake inhibitors, SSRIs = selective serotonin reuptake inhibitors
Swinson RP, et al. 2006. *Can J Psychiatry* 51(8 Suppl 2):9S-91S.

8.3 Psychosis

- Characterized by loss of contact with reality, manifesting as delusions and hallucinations[21,22] (see **DSM-IV** for specific criteria)

General Approach

- Evaluate patient's needs prior to interview (e.g. medication, bathroom, food/water)
- Ensure the environment is comfortable for the patient
- Ensure the safety of the interviewer and the patient (e.g. escape routes, presence of a third party, privacy, and confidentiality)
- Addressing confidentiality issues might be important for paranoid patients
- Engage the patient by inquiring about and understanding his/her expectations for the encounter
- Make the questions simple and brief, as the patient might have attention deficits
- Normalize questions: "When people are under stress, sometimes they might experience…Have you also had these experiences?"
- Explain the diagnosis and treatment approach

Interview Techniques

- Begin the interview by allowing the patient to talk freely for a few minutes while observing the patient's speech and behavior for the purpose of generating hypotheses for differential diagnosis
- In the HPI, the following points should be covered:
  - What is the reason/trigger for the consultation?

- o Clarify the details of symptoms reported: quality, onset/prodrome, progress, premorbid personality
  - o May not be therapeutic to challenge the patient's delusions
  - o Evaluate the nature of the patient's belief(s) against the criteria for delusions
  - o Ensure confidentiality is protected and consider gathering information from third parties in challenging interviews
  - o Current level of functioning and any changes in cognition
  - o Safety risks: caring for self and others, activities of daily living (ADLs)
  - o Harming self or others
- History and quantity of substance use
- Legal history in relation to neighbors, police, charges, crimes, and jail time
- Medical history, past, and family psychiatric history, medications
- MSE (see **Mental Status Examination**, p.322)

PSYCHIATRIC

Psychotic Symptoms

- Hallucinations and delusions (see **Mental Status Examination**, p.323)
- Common delusions and screening questions:
  - o **Delusion of Grandeur:** "Did you ever feel that you were especially important in some way, or that you had special powers or abilities?"
  - o **Persecutory/Paranoid Delusion:** "Have you felt afraid that people may be trying to hurt you or are out to 'get you'?"
  - o **Delusion of Reference:** "Did it ever seem that people were talking about you?" "When watching TV or listening to the radio, did you ever feel that there were special messages intended specifically for you?"
  - o **Thought Broadcasting:** "Did you ever feel as if your thoughts were being broadcast out loud so that other people could hear what you were thinking?"
  - o **Thought Insertion/Withdrawal:** "Did you ever feel that certain thoughts were put into or taken out of your head?"
  - o **Mind Reading:** "Did you ever feel as if people were able to read your mind and know what you're thinking?"
  - o **Delusion of Control:** "Did you ever feel like you were being controlled against your will by someone or some power from outside yourself?"
  - o **Delusion of Guilt:** "Did you ever blame yourself for bad things in the world?" "Did you ever feel like you had done something terrible and deserved to be punished?"
  - o **Somatic Delusion:** "Do you fear that something is terribly wrong with your body?"

Management Approach

- Rule out organic disorders (thyroid measures [TSH, T_3/T_4], glucose, vitamin B12, HIV, TB, ceruloplasmin, cortisol, autoimmune, etc.)
- Baseline blood work (CBC, liver and renal function tests, prolactin, fasting glucose, and lipids), weight, and ECG before starting antipsychotic medication
- Frequent monitoring of medication side effects

Pharmacological (see **Table 8**)

Table 8. Pharmacological Treatment of Psychotic Disorders

Class	Medications	Notes
Atypical (2nd Gen)	Olanzapine Risperidone Quetiapine Clozapine Ziprasidone Paliperidone Aripiprazole	• Fewer neurological side effects (e.g. EPS) • More effective in negative symptoms, cognitive impairment, and depressive symptoms
Typical (1st Gen)	Haloperidol Chlorpromazine Perphenazine Flupenthixol	• Increased risk of EPS and TD • Fewer metabolic side effects (weight gain, DM, dyslipidemia)

Note: Controversy currently exists about the differential efficacy and safety of different antipsychotic classes. For discussion, see Meyer JM, 2007.[23]
EPS = extrapyramidal symptoms, TD = tardive dyskinesia
Canadian Psychiatric Association. 2005. *Can J Psychiatry* 50(13 Suppl 1):7S-57S.

8.4 Substance-Related Disorders (SRD)

- Divided into two groups: those related to an aberrant pattern of use and those related to physiological effects (see **DSM-IV** for criteria)

General Approach

- ***Note:*** any psychiatric disorder can be caused by substance intoxication or withdrawal, so always include SRD in differential diagnosis
- Having a concurrent psychiatric illness increases prevalence of SRD[2]
- Investigations: urine toxicology; breathalyzer; CBC; and serum transaminase levels
- At first encounter, discuss the limits of confidentiality with the patient
  - The following situations require legal reporting: suspected child abuse or neglect; driving while impaired

Interview Techniques

- Most important thing is to be nonjudgmental[2]
  - Avoid "why" questions ("Why do you use substance X?")
  - Ask questions that bring out his/her motivation for using, his/her experiences while using, and what happens when he/she stops: "Help me understand the good things about drug use for you. How do you feel when you stop taking drugs? What worries you about coming off of substance X?"
  - Areas of questioning to screen for substance-related disorders
  - Substance use history: quantity and frequency (over lifetime and past 30 d)
  - Symptoms of substance intoxication/overdose, substance withdrawal, depression, and anxiety
  - SI
  - Consequences of use on functioning: school/work, social, legal, romantic
  - Medical consequences of use
  - Associated risky behaviors: using while operating a motorized vehicle; unprotected sexual activity; needle sharing; family violence; safety of children
  - Pain history and management
- Physical exam
  - Needle track marks

- Nasal septal perforation
- Conjunctival injury
- Tobacco-stained fingers, teeth
- Alcoholic odor to breath

Management Approach

Note: The following are general principles only; recommendations for treatment of substance-specific SRD can be found in the APA treatment guidelines (http://psychiatryonline.org/guidelines.aspx)

Nonpharmacological

- Motivate the patient to reduce or eliminate his/her use
- Assessing patient's motivation to change: the **5 R**'s model[2]
  - **Relevance:** is this an important issue for the patient? How confident does he/she feel he/she can change?
  - **Rewards:** what are the benefits of using for the patient?
  - **Risks:** what are the negative effects on health, family, social, and occupational functioning? Provide education if required
  - **Roadblocks:** explore obstacles to change, and allow patient to brainstorm possible solutions. Allow patient to set short- and long-term goals. Avoid being overly directive
  - **Repetition:** reassess relevance and confidence at each subsequent visit, and update goals as needed
- Harm reduction strategies: needle exchange programs; methadone therapy
- Next step may involve management of withdrawal symptoms (home, community, medically supervised)
- Prepare for minor relapses to prevent them from developing into full-blown relapses

Pharmacological

- Consult treatment guidelines for substance-specific therapy (http://psychiatryonline.org/guidelines.aspx)

8.5 Eating Disorders

- 3 identified eating disorders: anorexia nervosa, bulimia nervosa, and eating disorder not otherwise specified (see **DSM-IV** for specific criteria)

General Approach

- Patterns of disordered eating include both extreme caloric restriction, and unhealthy patterns of bingeing and purging
  - ***Note:*** some patients with eating disorders may have a normal, or even elevated, body weight; therefore, do not base suspicion of an eating disorder on appearance alone[2]
- Patients may deny/minimize the severity of his/her symptoms (i.e. he/she may have poor insight)
- Anticipate that it may take time to develop an alliance
- For children with eating disorders, parents, school officials, and the family doctor/pediatrician should be involved[2]
  - It is important to educate collateral sources about the origins of eating disorders to avoid blaming the patient
- Investigations
  - Recommended for all patients: CBC and differential; electrolytes; renal function tests (creatinine, BUN); ECG
  - Optional: thyroid measures (TSH, T_3/T_4); serum levels of phosphate, magnesium, and calcium; blood glucose; LFTs; serum amylase; urinalysis; stool analysis

PSYCHIATRIC

Interview Techniques

- Discuss why patient seeks help
- Ways to engage patients with eating disorders[2]:
  - Validate his/her apprehension and anxiety
  - Be empathic and nonjudgmental
  - Monitor your emotional reaction, and try to avoid showing anger, frustration, or helplessness
  - If patient is above age of consent, interview him/her alone
- The following items are critical to a comprehensive HPI:
  - Weight history: What is it now? How has it changed over time? If the patient has or had amenorrhea, at what weight did this occur?
  - History of disordered eating behaviors: food restriction; self-induced vomiting; laxative, diuretic, and diet pill use (number and type); herbal product use; thyroid medicine and ipecac use; abuse of insulin; illicit substances; exercise; food rituals; checking behavior (weight, calorie-counting); bingeing; pattern of eating (alone or with others? are there regular meal times? is the food the same or different from what the family eats?)
  - Other psychiatric symptoms: mood; anxiety; personality features; substance use; suicidal and homicidal ideation
- Physical Exam
  - **General:** height; weight; BMI; waist circumference; acetone odor on breath (sign of starvation)
  - **Vitals:** pulse rate (often bradycardic and irregular); pulse and blood pressure should be taken supine and seated because orthostatic changes are common
  - **Dermatological:** pallor; scars on dorsum of hand (Russell's sign); cyanosed fingers and toes; orange skin; sores and/or rashes around mouth; salivary gland swelling; periorbital petechiae; thin scalp hair; presence of lanugo hair
  - **Cardiovascular:** edema; weak peripheral pulses
  - **Gastrointestinal:** abdominal masses and/or tenderness; bowel sounds
  - **Neurological:** diminished peripheral sensation; hyporeflexia (electrolyte abnormalities); hyperreflexia (mineral deficiencies)

Management Approach

Anorexia Nervosa

- Often requires combination of inpatient, day patient, and outpatient settings
- Usually takes mo to yr
- Goal is to restore body weight
  - Inpatient: 0.5-1 kg/wk; outpatient: 0.2-0.5 kg/wk[24]
  - Should always try to motivate the patient to change his/her weight and behavior
  - Forced treatment should be avoided whenever possible
- Limited use for pharmacotherapy
  - Low-dose anxiolytics may be used for anxiety
  - Antidepressants may be used to treat comorbid depressive symptoms

Bulimia Nervosa

- Psychotherapy is the treatment of choice (minimum 25 sessions)
  - CBT (most evidence)
  - IPT
  - Psychodynamic therapy may be offered as an alternative
  - Some patients may benefit from self-help programs
- Limited use for pharmacotherapy
  - SSRIs are first choice for symptom reduction

8.6 Cognitive Impairment (CI)

- Different degrees of CI[25]
  - Mild cognitive impairment (MCI)/cognitive impairment, no dementia (CIND)
  - Dementia (mild, moderate, and severe)

General Approach

- Traditional office setting may not be appropriate, so be flexible
- Glasses and/or hearing aids should be worn if necessary
- Should have ready access to laboratory and imaging facilities to rule out general medical conditions and vitamin deficiencies
- 3 common causes of CI include dementia, delirium (see **Delirium**, p.336), and depression (see **Table 9**)

Table 9. Differentiating Causes of Cognitive Impairment

	Dementia	Delirium	Depression
Onset	Insidious	Acute	Subacute
Course	Progressive	Increased mortality	Recovery/ recurrent
Medical Status	Variable	Acute illness, drug toxicity (e.g. anticholinergic)	Variable
Family History	10%	Negative	Mood disorder, substance abuse

Goldbloom DS (Editor). *Psychiatric Clinical Skills*. Philadelphia: Mosby Elsevier; 2006.

Interview and Assessment

- Be patient
- Be alert to any spontaneous mention of impairment to memory and/or cognition and explore it
- Observe for difficulties in providing history (including chronology and details)
- Be sensitive when transitioning into cognitive assessment, and avoid using the word "test"[2]: "I'll now move to assess your concentration and memory"
- Cognitive screening (see **Table 3**)
- If patient has a caregiver, very useful to interview patient and caregiver separately

> **Clinical Pearl: Caregiver Beliefs**
> When caregiver believes that something is wrong, he/she is often correct.[2]

Management Approach

Note: not applicable to CI caused by other medical, neurological or psychiatric conditions

Nonpharmacological

- MCI or CIND[26]
  - Promotion of stimulating cognitive activities
  - Promotion of physical activity
  - Treatment of vascular risk factors: systolic BP <140 mmHg
  - Some evidence recommends against using NSAIDs, estrogen replacement therapy, and ginkgo biloba or vitamin E
- Mild to Moderate Dementia[27]
  - Address the needs of any family caregivers

- Individualized exercise program recommended
- Insufficient evidence for cognitive training, cognitive rehabilitation, or environmental interventions
- Severe Dementia/Alzheimer's Disease[28]
  - Patients should be assessed at least every 4 mo
  - Assess caregiver(s) for stress level
  - Use combination of MMSE and Global Deterioration Scale to monitor disease progression
  - Monitor medical and nutritional status
  - Discuss the possibility of long-term institutional care with caregivers, taking into account the patient's prior wishes when competent

PSYCHIATRIC

Behavioral and Psychological Symptoms of Dementia (BPSD) (see **Table 10**)
- Nonpharmacological therapy is the recommended first-line treatment
- Pharmacologic therapies should be given concurrently with nonpharmacologic therapies, initiated at the minimum dose, titrated slowly, and closely monitored for safety and efficacy
- Controversies about atypical antipsychotics in dementia include small but significant absolute increased risk of stroke or death, but typical antipsychotics (e.g. haloperidol, loxapine) have not been shown to be safer from that perspective and have a higher risk of extrapyramidal symptoms (EPS) and tardive dyskinesia (TD)

Table 10. Management of BPSD

Type	Examples
Nonpharmacological	**Patients:** controlled multisensory stimulation (Snoezelen); psychomotor, bright light, reminiscence, validation, aroma, or massage and touch therapy **Caregivers:** education and support groups
Pharmacological	For agitation, psychosis, or aggression, risperidone or olanzapine may be used (BZDs in emergencies)

BZDs = benzodiazepines
Hermann N, Gauthier S. 2008. *CMAJ* 179(12):1279-1287.

Pharmacological (see **Table 11**)
- For concurrent depression, SSRIs may be used
- For severe insomnia, short- to intermediate-acting BZDs may be used (at minimum dose and for minimum duration)

Table 11. Pharmacotherapy for Cognitive Impairment

Class	Examples	Notes
Cholinesterase Inhibitors	Donepezil Galantamine Rivastigmine	• Selection should be individualized and evaluated after 3-6 mo to monitor side effects and response ***Note:*** will not stop progression, but may delay decline, improve function or behavior
NMDA-R Antagonist	Memantine	• Monotherapy or adjunctive to cholinesterase inhibitors in moderate to severe cases of Alzheimer's disease • Not recommended for mild dementia

NMDA-R = N-methyl-D-aspartate receptor
Hermann N, Gauthier S. 2008. *CMAJ* 179(12):1279-1287.
Hogan DB, et al. 2008. *CMAJ* 179(10):1019-1026.

8.7 Delirium

- A syndrome of acute onset that includes CI accompanied by fluctuating consciousness/alertness[6]
- Very common in patients with dementia
- Often missed in clinical settings[3]

Etiology

- Very broad differential diagnosis[3,6]
- Always medical or substance-related (intoxication or withdrawal) in origin
- One case may have multiple etiologies

Diagnosis

- History (often collateral) and physical exam
  - Review all medications in detail
- Neurological assessment
- Cognitive assessment (see **Table 3**, p.326)
- Neuroimaging (CT or MRI) may be required if history cannot be completed, or if focal neurological deficits are found[3]
- Routine lab testing: blood work (electrolytes, glucose, calcium, serum creatinine, LFTs, and CBC)
- Other tests depend on suspected etiology: urinalysis; urine culture; toxicology screens; chest X-ray; ECG; pulse oximetry; arterial blood gases; CSF examination; syphilis or HIV serology; thyroid function; magnesium

Management Approach

- Resolution of underlying cause is the top priority
- ECT may be considered if other therapies have failed[3]

Nonpharmacological[3]

- Maximize safety and comfort of the environment: provide hearing aids/glasses when applicable; avoid placing patient in shared room; minimize noise
- Provide comfort and support: continuity of care providers; providing familiar and/or orienting items from home in patient's room
- Ensure adequate nutrition

Pharmacological (see **Table 12**)

- Aimed at reducing agitation associated with delirium

Table 12. Pharmacological Management of Delirium

Drug Class	Examples	Notes
TAPs	Haloperidol	• Haloperidol preferred over other TAPs • Preferred antipsychotic due to potency, and fewer anticholinergic and hypotensive side effects • Higher rate of EPS and TD • Monitor therapy closely
AAPs	Risperidone Olanzapine Quetiapine	• Useful for controlling aggression • Fewer EPS • Higher mortality • As a class, AAPs are generally preferred over TAPs

Table 12. Pharmacological Management of Delirium (continued)

Drug Class	Examples	Notes
BZDs	Lorazepam	• Treatment of choice when agitation is due to sedative-hypnotic withdrawal • Can worsen delirium

AAPs = atypical antipsychotics, TAPs = typical antipsychotics
Sadock BJ, Sadock VA, Ruiz P (Editors). *Kaplan and Sadock's Comprehensive Textbook of Psychiatry*, 9th ed. Philadelphia: Lippincott Williams & Wilkins; 2009.

8.8 Personality Disorders (PD)

- A personality profile that is considered maladaptive, long-standing, and inflexible
- See **DSM-IV** for specific criteria of paranoid, schizoid, schizotypal, antisocial, borderline, histrionic, narcissistic, avoidant, dependent, and obsessive-compulsive PD

General Approach

- Obtain a detailed developmental history, with special focus on childhood traits and temperament
- Focus on the functional impact of the symptoms more than the symptoms themselves
- If the patient has a history of negative experiences with clinicians, do not interview him/her alone[2]
- Be aware that it may take a long time to develop a true therapeutic relationship
- Be especially attentive at maintaining boundaries
- Abnormal personality may be due to a PD, or another psychiatric condition (see **Table 13**)

Table 13. Differentiating Personality Disorders from Psychiatric Conditions

	Personality Disorder	Other Psychiatric Disorder
Onset	Chronic	Recent (first onset, or relapse)
Progression	Presence of symptoms often strongly linked to interpersonal relationships	Variable
Presentation	Context-dependent (maybe)	Context-independent
Duration	Years	Variable
Relation to Life Events	Present even without stressors	Can show strong association with negative life event

Goldbloom DS (Editor). *Psychiatric Clinical Skills*. Philadelphia: Mosby Elsevier; 2006.

- Obtain collateral information whenever possible (with consent)
- Other factors to consider when making a diagnosis:
  - Why is the patient seeking help?
  - Is there a family history of PD?
  - What is the pattern of the patient's interpersonal interactions?
  - "Signal behaviors/symptoms"[1] (see **Table 14**)

Table 14. Signal Behaviors and Symptoms of Personality Disorders

Behavior or Symptom	Possible Personality Diagnoses*
Comment on Clinician Performance	Antisocial; Histrionic; Borderline
Complaints about Clinician/System	Antisocial; Borderline; Narcissistic; Paranoid
Flirtatious/Sexual Bragging	Antisocial; Histrionic; Narcissistic
Dramatic Behavior/Dress	Histrionic; Borderline
Helpless/Child-like	Dependent; Borderline; Histrionic
Manipulative	Narcissistic; Borderline; Histrionic
Self-Mutilation	Borderline
Extreme Perfectionism	Obsessive-Compulsive
Law Breaking	Antisocial
Dramatic Anger and Physical Fighting	Antisocial; Paranoid; Borderline; Narcissistic; Histrionic
Low Self-Esteem	Dependent; Borderline; Schizotypal; Avoidant
Intense Anxiety	Obsessive-Compulsive; Dependent; Avoidant
Poor Empathy	Antisocial; Histrionic; Narcissistic; Schizoid

*Signal behaviors or symptoms may be the result of a wide variety of psychiatric conditions. However, they increase the likelihood that the listed personality disorders are present.
Shea S. *Psychiatric Interviewing: The Art of Understanding*. Philadelphia: W.B. Saunders Company; 1988.

PSYCHIATRIC

Interview Techniques

- "Probe questions"[1] for specific PD can be useful (see Shea 1988,[2] chapter 6 for examples)
- Be flexible and willing to side-track when necessary
- Techniques to help elicit sensitive material[1]
  - **Shame Reversal:** reframe questions such that a positive answer is not an admission of failure (e.g. "Are any of your coworkers really difficult to work with?" or "Are you able to hold your liquor pretty well?")
    - Do not condone the behavior
  - **Symptom Amplification:** give patients options that, even if they minimize their behavior, uncover the behavior in question (e.g. "Do you drink about 5 drinks a d, a little less, a little more?" or "How many jobs would you say you've had in the last yr? 5, 10, 20?")
  - Maintain the same body language and tone of voice as when asking mundane questions
  - Normalize the patient's symptoms ("It's not uncommon for people in those circumstances to…")
  - Begin by assuming that the patient has engaged in/experienced the behavior
  - When appropriate, validate past positive behavior
- Techniques for engaging certain types of patients[2]
  - **Distrustful:** maintain professional demeanor; be as predictable as possible
  - **Socially Awkward:** tolerate silence; be aware of boundaries, and professional distance

- **Eccentric Patients:** carefully monitor your responses (verbal and nonverbal)
- **Distressed/Anxious:** validate feelings to prevent escalation; keep focused on the present
- **Narcissistic:** acknowledge and accept sense of entitlement

Management Approach

Note: be sure to involve the patient in every stage of treatment

- Establish a management framework early in treatment
  - Outline what is expected of the patient
  - If care involves multiple providers, determine who will assume primary responsibility
  - Have a crisis plan in place
  - Have a "low consultation threshold"[2]
  - Carefully monitor your emotional response to patients

> **Clinical Pearl: Personality Disorder and Remission**
> Maintain a sense of hope for remission in patients with PD. Evidence has shown these disorders to be more changeable than previously thought by both clinicians and patients.[2]

9. MENTAL HEALTH ISSUES IN CHILDREN

- See **Pediatric Exam**, Psychiatric and Behavioral Problems section, p.287

10. MENTAL HEALTH ACT FORMS (see **Table 15**)

- Basic Criteria for Certification:
  1. Serious bodily harm to the person; or
  2. Serious bodily harm to another person; or
  3. Imminent and serious physical impairment of the person

Table 15. Ontario Mental Health Act Forms

Form	Form Name/ Function	Purpose
FORM 1 (FORM 42 to patient)	Application by Physician for Psychiatric Assessment	Duration: 72 h from admission Reason: meets criteria for certification and for psychiatric assessment Issued: by examining physician within 7 d
FORM 2	Order for Examination under Section 16	Duration: 7 d to get patient to hospital Reason: hospitalization and psychiatric assessment Issued: by Justice of the Peace
FORM 3 (FORM 30 to patient)	Certificate of Involuntary Admission	Duration: first Form 3 lasts 2 wk from date signed Reason: meets criteria for certification Issued: by attending physician different from Form 1 physician
FORM 5	Change to Informal or Voluntary Status	Reason: when physician feels that patient does not require involuntary admission, but does not necessarily mean that patient is ready for discharge

Table 15. Ontario Mental Health Act Forms (continued)

Form	Form Name/ Function	Purpose
FORM 33	Notice to Patient that Patient is Incompetent	Reason: patient not mentally capable to consent to collection, use or disclosure of personal health information; patient not mentally capable to manage property; patient is not mentally capable to consent to treatment of mental disorder

PSYCHIATRIC

REFERENCES

1. Goldbloom DS (Editor). *Psychiatric Clinical Skills.* Philadelphia: Mosby Elsevier; 2006.
2. Shea SC. *Psychiatric Interviewing: The Art of Understanding.* Philadelphia: W.B. Saunders Company; 1988.
3. Sadock BJ, Sadock VA, Ruiz P (Editors). *Kaplan & Sadock's Comprehensive Textbook of Psychiatry*, 9th ed. Philadelphia: Lippincott Williams & Wilkins; 2009.
4. Dhalla S, Kopec JA. 2007. The CAGE questionnaire for alcohol misuse: A review of reliability and validity studies. *Clin Invest Med* 30(1):33-41.
5. Carlat DJ. *The Psychiatric Interview: A Practical Guide*, 2nd ed. London: Lippincott Williams & Wilkins; 2005.
6. Shader RI (Editor). *Manual of Psychiatric Therapeutics*, 3rd ed. Philadelphia: Lippincott Williams & Wilkins; 2003.
7. Borson S. 2000. The mini-cog: A cognitive "vital signs" measure for dementia screening in multi-lingual elderly. *Int J Geriatr Psychiatry* 15(11):1021-1027.
8. Shulman KI, Gold DP, Cohen CA, Zucchero CA. 1993. Clock-drawing and dementia in the community: A longitudinal study. *Int J Geriatr Psychiatry* 8(6):487-496.
9. Patterson CJ, Gauthier S, Bergman H, Cohen CA, Feightner JW, Feldman H, et al. 1999. The recognition, assessment and management of dementing disorders: Conclusions from the Canadian Consensus Conference on Dementia. *CMAJ* 160(12 Suppl):S1-S20.
10. Patterson WM, Dohn HH, Bird J, Patterson GA.1983. Evaluation of suicidal patients: The SAD PERSONS scale. *Psychosomatics* 24(4):343-349.
11. Bolton JM, Spiwak R, Sareen J. 2012. Predicting suicide attempts with the SAD PERSONS scale: A longitudinal analysis. *J Clin Psychiatry* 73(6):e735-e741.
12. Fawcitt J. Saving the suicidal patient: The state of the art. In: Ayd F, Taylor I (Editors). *Mood Disorders: The World's Major Public Health Problem.* Baltimore: Ayd Medical Communications; 1978.
13. Shea SC. *The Practical Art of Suicide Assessment: A Guide for Mental Health Professionals and Substance Abuse Counselors.* New York: John Wiley; 1999.
14. Reesal RT, Lam RW, CANMAT Depression Work Group. 2001. Clinical guidelines for the treatment of depressive disorders. II. Principles of management. *Can J Psychiatry* 46(Suppl 1):21S-28S.
15. English BA, Dortch M, Ereshefsky L, Jhee S. 2012. Clinically significant psychotropic drug-drug interactions in the primary care setting. *Curr Psychiatry Rep* 14(4):376-390.
16. Lam RW, Kennedy SH, Grigoriadis S, McIntyre RS, Milev R, Ramasubbu R, et al. 2009. Canadian Network for Mood and Anxiety Treatments (CANMAT) clinical guidelines for the management of major depressive disorder in adults. III. Pharmacotherapy. *J Affect Disord* 117(Suppl 1):S26-43.
17. Kennedy SH, Milev R, Giacobbe P, Ramasubbu R, Lam RW, Parikh SV, et al. 2009. Canadian Network for Mood and Anxiety Treatments (CANMAT) clinical guidelines for the management of major depressive disorder in adults. IV. Neurostimulation therapies. *J Affect Disord* 117(Suppl 1):S44-53.
18. Yatham LN, Kennedy SH, O'Donovan C, Parikh S, MacQueen G, McIntyre R, et al. 2005. Canadian Network for Mood and Anxiety Treatments (CANMAT) guidelines for the management of patients with bipolar disorder: Consensus and controversies. *Bipolar Disord* 7 Suppl 3:5-69.
19. Yatham LN, Kennedy SH, Parikh SV, Schaffer A, Beaulieu S, Alda M, et al. 2013. Canadian Network for Mood and Anxiety Treatments (CANMAT) and International Society for Bipolar Disorders (ISBD) collaborative update of CANMAT guidelines for the management of patients with bipolar disorder: Update 2013. *Bipolar Disord* 8(6):721-739.
20. Jain U, Lofchy J. Psychiatry. In: Panu N, Wong S (Editors). *MCCQE 2002 Review Notes.* 2002.
21. Canadian Psychiatric Association. 2005. Clinical practice guidelines: Treatment of schizophrenia. *Canadian Psychiatric Association.* 2005. 50(13 Suppl 1):7S-57S.
22. Feifel D. 2000. Rationale and guidelines for the inpatient treatment of acute psychosis. *J Clin Psychiatry* 61(Suppl 14):27-32.
23. Meyer JM. 2007. Antipsychotic safety and efficacy concerns. *J Clin Psychiatry* 68(Suppl 14):20-26.
24. Herpertz S, Hagenah U, Vocks S, von Wietersheim J, Cuntz U, Zeeck A, et al. 2011. The diagnosis and treatment of eating disorders. *Dtsch Arztebl Int* 108(40):678-685.
25. Feldman HH, Jacova C, Robillard A, Garcia A, Chow T, Borrie M, et al. 2008. Diagnosis and treatment of dementia: 2. Diagnosis. *CMAJ* 178(7):825-836.
26. Chertkow H, Massoud F, Nasreddine Z, Belleville S, Joanette Y, Bocti C, et al. 2008. Diagnosis and treatment of dementia: 3. Mild cognitive impairment and cognitive impairment without dementia. *CMAJ* 178(10):1273-1285.
27. Hogan DB, Bailey P, Black S, Carswell A, Chertkow H, Clarke B, et al. 2008. Diagnosis and treatment of dementia: 4. Approach to management of mild to moderate dementia. *CMAJ* 179(8):787-793.
28. Herrmann N, Gauthier S. 2008. Diagnosis and treatment of dementia: 6. Management of severe alzheimer disease. *CMAJ* 179(12):1279-1287.

The Respiratory Exam

Editors:
Mostafa Fatehi
Miranda Boggild

Faculty Reviewers:
Meyer Balter, MD, FRCP(C)
David Hall, MD, FRCP(C)

RESPIRATORY

TABLE OF CONTENTS

1. ESSENTIAL ANATOMY

Landmarks

- **Apex:** 2-4 cm above medial third of clavicle
- **Oblique Fissure (both lungs):** line from T3 spinous process, through 5th rib in the mid-axillary line, ending at the 6th rib in the mid-clavicular line
  - Right oblique fissure: separates the lower lobe from the upper and middle lobes
  - Left oblique fissure: separates the upper and lower lobes
- **Horizontal Fissure (right lung):** separates the upper and middle lobes; extends from the 5th rib in the right mid-axillary line to the 4th rib at the sternal border
- **Inferior Margins (both lungs):** extend from T10 posteriorly, through the 8th rib in the mid-axillary line to the 6th rib in the mid-clavicular line
- **Carina:** located at the level of the angle of Louis (T4)
- **Right Hemidiaphragm:** at the level of the 5th rib anteriorly and T9 posteriorly at end of respiration (higher than left due to liver)

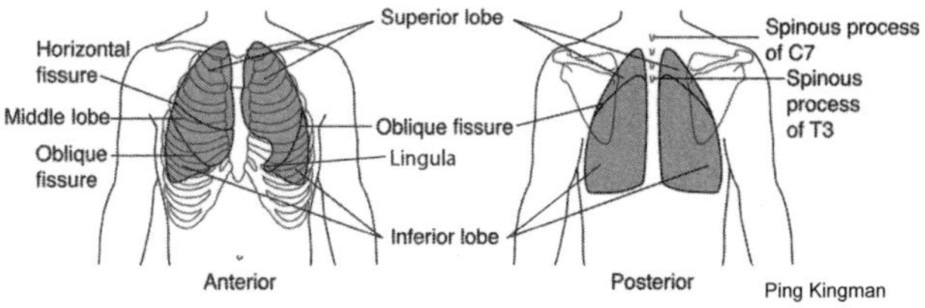

Figure 1. Locations of Lobes and Landmarks

RESPIRATORY

2. APPROACH TO THE RESPIRATORY HISTORY AND PHYSICAL EXAM

In addition to general history taking, important aspects of the respiratory history include:

- Cough ± sputum production
- Wheezing/stridor
- Dyspnea
- Hemoptysis
- Pleuritic chest pain
- Cyanosis, edema
- Past history of respiratory infections
- FHx of atopy
- Smoking
- Previous CXR or pulmonary function test results
- Animal exposure, allergies
- Environmental/occupational exposures
- Travel history/birthplace (TB endemic)
- Sexual history

3. COMMON CHIEF COMPLAINTS

- Cough
- Phlegm production (sputum)
- Wheezing
- Shortness of breath (dyspnea)
- Coughing up blood (hemoptysis)
- Chest pain
- Chest radiographic abnormalities (as reason for referral)

Overview of the Physical Exam

- **Inspection**
  - Rate and pattern of respiration
  - Signs of respiratory effort and distress (accessory muscle use, paradoxical breathing)
  - Cyanosis (central, peripheral)
  - Chest configuration (kyphosis, scoliosis, barrel chest)
  - Clubbing
  - Pursed-lip breathing
  - Presence of equipment (e.g. oximeter, supplementary oxygen)
- **Palpation**
  - General tenderness and deformities
  - Position of trachea
  - Chest expansion
  - Tactile fremitus
- **Percussion**
  - General percussion (resonance, dullness)
  - Diaphragmatic excursion
- **Auscultation**
  - Type of breath sounds (vesicular, bronchovesicular, bronchial, tracheal)
  - Symmetry of breath sounds
  - Presence of adventitious sounds (crackles, wheezes, stridor, pleural rub)

4. FOCUSED HISTORY

Cough

- Onset/Duration: acute/chronic, time of day, frequency, quality, progression, ± sputum (see **Table 1**)
- Aggravating/Alleviating Factors: body position, season, different environments
- Associated Symptoms: fever, chills, night sweats, weight loss, post-nasal drip, runny nose, hoarseness, wheezing, heartburn
- Risk Factors: smoking, sick contacts, travel history, pets, occupational history
- Common Causes of Cough: asthma, GERD, post-viral cough, upper airway cough syndrome

Table 1. Cough Descriptors and Possible Etiologies to Consider

Cough Descriptors	Possible Etiologies
Dry, hacking	Viral pneumonia, interstitial lung disease, tumor, laryngitis, allergies, anxiety
Chronic, productive	Bronchiectasis, chronic bronchitis, abscess, pneumonia, TB
Barking	Epiglottal disease (e.g. croup)
Morning	Smoking
Nocturnal	Post-nasal drip, CHF, asthma
Upon eating/drinking	Neuromuscular disease of the upper esophagus

Note: While the descriptions of a cough obtained by history may be helpful when considering the differential diagnosis of cough, these descriptions alone cannot determine the etiology of cough. A clinical anatomic-pathologic diagnostic approach and supportive tests, such as spirometry, pulmonary function tests, imaging, and 24 h esophageal pH monitoring, are crucial steps in diagnosis after taking a history.
Swartz M. *Textbook of Physical Diagnosis*, 6th ed. Philadelphia: Elsevier; 2010.

Sputum

- Onset/duration, frequency, progression, quantity, color, consistency, odor, hemoptysis
- Mucoid (uninfected) sputum is odorless, transparent, and whitish-gray
- Purulent (infected) sputum is yellow, green in bronchiectasis and COPD, yellow or green sputum in an asthmatic is more often due to eosinophilia than infection
- Foul-smelling sputum is suggestive of a lung abscess

Wheezing/Stridor

- A high-pitched sound caused by a partially obstructed airway
  - Wheezing: due to intrathoracic obstruction, on expiration
  - Stridor: due to extrathoracic tracheal obstruction, on inspiration
- Causes: bronchospasm (e.g. asthma), mucosal edema, loss of elastic support, tortuosity of airways
- Determine onset, frequency, progression, duration of episodes, alleviating factors, associated symptoms
- Aggravating/Precipitating Factors: food, odors, emotions, animals, allergens (e.g. dust, pollen)
- Risk Factors: history of nasal polyps, cardiac disease (e.g. CHF), smoking

RESPIRATORY

Dyspnea

- Onset: gradual vs. sudden, provoking/palliating factors, duration, body position (see **Table 2**)
- Dyspnea on exertion
  - Quantify with exercise tolerance (e.g. number of blocks walked or flights of stairs climbed before onset)
  - Compare dyspnea before and after exertion
- Progression of Symptoms: current symptoms vs. 6 mo prior
- Paroxysmal Nocturnal Dyspnea (PND): sudden onset of dyspnea that awakens an individual from sleep (patient classically describes needing to go to an open window for air)
- Associated Symptoms
  - Fever, chills, night sweats
  - Cough, hemoptysis, sputum
  - Fatigue, chest pain, palpitations, peripheral edema
- Risk Factors: sick contacts, industrial exposure (e.g. asbestos, sandblasting), travel history

Table 2. Types and Etiologies of Positional Dyspnea

Type	Etiology
Orthopnea (dyspnea when lying horizontally)	CHF Mitral valve disease Severe asthma (rare) COPD (rare) Neurological diseases (rare)
Trepopnea (dyspnea when lying on one side)	CHF
Platypnea (dyspnea when seated)	Status post-pneumonectomy Neurological diseases Cirrhosis (intrapulmonary shunts) Hypovolemia

Swartz M. *Textbook of Physical Diagnosis*, 6th ed. Philadelphia: Elsevier; 2010.

Hemoptysis

- Onset, number of episodes, quantity, quality (clots or blood-tinged sputum)
- Precipitating Factors: cough, N/V
- Associated Symptoms
  - Fevers, chills, night sweats, weight loss
  - Pleuritic chest pain, leg pain, leg edema
  - Persistent cough, dyspnea, palpitations, arrhythmias
- Risk Factors: recent surgery (DVT/PE), smoking, anticoagulants, clotting disorders, oral contraceptives, TB exposure
- Be sure to distinguish hemoptysis from hematemesis
  - Hemoptysis: associated with coughing and dyspnea; red, frothy, mixed with sputum, alkaline
  - Hematemesis: associated with N/V; red/brown, not frothy, may be mixed with food, acidic (unless on antacids/proton pump inhibitors)

Pleuritic Chest Pain

- Localized "knife-like" pain associated with inspiration or coughing
- Suggests involvement of parietal pleura
  - Primary diseases of the pleura: mesothelioma and pleuritis
  - Pulmonary diseases that can extend to the pleura: pneumonia and pulmonary thromboembolism

Exposure History
- Domestic exposures: pets, hobbies, pollution
- Occupational exposures (see **Table 3**)
- Recent travel and immigration history

Table 3. Occupational Exposures

Type	Etiology
Grain Dust, Wood Dust, Tobacco, Pollens, Many Others	Occupational asthma
Asbestos	Pleural mesothelioma Pulmonary fibrosis
Coal	Pneumoconiosis
Sandblasting and Quarries	Silicosis
Industrial Dusts	Chronic bronchitis

5. FOCUSED PHYSICAL EXAM

Inspection
- **Signs of Respiratory Distress**
  - General difficulty breathing (nasal flaring, stridor or wheezing, pursed-lip breathing on expiration)
  - Use of accessory muscles (trapezius, sternocleidomastoids, retraction of intercostal muscles)
  - Orthopnea: dyspnea that occurs when lying down and improves upon sitting up
  - Tripoding: sitting upright and leaning forward on outstretched arms
  - Paradoxical Breathing: inward movement of abdomen on inspiration
  - Use of O_2 therapy/respiratory equipment (e.g. nasal prongs, mask, transtracheal O_2, endotracheal/tracheostomy tube with ventilator, oximeter)
- **Cyanosis (Central or Peripheral)**
  - Signs of peripheral cyanosis include coolness and bluish color of extremities (fingers, toes, nose, ears)
  - Signs of central cyanosis include bluish mucous membranes (lips, frenulum, buccal mucosa)
  - Central cyanosis occurs when oxygen saturation falls below 85% (and patient is not anemic)
- **RR and Pattern** (assessed immediately after measuring pulse so patient is unaware of it being done)
  - Normal adults: RR = 12-16 breaths/min
  - Apnea: a period without breathing
  - Bradypnea: abnormally slow rate of respiration (RR <12)
  - Cheyne-Stokes Breathing: periods of deep breathing alternating with periods of apnea
  - Hyperpnea (Kussmaul's breathing): increased depth and rate of breathing
  - Tachypnea: abnormally fast rate of respiration (RR >16)
- **Chest Configuration (AP and Lateral)**
  - Masses, scars, lesions, lacerations
  - Normal: AP diameter < lateral diameter
  - Barrel chest: AP diameter equal to lateral diameter
  - Pectus excavatum (funnel chest): a depression of the sternum; associated with mitral valve disease
  - Pectus carinatum (pigeon chest): an anterior protrusion of the sternum

- Kyphosis: abnormal AP curvature of spine
- Scoliosis: abnormal lateral curvature and torsion of spine

- **Clubbing**
  - Loss of Lovibond's angle between the nail bed and the axial plane of the DIP
  - Look for Schamroth sign: loss of diamond-shaped window when dorsal surfaces of terminal phalanges on opposite fingers are opposed
  - Sponginess of nail bed

Palpation

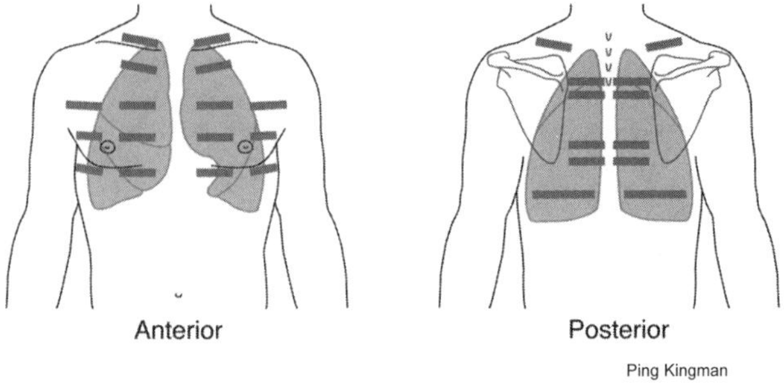

Figure 2. Sites of Lung Percussion, Palpation, and Auscultation

- **Chest Wall Tenderness**
  - Gently palpate all areas of chest for tenderness and deformities; check for MSK pain (beware of rib fractures)
- **Tactile Fremitus**
  - Place ulnar side of the hand against chest wall and ask patient to say "ninety-nine" or "boy-oh-boy"
  - The hand must be moved from side-to-side to compare left to right sides and from the top downward (see **Figure 2**)
  - Each lung field should be palpated both posteriorly and anteriorly (including the supraclavicular fossae, mid-axillary line, and anterior intercostal spaces beginning at the clavicle)

Table 4. Interpretation of Tactile Fremitus

Transmission	Pathologies
Increased	Consolidation (e.g. pneumonia)
Decreased: Unilateral	Atelectasis, bronchial obstruction, pleural effusion, pneumothorax, pleural thickening
Decreased: Bilateral	Chest wall thickening (muscle, fat), COPD, bilateral pleural effusion

Swartz M. *Textbook of Physical Diagnosis*, 6th ed. Philadelphia: Elsevier; 2010.

- **Evaluation of Position of Trachea**
  - Palpate the trachea in the suprasternal notch to determine if it is midline
  - Trachea is deviated to ipsilateral side in atelectasis, fibrosis, lung collapse
  - Trachea is deviated to contralateral side in pleural effusion, hemothorax, tension pneumothorax
  - Non-pulmonary causes: lateral tracheal deviation can be caused by neck mass or retrosternal goiter

- **Evaluation of Trachea Mobility**
  - A tracheal tug may be used to assess if the trachea is fixed in the mediastinum
  - With the patient's neck slightly flexed, support the back of the patient's head and position the middle fingers of the opposite hand into the cricothyroid space
  - Push the larynx upward
  - Normally, the trachea and larynx will move up 1-2 cm
  - Slowly lower the larynx before removing fingers
  - A fixed trachea may be due to mediastinal fixation (neoplasm or TB)
- **Chest Expansion**
  - Place hands flat on back with thumbs parallel to the midline at the level of the 10th rib and fingers gripping the flanks
  - Ask patient to exhale completely and then inhale deeply: look for symmetry in outward movement of hands
  - Asymmetrical with pleural effusion, lobar pneumonia, pulmonary fibrosis, bronchial obstruction, pleuritic pain with splinting, pneumothorax

Percussion

- Percussion is performed in the same areas as tactile fremitus (see **Figure 2**)
- Normally, chest is resonant everywhere except in the left 3rd-5th intercostal spaces anteriorly (cardiac dullness); loss of dullness suggests hyperinflation (e.g. emphysema) (see **Table 5**)

Table 5. Interpretation of Percussion Notes

Percussion Note	Pathologies
Dull	Lobar pneumonia, hemothorax, empyema, atelectasis, tumor, pleural effusion (can be flat/"stony dull")
Resonant	Simple chronic bronchitis
Hyperresonant	Emphysema, asthma, pneumothorax (can be tympanic)

Bickley LS, Szilagyi PG, Bates B. *Bates' Guide to Physical Examination and History Taking*, 10th ed. Philadelphia: Lippincott Williams & Wilkins; 2009.

- **Diaphragmatic Excursion**
  - Locate level of diaphragm during quiet respiration by percussing in an inferior direction for a change from resonant to dull
  - The level of the diaphragm may be stated in reference to the vertebral level by counting down the vertebrae starting with the vertebral prominence (C7)
  - Have the patient hold as full an inhalation as possible and locate the new (inferior) level of the diaphragm
  - Have the patient hold as full an exhalation as possible and relocate the level of the diaphragm (now superior)
  - Normal diaphragmatic excursion is 4-5 cm
  - Consider percussing bilaterally to compare excursion (i.e. check for hemiparalysis)

Auscultation

- Instruct patient to breath deeply through an open mouth and listen to breath sounds using the stethoscope's diaphragm in the same areas as for tactile fremitus (see **Figure 2**)
- Note intensity, pitch, and ratio of duration of inspiration to expiration (see **Table 6**)

- Silent gap between inspiratory and expiratory sounds suggests bronchial breath sounds
- Compare breath sounds on both sides
- Over peripheral lung fields:
  - Bronchial breath sounds usually indicate consolidation
  - Bronchovesicular breath sounds may indicate bronchospasm or interstitial fibrosis

Table 6. Interpretation of Breath Sounds

Characteristic	Tracheal	Bronchial	Broncho-vesicular	Vesicular
Description	Harsh	Air rushing through tube	Rustling but tubular	Gentle rustling
Normal Location	Extrathoracic trachea	Manubrium	Mainstem bronchi	Peripheral lung fields
Pitch	Very high	High	Moderate	Low
Inspiration: Expiration	1:1	1:3	1:1	3:1

Swartz M. *Textbook of Physical Diagnosis*, 6th ed. Philadelphia: Elsevier; 2010.

- **Adventitious Sounds**
  - Listen for sounds that are superimposed upon the usual breath sounds (see **Table 7**)

Table 7. Adventitious Sounds

Sound	Description	Mechanism	Causes
Crackles	Short, discontinuous, nonmusical sounds heard mostly during inspiration Fine: high-pitched Coarse: low-pitched	Often excess airway secretions (exception is pulmonary fibrosis)	Timing in inspiratory cycle can be important: atelectasis (early), pneumonia (mid), fibrosis (late), CHF (late), pulmonary edema
Wheezes	Continuous, musical, high-pitched sounds; usually heard on expiration	Rapid airflow through obstructed airway	Asthma, secretions, pulmonary edema, bronchitis, CHF, bronchiectasis, foreign body, tumor
Stridor	Inspiratory musical sounds best heard over trachea during inspiration	Upper airway extrathoracic obstruction	Partial obstruction of larynx or trachea
Pleural Rub	Grating or creaking sounds best heard at end of inspiration and beginning expiration	Inflammation of the pleura	Pneumonia, pulmonary infarction

Swartz M. *Textbook of Physical Diagnosis*, 6th ed. Philadelphia: Elsevier; 2010.
Bickley LS, Szilagyi PG, Bates B. *Bates' Guide to Physical Examination and History Taking*, 10th ed. Philadelphia: Lippincott Williams & Wilkins; 2009.

- **Consolidation**
  - Higher-pitched sounds are better transmitted through consolidated lung than air-filled lung
  - **Egophony:** when patient utters "E-E-E", sounds like "A-A-A" over area of consolidation
  - **Whispered Pectoriloquy:** whispered words (e.g. "one-two-three") by patient are auscultated more clearly over area of consolidation

6. COMMON INVESTIGATIONS

Pulse Oximetry

- LED device on finger, toe or earlobe measures oxygen saturation of hemoglobin
- Does not measure the oxygen tension (P_aO_2); interpret O_2 saturation with the oxyhemoglobin dissociation curve in mind
- Reads incorrectly high (100%) during hemoglobinopathies such as carbon monoxide poisoning
- Reads incorrectly low if there is movement, highly calloused skin, nail polish, hypoperfusion to extremity being used for monitoring (cold, use of vasopressor), or methemoglobinemia

RESPIRATORY

Arterial Blood Gases (ABGs)

- Arterial oxygen tension (P_aO_2), carbon dioxide tension (P_aCO_2) and pH are measured; bicarbonate concentration is calculated using Henderson-Hasselbalch equation
- Useful for assessing acid/base disturbances (see **Essentials of Fluids, Electrolytes, and Acid/Base Disturbances**, p.467)
- Alveolar air equation used to determine theoretical alveolar oxygen tension (P_AO_2)
- $P_AO_2 = PO_{2\,(inspired)} - (P_aCO_2/0.8) = 150 - (P_aCO_2/0.8)$
- The alveolar-arterial oxygen gradient (A-a D_{O2}) is the difference between the calculated P_AO_2 and the measured P_aO_2
  - Normally not >15 mmHg in healthy patients breathing room air
  - A-a D_{O2} increases with normal aging
  - Elevated A-a D_{O2} occurs with ventilation-perfusion (V/Q) mismatch or shunting

Ventilation Perfusion Scanning

- Radioactive gas is respired; radiolabeled albumin is injected intravenously and deposits in the pulmonary capillaries
- Radiation from both sources is measured simultaneously to visualize the distribution of both ventilation and perfusion

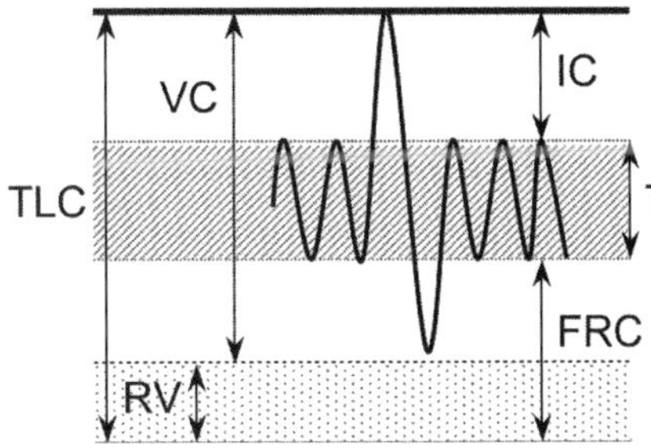

Figure 3. Lung Volumes
FRC = functional residual capacity, IC = inspiratory capacity, RV = residual volume, TLC = total lung capacity, TV = tidal volume, VC = vital capacity

RESPIRATORY

Pulmonary Function Tests (PFTs)

- Patient exhales into a spirometer from total lung capacity (TLC) down to residual volume (RV) with maximum effort; the maximum expiratory flow-volume envelope is plotted (see **Figure 5**, p.358)
  - FEV_1 = forced expired volume in first second
  - FVC = forced vital capacity
  - V50 = forced expired flow at 50% of vital capacity
  - V25 = forced expired flow at 25% of vital capacity
  - Response to bronchodilator and/or methacholine can be used to test for asthma
- A plethysmograph measures TLC, functional residual capacity (FRC) and RV; panting against a closed shutter allows total airway resistance (Raw) to be measured
- Carbon monoxide is used to measure diffusion capacity (D_{CO})

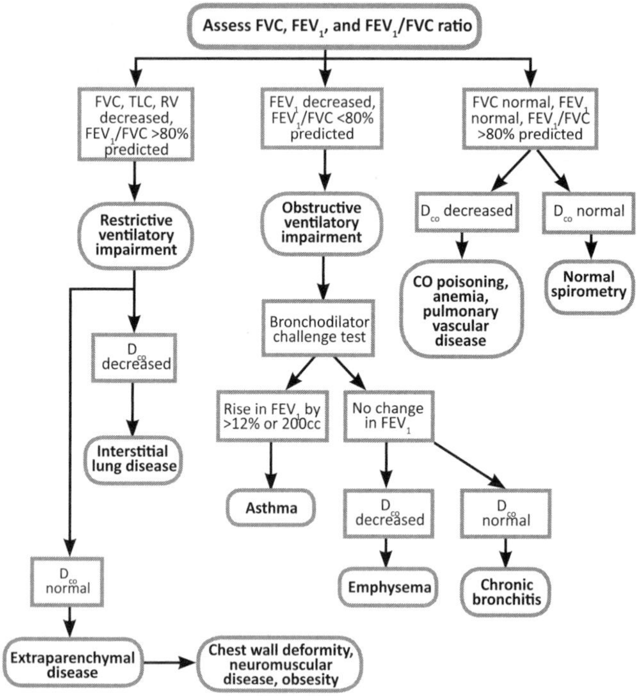

Figure 4. An Approach to Intepreting PFTs

Chest X-ray

- See **Essentials of Medical Imaging**, p.513

Table 8. Characteristic Results of Pulmonary Function Tests in Obstructive and Restrictive Lung Disease

		Obstructive	Restrictive
Lung Volumes	VC	Decreased or N	Decreased
	FRC	Increased	Decreased
	RV	Increased	Decreased
	TLC	Increased or N	Decreased
Flow Rates	FEV_1	Decreased	Decreased or N
	FEV_1/FVC	Decreased	Increased or N
	V50	Decreased	Increased, decreased or N
	V25	Decreased	Increased, decreased or N
Airway Resistance	Raw	Increased	N

N = normal

7. COMMON DISORDERS

Disorders marked with (✓) are discussed in **Common Clinical Scenarios**

✓ Asthma
✓ COPD (chronic bronchitis, emphysema)
✓ Infections (TB and pneumonia)
✓ Pulmonary embolism
- Interstitial lung disease
- Obstructive sleep apnea
- Pneumothorax
- Bronchogenic carcinoma
- Acute respiratory distress syndrome
- Bronchiectasis
- Occupational lung disease

8. COMMON CLINICAL SCENARIOS

8.1 Obstructive Lung Disease

- Characteristic "scooped-out" expiratory flow-volume curve (see **Figure 5**)
- Asthma
- COPD (emphysema, chronic bronchitis)
- Bronchiectasis

EBM: Obstructive Airway Disease (OAD)

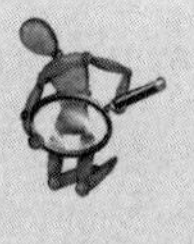

Four elements of history and physical exam are significantly associated with the diagnosis of OAD:

Finding	**Likelihood Ratio**
Smoking history >40 pack yr	8.3
Self-reported history of chronic OAD	7.3
Maximum laryngeal height of ≤4 cm	2.8
Age at least 45 yr	1.3

Patients with all 4 findings had LR+ of 220. Those with none had LR- of 0.13.

Straus SE, et al. 2000. *JAMA* 283(14):1853-1857.

8.2 Restrictive Lung Disease

- Generally decreased lung volumes (see **Figure 5**)
- Interstitial lung disease (e.g. idiopathic pulmonary fibrosis [IPF], pneumoconiosis, hypersensitivity pneumonitis, iatrogenic)
- Neuromuscular disease (e.g. polio, myasthenia gravis)

- Chest wall disease (e.g. kyphoscoliosis)
- Space-occupying lesions (e.g. tumors, cysts)
- Pleural disease (e.g. effusions, pneumothorax)
- Extrathoracic conditions (e.g. obesity, ascites, pregnancy)

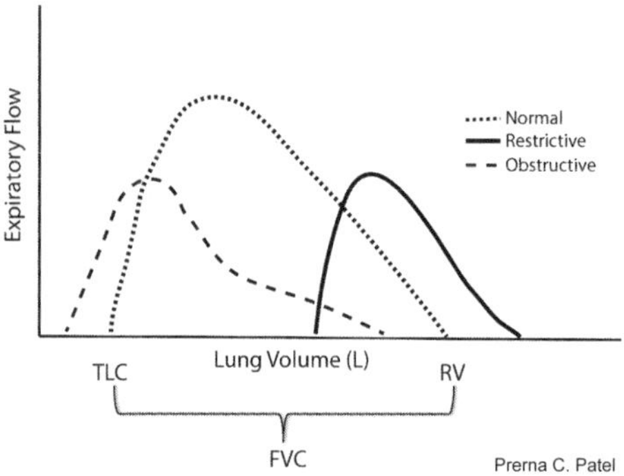

Figure 5. Flow-Volume Curves for Normal, Obstructed, and Restricted Lungs

8.3 Asthma

- Chronic inflammatory disorder of the airways
- Association with: atopy/allergy, ASA sensitivity, sinusitis, nasal polyps
- Signs and Symptoms
  - Dyspnea
  - Chest tightness
  - Wheezing
  - Sputum production (white, scant)
  - Cough (especially nocturnal)
  - Respiratory distress (nasal flare, use of accessory muscles, intercostal indrawing, pulsus paradoxus [drop in systoic BP (SBP) > 10 mmHg during inspiration when compared to SBP in expiration], inability to speak)
  - Life-threatening episodes include silent chest, fatigue, cyanosis, diminished respiratory effort and/or decreased LOC
- Investigations
  - Peak expiratory flow rate (PEFR) meter can be used at the bedside to monitor response to therapy
  - ABGs: only do if PEFR <25% predicted, cyanotic, or decreased LOC present
    - P_aO_2 decreased during attack
    - P_aCO_2 decreased in mild asthma due to hyperventilation
    - Normal or increased P_aCO_2 in severe attack (ominous sign)
  - PFTs showing obstructive pattern (may not be possible during severe attacks)[1-3]
- Management
  - Life-Threatening Episodes
    - ABCs: sit upright, O_2 by mask, cardiac monitor, oximetry, IV fluids
    - β2-agonists and anticholinergics (metered-dose inhaler through a spacer device)
    - Systemic corticosteroids PO or IV in emergency room
    - If episode continues to progress with decreased LOC, exhaustion, cyanosis, acidemia, silent chest consider magnesium sulfate, intubation, and intensive care unit (ICU) admission

- Short-Term Management
  - Bronchodilators (selective β2-agonists, anticholinergics)
  - Inhaled corticosteroids do not treat an acute exacerbation but should be initiated early to prevent subsequent exacerbations
  - Systemic corticosteroids
- Long-Term Management
  - Asthma education
  - Environmental control
  - Inhaled corticosteroids as first-line management and long-acting β2-agonists (LABAs) or leukotriene receptor antagonists (LTRAs) as add-on therapy
  - Short-acting β2-agonists PRN as reliever therapy

RESPIRATORY

8.4 Chronic Obstructive Pulmonary Disease

- Characterized by progressive, partially reversible airway obstruction, lung hyperinflation and increasing frequency and severity of exacerbations
- Includes chronic bronchitis ("blue bloaters") and emphysema ("pink puffers")

Chronic Bronchitis

- Signs and Symptoms
  - Clinical diagnosis of chronic cough and sputum production on most days for at least 3 consecutive months over 2 successive years
  - Mild dyspnea with onset noted after cough
  - Sputum often purulent
  - Crackles, wheeze
  - Hemoptysis
  - Often cyanotic due to V/Q abnormalities ("blue")
  - Peripheral edema from RV failure (cor pulmonale) may be present ("bloater")
  - Hypoxemia causes secondary polycythemia and pulmonary vasoconstriction with pulmonary hypertension and eventual cor pulmonale
  - Obesity is often part of the clinical picture
- Investigations
  - CXR (normal or increased bronchovascular markings, enlarged heart with cor pulmonale)
  - ABGs (hypoxemia with V/Q mismatch, hypercapnia with abnormal central respiratory drive and increased work of breathing)
  - PFTs (see **Table 8**)

Emphysema

- Signs and Symptoms
  - Exertional dyspnea with minimal cough
  - Tachypnea
  - Hyperinflation/barrel chest
  - Use of accessory muscles
  - Pursed-lip breathing
  - Hyperresonant on percussion (absent cardiac dullness)
  - Decreased diaphragmatic excursion
  - Decreased breath sounds
  - Pneumothorax due to bulla formation
- Investigations
  - CXR (hyperinflation, flat hemidiaphragm, increased AP diameter, increased restrosternal airspace, bullae, reduced peripheral vascular markings, small heart)
  - ABGs (P_aO_2 and P_aCO_2 are normal or mildly decreased)
  - PFTs (see **Table 8**)

Management of COPD (Emphysema and Chronic Bronchitis)

- Nonpharmacological
  - Smoking cessation
  - Multidisciplinary pulmonary rehabilitation
  - Exercise
- Pharmacological[4,5]
  - Aggressive treatment of respiratory infections
  - Influenza vaccine and Pneumovax to prevent pneumonia
  - Short-acting bronchodilators (anticholinergics and/or β2-agonists)
  - Long-acting bronchodilators (e.g. tiotropium, salmeterol or formoterol) with short-acting β2-agonists as needed and inhaled corticosteroids for patients with moderate to severe COPD
  - Oral theophylline in some patients
- Others
  - Home oxygen
  - Lung transplant
  - Lung volume reduction surgery

RESPIRATORY

8.5 Pneumonia

- Infection of the pulmonary parenchyma
- Separated into 4 classes: community-acquired (CAP), hospital-acquired (HAP), ventilator-associated (VAP), and healthcare-associated pneumonia (HCAP)

Table 9. Common Organisms in Community-Acquired and Hospital-Acquired Pneumonias and their Empiric Antibiotic Treatment

Sites of Pathogen Acquisition	Organism	Empiric Antibiotic Coverage
Community	*S. pneumoniae* *M. pneumoniae* *C. pneumoniae* *H. influenzae* Respiratory viruses: influenzas A and B, adenoviruses	**Outpatient:** Macrolide (no risk factors for MDR), respiratory fluoroquinolone (if comorbidities) **Inpatient:** Respiratory fluoroquinolone or beta-lactam + macrolide (such as ceftriaxone + azithromycin)
Hospital	Think about patient's risk of MDR pathogens (multidrug-resistant) *S. pneumoniae* *S. aureus* (commonly MRSA) *C. pneumoniae* *Legionella* spp. *H. influenzae* Gram-negative bacilli *Pseudomonas* (common MDR pathogen)	**No Risk Factors for MDR Infection:** Respiratory fluoroquinolone or ceftriaxone or ampicillin or ertapenem **Risk Factors for MDR Infection*:** Antipseudomonal cephalosporin (cefepime, ceftazidime) or antipseudomonal carbapenem or piperacillin-tazobactam PLUS respiratory fluoroquinolone or aminoglycoside PLUS vancomycin (for MRSA)

*Risk factors for multiple drug resistant (MDR) pathogen causing HAP, HCAP or VAP include: hospitalization >5 d, amtimicrobial therapy in preceding 90 d, immunosuppressive disease/therapy, residence in nursing home, dialysis, home wound care, hospitalization >2 d in preceding 90 d.

MRSA = methicillin-resistant *Staphylococcus aureus*

American Thoracic Society, Infectious Diseases Society of America. 2005. *Am J Respir Crit Care Med* 171(4):388-416.

- Signs and Symptoms
  - Cough:
    - Often sudden onset and productive in typical infections
    - Often insidious and dry in atypical infections
  - Pleuritic chest pain
  - Infectious symptoms (fevers, headache, chills, rigors, nausea, myalgia)
  - Dyspnea, tachypnea
  - Signs of consolidation (dullness to percussion, increased tactile and vocal fremitus, crackles, bronchial breath sounds, egophony, whispered pectoriloquy)
- Investigations
  - ABGs
  - Blood culture
  - CXR (infiltrate ± cavitations)
  - Sputum culture and Gram stain
  - Nasopharyngeal culture
  - Pleural fluid culture
  - Serology (*Legionella* urine antigen, induced sputum for TB acid fast bacilli [AFB] stain)
  - Bronchoalveolar lavage and bronchoscopy
- Management
  - For CAP, determine need for hospitalization with the use of a severity-of-illness score such as the CURB-65 criteria (confusion, uremia, respiratory rate, low BP, age >65 yr, and clinical judgment)
  - Empiric antibiotic therapy until cultures return (see **Table 9**)

EBM: Community-Acquired Pneumonia (CAP)

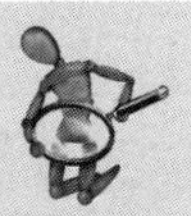

Recommendations for diagnostic testing remain controversial. The overall low yield and infrequent positive effect on clinical care argue against the routine use of common tests such as blood and sputum cultures. However, these cultures may have a major impact on the care of individual patients and are important for epidemiologic reasons. The most definite indication for extensive diagnostic testing is in the critically ill CAP patient. "Such patients should at least have blood drawn for culture and an endotracheal aspirate obtained if they are intubated."

Mandell LA, et al. 2007. *Clin Infect Dis* 44(Suppl 2):S27-S72.

8.6 Pulmonary Embolism

- Signs and symptoms depend on the size of the embolus and the patient's underlying cardiovascular status, but may include:
  - Dyspnea
  - Chest pain (pleuritic or nonpleuritic)
  - Tachypnea (the only physical exam finding reliably found in >50% of patients with PE)
  - Hemoptysis
  - Syncope
  - Stabbing pain on inspiration
  - Predisposition to venous thrombosis increases risk of PE (see **Peripheral Vascular Exam**, p.311)
  - Many substances other than thrombus can embolize to the pulmonary circulation including:
    - Air
    - Amniotic fluid (during active labor)
    - Fat (as a complication of long-bone fractures)
    - Foreign bodies (talc in IV drug users)
    - Parasite eggs (schistosomiasis)

    - Septic emboli (infectious endocarditis)
    - Tumor cells (renal cell carcinoma)
- Investigations
  - Use PERC (pulmonary embolism rule-out criteria) and Wells criteria to determine the pretest probability of PE and guide investigation
  - ABGs:
    - Arterial hypoxemia and elevated alveolar-arterial oxygen gradient
    - Acute respiratory alkalosis due to hyperventilation
    - These changes, along with a normal CXR in a patient with no pre-existing lung disease, are highly suspicious for PE
  - CXR helpful only in excluding other lung diseases and interpreting the V/Q scan
  - V/Q Scan:
    - Two or more lung segments with perfusion defects and normal ventilation are highly suggestive of PE
    - Defects in perfusion are interpreted in conjunction with ventilation and assigned either a high, low, or indeterminate probability that PE is the cause of the abnormality
  - Helical CT arteriography involves IV injection of radiocontrast dye; it is sensitive for detection of PE in the proximal pulmonary arteries, but not as much for the segmental and sub-segmental arteries
  - Venous thrombosis studies (see **Peripheral Vascular Exam**, p.312)
- Management
  - Anticoagulation: regimen of heparin followed by oral warfarin reduces risk of recurrent DVT and death from PE
    - Duration of anticoagulation will depend on potentially reversible risk factors including the patient's age, the likelihood of potential consequences of hemorrhage, and the patient's preferences
  - Thrombolytic therapy: streptokinase, urokinase or tissue plasminogen activator (tPA); shown to accelerate resolution of PE if administered within the first 24 h
    - Should be used in patients at high risk of death and for whom the faster resolution may be life-saving
  - Inferior vena cava filter: recommended for patients in whom anticoagulation is contraindicated or who have experienced repeated PEs in spite of anticoagulation

REFERENCES

1. Lemière C, Bai T, Balter M, Bayliff C, Becker A, Boulet LP, et al. 2004. Adult Asthma Consensus Guidelines update 2003. *Can Respir J* 11(Suppl A):9A-18A.
2. Lougheed M, Lemière C, Dell S, Ducharme D, Fitzgerald M, Leigh R, et al. 2010. Canadian Thoracic Society Asthma Management Continuum – 2010 Consensus Summary for children six years of age and over, and adults. *Can Respir J* 17(1):15-24.
3. Sin DD, Man J, Sharpe H, Gan WQ, Man SF. 2004. Pharmacological management to reduce exacerbations in adults with asthma: A systematic review and meta-analysis. *JAMA* 292(3):367-376.
4. O'Donnell DE, Aaron S, Bourbeau J, Hernandez P, Marciniuk D, Balter M, et al. 2003. Canadian Thoracic Society recommendations for management of chronic obstructive pulmonary disease – 2003. *Can Respir J* 10(Suppl A):11A-65A.
5. O'Donnell DE, Hernandez P, Kaplan A, Aaron S, Bourbeau J, Marciniuk D, et al. 2008. Canadian Thoracic Society recommendations for management of chronic obstructive pulmonary disease – 2008 update – Highlights for primary care. *Can Respir J* 15(Suppl A):1A-8A.
6. Mandell LA, Marrie TJ, Grossman RF, Chow AW, Hyland RH. 2000. Canadian guidelines for the initial management of community-acquired pneumonia: An evidence-based update by the Canadian Infectious Diseases Society and the Canadian Thoracic Society. The Canadian Community-Acquired Pneumonia Working Group. *Clin Infect Dis* 31(2):383-421.
7. Metlay JP, Kapoor WN, Fine MJ. 1997. Does this patient have community-acquired pneumonia? Diagnosing pneumonia by history and physical examination. *JAMA* 278(17):1440-1445.

The Urological Exam

Editors:
Sena Aflaki
Anna Krylova

Faculty Reviewers:
Michael Jewett, MD, FRCS(C)
Sender Herschorn, BSc, MDCM, FRCS(C)

TABLE OF CONTENTS

1. ESSENTIAL ANATOMY

Essential Male Anatomy

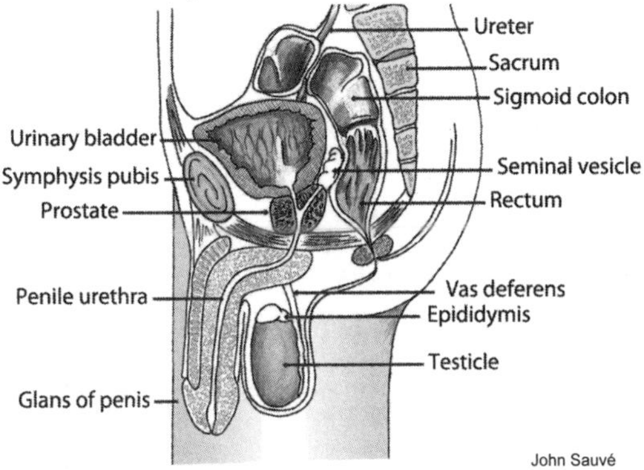

Figure 1. Anatomy of the Male Genitourinary Tract and Organs

Essential Female Anatomy

- See the **Gynecological Exam,** p.79 for a depiction of the external female genital anatomy

UROLOGICAL

2. COMMON CHIEF COMPLAINTS
- Pain (costovertebral angle, suprapubic, genitals)
- Blood in urine (hematuria)
- Pain or burning while urinating (dysuria)
- Urinary frequency ± polyuria
- Waking from sleep to pass urine one or more times (nocturia)
- Difficulty initiating urinary stream (hesitancy)
- Weak/intermittent flow or interrupted stream (intermittency)
- Low urine output (oliguria/anuria)
- Urinary urgency
- Incontinence
- Postvoid dribbling
- Discharge (penile or vaginal)
- Fever, chills, nausea
- Pain during intercourse or ejaculation (dyspareunia)

Male Specific

♂ Erectile dysfunction
♂ Blood in semen (hematospermia)
♂ Testicular mass
♂ Infertility

Female Specific

♀ Vaginal fullness

3. FOCUSED HISTORY
Lower Urinary Tract Symptoms (LUTS)

Storage Symptoms
- Frequency: How frequently do you urinate during the day?
- Nocturia: Do you wake up at night to urinate?
- Urgency: Do you ever have a strong, sudden impulse to urinate? Do you ever have such a strong urge to urinate that you fear not being able to make it to the toilet in time?
- Dysuria: Do you ever have pain or burning during urination? At which point in the stream do you feel pain: beginning, middle, end or throughout?
- Incontinence (see **Table 2**)

Voiding Symptoms
- Straining: Do you ever have to strain to fully empty your bladder?
- Hesitancy: Do you ever have difficulty starting urination?
- Intermittency: Is your stream continuous, or are there times when the flow stops and restarts?
- Postvoid dribbling: Do you ever notice a continued release of drops of urine after voiding?
- Decreased force of urination: Have you noticed a weaker stream?
- Incomplete emptying (sensation that urine retained): Do you ever feel as though there is residual urine remaining in your bladder after you urinate? Do you have to urinate again a second time ("double voiding")?

Genitourinary Pain (see **Table 1**)
- Onset, provoking/alleviating factors, quality, radiation, severity, duration, and location

Discharge
- Continuous discharge vs. intermittent discharge
- Bloody (urethral carcinoma) vs. purulent (infection)
- Gonococcal pus: thick, profuse, and yellow to gray (see **Essentials of Infectious Diseases**, p.494)
- Sexual history: ask about multiple partners, previous STIs, and UTIs

Gross Hematuria (see **Common Clinical Scenarios**, p.371)

- Timing: Is blood present at the beginning, middle, end or throughout the stream?
- Quantify: Is most of your stream bloody or is it only a few drops? Have you noticed any blood clots?
- Painful vs. painless

Past Medical History

- Previous urological problems
- Previous surgeries
- Ask about TB, DM, renal disease, malignancies

Family History

- FHx of urological illness (stones, cancer, polycystic kidney disease, congenital abnormalities)

Travel History

- Urological sequelae of schistosomiasis

Social History

- Smoking (bladder cancer, erectile dysfunction [ED]) and alcohol use (testicular atrophy)
- Occupational exposure

UROLOGICAL

Table 1. Approach to Genitourinary Pain by Region

Type of Pain	Location	Cause
Renal Capsule	Ipsilateral costovertebral angle (CVA) May radiate to upper abdomen/umbilicus	Distension of renal capsule (inflammation or obstruction)
Ureteral	Mid-ureter: referred to ipsilateral lower quadrant of abdomen Lower-ureter: referred to suprapubic area and genitals	Obstruction of ureter leading to distension and spastic peristalsis
Vesical	Suprapubic region	Cystitis, interstitial cystitis/bladder pain syndrome (IC/BPS), carcinoma, over-distension of bladder due to urinary retention
Prostatic	Referred to perineum, lower back, inguinal region or testes	Inflammation
Penile	Glans and shaft of penis	Flaccid: cystitis/urethritis, paraphimosis, trauma Erect: Peyronie's disease, priapism, trauma
Testicular	Scrotum	Epididymitis, torsion, mass, trauma

Table 2. Classification of Incontinence

Type of Incontinence	Definition	Possible Cause
Stress	Urine loss with increased intra-abdominal pressure (e.g. cough, sneeze, laugh) and not associated with the urgency to urinate	Postpartum, postmenopausal, or surgical loss of anterior vaginal support of bladder and proximal urethra, postoperative (e.g. prostatectomy) in men
Urgency	Urine loss due to uninhibited bladder contractions – precedes urgency to urinate	Overactive bladder, cystitis, neurogenic bladder (following stroke, dementia, cord lesion above sacral level)
Overflow	Urine loss due to chronically distended bladder – even after effort to void	Bladder outlet obstruction, weak detrusor muscle, impaired sensation (e.g. diabetic neuropathy)
Pharmacologic	Urine loss secondary to medication	Sedatives, tranquilizers, anticholinergics*, sympathetic blockers, potent diuretics

**Note:* anticholinergics lead to incontinence secondary to urinary retention

UROLOGICAL

3.1 Male-Focused Topics

Scrotal Swelling

- Onset, duration, provoking/alleviating factors, change over time, associated trauma

Table 3. Differential Diagnosis for Scrotal Swelling

Painful	Painless
Epididymitis	Hydrocele
Orchitis	Spermatocele
Testicular torsion	Varicocele
Tumor (hemorrhagic)	Tumor (nonhemorrhagic)
Hematocele	Nonstrangulated inguinal hernia
Strangulated inguinal hernia	Scrotal hematoma
Epididymal cyst	

Erectile Dysfunction (Impotence)

- Inability to achieve and/or maintain an erection adequate for intercourse
- Onset, alleviation/aggravation (constant problem vs. situational)
- Psychogenic vs. organic (presence or loss of morning erections)
- Differentiate from other male sexual disorders (loss of libido, failure to ejaculate, anorgasmia, premature ejaculation)

4. FOCUSED PHYSICAL EXAM[1]

General Inspection

- Inspect the patient at rest
- Look for signs of distress or restlessness (e.g. renal colic)
- Inspect for supraclavicular lymphadenopathy (metastases from GU malignancy)

Abdominal Exam
- Inspect for masses, scars, suprapubic distension (see **Abdominal Exam**, p.20)

Kidneys (see **Abdominal Exam**, p.26)
- Ballotment: place one hand under the patient's back and apply upward pressure near the 12th rib; attempt to 'catch' the kidney between your hands by placing the opposite hand firmly and deeply in the ipsilateral upper quadrant of the abdomen
- Costovertebral angle (CVA) tenderness: with a closed fist, percuss at the costovertebral angle (junction of the inferior margin of 12th rib and vertebral column)
  - Tenderness: capsular distension

Bladder
- Normal adult bladder (lies below pubic symphysis) cannot be palpated/percussed unless filled with at least 150 mL of urine
- Palpation: deeply palpate the midline of the suprapubic abdomen
- Percussion: percuss immediately above the symphysis pubis and move cephalad until there is a change in pitch from dull to resonant (over the bladder should be dull)

Femoral Hernias
- Inspect the femoral canal for bulging or mass
- Palpate on the anterior thigh in the femoral canal; attempt to reduce mass if present

Inguinal Lymph Nodes (see **Lymphatic System and Lymph Node Exam**, p.128)
- Inspect for inguinal lymphadenopathy
- Only the superficial inguinal lymph nodes can be palpated on physical exam (indicates infection or tumor at distal 1/3 of urethra, scrotum or vulva)
- Drainage of the testes and internal female genitalia is to the abdomen, pelvic and paraaortic nodes (not palpable on exam)

Genital Exam
- See **Male-Specific Exam Maneuvers** and **Female-Specific Exam Maneuvers** below

Additional Exams

♂ Digital Rectal Exam

♀ Urinary Stress Test

4.1 Male-Specific Exam Maneuvers

Penis
- Inspect prepuce (circumcised vs. uncircumcised), glans, shaft, and base for lesions, discoloration, masses, tumescence
- Inspect meatus: location (epispadias, hypospadias), blood, discharge, stricture/stenosis
- Open the urethral meatus by compressing the glans between the index finger and thumb; examine the inside for discoloration, inflammation, discharge, or lesions
- Ask patient to retract foreskin; if problematic: phimosis
- Ask patient to reduce foreskin; if problematic: paraphimosis
- Palpate the penis along the shaft from glans to base to assess for masses, nodularity, tenderness

UROLOGICAL

UROLOGICAL

Scrotum and Contents

- While supine, have the patient flex his leg on the side of the scrotum being examined
- Examine each side separately
- Inspect for size, shape, symmetry, swelling, erythema, skin changes, presence of rugae
- Lift the scrotum to examine the posterior surface
- Examine the scrotal sac by rolling the skin between the index finger and thumb
- Testicular exam
  - Palpate each testicle separately using both hands (left hand holding superior/inferior poles, right hand palpates and squeezes the anterior/posterior surfaces)
  - Note size, shape, and consistency (normal testicle: firm, rubbery consistency, smooth surface)
  - Abnormally small testicles suggests hypogonadism
  - Hard area or nodularity is malignant until proven otherwise
- Epididymis
  - Palpable ridge on superoposterior surface of each testicle
  - Palpate for tenderness, nodularity or masses
  - Epididymitis: epididymis is very tender or painful and indistinguishable from testis on palpation (*E. coli*, *C. trachomatis*, *N. gonorrhoeae*)
- Spermatic cord
  - Palpate both cords simultaneously with thumbs and index fingers
  - Note size, tenderness or beading
  - Cords should be firm from epididymis to superficial inguinal ring
  - Varicocele confirmed by pulsation when patient is asked to cough
  - Transilluminate scrotal masses to differentiate between solid and cystic
  - Darken room, apply light source to side of scrotal enlargement
  - Cystic masses (hydrocele, spermatocele) transilluminate
  - Solid masses (tumor, varicocele, hernia) do not transmit light
- Inguinal area (hernias)
  - With the patient standing, invaginate the scrotal skin with the index finger of one hand
  - Palpate the external inguinal ring by following the spermatic cord toward the inguinal canal using the finger
  - Place the fingertips of the other hand over the abdomen in the area of the ipsilateral internal inguinal ring and ask the patient to turn his head and cough (Valsalva)
  - Hernia is felt as a bulge that descends against index finger at the external inguinal ring

Digital Rectal Exam

Note: if urinalysis is required, collect specimen before performing DRE

- Position
  - Explain why and how examination is done, allow time for patient to prepare, relax, and be draped appropriately
  - Patient should either be in left lateral decubitus (if the examiner is right-handed), right lateral decubitus (if the examiner is left-handed) or standing bent over the examination table
  - Put on glove and lubricate the index finger thoroughly
- Inspection (anus)
  - Inflammation, excoriation
  - Anal carcinoma or melanoma
  - Hemorrhoids: ask patient to bear down while inspecting

- Palpation (see **Figure 2**)
  - Relax sphincter with pressure from palmar surface of gloved, lubricated finger
  - Gently and slowly insert index finger into anus by rotating finger
  - Estimate sphincter tone
    - Flaccid or spastic sphincter suggests similar changes in urinary sphincter and may be suggestive of neurogenic disease
  - Assess for the presence of any rectal masses
  - Palpation of the prostate:
    - Do not massage prostate in patients with acute prostatitis
    - Assess size, consistency, sensitivity, and shape (see **Table 4**)
  - Withdraw index finger gently and slowly
  - Note color of stool on glove and test for occult blood
  - Wipe the anal area of lubricant with a tissue and provide patient tissues to clean himself

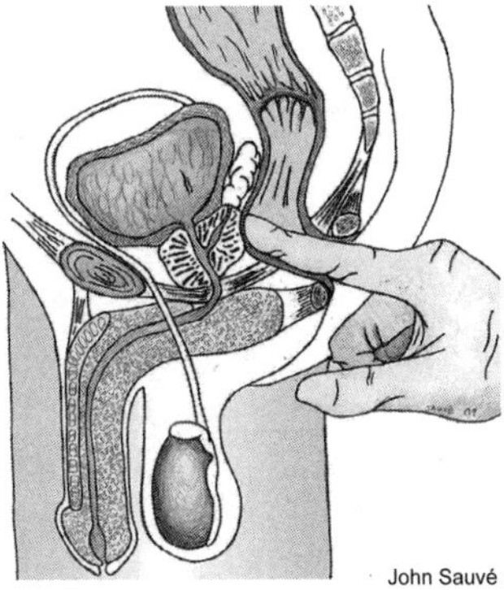

John Sauvé

Figure 2. Digital Rectal Examination and Palpation of the Prostate

Table 4. Features of the Prostate on DRE

Feature	Normal	Pathologic
Size	Approximately 4 cm in length and width (chestnut size)	Enlarged (benign prostatic hypertrophy [BPH], advanced prostate cancer)
Consistency	Rubbery	Firm/nodular (prostate cancer)
Mobility	Variable	Fixed
Sensitivity	Painless	Painful (prostatitis) Painless (prostate cancer)

4.2 Female-Specific Exam Maneuvers

Vagina

- Inspect the vulva/vagina for swelling, erythema, atrophy (degree of estrogenization), and lesions
- Pelvic exam (see **Gynecology Exam**, p.82)
  - Examine for cystocele: bulge in anterior vaginal wall
  - Examine for rectocele: bulge in posterior vaginal wall
  - Assess anterior wall mobility by having patient perform Valsalva
- Urethral orifice
  - Examine for caruncle: small, red, benign tumor in urethral opening (posterior portion)
  - Examine for urethral prolapse: swollen red ring of urethral mucosa protruding from urethral opening

UROLOGICAL

Hernias

- Occurrences in females are less common than in males; when occurring: indirect inguinal > femoral > direct inguinal
- Examination for inguinal hernias: palpate within the labia majora and move finger upward, ending just lateral to the pubic tubercle
- If a hernia is present, a bulge will be felt against finger tip when patient performs Valsalva

Urinary Stress Test

- Have patient assume the lithotomy position on the examining table with a full bladder; legs are spread and perineal area is relaxed
- Ask the patient to cough vigorously: if urine is lost, beginning and ending with the cough, the test is confirmatory for stress incontinence

5. COMMON INVESTIGATIONS

Urinalysis

- Should be performed in all urologic patients (see **Appendix 3**, p.606)
- A complete urinalysis includes both chemical and microscopic analyses (R&M)

Gram Stain and Culture

- Include susceptibility testing if urethritis is suspected

Cytology

- Urine should be screened for tumor markers in:
  - High risk individuals (e.g. environmental exposures)
  - Presence of painless hematuria
  - Evaluation for recurrence after bladder tumor resection

Cystoscopy

- Visualization of the bladder via insertion of fiberoptic instrument (rigid or flexible) through the urethra
- Aids in diagnosis of bladder tumors and calculi, management of urethral stricture or accessing bladder for visualization of ureters (with X-ray) and stent placement
- Caution should be exercised when performing in patients with an active UTI

Ultrasound

- Often used to determine postvoid residual volume, total bladder capacity, and bladder proprioception in the setting of incontinence
- Scrotal ultrasound is used to investigate for scrotal masses
- Abdominal or pelvic ultrasound for hydronephrosis, renal masses, and lymph nodes

Urodynamic Testing

- Uroflowmetry: patient urinates into device for catching and measuring urine and a computer calculates the flow rate
- Postvoid residual volume: the volume of urine remaining in the bladder after voiding; it can be measured via ultrasound or directly by inserting a catheter and measuring the output
- Cystometrogram: test to measure the response of the bladder filling
- Pressure/flow studies: can be used to test for outlet obstruction
- Video-urodynamics: use of X-ray contrast to obtain fluoroscopic images during urodynamic testing
- Catheter monitoring can be used to measure pressure during bladder filling and emptying

6. COMMON DISORDERS

Kidneys
- Renal colic (stones)
- Renal mass (benign or malignant)
- Pyelonephritis

Bladder
- Carcinoma
- Cystitis
- Interstitial cystitis/bladder pain syndrome (IC/BPS)

Prostate ♂
- Prostatitis
- Carcinoma
- Benign prostatic hyperplasia (BPH)

Penis ♂
- ED
- Phimosis (inability to retract foreskin over glans)
- Paraphimosis (inability to reduce foreskin: emergency)
- Priapism (low flow vs. high flow)
- Anterior urethral stricture
- Peyronie's disease (fibrous plaque at tunica albuginea)

Vagina ♀
- Cystocele (bladder prolapse into vagina)
- Urethrocele (urethral prolapse into vagina)

UROLOGICAL

7. COMMON CLINICAL SCENARIOS

Renal Colic
- Signs and Symptoms
  - Intense, sudden onset, unilateral pain in flank (or lower abdomen), restlessness, and vomiting
  - Blood may be seen or detected in urine
  - May be associated with infection (fever, chills, sweats)
- Physical Exam
  - Complete abdominal and urological exam (including DRE) → tenderness
  - Rule out aortic aneurysm by checking for pulsating mass
  - Rule out gallbladder by assessing for Murphy's sign
- Investigations
  - Urinalysis (R&M and C&S)
  - Non-contrast helical CT abdomen is diagnostic test of choice
  - Plain abdominal X-rays can track already detected stone

Hematuria
- Can be gross (visible in urine) or microscopic (>2-5 RBCs per high power field [RBCs/HPF])
- Signs and Symptoms
  - Timing: initial stream, terminal stream, total stream
  - Pain (inflammation or obstruction from calculi/clots)
  - Storage urinary symptoms (suggests UTI)
  - Voiding LUTS (fever, chills, N/V)
- Other important aspects of hematuria history:
  - Recent sexual history (STIs)
  - Recent instrumentation

- Drugs: anticoagulants, ASA, NSAIDs, phenytoin, chemotherapeutics
- Others: trauma, sickle cell anemia, hemophilia, glomerulonephritis, malaria/schistosomiasis (travel history)

• Physical Exam
  - Complete abdominal and urological exams (including DRE) → tenderness, masses, distension, and induration

> **Clinical Pearl: Clinical Suspicion of Hematuria**
> Hematuria of any degree should never be ignored and, in adults, should be regarded as a symptom of urologic malignancy until proven otherwise.

• Investigations (see **Figure 3**)
  - Urinalysis
  - Urine cytology
  - Cystoscopy
  - Imaging (ultrasound, spiral CT)

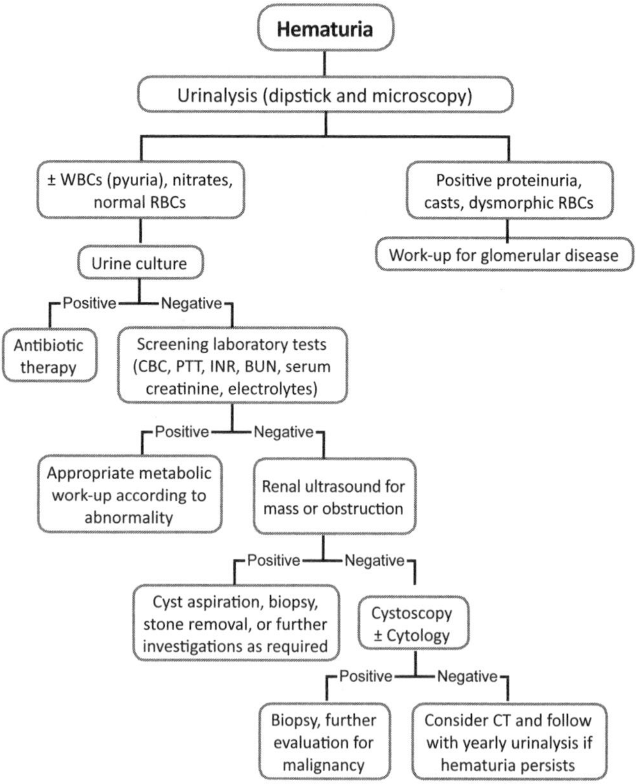

Figure 3. Investigations for Hematuria

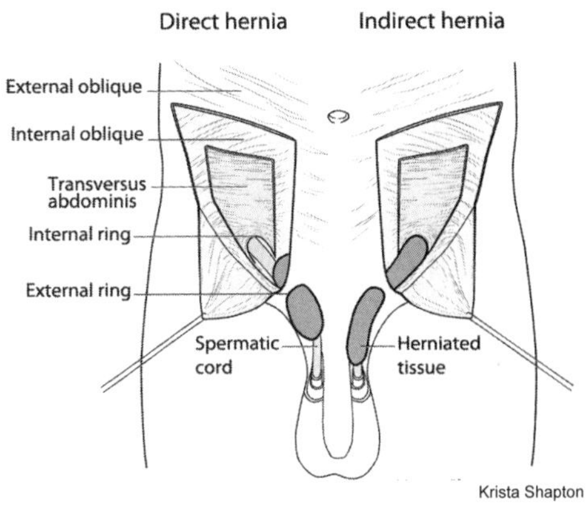

Figure 4. Direct and Indirect Hernias

Hernias (See **Figure 4**)

- Signs and Symptoms
  - Lump or swelling in groin or scrotum
  - Sudden pain in scrotum
  - Pain in scrotum while standing or moving
  - Heavy feeling in groin
- Physical Exam
  - Observe inguinal canal for bulge and size increased with cough
  - In male patients, the exam is best performed seated with patient standing; invaginate scrotum with finger, ask patient to cough and feel for impulse
  - In female patients, palpate within the labia majora and move finger superiorly, feel for bulge on Valsalva
  - Investigations are often not necessary to make diagnosis
  - Indicative of hernias if: masses return to the abdomen upon lying down, have bowel sounds on auscultation, and do not transmit light when transilluminated

7.1 Male-Specific Scenarios

BPH

- Clinically appears in 25% of men in their 50s, 33% of men in their 60s, and 50% of men in their 70s
- Signs and Symptoms
  - Storage/voiding LUTS
- Physical Exam
  - DRE: note size and consistency (average prostate ~20 g)
  - ***Note:*** BPH is not a risk factor for prostate cancer
  - With BPH, prostate should be smooth, firm, elastic, and enlarged
  - Induration found with DRE indicates further investigation for cancer
- Investigations
  - Urinalysis (to exclude infection/hematuria)
  - Creatinine
  - PSA (to exclude prostate cancer)
  - Transrectal ultrasound (TRUS) to assess size

Prostate Cancer

- Signs and Symptoms
  - Most are asymptomatic
  - Storage and voiding LUTS may suggest locally advanced or metastatic disease
  - Bone pain may be suggestive of metastases
  - Paresthesias, weakness of lower extremities, and urinary or fecal incontinence may be observed in advanced disease with cord compression
- Physical Exam
  - Induration found with DRE indicates further investigation to rule out cancer (i.e. PSA screen/TRUS/biopsy)
- Investigations
  - PSA screen
  - Percent free PSA (fPSA)
  - PSA velocity
  - TRUS (if appropriate)
  - Biopsy (if appropriate)

Screening for Prostate Cancer

- Males 50-75 yr with life expectancy of >10 yr should be informed of the risks/benefits of PSA testing
  - Men over 75 yr should not be tested
- Men at a higher risk for prostate cancer:
  - African-American descent
  - 1st generation relative with prostate cancer
  - High fat diet
  - Prostatic nodule found on DRE
  - Abnormal-feeling prostate
  - Discrete change either in texture, fullness or symmetry
- PSA has limited specificity because elevations also occur in men with benign disease (e.g. prostatic hyperplasia, prostatitis)
- PSA levels vary according to age and degree of hyperplasia, but cancer produces excess levels
- Consider tests such as PSA velocity or percent free PSA (fPSA) to supplement investigation

Clinical Pearl: PSA Measurements After Treatment of Prostate Cancer
PSA measurements become an integral part of follow-up visits post-treatment. The frequency and parameters of these measurements will depend on the modality of treatment and the physician's or hospital's protocol.

EBM: PSA as a Screening Test for Prostate Cancer

In long-term follow-up trials, the benefit of prostate cancer screening on mortality remains controversial. While some trials, such as the PCLO trial*, have shown no benefit of PSA testing on mortality, a large European study, the ERSPC trial[†], showed death rates to be reduced by 20%. However, the PLCO trial has been criticized for contamination of the control group*. The 20 yr Swedish trial showed a decrease in mortality with PSA screening but had a small sample[‡]. The ERSPC trial was found to have varying eligibility criteria and treatments[†]. The debate regarding the benefit of testing as a screening tool continues.

*Andriole GL, et al. 2009. *N Engl J Med* 360(13):1310-1319.
[†]Schröder FH, et al. 2009. *N Engl J Med* 360(13):1320-1328.
[‡]Hugosson J, et al. 2010. *Lancet Oncol* 11(8):725-732.

Varicocele

- Signs and Symptoms
  - o Most are asymptomatic
  - o May present as infertile patient
  - o May report scrotal heaviness
- Physical Exam
  - o Careful inspection, may appear as "bag of worms" in scrotum
- Investigations
  - o If unclear, then do high resolution Doppler ultrasonography
  - o Semen analysis to determine if surgery needed

Testicular Torsion

- Signs and Symptoms
  - o Sudden onset of severe testicular pain followed by inguinal and/or scrotal swelling
  - o Testicle retracted upward
  - o 1/3 have GI upset
  - o May be preceded by trauma
- Physical Exam
  - o Swollen, tender, high-riding, transverse testis
  - o Lifting the testicle will increase pain (in epididymitis it will relieve pain)
  - o Absence of cremasteric reflex supports diagnosis
- Investigations
  - o If physical exam suggests testicular torsion, refer patient to OR for immediate scrotal exploration

UROLOGICAL

7.2 Female-Specific Scenarios

Pelvic Organ Prolapse

- Descent or herniation of pelvic organs from their normal positions/ attachment sites in the pelvis
  - o Urethral prolapse
  - o Uterine prolapse
  - o Vault prolapse (after hysterectomy)
  - o Anterior vaginal wall prolapse: cystocele
  - o Posterior vaginal wall prolapse: rectocele
- Signs and Symptoms
  - o Often asymptomatic
  - o Vaginal bleeding (from exposed/ulcerated mucous membrane)
  - o Sensation of vaginal fullness/pressure
  - o History of coital difficulties
  - o History of voiding or defecation difficulty
  - o Sacral back pain
  - o Bulge protruding into vagina or through vaginal introitus
- Other important aspects of history with pelvic organ prolapse include:
  - o Multiparous (higher risk for prolapse)
  - o Other signs and symptoms of vaginal atrophy/hypoestrogenism
  - o Increased intra-abdominal pressure (obesity, COPD, etc.)
  - o Connective tissue disease (e.g. Marfan disease)
- Physical Exam
  - o Examine the patient in lithotomy position as well as standing, both while relaxed and during maximal straining
  - o Urethral prolapse: swollen, red, ring around urethral meatus
  - o Cystocele if bulge in anterior vaginal wall
    - » 1st Degree: protrusion to upper vagina
    - » 2nd Degree: protrusion to the introitus
    - » 3rd Degree: protrusion external to the introitus
  - o Rectocele if bulge in posterior vaginal wall

- Uterine (or vault) prolapse (may be associated with cystocele and/or rectocele): progressive retroversion of uterus and descent into vagina with lowering of cervix:
  - 1st Degree: cervix remains within vagina
  - 2nd Degree: cervix is at the introitus
  - 3rd Degree: cervix and vagina are outside the introitus
- Investigations
  - Assess for urinary retention: postvoid residual volume (ultrasound)
  - Assess strength of pelvic floor musculature
  - If patient is asymptomatic and there is no urinary retention, may do nothing

Urinary Tract Infection (UTI)

- Definition: >100,000 bacteria/mL in midstream urine (MSU); can be less if patient is symptomatic
- May be pyelonephritis, cystitis, and/or urethritis
- Uncomplicated if infection in a healthy patient with structurally and functionally normal urinary tract
- Complicated if infection in advanced age, chronic renal disease, DM, immunodeficiency, pregnancy, recurrent instrumentation, urological abnormalities
- Most commonly due to ascending GI organisms (*E. coli*, entercocci), but also commonly due to *Klebsiella spp.*, *Proteus spp.*, *Pseudomonas spp.*, *S. saprophyticus*, *S. fecalis*
- Signs and Symptoms
  - Storage/voiding LUTS
  - Hematuria
  - Cloudy/malodorous urine
  - Pain/tenderness (costovertebral angle: pyelonephritis, suprapubic, back)

EBM: Acute Uncomplicated UTI in Women

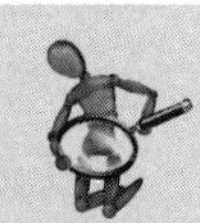

Approximately 1/3 of women will develop at least one urinary tract infection over the course of their lives. The diagnosis of acute uncomplicated UTI can be made primarily by history; women with dysuria AND urgency or frequency will have a diagnosis of UTI 80% of the time and should be treated with empiric antibiotics. If a woman presents with vaginal symptoms in addition to urinary symptoms, the likelihood of UTI is significantly decreased. Consider C&S testing only in the setting of pyelonephritis symptoms, complicating factors, persistence of symptoms, or history of recurrent UTIs.

University of Michigan Health System. *Urinary Tract Infection.* Ann Arbor: University of Michigan; 2011.

7.3 Pediatric Male-Specific Scenarios

Hypospadias

- Signs and Symptoms
  - Asymptomatic, signs present at newborn exam
  - Foreskin has dorsal hooded prepuce
  - Two apparent urethral openings, with blind meatus in normal location and displaced true meatus
  - Abnormal penile curvature: chordee
- Physical Exam
  - Meatal location
  - Glans configuration
  - Penile curvature
  - Penile length assessment
  - Scrotal exam

- Investigations
  - Investigations not needed; surgery necessary to correct meatal opening and foreskin

Cryptorchidism

- Signs and Symptoms
  - A testicle not found within the scrotum
  - The scrotum may be small and minimally rugated
- Physical Exam
  - Genital exam to assess for other abnormalities
  - Two-handed exam is needed: one soapy or lubricated hand making sweeping movements along anterior inguinal canal and the other over the scrotum assessing for a retractile or ectopic testis
    - » The child should be in squatting position
  - Testicular position: inguinal canal vs. scrotum vs. typical ectopic sites
  - Testicular consistency
  - Size of testicle in relation to opposite testis
  - Evaluation for a nonpalpable testis
- Investigations
  - Radiologic examination is not warranted, aside from cases in which presence of uterus needs to be excluded or in assessment of obese boys

REFERENCES

1. Wein AJ, Kavoussi LR, Novick AC, Partin AW, Peters CA (Editors). *Campbell-Walsh Urology*, 10th ed. Philadelphia: Saunders Elsevier; 2012.
2. Andriole GL, Crawford ED, Grubb RL 3rd, Buys SS, Chia D, Church TR, et al. 2009. *N Engl J Med* 360(13):1310-1319.
3. Hugosson J, Carlsson S, Aus G, Bergdahl S, Khatami A, Lodding P, et al. 2010. *Lancet Oncol* 11(8):725-732.
4. Schröder FH, Hugosson J, Roobol MJ, Tammela TL, Ciatto S, Nelen V, et al. 2009. *N Engl J Med* 360(13):1320-1328.
5. University of Michigan Health System. *Urinary Tract Infection*. Ann Arbor: University of Michigan; 2011.

The Essentials of Clinical Pharmacology and Toxicology

Editors:
Tenneille T. Loo
Kaspar Ng

Faculty Reviewer:
David Juurlink, BPhm, MD, PhD, FRCP(C)

TABLE OF CONTENTS

1. DRUG PRESCRIBING PRACTICES

The following chapter provides a brief overview of common topics in practical drug prescribing, and clinical pharmacology and toxicology. Please refer to the *Compendium of Pharmaceuticals and Specialties* (CPS), *United States Pharmacopeia Drug Information* (USP DI) or other pharmacology textbooks for more detailed information on the topics reviewed.

1.1 Common Abbreviations

Always consult the hospital formulary for approved abbreviations that are specific to each institution. To correct for common error-prone abbreviations, write out the order in full or use the correct abbreviation(s) (see **Table 1** and **Table 2**).

Table 1. Common Abbreviations for Medication Directions and Route of Administration

Abbreviation	Interpretation
ac	Before meals
Amp	Ampule
BID	Twice a day
Cap	Capsule
cc	With meals

Table 1. Common Abbreviations for Medication Directions and Route of Administration (continued)

Abbreviation	Interpretation
CVL	Central venous line
D5W	Dextrose 5% in water
GT	Gastrostomy tube
gtt	Drop
hs	At bedtime
IM	Intramuscular
IT	Intrathecal
IV	Intravenous
M or Mitte	Dispense this amount
mcg	microgram
mEq	milliequivalent
mg	milligram
mL	millilitre
NG tube	Nasogastric tube
NPO	Nothing by mouth
OTC	Over-the-counter
NS	Normal saline
pc	After meals
po	Oral route
pr	Rectal route
pv	Vaginal route
prn	When required
q()h	Every () hour(s)
qAM	Every morning
SC	Subcutaneous
SL	Sublingual
STAT	At once
Supp	Suppository
Susp	Suspension
Tab	Tablet
TID	3 times a day
TPN	Total parenteral nutrition
v/v	Volume in volume
w/v	Weight in volume
w/w	Weight in weight

Chabner DE. *Language of Medicine*. Missouri: Saunders Elsevier; 2004.

Table 2. Common Error-Prone Abbreviations

Full Order	Avoid Writing	Misinterpretations
Each ear	au	ou (each eye)
Each eye	ou	au (each ear)
Every other day	q.o.d.	QID (4 times a day)
Four times a day	QID	qd or q1d (once daily)
International units	IU	IV or number 10
Intranasal	IN	IM (intramuscular)
Left ear	as	os (left eye)
Left eye	os	as (left ear)
Microgram	μg	mg (milligram)
Once daily	qd or q1d OD	QID (4 times a day) right eye
Right ear	ad	od (right eye)
Right eye	od	ad (right ear) once daily
Units	U	number 0

Institute of Safe Medication Practices. List of Error-Prone Abbreviations, Symbols, and Dose Designations. 2013. http://www.ismp.org/tools/errorproneabbreviations.pdf

PHARMACOLOGY

1.2 Essentials of Writing a Prescription

Essential Components of a Drug Prescription:

- Name, address, and phone number of prescriber (and institution if applicable)
- Date of the written prescription
- Patient information: name and address
- Drug information: name, strength, and dosage form
- Instructions for the patient
- Quantity to dispense
- Refill information
- Prescriber signature: write down the prescriber name if using an institution prescription note
- May include allergies, date of birth/age, and weight of the patient, which can be helpful for verifying prescription

Other points to consider when writing a prescription:

- Do not follow a decimal point with a zero (i.e. use 2 mg NOT 2.0 mg)
- Use zero before a decimal point when the dose is less than one whole unit (i.e. use 0.125 mg NOT .125 mg)
- Place adequate space between the drug name, dose, and unit of measure
- Use commas for dosing units at or above 1,000 or use words to improve readability
- Use complete drug names; do not abbreviate them
- Write in ink
- If worried about a patient altering a prescription (i.e. for controlled substances), then the quantity of medication and any repeats should be written in words
- Record in the chart, or keep a copy of which prescriptions were written for the patient
- May include reason for prescribing drug to help avoid prescribing the wrong drug with a similar name
- Ensure that the prescription is written legibly

> **Clinical Pearl: Narcotics and Controlled Substances**[1]
> Since November 1, 2011, narcotics and controlled substances prescriptions in Ontario must include:
> - The physician's College of Physicians and Surgeons of Ontario (CPSO) number
> - The patient's government-issued ID number (same ID must be presented to pharmacist)

2. CLINICAL PHARMACOLOGY AND TOXICOLOGY

2.1 Factors Modifying Drug Actions and Localization

Individual factors may alter the effect of how the body absorbs, distributes, metabolizes, and eliminates a drug. The following are common modifying factors (see **Table 3**); for a complete list, a pharmacology text should be consulted.

Table 3. Factors Modifying Drug Actions and Localization

Modifying Factor	Effect
Concurrent Illnesses	Renal disease, liver disease, cardiac failure, shock, and protein loss may alter pharmacokinetics
Concurrent Medications	May inhibit or induce absorption, metabolism, and/or elimination May produce additive, synergistic, or antagonistic pharmacodynamic effects
Food Intake	May alter the absorption of medications taken by mouth
Genetics	Genetic variations in drug metabolizing enzymes or target sites may increase toxicity or decrease effect
Pregnancy	Increased plasma volume, decreased protein binding, and changes in glomerular filtration rate may alter pharmacokinetics
Route of Administration	Each differs in rates or amounts of absorption and distribution: • Oral (passive intestinal absorption, then first pass effect) • Rectal (local or systemic effects; hepatic portal circulation is bypassed, which minimizes first pass effect) • SL (rapid diffusion into blood for direct systemic effects; no first pass effect) • IV (no absorption barriers; no first pass effect; rapid effect; useful in continuous administration and in large volumes) • IM (speed and duration of effect is dependent on formulation: aqueous [fast] or depot [sustained]) • SC (slower than IV, similar to IM) • Inhalation (rapid delivery across mucous membranes) • Topical (local and direct effects) • Transdermal (systemic effects)
Smoking	May affect drug absorption, distribution, metabolism and/or elimination

Lew-Sang E. 1975. *Aust Nurses J* 4(10):21-22.

PHARMACOLOGY

2.2 Common Drug Interactions

Interacting agents can increase or decrease the actions of the following drugs (see **Table 4**). This list is not exhaustive (refer to drug monographs and other references for specific details and complete lists). Drug interactions may increase the risk for toxicity/overdose or may decrease the therapeutic response. Pharmacokinetic drug interactions commonly result from changes in absorption, distribution, metabolism, or elimination. Pharmacodynamic drug interactions may be additive, synergistic, or antagonistic. Changes in drug metabolism can often be predicted by consulting a table of known cytochrome P450 substrates (see **Online Resources**, p.393). Therapeutic drug monitoring may be required.

Table 4. Common Drug Interactions[2-5]

Object Drug or Drug Class	Change in Drug Level or Effect	Precipitant Agent
ACEIs and ARBs	↑	Amiloride, cotrimoxazole, NSAIDs, spironolactone (additive hyperkalemia)
	↓	NSAIDs (antagonize hypotensive effect)
Azole Antifungals	↓	Antacids, H2-blockers, PPIs (increased gastric pH decreases absorption)
	↓	Barbiturates, rifampin (CYP3A4 induction)
Benzodiazepines	↑	Alcohol, opioids and other CNS depressants (additive CNS depression)
β-blockers (CYP2D6 metabolism) (e.g. carvedilol, labetalol, metoprolol)	↑	Fluoxetine, paroxetine (CYP2D6 inhibition)
Calcium Channel Blockers	↑	Azole antifungals, clarithromycin, erythromycin (CYP3A4 inhibition)
	↓	Barbiturates, carbamazepine, rifampin (CYP3A4 induction)
Carbamazepine	↑	Azole antifungals, cimetidine, clarithromycin, diltiazem, erythromycin, fluoxetine, fluvoxamine, isoniazid, verapamil (CYP3A4 inhibition leading to CBZ toxicity)
	↓	Rifampin, SJW (CYP3A4 induction)
Codeine (prodrug of morphine)	↓	Amiodarone, bupropion, fluoxetine, paroxetine (CYP2D6 inhibition leading to impaired morphine synthesis and reduced analgesia)
Cyclosporine	↑	Azole antifungals, clarithromycin, diltiazem, erythromycin, ritonavir, verapamil (CYP3A4 inhibition)
	↓	Barbiturates, carbamazepine, rifampin (CYP3A4 induction)
Dextrometho-rphan	↑	MAOIs (risk of serotonin syndrome): contraindicated

Table 4. Common Drug Interactions[2-5] (continued)

Object Drug or Drug Class	Change in Drug Level or Effect	Precipitant Agent
Digoxin	↑	Amiodarone, clarithromycin, diltiazem, erythromycin, verapamil (inhibition of PGP leading to increased absorption and reduced renal clearance)
	↓	Rifampin (induction of PGP clearance)
Diuretics	↓	NSAIDs (antagonistic)
HMG-CoA Reductase Inhibitors (CYP3A metabolism), does not include pravastatin and rosuvastatin	↑	Azole antifungals, clarithromycin, cyclosporine, erythromycin, grapefruit juice (CYP3A4 inhibition)
Lithium	↑	ACEIs, diuretics, NSAIDs (decreased renal clearance)
	↓	Theophylline (increased clearance: unknown mechanism)
MAOIs	↑	Anorexiants (e.g. amphetamines), other antidepressants (risk of serotonin syndrome): contraindicated
	↑	Sympathomimetics (risk of hypertensive crisis)
Nitrates	↑	Sildenafil, tadalafil, vardenafil (additive hypotensive effect): contraindicated
NSAIDs	↑	Anticoagulants, antiplatelets, ASA, SSRIs, warfarin (bleeding risk)
Phenytoin	↑	Amiodarone, co-trimoxazole, metronidazole (CYP2C9 inhibition)
	↓	Carbamazepine, rifampin (CYP2C9 induction)
Quinolones	↑	Drugs that can prolong QT interval (see p.385)
	↓	Antacids, calcium, iron, sucralfate: separate oral administration times by 2 h
SSRIs	↑	MAOIs (risk of serotonin syndrome): contraindicated
	↑	NSAIDs (bleeding risk)
Sulfonylureas	↑	Amiodarone, co-trimoxazole, fluconazole, fluoxetine, fluvoxamine, metronidazole (CYP2C9 inhibition)
Sympathomimetics	↓	β-blockers (antagonistic)
	↑	MAOIs, TCAs (additive)
TCAs	↑	MAOIs (risk of serotonin syndrome): contraindicated
	↑	Amiodarone, cimetidine, haloperidol, SSRIs, terbinafine (CYP2D6 and 3A4 inhibition)
	↓	Barbiturates, rifampin (CYP3A4 induction)

Table 4. Common Drug Interactions[2-5] (continued)

Object Drug or Drug Class	Change in Drug Level or Effect	Precipitant Agent
Theophylline	↑	Cimetidine, ciprofloxacin, fluvoxamine (CYP1A2 inhibition)
	↓	Rifampin, smoking (CYP1A2 induction)
Thiopurines	↑	Allopurinol (decreased metabolism and elimination)
Warfarin	↑	Acetaminophen, acute alcohol intake, allopurinol, amiodarone, azole antifungals, cimetidine, co-trimoxazole, fibrates, metronidazole (decreased metabolism)
	↑	Antibiotics (disrupts Vitamin K biosynthesis by gut flora)
	↑	ASA, antiplatelets, NSAIDs (bleeding risk)
	↓	Barbiturates, carbamazepine, phenytoin, rifampin (increased metabolism)

ACEI = angiotensin conversion enzyme inhibitor, ARB = angiotensin receptor blocker, CBZ = carbamazepine, PGP = P-glycoprotein, PPI = proton pump inhibitor, SJW = St. John's wort

Clinical Pearl: β-Blockers and Hypoglycemia
β-blockers will mask symptoms of hypoglycemia except for sweating.

Clinical Pearl: Histamine H2-Receptor Antagonists and Warfarin
Less problematic alternatives to cimetidine from the same class are ranitidine and famotidine.

2.3 Drugs That Can Prolong QT Interval

The following are selected medications that can prolong the QT interval with risk of inducing torsade de pointes arrhythmia when used according to labeling[6,7] (for more drugs, see **Online Resources**, p.393). Prior to prescribing these drugs, consideration should be given to duration of therapy, concurrent QT-prolonging drugs, and drug interactions. The patient should be assessed for risk factors including electrolyte abnormalities, congenital long QT interval, female gender, age, bradycardia, and myocardial injury. Consultation with a specialist or drug information service for use and monitoring guidelines is recommended.

- Amiodarone
- Azithromycin
- Chloroquine
- Chlorpromazine
- Citalopram
- Quinolones
- Domperidone
- Macrolides
- Methadone
- Moxifloxacin
- Pentamidine
- Pimozide
- Procainamide
- Sotalol
- Thioridazine

2.4 Special Populations

Important Variations to Consider when Deciding on Drug Therapy in the Pediatric, Adult, and Geriatric Populations

- Changes in body composition as a percentage of weight (e.g. fat, total body water)
- Changes in protein binding
- Physical size: body surface area
- Maturation and degeneration: hepatic metabolism, renal clearance

These factors affect the absorption, distribution, metabolism, and elimination of drugs, as well as their localization. Refer to drug monograph or pediatric drug references for guidelines on pediatric dose adjustments[8].

General Considerations for Geriatric Patients

- Assess for non-drug alternatives
- Define goal for drug therapy
- Take a detailed drug history including OTC and herbal products; rule out drug-induced symptoms
- Refer to the Beers Criteria that lists medications to avoid in the geriatric population, particularly those with certain diseases or syndromes[9] (see **Online Resources**, p.393)
- Simplify the number of drugs taken and number of administration times to increase compliance
- Ensure the drug is at steady state before changing dosing

PHARMACOLOGY

Pregnancy

Proper counseling should be provided to pregnant women who use medications. When considering therapeutics in pregnancy, the baseline risk for congenital abnormalities, the risks of the medication (teratogenic and perinatal), the risk of foregoing treatment, and the benefit of treatment must be weighed. Please consult a teratogen information service for more information, such as Motherisk (Canada) or the Organization of Teratology Information Specialists (USA).

One commonly used drug cataloging system is the US Food and Drug Administration (FDA) risk classification system. This arrangement classifies medications into Category A, B, C, D, or X. In brief, drugs in Category A have failed to demonstrate fetal harm at certain doses, whereas drugs in Categories B to X are considered to be teratogenic in increasing levels. Category X is most likely to cause fetal harm[10]. See **Online Resources**, p.393 for specific definitions for each category. Not all teratogenic medications are absolutely contraindicated in pregnancy. Pre-pregnancy planning is advised for all patients using these medications. The following are select medications in each category[11].

- **Category X**
  - Danazol, methyltestorenone, isoretinoin, etretinate, diethylstilbestrol
- **Category D**
  - Coumadin derivative (warfarin; under classification X as per manufacturer)
  - Oxytetracycline, tetracycline, phenytoin, valproic acid, clonazepam, carbamazepine
  - Azathioprine, cyclophosphamide, vincristine
  - ACE inhibitors in 2nd and 3rd trimesters
- **Category C**
  - Ethosuximide, lamotrigine, mephenytoin
  - ACE inhibitors in 1st trimester

- **Category B**
  - Acetaminophen, ranitidine
- **Category A**
  - Doxylamine/pyridoxine

Note: These classifications do not always distinguish between human versus animal data, doses, or differences in frequency, severity, and type of fetal developmental toxicities. Differences in these aforementioned factors will pose different risks (see **Online Resources**, p.393 for further details).

In general, the following are considered safe at their recommended doses in pregnancy:

- Acetaminophen[12]
- Antacids[13]
- Antihistamines (e.g. diphenhydramine, hydroxyzine)[13]
- Beta-lactams (penicillins)[13]
- Doxylamine/pyridoxine[14]
- Flu vaccine[13]
- Ranitidine[15]

> **Clinical Pearl: Codeine and Breastfeeding[16]**
> Controversy: Should the use of codeine be avoided in breastfeeding mothers who are known ultrametabolizers of CYP2D6 or whose CYP2D6 polymorphism is unknown? Patients who are CYP2D6 ultrametabolizers biotransform higher levels of codeine into morphine, thus exposing the neonate to excessive morphine levels. However, the severity and prevalence of this issue is under debate.

2.5 Approach to the Toxic or Poisoned Patient

Drug toxicity can result from drug overdose; altered drug absorption, distribution, metabolism, and elimination; drug-drug interactions; and idiosyncratic hypersensitivity. Altered mental status, seizures, or cardiovascular changes are a few of the many symptoms that may lead to the suspicion of poisoning. Contact the local poison control center for consultation. The following includes an approach to a poisoned patient after airway, breathing, circulation, and glucose level have been assessed.

- Take the history from family/friends, police officers, paramedics about what substance(s) were taken; often the history is unreliable and if possible, ask for any bottles, syringes, or household products that were found around the patient
- To aid in the differential of possible poisons, assess the following and determine any characteristic toxic syndrome (see **Table 5**)
- Assess vital signs including pulse, RR, BP, and temperature:
  - Observe the eyes for miosis, mydriasis, nystagmus, or ptosis
  - Assess the color, dryness, and temperature of the skin
  - Auscultate for bowel sounds to determine ileus or increased sounds
  - Perform a neurological exam
- Order a broad toxicology screen (blood and urine)
- Decontamination procedures (including administration of activated charcoal and whole bowel irrigation) should be individualized according to age, properties of substance(s) ingested, and the time elapsed since ingestion

Table 5. Common Toxic Syndromes and Treatments

Agents	Signs and Symptoms	Treatment
Acetaminophen	GI upset, hepatotoxicity	N-acetylcysteine to prevent liver injury; consult Rumack-Matthew Nomogram for acetaminophen toxicity
Amphetamines and Other Stimulants	Agitation, acute psychosis, HTN, tachycardia, hyperthermia, seizures, serotonergic effects (see below)	Benzodiazepines for seizure; phentolamine for HTN if needed; manage serotonergic effects (see below)
Anticholinergic Agents	Blurred vision, dry skin and mucous membranes, confusion, hyperthermia, flushing, urinary retention (see **Table 12**, **Essentials of Emergency Medicine**, p.436)	General support; physostigmine in selected patients: rule out tricyclic antidepressants before using (see below)
Antipsychotics	CNS depression, anticholinergic effects (see above), miosis (sometimes mydriasis), dystonia, akathisia, cardiac conduction delays with ventricular tachydysrhythmias	Sodium bicarbonate for ventricular tachydysrhythmias; magnesium for torsade de pointes
Aspirin (salicylate)	Initial hyperventilation and respiratory alkalosis, followed by AGMA	IV fluids; sodium bicarbonate; dialysis
Benzodiaz-epines	Amnestic effects, confusion, respiratory depression	General support
β-blockers	AV block, bradycardia, hypotension, hyperkalemia, hypoglycemia	Catecholamines; insulin with dextrose; dialysis for select β-blockers
Calcium Channel Blockers	AV block, bradycardia, hyperglycemia	Calcium; high dose insulin with dextrose
Carbon Monoxide	Confusion, headache, nausea, tachypnea	Oxygen
Cholinesterase Inhibitors	**Muscarinic:** Abdominal cramps, diaphoresis, diarrhea, lacrimation, salivation **Nicotinic:** Fasciculations, HTN, tachycardia, seizure	Atropine for muscarinic symptoms; pralidoxime can be considered for patients with organophosphate poisoning (not carbamate poisoning)
Digoxin	Hyperkalemia (with acute overdose), variety of cardiac rhythm disturbances, visual changes (yellow-green predominance), vomiting	Digoxin antibodies; avoid calcium except with severe hyperkalemia (usually chronic toxicity with renal failure)
Ethylene Glycol and Methanol	AGMA, osmolar gap, respiratory depression, visual disturbances	Sodium bicarbonate to correct acidemia; fomepizole or ethanol to prevent toxicity; dialysis

Table 5. Common Toxic Syndromes and Treatments (continued)

Agents	Signs and Symptoms	Treatment
Iron Salts	Vomiting, diarrhea, abdominal pain, GI bleeding, hepatotoxicity, coagulopathy, AGMA, seizure; radio-opaque tablets on abdominal X-ray	Sodium bicarbonate to correct acidemia; deferoxamine for systemic toxicity
Opioids	N/V, constipation, respiratory depression, bradycardia, lethargy	Naloxone (start with small initial doses to patients with opioid-dependence)
Serotonin Syndrome	Agitation, confusion, hyperreflexia, rigidity, tremors, diarrhea, diaphoresis, HTN, tachycardia, hyperthermia	Aggressive cooling; benzodiazepines; consider cyproheptadine; discontinue offending agent
Tricyclic Antidepressants	Initial HTN, followed by hypotension in severe overdose, tachycardia, arrhythmia, anticholinergic effects (see above)	Sodium bicarbonate for arrhythmia; avoid physostigmine

AGMA = anion gap metabolic acidosis, AV = atrioventricular
Longo DL, et al. (Editors). *Harrison's Online*, 18th ed. 2012.
Micromedex Online: POISINDEX Database. Greenwood Village: Thomson Reuters (Healthcare) Inc.; 2013.

PHARMACOLOGY

2.6 Common Recreational Drugs

It is not uncommon for patients to be using street drugs in addition to prescribed medications. Knowledge about the health effects produced by these drugs along with some of the various street terms is useful (see **Table 6**).

Table 6. Common Recreational Drugs

Drug	Alternative Street Names	Short-Term Health Effects
Amphetamine family (e.g. amphetamines, methamphet-amines, dextro-amphetamine)	Amphetamine family: speed, bennies, glass, crystal, crank, uppers, pep pills Methamphetamines: speed, crystal meth, meth, chalk, ice, crystal, jib	CNS stimulant drug; increased alertness, energy, restlessness; increased blood pressure, respiratory rate; paranoia, hallucinations
Benzodiaz-epines	Benzos, tranks, downers	CNS depressant; often used in conjunction with opioids or stimulants (to decrease their effect); produces calming and relaxing effect
Cannabis: includes marijuana, hashish, and hash oil	Marijuana: grass, weed, pot, dope, ganja Hashish: hash Hash oil: weed oil, honey oil	Perceptual distortions, drowsiness, spontaneous laughter, euphoria, relaxation or anxiety; increased appetite and heart rate; decreased blood pressure and balance; apathy

Table 6. Common Recreational Drugs (continued)

Drug	Alternative Street Names	Short-Term Health Effects
Cocaine	Blow, C, coke, flake, rock, snow, marching powder, nose candy	CNS stimulant drug; increased alertness and energy, awareness of senses; decreased sleep and hunger; increased heart rate, temperature, blood pressure, restlessness, anxiety; cardiac toxicity
Crack	Freebase, rooster, tornado	Smoking form of cocaine; see cocaine (above)
Ecstasy/Methylenedioxymethamphetamine (MDMA)	E, XTC, Adam, the love drug	Effects of both a stimulant and a hallucinogen; stimulant effects include increased blood pressure, heart rate, temperature, sense of euphoria; hallucinogen effects include hallucinations, distortion of perception
Gamma Hydroxybutyrate (GHB)	Goop, G, liquid ecstasy, liquid x	CNS depressant; at low doses, can allow user to feel euphoric, less inhibited, and more sociable; at higher doses, dizziness, memory loss, decreased consciousness, breathing, heart rate; loss of coordination; chronic use can lead to severe withdrawal syndrome
Gravol® (Dimenhydrinate)		Antinausea medication available over-the-counter; can cause euphoria and hallucinations
Jimson Weed	Jamestown weed, angel's trumpet, devil's trumpet, devil's snare, devil's seed, mad hatter, zombie cucumber	Plant that contains atropine and scopolamine; may lead to confusion, euphoria, hallucinations, delirium, and an anticholinergic toxidrome
Ketamine	K, special K, ket, vitamin K, cat tranquilizers	Anesthetic drug and hallucinogen; produces intense hallucinations and sense that mind is detached from body (dissociation); also loss of coordination, confusion, memory loss, increased sleepiness
Heroin	Big H, China white, Mexican brown, smack, junk, dope	Opioid type of drug; sedative effect; euphoria; detachment from physical and emotional pain; respiratory depression, constipation, miosis
Lysergic Acid Diethylamide (LSD)	Acid, blotter, microdot, windowpane	Hallucinogen; can experience sense of joy, confusion, anxiety; vivid visual effects and altered sense of hearing, smelling, taste; GI upset, tremors, tachycardia

Table 6. Common Recreational Drugs (continued)

Drug	Alternative Street Names	Short-Term Health Effects
Mescaline	Cactus, cactus heads, cactus buttons, buttons, mesc, mese	Hallucinogen; abnormal visual perception, anxiety, paranoia; hyperreflexia
Opioids (such as oxycodone, fentanyl)	Hillbilly heroin, killers, OC, oxy, oxycotton, oxy80	Opioid, sedative effect; respiratory depression (may be fatal); euphoria
Phencyclidine (PCP)	Angel dust, dust, crystal joint, tic tac, zoom, boat	Hallucinogen; hallucinations, anxiety, panic, increased heart rate, blood pressure, drowsiness, lack of coordination; agitation, hostility
Psilocybin	Mushrooms, shrooms, magic mushrooms, musk, magic	Hallucinogen; hallucinations, calming effect, anxiety, panic, increased heart rate, blood pressure, drowsiness, lack of coordination
Rohypnol	Roofies, roachies, rope, rophies, ruffies, "date rape" drug	CNS depressant (part of the benzodiazepine family); calming effect, drowsiness, loss of consciousness at higher doses
Steroids	Juice, pumpers, weight trainers, roids	Increased muscle bulk, energy, irritability, anxiety, aggression; reduced fertility

Longo DL, et al. (Editors). *Harrison's Online*, 18th ed. 2012.
Hindmarsh WK. *Drugs: What your Kid Should Know*. Gauteng: Pharmacy and Apotex Continuing Education; 2000.

PHARMACOLOGY

2.7 Important Pharmacokinetic Formulae

Clearance

$$Cl = \frac{\text{rate of drug elimination}}{\text{plasma drug concentration}}$$

Creatinine Clearance (measured)

$$CrCl = \frac{U_{Cr} \times V}{P_{Cr}}$$

where CrCl = creatinine clearance, U_{Cr} = creatinine concentration in collected urine sample, V = urine flow rate, P_{Cr} = plasma creatinine concentration

Estimated CrCl (Cockcroft Gault)

$$CrCl = \frac{1.23 \times wt \times (140 - age)}{Cr} (\times 0.85 \text{ for females})$$

where CrCl = estimated creatinine clearance [mL/min], wt = weight in kg, age = years, Cr = serum creatinine [μM]

Volume of Distribution

$$V_d = \frac{\text{amount of drug in body}}{\text{plasma drug concentration}}$$

Elimination Half-life

$$t_{1/2} = \frac{(0.693)(V_d)}{Cl}$$

Ideal Body Weight (IBW)

- For Males: IBW = 50kg + [2.3kg x (# of inches>5ft)]
- For Females: IBW = 45.5kg + [2.3kg x (# of inches>5ft)]

Doses for certain drugs (e.g. acyclovir) should be calculated with IBW to avoid toxicity

Steady State Drug Concentration (Css)

$$C_{ss} = \frac{(F)(\text{rate of drug administration})}{Cl}$$

where F = bioavailability fraction of dose, rate of drug administration = dose/time

PHARMACOLOGY

Loading Dose (LD)

$$LD = \frac{(C_p)(V_d)}{F}$$

where Cp = target plasma drug concentration, F=1 for IV drug and F<1 for oral drug

Maintenance Dose (MD)

$$MD = \frac{C_p \times Cl \times \tau}{F}$$

where τ = dosing interval

- With Renal Impairment

$$MD = \frac{\text{CrCl (patient)}}{\text{CrCl (normal)}} \times \text{Standard Dose of Drug}$$

where CrCl = creatinine clearance (when drug is renally excreted)

2.8 Online Resources

- Cytochrome P450 Drug Interaction Table. Indiana University School of Medicine. www.drug-interactions.com
- QT Prolongation Drugs. Arizona Center for Education and Research on Therapeutics. http://www.azcert.org
- Beers Criteria. American Geriatrics Society. http://www.americangeriatrics.org/health_care_professionals/clinical_practice/clinical_guidelines_recommendations/2012
- FDA Pregnancy Categories. http://depts.washington.edu/druginfo/Formulary/Pregnancy.pdf
- FDA Summary of Proposed Rule on Pregnancy and Lactation Labeling. http://www.fda.gov/Drugs/DevelopmentApprovalProcess/DevelopmentResources/Labeling/ucm093310.htm

REFERENCES

1. Ontario Ministry of Health and Long-Term Care. Ontario Public Drug Programs: Narcotics Monitoring System (NMS) Pharmacy Reference Manual. 2012. Available from: http://www.health.gov.on.ca/english/providers/program/drugs/resources/pharmacy_manual.pdf
2. Katzung B, Masters S, Trevor A. *Basic and Clinical Pharmacology*. New York: Lange Medical Books/McGraw-Hill, Medical Publications Division; 2012.
3. Regal R, Ong Vue C. 2004. Drug interactions between antibiotics and select maintenance medications: Seeing more clearly through the narrow therapeutic window of opportunity. *Consult Pharm* 19(12):1119-1128.
4. Lesher BA. 2004. Clinically important drug interactions. Detail-Document #200601. *Pharmacist's Letter* 20(6):200601.
5. Juurlink D. 2011. *Drug Interactions for the Front-Line Clinician*. Oral Presentation. Toronto, Ontario, Canada.
6. Arizona Center for Education and Research on Therapeutics (CERT). Drug Lists by Risk Groups: Drugs that Prolong the QT Interval and/or Induce Torsades de Pointes. 2013. Available from: http://www.azcert.org/medical-pros/drug-lists/drug-lists.cfm
7. Gowda RM, Khan JA, Wilbur SL, Vasavada BC, Sacchi TJ. 2004. Torsade de pointes: The clinical considerations. *Int J Cardiol* 96(1):1-6.
8. Allegaert K, Verbesselt R, Naulaers G, van den Anker JN, Rayyan M, Debeer A, et al. 2008. Developmental pharmacology: Neonates are not just small adults... *Acta Clin Belg* 63(1):16-24.
9. American Geriatrics Society 2012 Beers Criteria Update Expert Panel. 2012. American Geriatrics Society Updated Beers Criteria for potentially inappropriate medication use in older adults. *J Am Geriatr Soc* 60(4):616-631.
10. Bánhidy F, Lowry B, Czeizel A. 2005. Risk and benefit of drug use during pregnancy. *Int J Med Sci* 2(3):100-106.
11. Briggs GG, Freeman RK, Yaffe SJ. *Drugs in Pregnancy and Lactation: A Reference Guide to Fetal and Neonatal Risk*. London: Lippincott Williams & Wilkins; 2008.
12. Babb M, Koren G, Einarson A. 2010. Treating pain during pregnancy. *Can Fam Physician* 56(1):25,27.
13. Schaefer C, Peters PWJ, Miller RK. *Drugs During Pregnancy and Lactation*. Amsterdam: Elsevier; 2007.
14. Einarson A, Maltepe C, Boskovic R, Koren G. 2007. Treatment of nausea and vomiting in pregnancy: An updated algorithm. *Can Fam Physician* 53(12):2109-2111.
15. Law R, Maltepe C, Bozzo P, Einarson A. 2010. Treatment of heartburn and acid reflux associated with nausea and vomiting during pregnancy. *Can Fam Physician* 56(2):143-144.
16. Madadi P, Koren G, Cairns J, Chitayat D, Gaedigk A, Leeder JS, et al. 2007. Safety of codeine during breastfeeding: Fatal morphine poisoning in the breastfed neonate of a mother prescribed codeine. *Can Fam Physician* 53(1):33-35.
17. Kalant H, Grant DM, Eds MJ. *Principles of Medical Pharmacology*. Toronto: Elsevier; 2007.
18. Motherisk. Pregnancy and Breastfeeding Resources. 2013. Available from: http://www.motherisk.org/women/index.jsp

The Essentials of Dermatology

Editors:
Thanh-Cat Ho
Theodore W. Small

Faculty Reviewers:
Yvette Miller-Monthrope, MD, FRCP(C)
James Shaw, MD, FRCP(C)

TABLE OF CONTENTS

1. ESSENTIAL ANATOMY

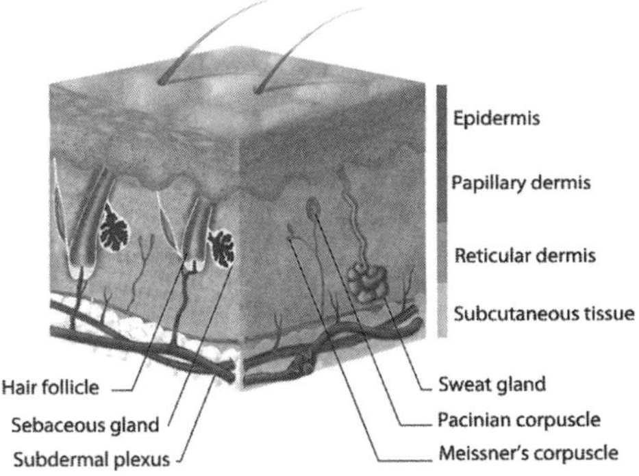

Figure 1. Layers of the Skin
Douglas G, Nicol F, Robertson C. *Macleod's Clinical Examination*, 12th ed. Philadelphia: Churchill Livingstone; 2009.
Chiang N, Verbov J. *Dermatology: A Handbook for Medical Students and Junior Doctors*. Liverpool: British Association of Dermatologists; 2009.

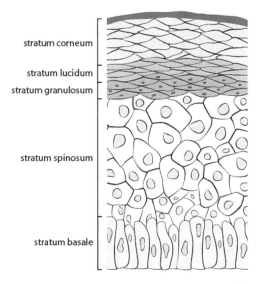

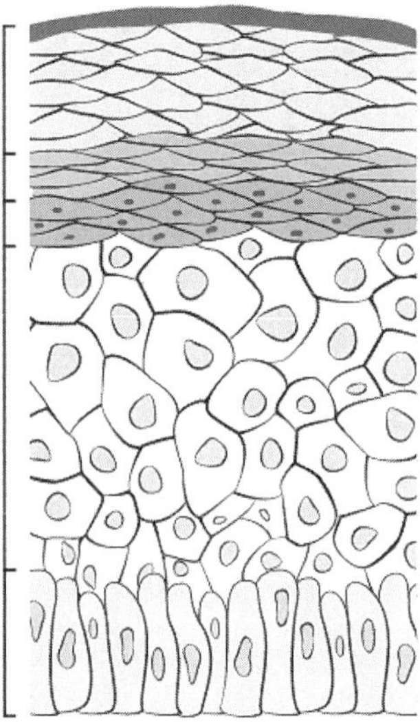

Figure 2. Layers of the Epidermis
Chiang N, Verbov J. *Dermatology: A Handbook for Medical Students and Junior Doctors.* Liverpool: British Association of Dermatologists; 2009.

DERMATOLOGY

> **Clinical Pearl: Epidermis Turnover**[1]
> The epidermis turns over every 40-56 days.

2. FOCUSED HISTORY

- In contrast to most areas of medicine, it can be helpful in dermatology to do a physical exam before taking a detailed history; this allows for interpretation of the lesion without predetermined ideas and for a more objective interpretation of the history

History of Presenting Illness: OPQRST

- **O**nset: how long has the eruption/lesion been present?
- **P**osition: where is the eruption/lesion located?
- **Q**uality: are there any symptoms such as pruritus (itch), pain, or numbness?
- **R**elevant exposures: sun, tanning beds, plants, contact allergens, chemicals, contact with people with similar lesions, travel, animals/pets
- **S**ystems review: fever, joint pain, weight loss, malaise
- **T**iming (course): is this eruption/lesion recurrent or persistent?
    - Emphasis on change over time
- Aggravating Factors: are there any things that make/have made it worse (e.g. sunlight, temperature)
- Alleviating Factors: have any treatments been tried? Has anything helped?
- Specific questions for hair loss:
    - Symmetric/asymmetric
    - Focal/diffuse
    - Rash/no rash

- Specific questions for nails:
    - Recent illnesses or stressors
    - Exposure (e.g. toxins, commercial nail products, chemicals)

Past Medical History
- History of skin disease or skin cancer (e.g. non-melanoma skin cancer, melanoma)
- Inflammatory skin disorders (e.g. psoriasis, atopic dermatitis)
- Chronic disease (e.g. DM, rheumatologic, thyroid, collagen vascular)

Medications and Allergies
- Complete list of medications and allergies with resulting symptoms

Family History
- Atopy, autoimmunity, skin cancer, etc.

3. FOCUSED PHYSICAL EXAM
- The focused physical exam includes:
    1. A general examination of the skin
    2. Inspection of skin lesion(s); confirm location, distribution, and characteristics of the lesion
    3. Palpation of lesion
    4. Examination of secondary sites such as the nails, hair, and mucosal sites
- Ensure appropriate lighting for this exam

> **Clinical Pearl: Lesion Interpretation**
> Some skin eruptions are so characteristic that they do not require an initial history; seeing the lesion first can allow for more objective interpretation of the complaint.

General Skin Inspection
- General inspection: Does the patient look sick or not sick?
- Skin color: erythema (red), cyanosis (pale), jaundice (yellow), pigmentary abnormalities
- State of skin: dry, normal, moist

Inspection of Skin Lesions
- The ability to correctly characterize the lesion is half the challenge in dermatology; when characterizing the lesion, avoid the word "rash" and apply this mnemonic: **SCALDA**
    - **S**ize/**S**urface area
    - **C**olor
    - **A**rrangement (see **Figure 3** and **Table 1**)
    - **L**esion morphology (see **Table 2** and **Figure 4**)
    - **D**istribution
    - **A**lways check hair, nails, mucous membranes, and intertriginous areas

> **Clinical Pearl: Scaling and Crusting**
> Scaling and crusting may obscure diagnostic features; careful physical removal of surface crusts may be helpful (use appropriate sterile techniques such as wiping the lesion with rubbing alcohol prior to inspection).

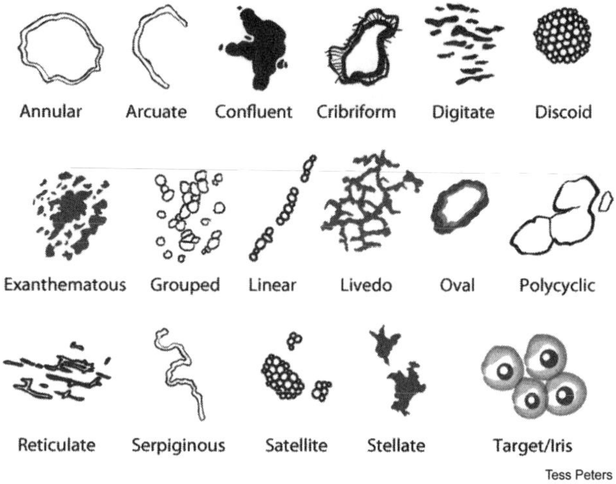

Figure 3. Common Arrangements and Patterns of Skin Lesions
Burns DA. *Rook's Textbook of Dermatology*, 8th ed. New York: Blackwell Publishing; 2009.

Table 1. Arrangements and Patterns of Skin Lesions

Shape/Pattern	Examples
Annular	Granuloma annulare (non-scaling), tinea corporis (scaling)
Arcuate	SLE, urticaria
Confluent	Psoriasis plaques, scaly macules of pityriasis versicolor (yeast), serious drug or viral reaction
Cribriform	Pyoderma gangrenosum heals with this pattern
Dermatomal	Shingles (herpes zoster)
Digitate	Digitate dermatosis
Discoid/ Nummular	Discoid eczema, psoriasis
Exanthematous	Viral infections, drug eruptions
Grouped	Insect bites, herpes simplex
Linear	Striae, scabetic burrows, insect bites, excoriations
Livedo	Cutis marmorata, erythema ab igne, vasculitis
Oval	Pityriasis rosea
Polycyclic	Psoriasis, tinea corporis
Reticulate	Wickham's striae in lichen planus
Serpiginous	Track left by hookworm in cutaneous larva migrans
Satellite	Local malignant spread, candida diaper dermatitis
Scattered and Disseminated	Varicella, disseminated metastases, cutaneous lymphoma, benign nevi
Stellate (rare)	Meningococcemia
Target/Iris	Erythema multiforme

Burns DA. *Rook's Textbook of Dermatology*, 8th ed. New York: Blackwell Publishing; 2009.

Table 2. Primary Lesion Morphology

Classification	General Size	
	<1 cm Diameter	>1 cm Diameter
Flat, Smooth	Macule (e.g. freckle)	Patch (e.g. vitiligo)
Raised, Superficial	Papule (e.g. wart)	Plaque (e.g. psoriasis)
• ***If purulent***	Wheal (e.g.urticaria)	
Raised, Fluid-Filled	Vesicle (e.g. HSV)	Bulla (e.g. bullous pemphigoid)
• ***If purulent***	Pustule	
Palpable Deep (dermal)	Nodule (e.g. dermatofibroma)	Tumor (e.g. lipoma)
• ***If Semi-Solid or Fluid-Filled***	Cyst	

Secondary Skin Lesion Morphology

- **Scaling:** increase in keratin, dead cells on surface of skin (e.g. dermatitis, psoriasis)
- **Crust:** dried fluid (pus, blood, serum) originating from lesion (e.g. impetigo)
- **Lichenification:** thickening of skin with accentuated skin markings (e.g. chronic atopic dermatitis, lichen simplex chronicus)

Other Morphology

- **Purpura:** bleeding into dermis
  - Petechiae <3 mm diameter
  - Ecchymoses (bruises) >3 mm diameter
- **Telangiectasia:** dilated superficial blood vessels; blanchable
- **Excoriation:** a scratch mark
- **Erosion:** disruption of skin involving epidermis alone; heals without scarring
- **Ulcer:** disruption of skin into the dermis or beyond; heals with scarring
  - Can form dark colored crust called eschar

Palpation

- It is recommended to wear gloves when palpating a lesion; however, many clinicians do not wear gloves as it is more difficult to assess (most only wear gloves if there is a concern of infection)
- Assess for texture, consistency, fluid, adjacent edema, tenderness, blanching
- Texture:
  - Superficial (largely epidermal) or deep (more likely in dermis)
  - Soft (e.g. lipoma) or doughy (e.g. hypothyroidism) vs. hard (e.g. scleroderma, calcification), firm (e.g. lichen planus, sarcoid, amyloid) or indurated (e.g. pretibial myxedema)
  - Dry (e.g. hypothyroidism) vs. wet
  - Velvety (acanthosis nigricans, Ehlers-Danlos syndrome)
  - Leathery and "bark-like" (lichenification): epidermal hypertrophy from prolonged rubbing/scratching, pruritic cutaneous disorder (e.g. lichen simplex chronicus, neurodermatitis)

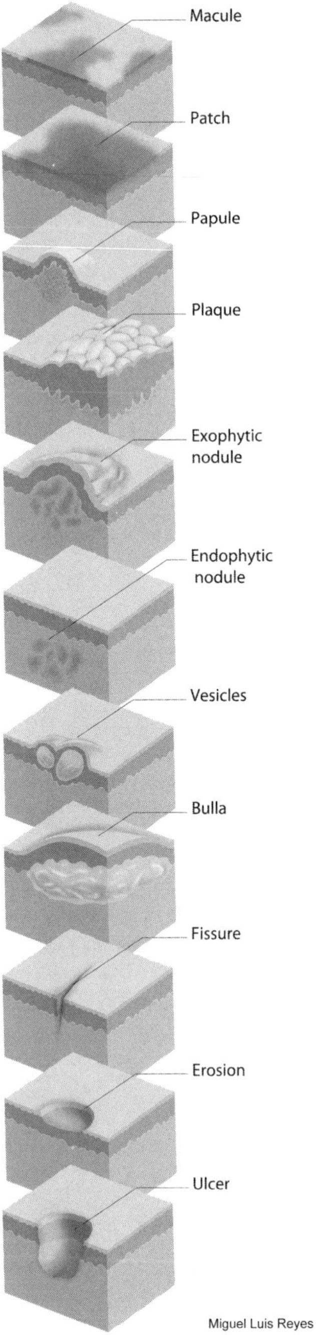

Figure 4. Primary Lesion Morphology
Chiang N, Verbov J. *Dermatology: A Handbook for Medical Students and Junior Doctors.* Liverpool: British Association of Dermatologists; 2009.

Hair

- Texture should be examined (e.g. coarse: hypothyroidism, fine: hyperthyroidism)
- Alopecia (loss of hair) (see **Alopecia**, p.411)
- Hirsutism (abnormally exuberant hair growth) should be examined (e.g. polycystic ovarian disease, neoplasm of the adrenals and gonads)

Nails

- Shape, size, color, and brittleness should be noted
- Hemorrhages under the nail (e.g. splinter hemorrhages in bacterial endocarditis)
- Grooves in the nail (e.g. trauma, Beau's lines)
- Increased white area under the nail bed (e.g. renal disease, liver disease)

Table 3. Typical Nail Changes Associated with Medical Conditions

Abnormality	Characteristics	Common Associations
Clubbing	**Nail-Fold Angles:** nail projects from nail bed (hyponychial angle) ~160° (normal), approaches 180° in clubbing **Phalangeal Depth Ratio:** distal phalangeal depth smaller than interphalangeal depth (normal), reversed in clubbing **Schamroth Sign:** diamond-shaped window when dorsal surfaces of terminal phalanges of similar fingers are opposed (normal), no diamond-shaped window in clubbing **Palpation:** clubbed nails perceived as "floating" within soft tissues, in advanced cases may be able to feel proximal edge of the nail, elicited by rocking the nail	**Lungs:** bronchial cancer, bronchiectasis, lung abscess, CF, idiopathic pulmonary fibrosis, asbestosis **Heart:** congenital cyanotic heart disease, infective endocarditis **GI:** cirrhosis (especially primary biliary cirrhosis), IBD, celiac disease **Others:** hyperthyroidism, subclavian artery stenosis, familial, idiopathic
Splinter Hemorrhages	Longitudinal red-brown flecks on nail bed	<1 mm, in nail itself (i.e. will grow out): trauma (e.g. manual work) >1 mm, in nail bed: infections (e.g. endocardiditis, septicemia)
Leukonychia	White marks across nail bed	Fungal infections TB Chemotherapy Cirrhosis
Koilonychia	Spoon-shaped nails	Iron deficiency anemia
Onycholysis	Separation of nail from nail bed	Fungal infection Thyrotoxicosis Psoriasis Drugs
Pitting	Slight depression (<1 mm diameter) in nail bed	Psoriasis Psoriatic arthritis

Table 3. Typical Nail Changes Associated with Medical Conditions (continued)

Abnormality	Characteristics	Common Associations
Beau's Lines	Single transverse, non-pigmented ridge	Past debilitating illness: distance from cuticle corresponds to time since recovery from illness
Mees' Band	White lines across pink nail bed	Arsenic poisoning
Lindsay's Nails	"1/2 and 1/2 nails", pink-white proximally and brown distally	Chronic liver disease Azotemia
Terry's Nails	White nail beds with 1-2 mm of distal border of the nail	Cirrhosis Hypoalbuminemia

CF = cystic fibrosis

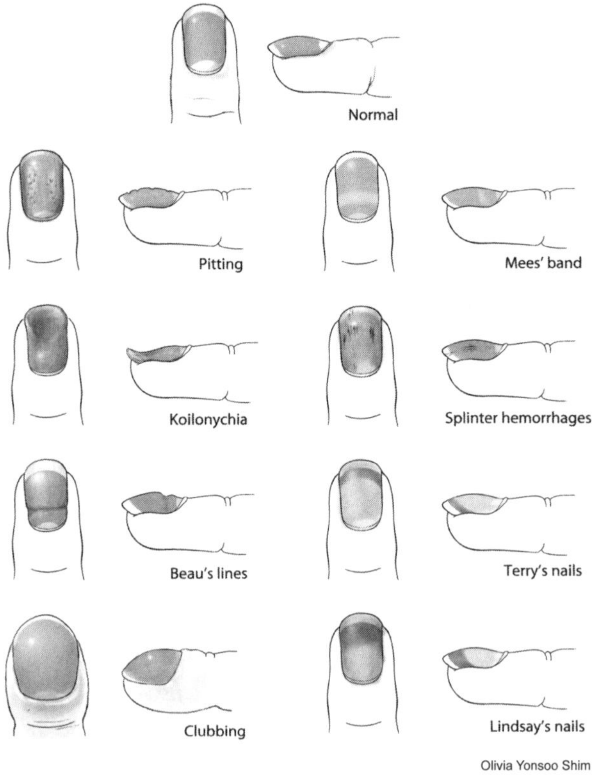

Figure 5. Common Nail Changes Associated with Systemic Disease

4. COMMON CLINICAL SCENARIOS

- The type, prevalence, and incidence of many skin diseases varies with age, gender, race, geographic location, culture, and socioeconomic status

- Appropriate management includes psychosocial interventions as skin diseases can have a major impact on the quality of life of the patient

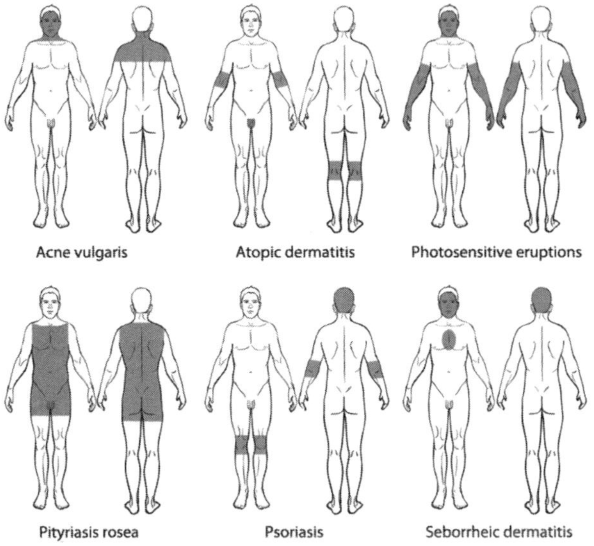

Figure 6. Distribution Patterns of Skin Lesions

4.1 Acne

- A common disease of the pilosebaceous unit
- Epidemiology[2]: age of onset 10-17 yr in females, 14-19 yr in males; however, can continue into 40s and beyond
- Presentation[2]: erythematous papules and pustules
  - Not usually pruritic, can be sore
- Distribution: face, chest, and back
  - Hormonal acne: along jaw line

Types of Lesions

- Inflammatory: discrete papules, pustules, nodules
- Noninflammatory (comedones):
  - Open comedones (blackheads)
  - Closed comedones (whiteheads)

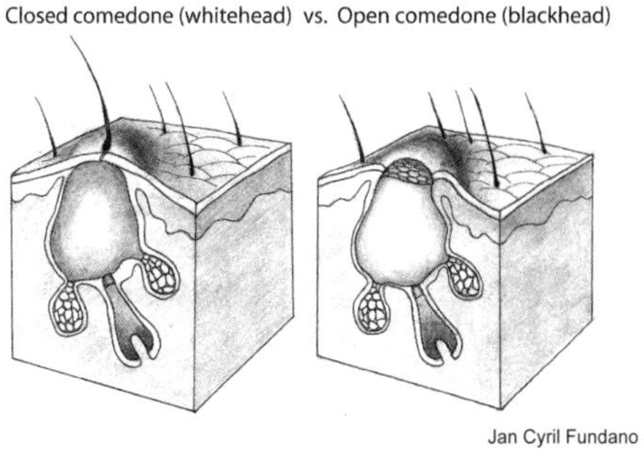

Figure 7. Closed vs. Open Comedones

Specific Investigations

- Most cases do not require any investigations; diagnosis can be made based on history and inspection
- Investigations to rule out other conditions may include:
  - Testosterone
  - DHEAS
  - Sex-hormone binding globulin, prolactin, FSH/LH

Pathogenesis

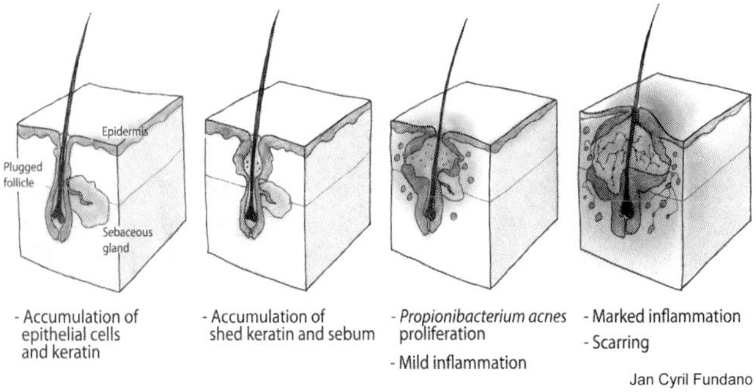

Figure 8. Pathogenesis of Acne Vulgaris
Fitzpatrick T, Johnson RA, Wolff K, Suurmond R. *Color Atlas & Synopsis of Clinical Dermatology: Common and Serious Conditions*. New York: McGraw-Hill; 2001.

> **Clinical Pearl: Acne**
> Emotional stress and mechanical pressure can exacerbate acne; contrary to popular belief, chocolate and fatty foods do not.

Treatment

First Line

- Behavioral changes
  - Cleanse face daily, but not aggressively
  - Use noncomedogenic sunblocks and facial products
- Topical agents
  - Benzoyl peroxide: 2.5-10%
  - Azelaic acid
  - Antibiotic: clindamycin, erythromycin
  - Topical retinoids (Vitamin A acid derivatives; unplugs sebaceous gland)
  - Contraindicated in pregnancy
  - Some deactivated by the sun
  - Benzoyl peroxide, azelaic acid, and a topical antibiotic can be used in combination

Second Line

- Anti-inflammatory oral antibiotics: tetracycline, doxycycline, minocycline, erythromycin
- In women
  - Oral contraceptive
  - Androgen-blocking medication: spironolactone
- Red and blue light therapy is controversial

Third Line

- Systemic isotretinoin (Accutane®)
  - 16-20 wk course

- 70-80% clear after single course
- Teratogenic; female patients must use two forms of contraception
- Monitor monthly: CBC, triglycerides, liver function tests
- Especially important to monitor β-hCG monthly

Variants of Acne

- **Hormonal Acne**
  - Women in high-androgen state
  - Acne along jaw line
  - Associated with: hirsutism, polycystic ovarian syndrome, irregular periods, metabolic syndrome, infertility
- **Neonatal Acne**
  - 20% of newborns
  - Appears at 2 wk, clear by 3 mo
- **Infantile Acne**
  - Appears at 3 mo, clear by 6 mo
- **Acne Conglobata**
  - Acne with systemic symptoms: fever, myalgias, arthralgias
  - Severe, explosive, inflammatory, and nodular acne

> **Clinical Pearl: Psychosocial Effects of Acne[3]**
> The social, psychological, and emotional impairment that can result from acne has been reported to be similar to that associated with epilepsy, asthma, diabetes, and arthritis.

DERMATOLOGY

4.2 Rosacea

- A chronic condition characterized by facial erythema, typically beginning across the cheeks, nose, and forehead. It can also affect the ears, scalp, or neck. In most cases it is a medically harmless condition, although it may greatly affect quality of life

> **Clinical Pearl: Acne vs. Rosacea[4]**
> Compared to acne, rosacea usually occurs in older patients and lacks comedones, nodules, cysts, or scarring. Patients may have both rosacea and acne. The presence of facial flushing, which is provoked by heat, alcohol, or spicy food helps distinguish rosacea from acne.

- Epidemiology[2]: found in all skin types, but most common in those with fair skin; female > male, usual age of onset is 30-50 yr, with peak incidence between 40-50 yr
- Exacerbating Factors[2]: hot food/drink, spices, alcohol (especially red wine), sun exposure

> **Clinical Pearl: Rosacea and Social Stigma**
> Common misconception that both the facial redness and the rhinophyma associated with rosacea are due to excessive alcohol consumption makes rosacea a socially stigmatizing condition for many patients.

- Lesion[2]:
  - Vascular component: erythema, flushing, blushing, and telangiectasia (visible dilatation of dermal venules)
  - Eruptive component: papules and pustules
- Distribution[2]: eruptions on the forehead, cheeks, nose, chin
- Associated Symptoms[2]: mild conjunctivitis with soreness, grittiness, and lacrimation; chronic, deep inflammation of the nose leading to irreversible hypertrophy in men (known as rhinophyma)

> **Clinical Pearl: Rosacea and Ocular Changes[1]**
> Ocular changes are present in more than 50% of patients.

- Clinical Diagnosis[2]: bacterial culture to rule out folliculitis, KOH test to rule out tinea, biopsy to rule out SLE if not responsive to standard therapy

4.3 Dermatitis/Eczema

- Noninfectious inflammation of the skin accompanied by edema and blistering

Contact Dermatitis

- Generic term for acute or chronic inflammatory reaction to substances which contact the skin (endogenous and exogenous agents)
- **Irritant Contact Dermatitis:** caused by exposure to chemical irritant; given enough exposure, all individuals react to irritants
- **Allergic Contact Dermatitis:** caused by antigen with type IV (cell mediated/delayed-type) hypersensitivity reaction (e.g. reaction to poison ivy)
- Common Allergens: nickel, chromate, cobalt, rubber additives in gloves and shoes, preservatives in water-based cosmetics, fragrances, dyes
- Lesion:
  - Vesicles, edema, erythema, extreme pruritus, papules, scale
  - Bullae may be present
- Distribution (for both irritant and allergic contact dermatitis):
  - Appearance at a specific site suggests contact with certain objects
  - Hands, forearms, and face
  - Usually first confined to the area of exposure
  - Distributed in linear streaks if caused by plants
  - May be patchy and asymmetric if caused by topical products
  - In chronic exposure, may spread beyond the area of contact

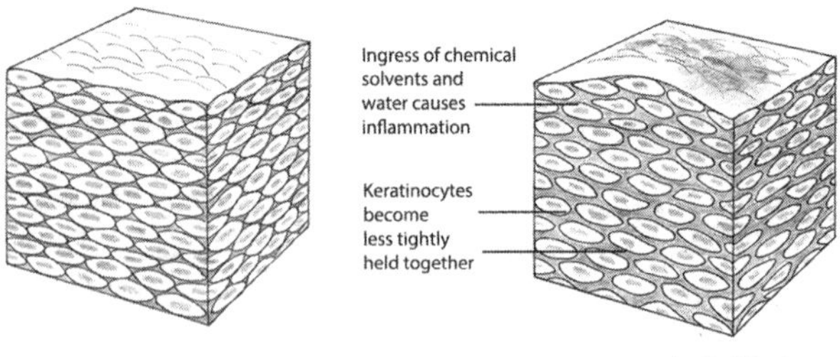

Figure 9. Skin Changes in Eczematous Skin

Atopic Dermatitis/Eczema

- A skin disorder defined by the presence of 4 of the following major diagnostic criteria:
  - Pruritus
  - Young age of onset
  - Typical morphology and distribution
  - Chronic and relapsing course
  - Personal or family history of atopy: asthma, allergic rhinoconjunctivitis

DERMATOLOGY

- Aggravated by contact irritants, allergens, perspiration, excessive heat, stress
- Lesion:
  - Papular lesions with erythema, scale, and severe pruritus
  - Acute lesions may be oozing and vesicular
  - Subacute lesions: scaly and crusted
  - Chronic lesions: dull red and lichenified
- Distribution (varies with age):
  - **Infantile** (2 mo-2 yr): often exudative lesions: cheeks, perioral area, scalp, around ears, extensor surfaces of feet and elbows; spares the diaper area if present on the body
  - **Childhood** (2-12 yr): flexural involvement: antecubital and popliteal fossae, neck, wrists, and ankles
  - **Adult:** flexural involvement, hands, face

4.4 Psoriasis

- Chronic, noninfectious, inflammatory condition with increased epidermal cell proliferation (epidermal turnover reduced to 4 days)
- Recurrent exacerbations and remissions; may be associated with arthritis
- Epidemiology[2]: equal sex incidence; onset at any age but has bimodal peaks in 20s/30s and 50s/60s
- Etiology: recognized familial genetic component (FHx is important)
- Lesion:
  - Well-demarcated, erythematous (red or salmon-pink) plaques topped with silvery scales; redness is constant
  - May bleed when scales detached (Auspitz's sign)
  - Symmetrical distribution
  - Classical presentation involves elbows, knees, sacrum, and scalp
- Margins:
  - Extensor > flexor surfaces
  - Scalp: scaling is very dense and may be very thick
  - Nails (matrix or nail bed involvement): pitting, onycholysis (separation of nail from nail bed), discoloration (oily or salmon-pink)
  - Nail changes support diagnosis if skin changes are questionable or absent

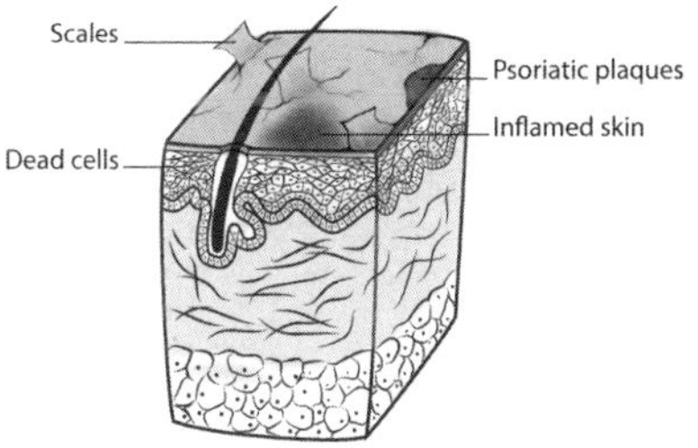

Figure 10. Skin Changes in Psoriasis

- Precipitating Factors:
  - **Koebner Phenomenon:** trauma to epidermis and dermis (e.g. scratching)
  - Infection: streptococcal pharyngitis (for guttate psoriasis)
  - Drugs: β-blockers, lithium, antimalarials
  - Stress, dry winter weather, possibly alcohol and smoking
- Associated Conditions: psoriatic arthritis, increased cardiovascular disease risk factors, DM, obesity, depression, IBD

DERMATOLOGY

Eruptive/Guttate Psoriasis (Youths and Adolescents)

- Acute symmetrical appearance of small, bright red, well-demarcated "drop-like" lesions on trunk and limbs
- Streptococcal pharyngitis may stimulate first episode: confirm presence of streptococci; may be widespread
- May develop rapidly; may disappear spontaneously in 2-3 mo
- DDx: secondary syphilis (no malaise, lymphadenopathy, or may see lesions on palms and soles), pityriasis rosea (light pink, scaling only around the edge of plaques)

Flexural Psoriasis (Elderly)

- Located in the axillae, submammary flexures, or other intertriginous areas
- Scales may only be present on the edge

Pustular Psoriasis

- In contrast to regular psoriasis, pustules, not papules are predominant in two subtypes:
  - Localized pustular psoriasis (*pustulosis palmaris et plantaris*)
    - Palmoplantar pustules: chronic, relapsing eruption on palms and soles
    - Pustules can be white, yellow, orange, or brown; do not rupture – turn brown and scaly as they reach the surface
  - Generalized pustular psoriasis (Von Zumbusch)
    - Life threatening, rare, and serious: requires immediate hospitalization
    - Small, sterile, yellow pustules on bright red, burning erythematous background
    - Rapid spread
    - Accompanied by acute fever, malaise, leukocytosis, "toxic" appearance

> **Clinical Pearl: Psoriasis**
> In psoriasis, pustules on the palms and soles vary in color; this can help distinguish localized psoriasis from both tinea and eczema (which have uniform color).

4.5 Fungal Infections

Cutaneous Fungal "Ringworm" Infections

- Due to dermatophytes (*Trichophyton*, *Microsporum*, *Epidermophyton*)

Table 4. Forms of Cutaneous Fungal Infections

Infection	Lesion Description	Lesion Location
Tinea Capitis	Annular patches of alopecia with surface scaling	Invasion of stratum corneum and hair shaft on scalp
Tinea Corporis	Annular lesions in a classic ringworm pattern begin as flat scaly spots; develop a raised advancing border extending in all directions with central clearing; lesions can coalesce	Trunk and limbs, face (Tinea faciei), beard (Tinea barbae)
Tinea Cruris (Jock Itch)	Often bilateral beginning in the crural fold; half-moon red plaque with a well-defined scaling border advancing onto thigh	Groin: moist environment with excessive sweating/itching

Table 4. Forms of Cutaneous Fungal Infections (continued)

Infection	Lesion Description	Lesion Location
Tinea Pedis (Athlete's Foot)	Classic ringworm pattern: scaly advancing border, may present with an acute vesicular eruption	Plantar surface/dorsum of foot, soles of feet, interdigital: toe webs between 4th and 5th digits

Fitzpatrick T, Johnson RA, Wolff K, Suurmond R. *Color Atlas & Synopsis of Clinical Dermatology: Common and Serious Conditions*. New York: McGraw-Hill; 2001.

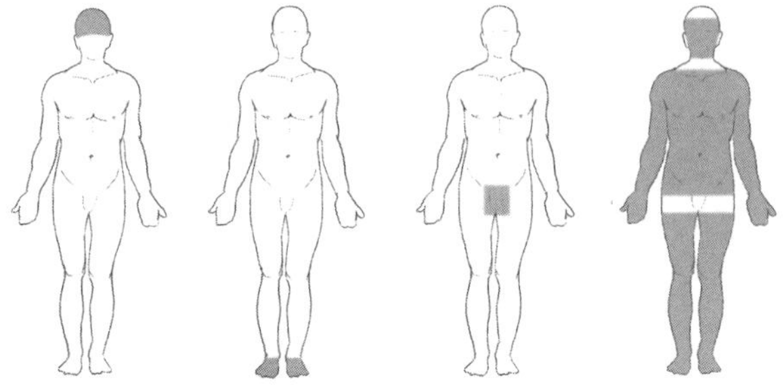

Figure 11. Distribution of Tinea Infections

Tinea Versicolor
- Common infection caused by the yeast *Malassezia spp.* (commensal flora)
- Epidemiology: adolescents and young adults, often first noticed after sun exposure
- Characteristics: pruritic but usually asymptomatic; may be infectious
- Risk Factors: adrenalectomy, Cushing's disease, pregnancy, malnutrition, burns, corticosteroid therapy, immunosuppression, oral contraceptives
- Lesion:
  - Multiple, small, circular macules with superficial, subtle scale
  - Hypopigmented or hyperpigmented, minimally scaly papules
- Distribution: upper trunk, upper arms, neck, abdomen
- Clinical Diagnosis: scale scrapings for culture; Wood's light: irregular, pale, yellow-to-white fluorescence which in some cases fades with improvement

4.6 Cysts
- Cysts can contain air, fluid, or semi-solid material; if pus is present then considered an abscess
- Most cysts in body are benign; however, a few have potential to become malignant (e.g. dermoid cysts)

> **Clinical Pearl: Scraping vs. Biopsy**
> If it scales, scrape it. Biopsy *thick* skin.

DERMATOLOGY

Table 5. Differentiating Cysts

Type	Description	Signs and Symptoms
Epidermal	Cyst from follicular origin; keratin-containing cyst lined by squamous epithelium; most common cutaneous cyst; youth to middle age	Present on parts of body with little hair; round, flesh-colored and slow growing, firm and mobile nodule; punctum often visible
Pilar	Keratin-containing cysts that form in hair follicles; second most common	Present most often on scalp; smooth, hard and mobile, can be tender; do not have central punctum
Dermoid	Cystic lesion often filled with skin and/or skin appendages and other mature tissue	Most common location is at the lateral third of eyebrow or midline under nose (along embryonal cleft closure lines); grow slowly and nontender
Ganglion	Cyst filled with clear, gelatinous fluid that originated from joint or tendon sheath; female > male; usually found in older patients	Around joints and tendons; solitary, rubbery, and translucent

Fitzpatrick T, Johnson RA, Wolff K, Suurmond R. *Color Atlas & Synopsis of Clinical Dermatology: Common and Serious Conditions*. New York: McGraw-Hill; 2001.

4.7 Scars

- Scars are a natural part of the healing process (**Figure 12** illustrates a simple scar that is flat and pale)
- Two additional types of scars can result from the overproduction of collagen (see **Table 6**)
- Epidemiology: keloid scars are more common in people with darker skin types and there may be a familial tendency
- Can be caused by surgery, trauma, or body piercing

Table 6. Hypertrophic vs. Keloid Scars

Scar Type	Description	Distinguishing Features
Hypertrophic	Erythematous, pruritic, raised lesion	Does not grow beyond boundaries of original wound
Keloid	Dense, thick nodules, can be single or multiple	Grows beyond boundaries of original wound

Fitzpatrick T, Johnson RA, Wolff K, Suurmond R. *Color Atlas & Synopsis of Clinical Dermatology: Common and Serious Conditions*. New York: McGraw-Hill; 2001.

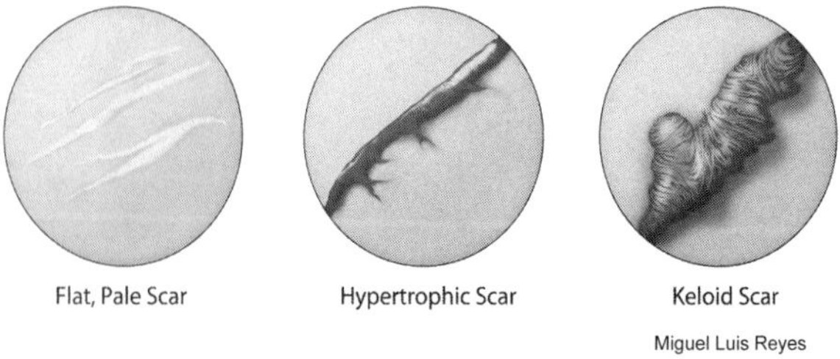

Figure 12. Type of Scar
Fitzpatrick T, Johnson RA, Wolff K, Suurmond R. *Color Atlas & Synopsis of Clinical Dermatology: Common and Serious Conditions*. New York: McGraw-Hill; 2001.

4.8 Nevi

- Epidemiology: nevi (which are often referred to as moles) are very common (most people have 10-40 nevi)
- Lesion:
  - Color: pink, tan, brown, or flesh-colored; may darken with sun exposure
  - Shape: flat or raised
  - Can change over time
- Distribution: over entire body
- Classification (see **Figure 13**):
  - **Junctional Nevi:** usually flat with dark brown color; appear in childhood and adolescence; nevus cells are found at the dermal-epidermal junction
  - **Compound Nevi:** slightly raised with less intense color than junctional nevi; the nevus cells are migrating into the dermis
  - **Dermal Nevi:** dome-shaped papules with even less pigmentation; nevus cells are completely within the dermis
  - **Melanocytic Nevi:** usually appear in adolescence and have dysplastic features

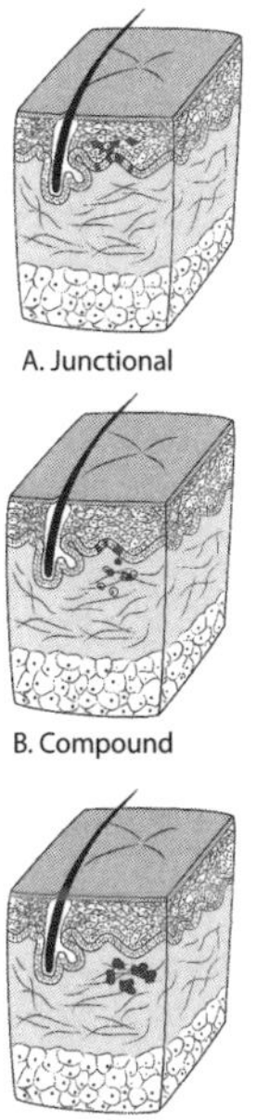

Bonnie Tang

Figure 13. Types of Nevi

4.9 Alopecia

- Definition: hair loss
- Investigative Blood Tests: CBC, thyroid function tests, ferritin
- Hair Pull Test: Pull gently on a group of hairs (40-60) from proximal to distal end. Normally less than 3 hairs come out with each pull. If more than 10% come out, the pull test is positive

> **Clinical Pearl: Telogen Hair Loss[5]**
> The scalp loses approximately 100 telogen hairs per day.

Nonscarring Alopecias
- Usually no scalp symptoms
- Follicular openings can all be seen

Androgenic Alopecia
- Epidemiology: males may begin any time after puberty, females later (40% of cases occur in 60s)[2]
- Pull test: negative
- With dermatoscope: progressive miniaturization (thinning) of hair shafts
- Males: androgens have essential role
  - Hair loss starts in temples and/or vertex
- Women: androgens do not have same defined role
  - Slow thinning over frontal and mid-scalp (front hair line usually not lost)
- Treatment:
  - Males:
    - Minoxidil 2-5%
    - Oral finasteride
    - Hair transplantation
  - Females:
    - Minoxidil 2-5%
    - Androgen-blocking medication (spironolactone, oral contraceptive)
    - Hair transplantation

Alopecia Areata
- Epidemiology: young onset (<25 yr), equal in both sexes
- Relatively common; about 1% of population has at least one episode by age 50 yr
- Circular areas of scalp hair loss for >5 mo
- Pull test: positive early on
- Etiology: autoimmune attack at level of hair
  - Can be associated with other autoimmune diseases (thyroid disease, vitiligo)
- Treatment: none (can resolve on its own), topical steroids, intralesional steroid injections

Telogen Effluvium
- Diffuse loss all over scalp for many mo
- Pull test: positive
- Etiology:
  - Hair follicles shifted into telogen/shedding stage
  - Three months after some trigger (e.g. surgery, pregnancy, endocrine, nutritional, drugs)
- Treatment: treat underlying cause, reassure patient that hair will grow back

Scarring Alopecias
- Usually has scalp symptoms (itching, burning, pain)
- Follicular openings cannot be seen

Central Centrifugal Cicatricial Alopecia
- Almost always occurring in African-American patients
- No scalp symptoms
- Central hair loss, starting at vertex and moving outward
- Possible contributing factors are styling techniques such as tight braids, extensions, and relaxing chemicals
- Treatment: steroids (topical and injections), immunomodulators

4.10 Common Pediatric Dermatologic Skin Conditions
- See **Pediatric Exam**, p.285

4.11 Common Skin Malignancies

Basal Cell Carcinoma (BCC)

- Most common primary skin malignancy (>75% of skin malignancies)[2]
- Increased prevalence in patients >40 yr, male > female
- Clinical variants: sclerosing, noduloulcerative, superficial, and pigmented
- Characterized by local destruction and slow growth
- Risk Factors: chronic sun exposure, ionizing radiation
- Rarely metastatic but local tissue destruction can be debilitating
- Distribution: face (80%), scalp, ears, neck; less often on sun-exposed areas of the trunk and extremities; rarely on the dorsum of the hand

Squamous Cell Carcinoma (SCC)

- Second most common primary skin malignancy
- Primarily in elderly, male > female
- Clinical variants: keratoacanthoma (low-grade SCC), SCC *in situ* (Bowen's disease)
- Risk Factors: chronic sun exposure, immunosuppression, HPV
- More rapid enlargement and more likely to metastasize than BCC
- Clinically looks like crusted nodule with erythematous base

Malignant Melanoma (MM)

- Most serious cutaneous malignancy
- Potentially curable, thus early diagnosis is important
- All pigmented lesions should be examined periodically: 30% of melanomas develop from a pre-existing nevus, 70% develop *de novo*[6]
- Early signs (see **Table 7** and **Figure 14**)
- Early Symptom: nonspecific pruritus
- Later Symptoms: tenderness, bleeding, ulceration
- Associated Symptom: regional lymphadenopathy; sentinel node biopsy is an important factor in determining prognosis

Table 7. Two Scales for Assessing Signs of Melanoma and When to Refer

Checklist	ABCD(E)	7-Point
Criteria	**A**symmetry: Overall shape is asymmetrical **B**order: Uneven edges **C**olor: Heterogenous color, two or more shades **D**iameter: >6 mm **E**volution: Changes or grows over time	Major (2 points each): • Irregular color • Irregular shape • Change in size Minor (1 point each): • Diameter >7 mm • Inflammation • Crusting/bleeding • Sensory changes
Refer	When one or more of the above is present	Point score of 3 or more
Sensitivity	92-100%	79-100%
Specificity	98%	30-37%

Goldstein BG, Goldstein AO. 2001. *Am Fam Physician* 63(7):1359-1368.
Whited JD, Grichnik JM. 1998. *JAMA* 279(9):696-701.

Superficial Spreading Melanoma (>50%)

- Most common form of melanoma
- Affects mainly caucasians
- Distribution on trunk and extremities; spreads laterally
- Lesions >6 mm, flat, asymmetric with varying coloration: ulcerate and bleed with growth

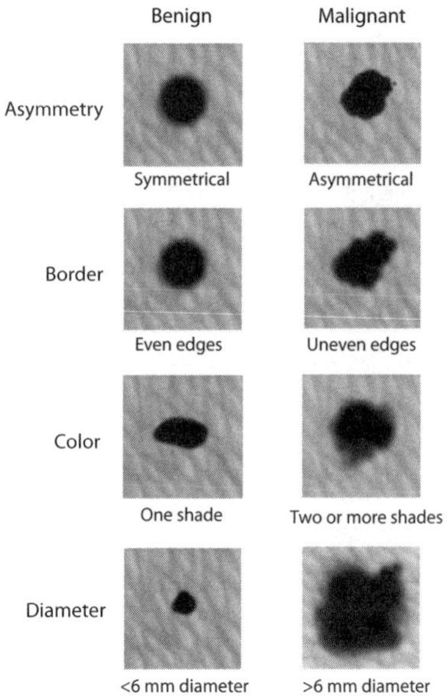

Bonnie Tang

Figure 14. Visual Depiction of ACBD Checklist
Whited JD, Grichnik JM. 1998. *JAMA* 279(9):696-701.

Nodular Melanoma (30%)
- Extremities; extends vertically: rapidly fatal
- Lesions are elevated, appear rapidly, and develop papules
- May be accompanied by local hemorrhage

Lentigo Maligna Melanomas (15%)
- Affects older Caucasian patients with a history of chronic sun exposure
- Distribution: face, neck, dorsal arms
- Lesions: flat and irregular in shape, brown in color but mottled; nodules and ulceration may indicate local invasion

Acral Lentiginous Melanoma (5%)
- Occurs mainly on the extremities
- Most common type of melanoma in darker skinned individuals

> **Clinical Pearl: Melanoma[5]**
> Not all black-blue pigmentation is due to melanoma (e.g. benign blue nevus).

Premalignant Skin Tumors
- May transform into malignancies and should be carefully monitored

Table 8. Precursors to Malignant Tumors

Malignant Tumor	Precursors
Basal Cell Carcinoma	Actinic keratosis, rarely nevus sebaceous
Squamous Cell Carcinoma	Actinic keratosis
Melanoma	Multiple "dysplastic" nevi or giant/congenital hairy nevi (>20 cm in diameter)
Melanoma	Lentigo maligna

Skin Cancer Risk Factors

1. Personal or FHx of skin cancer
2. Immunosuppression
3. Sun exposure, tanning bed use
4. Nevi[7]
   - 1+ giant congenital nevi (>20 cm)
   - >5 atypical nevi
   - >50 normal nevi
5. Skin phenotype: Fitzpatrick Skin Type I or II

Table 9. Fitzpatrick Skin Phenotypes

Skin Type	Skin Color	Characteristics
I	White, very fair; red/blond hair; blue eyes	Always burns, never tans
II	White, fair; red/blond hair; blue/hazel/green eyes	Usually burns, tans with difficulty
III	Cream white; fair with any eye or hair color	Sometimes mild burn, gradually tans
IV	Brown	Rarely burns, tans with ease
V	Dark brown	Very rarely burns, tans very easily
VI	Black	Never burns, tans very easily

Erian A. *Advanced Surgical Facial Rejuvenation: Art and Clinical Practice*. New York: Springer; 2012.

4.12 Sun Safety

UVA vs. UVB

- Mnemonic: UV**A** = aging, UV**B** = burning
- UVA
  - Penetrates deep into the dermis
  - Rays go through windows
  - Leads to premature skin aging (lentigines, wrinkles, leathery skin)
  - Lentigines are commonly known as sunspots, age spots, or liver spots
  - Suppresses immune system
  - Indirectly leads to skin cancer
- UVB
  - Burns the superficial layers of the epidermis, leading to traditional erythematous sunburn
  - Intensity of rays vary by season, location, and time of day
  - Directly leads to skin cancer

Sunscreen

- Broad-spectrum sunscreen (both UVA and UVB protection) of SPF (Sun Protection Factor) 30 or higher[8]
- SPF measures protection from UVB only (not UVA)
- Moisturizers and cosmetics with SPF protect from UVB only
- Sunscreen application:
  - Best applied liberally (1 teaspoon for face, 1 shot glass full for body)
  - Best reapplied every 2 h

> **Clinical Pearl: Sun Protection**
> In addition to using sunscreen, sun protection includes wearing sun-protective clothing (such as a hat, long-sleeved clothing, and sunglasses), avoiding direct exposure to the sun between 9 AM and 3 PM, and avoiding tanning.

Clinical Pearl: Skin Cancer and Tanning Beds[9]
Skin cancer risk increases over 75% when tanning bed use occurs before age 30.

4.13 Dermatologic Emergencies

Dermatologic Emergencies with Key Features

Clinical Pearl: Dermatologic Emergencies[5]
Suspect dermatologic emergency with skin pain, fever, mucosal blisters and lesions, or if patient is systemically unwell.

Angioedema: well-circumscribed areas of edema[9-11]

- Acute swelling usually of the face, extremities, or genitalia
- 10-25% of cases due to ACE inhibitor (ACEI) drugs
- Management: airway patency; cool, moist compresses; antihistamines

Exfoliative Erythroderma: erythematous skin eruption involving more than 90% of the cutaneous surface[9-11]

- Fluid and protein loss through the skin can lead to life-threatening hypotension, electrolyte imbalance, CHF, and enteropathy
- Management: supportive therapy, skin care involves emollients and compresses as well as topical corticosteroid therapy and antihistamines for pruritus

DERMATOLOGY

Meningococcemia: abrupt onset of morbiliform (maculopapular) or petechial rash and "flu-like" symptoms (fever, chills, malaise, and disorientation)[9-11]

- Altered mental status
- Petechial rash on the extremities and trunk (50-60% of cases)
- Irritability
- Neck stiffness
- Pustules, bullae, and hemorrhagic lesions with central necrosis
- Stellate purpura with characteristic central gunmetal-gray hue
- Upper respiratory tract infection
- Management: obtain blood cultures; supportive management and therapy with third generation cephalosporin or intravenous penicillin G therapy (chloramphenicol if patient allergic to penicillin)

Necrotizing Fasciitis: diffuse swelling of affected skin area followed by the development of bullae which becomes burgundy in color[9-11]

- Suspect if signs of severe sepsis are present or local symptoms and signs (severe pain, indurated edema, skin hyperesthesia, crepitation, muscle weakness, and foul-smelling exudate)
- Erythema, edema, and tenderness beyond lesion borders
- Smooth, swollen area that evolves into dusky plaques and late-stage full thickness necrosis with hemorrhagic bullae
- Black eschar that sloughs off
- Crepitus
- Dusky blue discoloration
- Fever and chills
- Hypotension; numbness over affected area
- Pain out of proportion to physical findings and precede skin findings by 24-48 h
- Violaceous bullae
- Management: aggressive management of sepsis and surgical debridement of necrotic tissue

Rocky Mountain Spotted Fever: petechial lesions that start on ankles and wrists, and then spread centrally to trunk and face

- 60% of patients present with fever, headache, and rash following tick bite
- Abdominal pain (mainly in children), fever, headache (almost all adults)
- Involvement of palms and soles
- Maculopapular rash
- Management: symptomatic support and antibiotic treatment (doxycycline); tick should be removed if embedded in the skin

Stevens-Johnson Syndrome (<10% Body Surface Area) and Toxic Epidermal Necrolysis (>30% Body Surface Area): skin tenderness, erythema, epidermal necrosis, and desquamation[9-11]

- Prodrome: fever, stinging eyes, and pain on swallowing followed by development of dusky erythematous macules that form into flaccid blisters
- Erythema and erosion of mucous membranes (buccal, genital, and ocular)
- Epidermal detachment is common
- Erythroderma and hypotension
- Atypical target lesions with central dusky purpura
- Bullae and blister formation
- Fever, malaise, headache, cough, and conjunctivitis 3 d before rash
- Mucosal and conjunctival findings are red flags
- Involvement of palms and soles
- Painful burning
- Positive Nikolsky sign (exfoliation of skin when rubbed)
- Sloughing and erosion; spreads from face downward to entire body
- Tachycardia
- Rapid progression
- Can present at any age
- Common Triggers: allopurinol, antiepileptics, penicillins, tetracyclines, sulfonamides, and NSAIDs
- Management: supportive measures including removal of offending agent and admission to burn unit

Toxic Shock Syndrome: rapid onset of generalized erythema with desquamation[9-11]

- Prodrome: 2-3 d of malaise and patient presents usually with fever, chills, nausea, and abdominal pain
- Rash initially appears on trunk and spreads peripherally to palms and soles
- Erythema and edema of palms and soles
- Diffuse "sunburn" rash with desquamation over one to two wk
- High fever
- Hyperemia of conjunctiva and mucous membranes
- Hypotension
- Strawberry tongue (inflamed red papillae on tongue)
- Occurs in menstruating women who use tampons and in postsurgical settings
- Management: supportive management and obtain culture specimens; treat with β-lactamase-resistant anti-staphylococcal antibiotic

Clinical Pearl: Disseminated Varicella
Disseminated varicella presents as widespread, discrete vesicles or papulovesicles. Early treatment with I.V. acyclovir is life-saving.

Conditions that Mimic Dermatologic Emergencies

Red Skin

- More itchy than painful: allergic contact dermatitis
- Itchy, lower extremities: stasis dermatitis
- Sun-exposed area: sunburn
- Emergencies: necrotizing fasciitis; Stevens-Johnson syndrome and toxic epidermal necrolysis; toxic shock syndrome[9-11]

Desquamation

- Localized with no systemic manifestations: bullous impetigo
- Emergencies: Stevens-Johnson syndrome and toxic epidermal necrolysis; toxic shock syndrome[9-11]

Petechiae and Purpura

- Trauma
- Healthy appearance: pigmented purpuric dermatosis; viral exanthema
- Emergencies: meningococcemia; Rocky Mountain spotted fever[9-11]

Generalized Pruritus

- In the absence of rash and dry skin may be due to a systemic cause[12]:
  - **Hematologic Disorders:** iron deficiency anemia, myeloproliferative disorders, monoclonal gammopathy, and multiple myeloma and lymphoma
  - **Renal Disorders:** uremia
  - **Liver Disorders:** cholestasis
  - **Endocrine Disorders:** hyperthyroidism or hypothyroidism

> **Clinical Pearl: Scabies and Pruritus[5]**
> Always suspect scabies in any patient with severe pruritus.

DERMATOLOGY

Erythema Nodosum

- Symmetric, tender, hot, erythematous nodules over the extensor legs
- Commonly affects young women
- Potential causes: think **NODOSUMM**[9-11]
  - **NO** cause in 50%
  - **D**rugs (bromides, iodides, sulfur drugs)
  - **O**CP (most common drug)
  - **S**arcoidosis
  - **U**lcerative Colitis and Crohn's Disease
  - **M**any Infections (e.g. TB)
  - **M**alignancies (leukemia)
  - Other: pregnancy, Beçhet's disease

> **Clinical Pearl: Sarcoidosis and Erythema Nodosum[5]**
> Consider and exclude sarcoidosis in all cases.

Systemic Diseases (see **Table 10**)

Table 10. Dermatological Manifestations of Systemic Diseases

Systemic Disease	Skin Manifestations
Addison's Disease	Generalized hyperpigmentation
Paget's Disease (Breast)	Persistent unilateral dermatitic-looking lesion on the breast
Cushing's Syndrome	Moon facies, purple striae, acne, hyperpigmentation, hirsutism, atrophic skin with telangiectasias

Table 10. Dermatological Manifestations of Systemic Diseases (continued)

Systemic Disease	Skin Manifestations
Hepatitis C Infection	Cutaneous vasculitis, polyarteritis nodosa, porphyria cutanea tarda, lichen planus, necrolytic acral erythema
HIV	Kaposi's sarcoma, seborrheic dermatitis, psoriasis
Hyperthyroidism	Moist warm skin, seborrheic dermatitis, acne, hirsutism, nail atrophy, onycholysis
Hypothyroidism	Cool dry scaly thickened skin, toxic alopecia, coarse hair, brittle nails
Liver Disease	Spider nevi, palmar erythema, alopecia
Rheumatic Fever	Nodules over bony prominences, erythema marginatum
SLE	Malar erythema, discoid rash, patchy/diffuse alopecia, photosensitivity
Thyroid Carcinoma	Sipple's syndrome: multiple mucosal neuromas
Inflammatory Bowel Disease	Pyoderma gangrenosum, erythema nodosum

Fitzpatrick T, Johnson RA, Wolff K, Suurmond R. *Color Atlas & Synopsis of Clinical Dermatology: Common and Serious Conditions*. New York: McGraw-Hill; 2001.

DERMATOLOGY

4.14 Drug-Induced Skin Reactions

Stevens-Johnson Syndrome and Toxic Epidermal Necrolysis (see **Dermatologic Emergencies**, p.417)

Exanthematous Reactions: bright red rash and skin may feel hot, burning or itchy

- Erythema, or morbilliform (maculopapular) lesions
- Location: often start on the trunk and also often involve extremities and intertriginous areas; face may be spared
- Common Causative Drugs: allopurinol, antimicrobials, barbiturates, captopril, carbamazepine, furosemide, gold salts, lithium, phenothiazines, phenylbutazone, phenytoin, thiazides

Urticaria: hives present as raised, itchy, red blotches or wheals that are pale in the center and red around the outside

- Common Causative Drugs: NSAIDs including Aspirin® and pharmaceutical excipients
- Urticaria has many causes that do not include medications

Erythroderma and Exfoliative Dermatitis: widespread confluent erythematous rash often associated with desquamation

- Systemic symptoms may be present such as fever, lymphadenopathy, and anorexia
- Common Causative Drugs: chloroquine, isoniazid, penicillin, phenytoin, sulfonamides

Fixed Drug Eruption: erythematous round or oval lesions of a reddish, dusky purple or brown color, sometimes featuring blisters, either bullae or vesicles

- Location: within hours at the same site; frequently hands, feet, tongue, penis, or perianal areas
- Common Causative Drugs: ACEIs, allopurinol, antimicrobials, barbiturates, benzodiazepines, calcium channel blockers, carbamazepine, dextromethorphan, diltiazem, fluconazole, lamotrigine, NSAIDs, proton pump inhibitors

Acne: papulopustular but comedones are often absent

- Common Causative Drugs: think "**B PIMPLES**"
  - **B**romides (halides, iodides)
  - **P**henytoin
  - **I**soniazid
  - **M**oisturizers
  - **P**rednisone
  - **L**ithium
  - **E**GFR inhibitors
  - **S**ystemic hormones (androgens, OCPs)

Psoriasis: erythematous plaques with large dry silvery scales

- Common Causative Drugs: ACEIs, β-blockers, chloroquine and hydroxychloroquine, digoxin, lithium, NSAIDs, tetracyclines, TNF-α antagonists

Management of Drug-Induced Reactions

- Accurate medication history including all recent medications and OTC medicines, herbal and homeopathic preparations
- Note the times when medications taken and if patient has taken medications before
- Note proprietary and generic name in order to have a record of pharmaceutical excipients
- Record any known or suspect adverse drug reactions with details of cause; advise that future exposure can be avoided and report to relevant regulatory authority

DERMATOLOGY

REFERENCES

1. Koster MI. 2009. Making an epidermis. *Ann N Y Acad Sci* 1170:7-10.
2. Fitzpatrick T, Johnson RA, Wolff K, Suurmond R. *Color Atlas & Synopsis of Clinical Dermatology: Common and Serious Conditions*. New York: McGraw-Hill; 2001.
3. Mallon E, Newton JN, Klassen A, Stewart-Brown SL, Ryan TJ, Finlay AY. 1999. The quality of life in acne: A comparison with general medical conditions using generic questionnaires. *Br J Dermatol* 140(4):672-676.
4. Powell FC. 2005. Clinical practice – Rosacea. *N Engl J Med* 352(8):793-803.
5. Shapiro J. 2007. Clinical practice – Hair loss in women. *N Engl J Med* 357(16):1620-1630.
6. Goldstein BG, Goldstein AO. 2001. Diagnosis and management of malignant melanoma. *Am Fam Physician* 63(7):1359-1368.
7. Jerant AF, Johnson JT, Sheridan CD, Caffrey TJ. 2000. Early detection and treatment of skin cancer. *Am Fam Physician* 62(2):357-368.
8. Moyal DD, Fourtanier AM. 2008. Broad spectrum sunscreens provide better protection from solar ultraviolet-simulated radiation and natural sunlight-induced immunosuppression in human beings. *J Am Acad Dermatol* 58(5 Suppl 2):S149-154.
9. Freiman A, Borsuk D, Sasseville D. 2005. Dermatologic emergencies. *CMAJ* 173(11):1317-1319.
10. Usatine RP, Sandy N. 2010. Dermatologic emergencies. *Am Fam Physician* 82(7):773-780.
11. McQueen A, Martin SA, Lio PA. 2012. Derm emergencies: Detecting early signs of trouble. *J Fam Pract* 61(2):71-78.
12. Lee A. 2009. Skin manifestations of systemic disease. *Aust Fam Physician* 38(7):498-505.
13. Lee A, Thomson J. Drug-induced skin reactions. In: Lee A. (Editor). *Adverse Drug Reactions*, 2nd ed. London: Pharmaceutical Press; 2006.
14. Lebwohl MG, Haymann WR, Berth-Jones J, Coulson I. *Treatment of Skin Disease: Comprehensive Therapeutic Strategies*, 2nd ed. London: Elsevier; 2004.

The Essentials of Emergency Medicine

Editors:
William K. Chan
Khaled Ramadan

Faculty Reviewers:
Sev Perelman, MD, MSc, CCFP(EM)
Lisa Thurgur, MD, MSc, MCFP

TABLE OF CONTENTS

EMERGENCY

1. RAPID PRIMARY SURVEY (RPS) OF TRAUMA

In order of priority, **ABCDE**:

- **Airway**
  - Assume cervical spine injury for trauma patient and use collar for immobilization
  - Assess airway (stridor, ability to speak, labored breathing, indrawing, cyanosis, decreased LOC and O_2 desaturation)
  - Basic Airway
    - To open airway: head-tilt or if C-spine injury suspected, use jaw thrust
    - To remove foreign material, sweep and suction
    - Maintain airway: nasopharyngeal airway (contraindicated if suspected basal skull fracture or severe facial trauma) or oropharyngeal airway (contraindicated if gag reflex present)
  - Definitive Airway
    - Indications for intubation:
      - Respiratory failure (e.g. apnea)
      - Airway obstruction/trauma
      - Inability to protect airway (e.g. altered mental status, GCS<8)
      - Potential airway compromise (e.g. profound shock, respiratory fatigue)
      - Intubation must be confirmed with end-tidal CO_2 detector and CXR if possible
    - If intubation not successful:
      - Bag valve mask, laryngeal mask airway (LMA), combitube/King-LTD, bougie

- Consider advanced airway intervention such as GlideScope® bronchoscope
  - » If intubation and ventilation not possible:
    - Cricothyroidotomy or jet ventilation

> **Clinical Pearl: Indications for Intubation (6 P's)**
> **P**atency, **P**rotection, **P**PV (positive pressure ventilation), **P**ulmonary Toilet, **P**harmacology, **P**rolonged Transport.

- **Breathing**
  - Inspect: RR, decreased LOC, anxiety, cyanosis, nasal flaring, pursed-lip breathing, tracheal tug, intercostal indrawing
  - Auscultate: equal breath sounds (including signs of upper airway obstruction: stridor, gurgling), wheezes, crackles
  - Palpate: air flow, tactile fremitus, tracheal shift, chest tenderness, flail segments, sucking chest wound, subcutaneous emphysema
- **Circulation**
  - Shock: insufficient perfusion of organs and tissue with oxygenated blood
  - Treat cause of shock and replace fluids based on % blood volume lost
    - » For details on fluid replacement (see **Essentials of Fluids, Electrolytes, and Acid/Base Disturbances**, p.471)

> **Clinical Pearl: Hypovolemic Shock**
> Hypovolemic shock is the most common type of shock in trauma (early signs include orthostatic changes in HR and BP).

Table 1. Classes of Shock

Class	I	II	III	IV
Respiratory Rate	20	30	35	>45
Pulse	<100	100-120	>120	>140
Blood Pressure	Normal	Normal	↓	↓
Capillary Refill	Normal	↓	↓	↓
% Blood Volume	<15%	15-30%	30-40%	>40%
Fluid Replacement	Crystalloid	Crystalloid	Crystalloid and blood	Crystalloid and blood

- **Disability**
  - Assess LOC using Glasgow coma scale (GCS) or **AVPU** (**A**lert, responds to **V**oice, responds to **P**ain, **U**nresponsive) (see **Table 2**)
  - GCS score: "numbers go low to high with head-to-toe" – eyes (1-4), verbal (1-5), motor (1-6)
    - » Mild disability (13-15)
    - » Moderate disability (9-12)
    - » Severe disability (≤8): "less than 8, intubate"
- **Exposure/Environment**
  - Expose entire body and assess for injuries
  - Avoid hypothermia with warm blankets, warm IV blood/fluids
  - Focused abdominal sonography in trauma (FAST) or emergency department echocardiogram (EDE)

Table 2. Glasgow Coma Scale

Eye Opening		Verbal Response		Motor Response	
Spontaneous	4	Oriented	5	Obeys commands	6
To verbal command	3	Confused	4	Localizes to pain	5
To pain	2	Inappropriate words	3	Withdraws from pain	4
None	1	Incomprehensible sounds	2	Flexion (decorticate)	3
		No verbal response	1	Extension (decer-ebrate)	2
				No response	1

2. SECONDARY SURVEY

A more detailed head-to-toe exam to identify significant injuries and concerns.

2.1 Sample History

- **S**igns and symptoms
- **A**llergies
- **M**edications
- **P**ast medical history
- **L**ast meal
- **E**vents surrounding episode

2.2 Focused Physical Exam

Neurological and Head & Neck

- Evaluate GCS or AVPU
- Evaluate for spinal cord injury: sensory level and motor exam
- Cranial nerve exams
  - Pupillary reactivity and reflex
    - Reactive pupils (symmetrical) + decreased LOC: metabolic/structural cause
    - Nonreactive pupils (or asymmetrical) + decreased LOC: structural cause
  - Extraocular movements, nystagmus
- Fundoscopy
- Assess tympanic membrane for CSF leakage/hemotympanum
- Evaluate for facial trauma
  - Signs of basal skull fracture:
    - Hemotympanum, CSF rhinorrhea, CSF otorrhea
    - Battle's sign (retroauricular hematoma), raccoon eyes (periorbital ecchymosis) (see **Figure 1**)

Chest

- Inspection: contusions, flail segments, symmetrical chest expansion, paradoxical breathing (seesaw respiration in children)
- Palpation: subcutaneous emphysema
- Auscultation: all lung fields

Abdomen/Pelvis

- Assess for intraperitoneal bleeding, acute abdomen (consider acute abdomen if abdominal wall does not move with breathing)
- DRE (look for high-riding or mobile prostate), blood at urethral meatus, bimanual exam

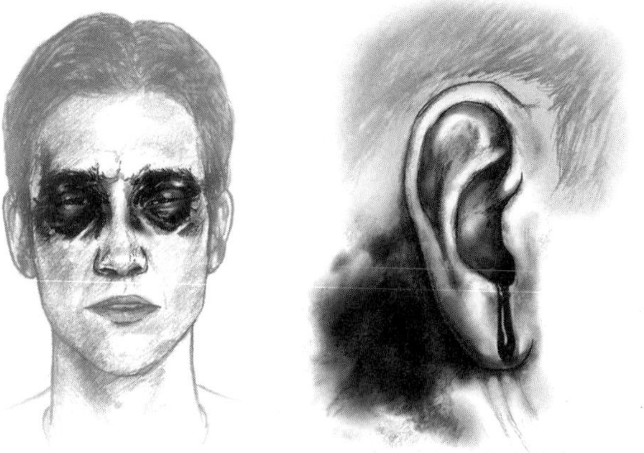

Periorbital ecchymosis Periauricular ecchymosis

Jan Cyril Fundano

Figure 1. Common Signs of a Basal Skull Fracture

MSK

- Log-roll and palpate cervical, thoracic, and lumbar spines for fractures
- Palpate pelvic girdle, pubic symphysis for instability indicating "open-book" fracture
- Extremity exam for fracture and neurovascular status

Investigations

- X-rays: C-, T-, and L-spine, chest, pelvis
- CT scans: head, chest, abdomen, pelvis

> **Clinical Pearl: Canadian CT Head Rules**[1]
> Risk criteria where CT head required
> - High Risk: GCS <15 two h after injury, suspected open/depressed skull fracture, signs of basilar skull fractures, vomiting >2 episodes, age >65 yr
> - Medium Risk: amnesia >30 min, dangerous mechanism (e.g. pedestrian struck by motor vehicle, occupant ejected, fall >3 ft (0.9 m) or 5 stairs)

3. COMMON CLINICAL SCENARIOS

3.1 Anaphylaxis/Anaphylactoid Reaction

Immune response mediated by massive release of histamine, leukotrienes, prostaglandins and tryptase resulting in severe systemic reaction occurring within minutes

- Common agents causing anaphylaxis:
  - IgE-mediated: medications (usually antibiotics), food (e.g. peanuts, tree nuts, shellfish, wheat, milk, eggs, soybeans, nitrates/nitrites), latex, hormones, animal/human proteins, exercise, venom, allergen vaccines, enzymes, polysaccharides, colorants
  - Non-IgE-mediated: intravenous immunoglobulin (IVIg), opioids, physical factors (temperature, exercise), radiocontrast media, ACE inhibitor, quaternary ammonium muscle relaxants, ethylene oxide gas on dialysis tubing, transfusion reaction to cellular elements, psychogenic, idiopathic

History
- Exposure to anaphylactic agent and time of exposure
- Symptoms from exposure
- Past history of allergic/systemic reactions, previous ICU admissions
- Check for allergy-identifying jewellery items and wallet

Clinical Features
- **General:** marked anxiety, tremor, weakness, cold sensation
- **CNS:** weakness, syncope, dizziness, seizures
- **Eyes:** lacrimation, ocular pruritus, conjunctival injection, mydriasis
- **Respiratory:** tachypnea, accessory muscle use, cyanosis, laryngeal edema (lump in throat, hoarseness, stridor), bronchospasm (cough, wheezing, chest tightness, respiratory distress)
- **CVS:** tachycardia, hypotension, chest pain
- **GI:** N/V, crampy abdominal pain, bloody diarrhea
- **Derm:** pruritic urticaria, edema, erythema

Table 3. Clinical Features and Management of Anaphylaxis

Type	Clinical Features	Management
All (General Approach)	• Key presenting features: bronchospasm, upper airway obstruction or laryngeal edema, urticaria or angioedema, vasodilation (e.g. hypotension)	• Prehospital care: Epi-pen and oral antihistamines • IV normal saline • Diphenhydramine • If bronchospasm, β-agonist aerosol (salbutamol) via nebulizer • Histamine blockers • Epinephrine
Mild to Moderate	• Minimal airway edema • Mild bronchospasm • Cutaneous reactions	• Diphenhydramine only • Adults: 50 mg IM or IV q4-6h; Children: 1 mg/kg IM or IV q4-6h
Moderate to Severe	• Laryngeal edema • Severe bronchospasm • Respiratory distress/ arrest • Shock • MI • Arrhythmia	• Diphenhydramine • IM/SC epinephrine: 0.3-0.5 mL of 1:1000 (adults); 0.01-0.4 mL of 1:1000 (children) • Histamine blockers:ranitidine • IV epinephrine if severe: 1 mL of 1:10000 (adult); 0.01 mL/kg (child); repeat every 5-10 min until symptoms resolve • Glucocorticoids as adjunct to epinephrine

IM = intramuscular, SC = subcutaneous

Management
- ABCDE
- Identify and treat responsible agent as soon as anaphylaxis is suspected
  - Should stop all IV meds until responsible agent identified
- IV normal saline
- Medications (see **Table 3**)
  - If administered epinephrine, must also be given steroids and remain 4 h for observation

EMERGENCY

Clinical Pearl: Rule of 5's for Adult Dosing

- Epinephrine: 0.5 mg, 1:1000 IM
- H1 Histamine blockers (diphenhydramine): 50 mg IV
- H2 Histamine blockers (ranitidine): 50 mg IV
- Glucocorticoids (methylprednisolone): 125 mg IV
- β-agonist aerosol (salbutamol): 5 mg in 3 cc normal saline IH

3.2 Hypothermia

Decline in core temperature below 35°C due to increased heat loss (convection, radiation, conduction, evaporation) or decreased heat production (metabolic, toxic, catatonic state)[2,3]

- Primary hypothermia from environmental exposure
- Secondary hypothermia from underlying medical condition which disrupts thermoregulatory mechanism (e.g. bacterial infection, thyroid disease, malnutrition, stroke, DM, spinal cord injury, use of medication or substance which affects CNS)

History

- Age (extremes of age at greatest risk)
- Duration of exposure
- Predisposing Factors: drug or alcohol overdose, toxins, cold water immersion, trauma, outdoor sports, impaired CNS-mediated thermoregulation (hypothalamus, spinal cord injury or surgery), malnutrition, endocrine failure

Table 4. Clinical Features of Hypothermia

Type	°C	Clinical Features	Management
Mild	32-34.9	Lethargy, shivering, tachypnea, tachycardia, altered judgment, ataxia, shivering	Passive rewarming (since thermoregulatory mechanism intact)
Moderate	28-31.9	Stupor, delirium, loss of shiver, dilated pupils, arrhythmias, slowed reflexes, muscle rigidity	Active external rewarming
Severe	<28	Unresponsive, coma, hypotension, fixed pupils, ventricular fibrillation, apnea, areflexia	Active core rewarming

Biem J, Koehncke N, Classen D, Dosman J. 2003. *CMAJ* 168(3):305-311.

Investigations

- ECG: wide QRS, prolonged QT, atrial fibrillation, J or Osborne wave (positive deflection at the J point)
- Blood work: hypoglycemia, hypomagnesemia, hypophosphatemia

Management

- ABCDE
- Secondary survey
- Monitor core temperature: rectal or esophageal temperature probes are most accurate
- Rewarming:
  - Passive
  - Active external (forced air blankets/"bear hugger", heated blanket, heating lamp, warm baths)
  - Active core (warmed humidified oxygen, IV fluids, peritoneal dialysis, irrigation of cavities, cardiopulmonary bypass: most effective and rapid but not readily available)

3.3 Hyperthermia

Increase in core temperature >37.5°C without a change in the body's temperature set-point[2]. This may lead to:

- Dilation of peripheral venous system, increased blood flow to skin, stimulation of sweat glands
- Severe hyperthermia: dehydration with electrolyte abnormalities → dysfunction of thermoregulatory mechanism → multi-system organ failure

Caused by:

- Increased heat production
  - Muscular activity, metabolism, drugs, severe infection
- Decreased heat loss
  - ↓ sweating, ↓ CNS response, ↓ cardiovascular reserve, drugs

History

- Peak ambient temperature
- Insidious onset of symptoms: fatigue, dizziness, irritability, weakness, headache, N/V, myalgias, muscle cramps
- Susceptible individuals have circulatory insufficiency: extremes of age, obesity, dehydration, CHF, diuretics, laxatives
- Excessive heat load: fever, environment, lack of acclimatization, exertional
- Medications: sympathomimetics (e.g. cocaine, ecstasy), lysergic acid diethylamide (LSD), anticholinergics, antihistamines, MAOIs, phencyclidine (PCP), drug or alcohol withdrawal, β-blockers, sympatholytics, anesthetic gases (i.e. malignant hyperthermia)

Table 5. Clinical Features of Heat Disorders

Heat Disorder	Clinical Features	Management
Heat Edema	Vasodilation and venous stasis → swelling of feet and ankles	Elevation of limbs
Heat Syncope	Peripheral pooling of intravascular volume → ↓ preload → orthostatic hypotension → syncope	Rest, cooling, and rehydration
Heat Cramps	Dehydration → salt depletion (Na^+/K^+ shifts) → spasms of voluntary muscles of abdomen and extremities	Fluid and salt replacement
Heat Exhaustion	Prolonged heat exposure → primary water loss or primary sodium loss → dehydration signs; no CNS symptoms	Rehydration and cooling
Heat Stroke	Extremely high body temperature (>40.5°C) → multiorgan dysfunction (e.g. rhabdomyolysis and hepatic damage) including CNS symptoms → altered mental status, confusion, bizarre behavior, hallucinations, disorientation, coma	Rapid reduction in body temperature

Barrow MW, Clark KA. 1998. *Am Fam Physician* 58(3):749-756, 759.

Focused Physical Exam (for Heat Exhaustion and Heat Stroke)

- **General:** fatigue, malaise, sweating (anhidrosis when severe), fever
- **CNS:** confusion/lethargy, weakness, headache, agitation, delirium, seizure, ataxia, coma
- **H&N:** fixed dilated pupils (heat stroke), subconjunctival hemorrhage
- **CVS:** tachycardia, hypotension, dehydration
- **Respiratory:** tachypnea, alkalosis, hemoptysis
- **GI:** N/V, diarrhea ± bright red blood or melena
- **GU:** oliguria or anuria (acute renal failure), hematuria
- **Derm:** dry, warm, diaphoretic, piloerection

Management

- ABCDE
- Cooling measures: convection (fan), evaporation (spray bottle), conduction (ice packs to groin and axillae, gastric lavage, iced peritoneal lavage), cooling blanket

3.4 Burns

History

- Age
- Exposure: duration, type (thermal, chemical, UV, electrical, inhalation), environment (e.g. enclosed space), materials involved (e.g. smoke, fire, carbon monoxide, cyanide poisoning, UV)
- Onset, course, location, and quality of pain
- Associated Symptoms: respiratory illness (persistent cough, wheeze, hoarseness from respiratory burns, soot-stained sputum)
- Comorbid conditions for high risk of secondary infections: immunodeficiency, DM, respiratory illness, renal disease
- Associated injuries (e.g. electrical, blast injury, etc.)

Focused Physical Exam

- Degree of burn assessed by:
  - Burn size: rule of nines for percentage of affected body surface area (BSA) in 2° and 3° burns (see **Figure 2**)
    - Add up all the burned areas of the body that have blisters or worse
  - Burn site: serious injuries if hands/feet, face, eyes, ears, perineum affected

Table 6. Classification of Burns

Burn Depth	Layers Involved	Signs and Symptoms
First Degree	Epidermis	Local erythema, pain
Second Degree	A: Superficial partial thickness B: Deep partial thickness	Blisters and bullae-covered skin that is erythematous, moist, and swollen (intact sensation); hair follicles are preserved
Third Degree	All layers of skin	No sensation, charring if severe/ eschar formation
Fourth Degree	Fat, muscle, bone	

- **H&N:** corneal damage, singed nasal hair, facial charring, mucosal burns
- **Respiratory:** hypoxic, stridor, wheezing, respiratory obstruction (due to inhalational injury), circumferential burns (i.e. eschar)
- **CVS:** cardiac irritability (electrical burns)
- **CNS:** neurologic dysfunction (electrical burns)
- **GU:** genital or perineal burns in children (suspect child abuse)
- **MSK:** reduced joint movement due to scarring over joints, mobility
- **Derm:** minimal surface wounds with extensive deep damage (electrical burns)

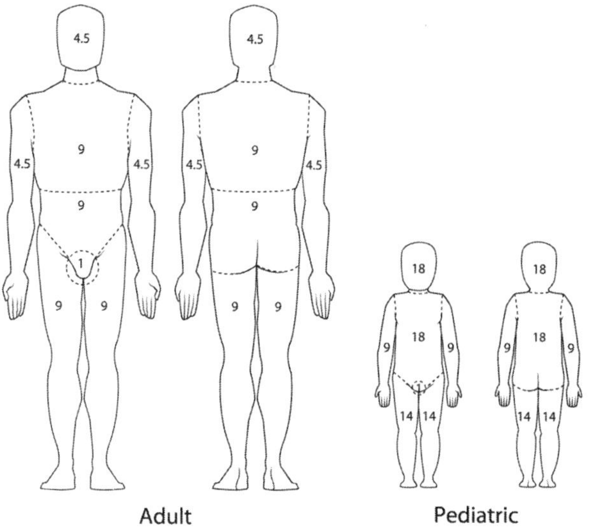

Caitin O'Connell

Figure 2. Rule of Nines

Management

- Airway: Control early with endotracheal tube (ETT) if:
  - Signs of upper airway and laryngeal edema (severe burns to lower face and neck, inhalation of superheated air in confined space, carbonaceous sputum, associated chemical inhalation)
  - Full thickness circumferential chest wall or abdomen involvement: emergency escharotomy if circumferential burns constrict chest movements
- Breathing: O_2 saturation
- Circulation: if hemodynamically unstable, initial fluid resuscitation with NS, then:
  - IV Ringer's lactate using **Parkland** formula:[4]
    - Fluid for first 24 h = Total body surface area burn (%) × Weight (kg) × 4 (mL); give ½ over first 8 h, ½ over next 16 h
    - Target urine output of 0.5-1.0 mL/kg/h
- Correct hyponatremia and hyperkalemia (check ECG for peaked T waves)
- Disposition/drugs/draw bloods/drains: assess GCS, routine bloods and arterial blood gas (ABG)/CO levels, CK if concern for tissue damage/ rhabdomyolysis, lactate if cyanide toxicity is a concern, sedatives/ narcotics as needed, tetanus, Foley catheter, nasogastric (NG) tube
- Expose and secondary survey: dress wounds (irrigation with sterile saline ± dressing to prevent heat loss and infection), evaluate for other associated injuries (e.g. fractures)
- Imaging as needed

3.5 Wound Care

- Establishment of absolute hemostasis (prevent further blood loss and formation of hematoma) before wound care through indirect and direct methods
  - Indirect: elevation of injured part above level of heart, direct pressure over wound or tourniquets for complex injuries, epinephrine-containing solutions (contraindicated in wounds on penis, digits, tip of nose)
  - Direct: ligation, electrocautery, chemical cautery
- Types of injuries: lacerations, bites, puncture wounds, stretch injuries, compression or crush injuries

History

- Time of injury (increased risk of infection if sutured >6 h after time of injury)
- Site of injury, contact with contaminants
  - Less infectious: face, hands
  - More infectious: back, buttocks
- Mechanism of injury, especially crush injuries
- Tetanus immunization status

Focused Physical Exam

- ABCDE
- **MSK:** loss of function in injured part, involvement of underlying structures (e.g. nerves, major blood vessels, ligaments, bones), degree of contamination, foreign body
- **Neuro:** use two-point discrimination on the finger to document nerve status (<4 mm is normal) on each side of the digits

Management

- Assess neurovascular status before using anesthetic agents (lidocaine ± epinephrine) via local infiltration
- Cleansing: irrigation (normal saline), cleaning agent (e.g. iodine, chlorhexidine), mechanical scrubbing
- Debridement
- Wound closure (absorbable or nonabsorbable sutures, steri-strips, steel and metallic clips or staples, wound tapes, wound staples, tissue adhesives)

3.6 Abdominal Pain

Focused History

- Age: related prevalence of different etiologies
- OPQRSTUVW
  - Location and radiation of pain vital for differential (see **Figure 3**)
- Anorexia, N/V
- Constipation, diarrhea
- Fever, rigors
  - Consider referred pain (e.g. cholecystitis causing subscapular pain)

> **Clinical Pearl: Abdominal Pain**
> - Abrupt, severe onset is suggestive of a vascular cause or viscus rupture
> - Gradual onset is more suggestive of inflammatory or infectious causes
> - Crampy, cyclic pain occurring in crescendo-decrescendo cycles may indicate small bowel obstruction
> - Renal colic is NOT a colicky, but rather a constant pain

Focused Physical Exam

- See **Abdominal Exam**, p.20

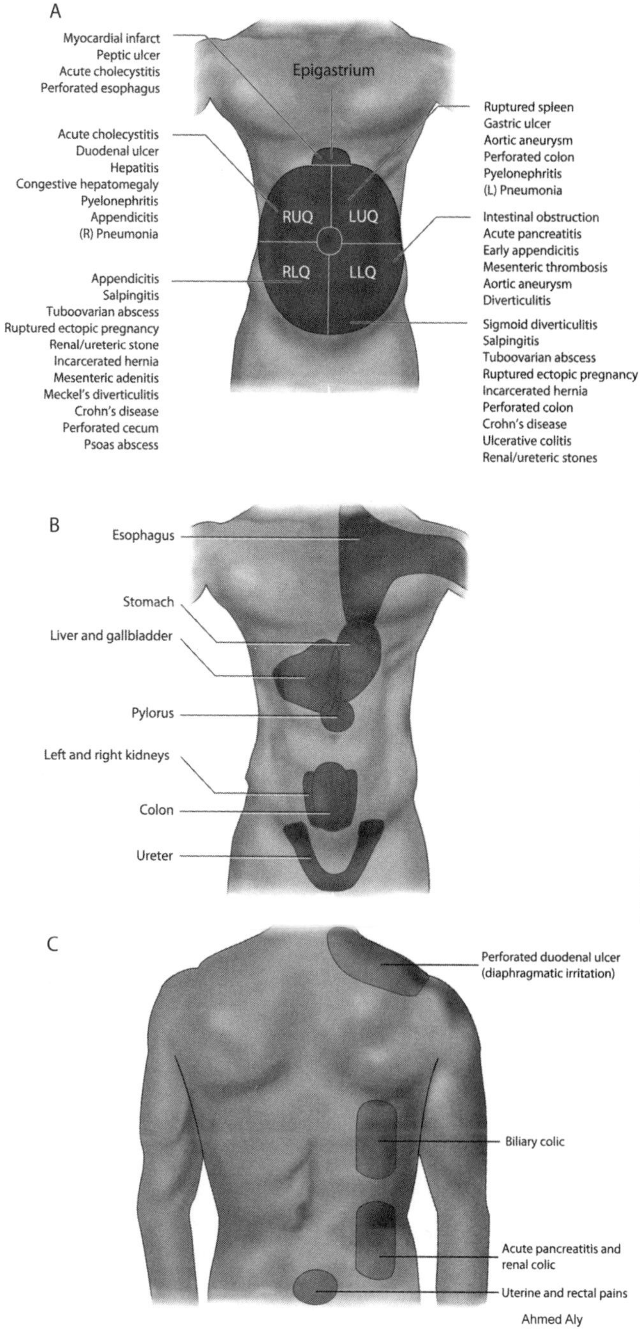

Figure 3. (A) Differential Diagnoses for Pain in Abdominal Quadrants (B) Localizations of Pain for Common Abdominal Pathologies, Anteriorly and (C) Posteriorly

EMERGENCY

Table 7. Signs and Symptoms and Imaging of Selected Causes of Abdominal Pain

Diagnosis	Signs and Symptoms	Investigations/Imaging
Appendicitis	Initial vague, colicky central abdominal pain; progresses to localized right lower quadrant (RLQ) pain over McBurney's point; anorexia; N/V; fever (50% of patients); leukocytosis (50% of patients); guarding, tenderness, psoas sign, obturator sign	Contrast-enhanced CT if diagnosis uncertain (diagnostic accuracy of 95-98%); U/S in females of reproductive age (sensitivity and specificity of 77% and 86%, respectively); MRI (diagnostic accuracy of 91-95%)
Abdominal Aortic Aneurysm	Pulsatile abdominal mass; if ruptured, then shock, HTN, mottled abdominal wall	CT if diagnosis uncertain; U/S in females of reproductive age
Acute Ischemic Bowel	Tachycardia; hypotension; fever; lactic acidosis; bloody diarrhea; abdominal pain out of proportion with physical exam (hallmark finding)	Contrast CT: thickened bowel wall loops (thumb-printing); abdominal angiography: may show embolus or thrombus
Cholecystitis	Right upper quadrant (RUQ) pain; anorexia; N/V; positive Murphy's sign	U/S: gallstones, gallbladder wall thickening (inflammation)
Ectopic Pregnancy	Adnexal mass	Transvaginal U/S: blood or mass in adnexa, ectopic cardiac activity or gestational sac; β-hCG >1500 and no intrauterine pregnancy
Obstruction	Abdominal distension; N/V	Abdominal X-ray: dilated bowel, air fluid levels
Splenic Rupture	Hypotension; peritonitis	CT (only in a stable patient): rupture seen, blood detected; U/S: free fluid around spleen

Investigations
- Vitals (temperature, HR, RR)
- CBC, differential, electrolytes
- Serum creatinine/BUN, lactate, LFTs, lipase
- Urinalysis
- β-hCG in all women of reproductive age
- ECG (especially if >40 yr)
- Abdominal X-ray (AXR), CXR, CT, U/S as needed

Management
- *Nil per os* (NPO), NG tube, IV fluids
- Treat shock
- Analgesia: judicious use of IV narcotics has been shown to aid the diagnostic process by making the physical exam more reliable
- Antiemetics and NG suction if necessary
- Consider holding back antibiotics unless sepsis/infection is obvious or until diagnosis is established
- Immediate surgical consult if hemodynamically unstable, acute abdomen, pulsatile abdominal mass

3.7 Chest Pain

Focused History

- OPQRSTUVW
- N/V, diaphoresis
- Dyspnea, palpitations, syncope
- Cardiac or other risk factors (e.g. travel, oral contraceptive, DVT/PE)
- Trauma
- Sense of doom

> **Clinical Pearls: Postemesis Chest Pain**
> - Onset of postemesis chest pain is suggestive of Boerhaave's syndrome
> - Consider drug use, especially cocaine and other sympathomimetics

Focused Physical Exam

- See **Cardiovascular Exam**, p.52

Table 8. Differential Diagnosis of Chest Pain by Organ System

Differential Diagnosis of Chest Pain	
Cardiovascular • **Aortic dissection** • **Cardiac tamponade** • **ACS (STEMI, NSTEMI, unstable angina)** • Pericarditis, myocarditis • Stable angina • Aortic stenosis, aortic insufficiency, mitral prolapse • Sickle cell crisis • Cocaine use	**Gastrointestinal** • **Boerhaave's syndrome/esophageal rupture** • Cholecystitis • Esophagitis • GERD • Gastritis • Peptic ulcer disease • Pancreatitis
Respiratory • **Pulmonary embolism** • (Tension) pneumothorax • Pleurisy • Pneumonia	**Musculoskeletal** • Costochondritis • Intercostal muscle strain • Rib fractures • Thoracic outlet syndrome
Neurological & Psychogenic • Spinal nerve root compression • Anxiety	**Dermatological** • Herpes zoster

Note: life-threatening conditions that always need to be ruled out are in bold
ACS = acute coronary syndrome, NSTEMI = non-ST segment elevation myocardial infarction, STEMI = ST segment elevation myocardial infarction

Investigations

- Vitals (temperature, HR, RR)
- CBC, electrolytes, serum glucose
- Serum creatinine, BUN
- Lipase, amylase
- Cardiac enzymes: creatine kinase isoform (CK-MB), troponins I/T, brain naturietic peptide (BNP)
- Consider D-dimer to rule out PE
- ECG
- CXR, EDE

Management

- Supplemental oxygen by facemask, nasal prongs
- Establish IV access (saline lock)
- Continuous cardiac monitoring (i.e. serial ECG)

- Evaluate for hypotension/shock
  - If hypovolemic: IV crystalloids, type and crossmatch 6-8 units pRBCs
- Aspirin and nitroglycerin if not contraindicated for suspected acute coronary syndrome (ACS)
- Other antiplatelet drugs
- IV analgesia
- Correct arrhythmias if present
- Consider thrombolytics or catheterization in event of ST segment elevation myocardial infarction (STEMI)
- Percutaneous coronary intervention (PCI) is treatment of choice

Table 9. Signs and Symptoms of Selected Causes of Chest Pain

Diagnosis	Signs and Symptoms	Investigations/Imaging
ACS (STEMI, NSTEMI, unstable angina)	Pain: retrosternal or radiating to arms, neck, epigastrium; N/V; diaphoresis; restlessness; dyspnea; heart failure; shock	CK-MB; troponin: may be elevated; ECG: can be diagnostic or normal
Aortic Dissection	Retrosternal pain: often described as tearing, often presents atypically; absent pulses, limb ischemia; myocardial infarction, stroke; hematuria	CXR: widened aortic silhouette (>80% but 12-15% will be normal)[5]; ECG: acute MI (only 1-2%); CT, angiography, and echo are investigations of choice
Cardiac Tamponade	Beck's triad: hypotension, increased JVP, muffled heart sounds	Echo and U/S are diagnostic; pericardiocentesis: used to confirm and treat
Aortic Stenosis	Triad of heart failure, angina, and syncope; crescendo-decrescendo systolic ejection murmur	ECG: left ventricular hypertrophy; echo is diagnostic
Mitral Prolapse	Palpitations; dyspnea; dizziness; late systolic click; mitral regurgitation murmur; arrhythmia possible	ECG: nonspecific T-wave abnormalities; echo is diagnostic
Pulmonary Embolism	Abrupt onset of pleuritic chest pain; dyspnea, tachypnea, hemoptysis (in some instances); friction rub (rare); hypoxemic, hypocapneic	ECG: sinus tachycardia or nonspecific ST-T changes most common, S1, Q3, T3 are the classic signs but uncommon; CT pulmonary angiography; V/Q scan if young female: areas of lung ventilated but not perfused; D-dimer: elevated under the ECG entry
Pneumothorax	Dyspnea; tachycardia; lung collapse; if tension pneumothorax: shock, tracheal deviation	CXR: absence of lung markings peripheral to visceral pleural line; if tension: mediastinal shift; EDE (absence of comet tails or lung sliding makes diagnosis)
Esophageal Rupture	Retrosternal pain; subcutaneous emphysema; history of frequent vomiting; esophageal instrumentation	CXR: pneumomediastinum, pleural effusion; esophagoscopy is diagnostic

ACS = acute coronary syndrome, EDE = emergency department echocardiogram, NSTEMI = non-ST segment elevation myocardial infarction, STEMI = ST segment elevation myocardial infarction, V/Q = ventilation-perfusion

3.8 Headache

Focused History

- OPQRSTUVW
  - Onset: acute onset or sudden change in pattern is serious
  - Quality:
    - Shooting pain in V1, V2 distribution indicative of trigeminal neuralgia
    - Steady, band-like pain indicative of tension headaches
  - Timing: headaches secondary to raised intracranial pressure (ICP) are often worst on awakening (prolonged supine position)
- Vomiting with no nausea, myalgia, jaw claudication, scalp tenderness
- Photopobia, phonophobia, aura, vision changes
- Meningeal signs
- History of recent head trauma
- Pregnancy status
- Highest risk for traumatic bleed: alcoholics, elderly, patients on antithrombotics

Focused Physical Exam

- Establish stability of patient: evaluate appearance, LOC and responsiveness, vital signs (especially BP and temperature)
- Inspection: neurofibromas, café-au-lait spots, cutaneous hemangiomas, purpuric rash
- Neurological exam and fundoscopy: neurological deficits or papilledema are suggestive of intracranial lesion
- Meningeal signs
- Palpate for scalp tenderness (temporal arteritis) and nuchal line tenderness (occipital neuralgia)
- Measure intraocular pressure to rule out glaucoma

Table 10. Differential Diagnosis of Headache

Differential Diagnosis of Headache (H/A)		
Acute Onset H/A	**Subacute H/A**	**Chronic H/A**
• **Cerebrovascular accident** • **Meningitis** • **Subarachnoid hemorrhage** • Migraine • Trauma • Venous sinus thrombosis	• **Preeclampsia/ hypertensive crisis** • **Temporal arteritis** • Intracranial mass/ pseudotumor or increased ICP • Meningitis/CNS infection • Trigeminal neuralgia • Polymyalgia rheumatica • Toxin exposure (e.g. CO) • Migraine	• Cervical spine disease • Cluster headache • Migraine • Tension headache • Sinusitis • Temporomandibular joint disease • Iritis • Glaucoma • Occipital neuralgia

Note: causes that are bold are most common

Table 11. Signs and Symptoms of Selected Causes of Headache

Diagnosis	Signs and Symptoms	Investigations/Imaging
Increased ICP	Worst on awakening and during coughing, sneezing; focal neurological deficits develop over time; papilledema: loss of venous pulsations (early sign)	CT or MRI are diagnostic
Meningitis	Fever; N/V; decreased LOC; meningismus; purpuric rash	Lumbar puncture for CSF profile, gram stain, C&S, polymerase chain reaction (PCR)

EMERGENCY

Table 11. Signs and Symptoms of Selected Causes of Headache (continued)

Diagnosis	Signs and Symptoms	Investigations/Imaging
Subarachnoid Hemorrhage	Sudden onset headache, "worst headache ever"; N/V; meningismus; focal neurological deficits; decreased LOC	CT: 90-95% sensitivity, 5-10% will be negative 12 h after event; lumbar puncture if CT negative but diagnosis still suspected: elevated opening pressure, xanthochromia, total RBCs in tubes 1 and 4
Temporal Arteritis	>50 yr; scalp tenderness; jaw claudication; fever; malaise; myalgia; weight loss; visual loss/disturbance	ESR: elevated (>50 mm/h); temporal artery biopsy is definitive

Investigations
- CBC, electrolytes, ESR
- If focal neurological symptoms: CT, MRI or angiography/magnetic resonance angiography (MRA)
- For subarachnoid hemorrhage, CT is 90-95% sensitive (5-10% will be false negative 12 h after onset of headache)
- If meningismus present: blood culture, lumbar puncture (LP)
- If temporal arteritis suspected: temporal artery biopsy

Management
- Varies depending on diagnosis:
  - Intracranial mass/subarachnoid hemorrhage: urgent neurosurgery consult
  - Meningitis: do not delay IV antibiotics for LP
  - Temporal arteritis: high-dose steroids

3.9 Toxicology/Acute Poisonings

Toxidrome: a constellation of signs and symptoms that suggest a specific type of poisoning (i.e. a set of physiologically-based abnormalities that typically occur due to a specific class of substances)

Table 12. Common Toxidromes

Toxidrome	Signs and Symptoms	Etiology
Anticholinergics	"Mad as a hatter": agitation/hallucinations; "Blind as a bat": dilated pupils; "Dry as a bone": dry skin; "Hot as a hare": fever; "Red as a beet": vasodilation; "The bowel and bladder lose their tone and the heart goes on alone": ileus, tachycardia, urinary retention	Antihistamines; antipsychotics; antiemetics; antispasmodics; atropine and belladonna (Jimson weed); tricyclic antidepressants
Cholinergics	**DUMBELS** **D**ecreased blood pressure/diaphoresis/defecation **U**rination **M**iosis **B**radycardia/bronchorrhea/bronchospasm **E**mesis **L**acrimation **S**alivation/seizures	Carbamates; nerve gases; organophosphates (i.e. pesticides)

Table 12. Common Toxidromes (continued)

Toxidrome	Signs and Symptoms	Etiology
Sympatho-mimetics	CNS excitation; diaphoresis; dilated pupils; HTN; increased temperature; N/V; tachycardia	Amphetamines; ASA; cocaine; LSD; PCP; theophyllines; sedative and alcohol withdrawal
Narcotics & Sedatives	CNS depression; respiratory depression; hypotension; miosis	Barbiturates; benzodiazepines; ethanol; GHB; opioids

Note: other common toxidromes include hallucinogens, and heart-blocking agents (β-blockers, calcium channel blockers, digoxin)

Focused History

- Time of exposure
- Type of exposure
- Amount/dose of exposure
- Route of exposure: inhalation, ingestion, mucous membrane exposure, cutaneous exposure, or injection
- Intent of poisoning (e.g. suicide)
- History of suicide attempts, suicidal ideation or other psychiatric illness
- In children, focus on potential environmental/household substances

Focused Physical Exam

- **Vitals:** BP, pulse, RR, O_2 saturation, temperature, capillary glucose
- **General:** fever, agitation, confusion, obtundation, somnolence, level of consciousness, sweating, hypothermia, hyperthermia
- **CNS:** seizures, LOC, altered deep tendon reflexes, coordination, cognition, tremor, fasciculations, cranial nerve assessment, slurred speech, psychosis, hallucinations
- **H&N:** eyes (nystagmus, constricted/dilated pupils, pupil reactivity, dysconjugate gaze, excessive lacrimation); oropharynx (hypersalivation, burning in the mouth, excessive dryness)
- **CVS:** assess rhythm, rate, regularity (e.g. arrhythmias, tachycardia, bradycardia)
- **Respiratory:** bronchorrhea, wheezing, pulmonary edema, bronchoconstriction, apnea, pneumothorax, alveolar hemorrhage, hypoventilation, tachypnea
- **GI:** N/V, diarrhea, abdominal tenderness/rigidity, bowel sounds, cramps
- **Derm:** flushing, diaphoresis, dryness, signs of injury/injection, ulcers, bullae, staining, bruising
- **GU:** discolored urine, urinary retention

Management

- Stabilize vital functions: ABC, appropriate monitoring
- If mental status depressed, administer universal antidotes (naloxone, dextrose, oxygen, thiamine)
- Obtain history and perform physical exam
- Identify agent(s) and/or toxidromes
- Apply methods to decrease absorption of toxin: decontamination (see **Table 13**)
- Obtain general labs and specific drug identification or levels as indicated, use ancillary tests as needed
- Continuous reevaluation, administer symptomatic and supportive care, correct fluid/electrolyte imbalances
- Perform enhanced metabolism and elimination
  - Administer sodium bicarbonate to facilitate elimination of weak acids (i.e. ASA and barbiturates): drug in anionic form becomes "ion trapped" in lumen

- **Hemodialysis** to remove chemical (not possible with digoxin)
- Use physiological antagonist or antidotes/chelators (see **Table 14**)

Table 13. Decontamination Agents

Decontamination Agents	Mechanism/ Procedure	Advantages	Disadvantages
Gastric Lavage	• Orogastric tube inserted through mouth • Saline or water added • Solution of poison and liquid aspirated back up through tube • Repeated until returning fluids are clear	• Compound is very toxic chemical; compound has not yet been absorbed (i.e. recent ingestions <1 h); no antidotes; patients have protected airways	• May not work for large tablets/ concretions; can damage/ tear esophagus; unpleasant for patient
Activated Charcoal	• Fine black carbon powder with a very large surface area that absorbs substances well • Administer at 10:1 ratio (charcoal:estimated dose of toxicant by weight)	• Patients who present within 1-2 h	• Ineffective: polar compounds with low molecular weights: methanol, ethylene glycol; metals: Fe, Pb; highly ionized salts: Li, CN • Contraindicated: patients with unprotected airways (risk of aspiration); patient with GI obstructions
Whole Bowel Irrigation	• Flush GI lumen with polyethylene glycol-electrolyte solution to speed up elimination of compound; takes 1-2 L/h for several hours until rectal effluent is clear	• Large ingestions; ingestions of sustained release or enteric-coated preparation; metal poisonings (e.g. Fe)	• Messy procedure, labor-intensive, time-consuming, and procedure often not tolerated well by patients[6]

Table 14. Antidotes/Chelators

Antidote	Indication for Poisoning	Mechanism
N-acetylcysteine (NAC)	Acetaminophen	Provides cysteine for production of glutathione; forms adduct with toxic metabolite of acetaminophen (NAPQI)
Naloxone	Opioids	Opioid competitive antagonist
Ca^{2+}	Calcium channel blocker (CCB); hydrofluoric acid	Floods Ca^{2+} channels with Ca^{2+} to improve myocardial contractility
Glucagon	β-blocker; CCB	Activates cAMP to improve myocardial contractility
Fomepizole	Methanol; ethylene glycol	Inhibits alcohol dehydrogenase
Digoxin Ab, Fab fragments	Digoxin	Binds digoxin
Deferoxamine	Iron	Chelates iron
Atropine + Pralidoxime	Organophosphates and carbamates in pesticides; cholinesterase inhibitors	Noncompetitive antimuscarinic antagonist; cholinesterase activating agent
Hydroxocobalamin	Cyanide (from industrial sources, sodium nitroprusside, amygdalin): chemical asphyxiant that binds to Fe^{3+} (i.e. cellular cytochrome oxidase) and prevents oxidative metabolism in the mitochondria of all tissues	Binds with cyanide to create cyanocobalamin (i.e. B12), which is excreted in urine
Flumazenil **"Ben is off with the flu":** **Benzodiazepine effects off with Flumazenil**	Benzodiazepines	Competitive antagonist at GABA receptors
Oxygen (in decompression chamber)	Carbon monoxide	Competitive antagonist for Hb

REFERENCES

1. Stiell IG, Wells GA, Vandemheen K, Clement C, Lesiuk H, Laupacis A, et al. 2001. The Canadian CT Head Rule for patients with minor head injury. *Lancet* 357(9266):1391-1396.
2. Barrow MW, Clark KA. 1998. Heat-related illnesses. *Am Fam Physician* 58(3):749-756, 759.
3. Biem J, Koehncke N, Classen D, Dosman J. 2003. Out of the cold: Management of hypothermia and frostbite. *CMAJ* 168(3):305-311.
4. Cartotto RC, Innes M, Musgrave MA, Gomez M, Cooper AB. 2002. How well does the Parkland formula estimate actual fluid resuscitation volumes? *J Burn Care Rehabil* 23(4):258-265.
5. Hagan PG, Nienaber CA, Isselbacher EM, Bruckman D, Karavite D, Rumman PL, et al. 2000. The International Registry of Acute Aortic Dissection (IRAD): New insights into an old disease. *JAMA* 283(7):897-903.
6. Ellenhorn MJ. *Ellenhorn's Medical Toxicology: Diagnosis and Treatment of Human Poisoning.* London: Williams and Wilkins; 1997.
7. Tintinalli JE, Kelen GD, Stapczynski JS (Editors). *Emergency Medicine: A Comprehensive Study Guide.* New York: McGraw-Hill Medical Publications Division; 2003.

The Essentials of Endocrinology

Editors:
Sabrina Nurmohamed
Jane Hsieh

Faculty Reviewer:
Jeannette Goguen, MD, FRCP(C)

TABLE OF CONTENTS

1. DISORDERS OF CARBOHYDRATE METABOLISM

1.1 Diabetes Mellitus (DM)

Classification

1. **Types 1 and 2 DM** (see **Table 1**)

Table 1. Types 1 and 2 Diabetes Mellitus

Condition	Type 1 DM (T1DM)	Type 2 DM (T2DM)
Definition	Lack of insulin due to autoimmune destruction of β-cell mass	Three-step pathophysiology: 1) insulin resistance, 2) β-cell failure, 3) increased hepatic glucose tolerance
Etiology	Multifactorial: genetic predisposition, autoimmune, environment	Multifactorial: genetic predisposition; obesity is major environmental risk factor
Age of Onset	Usually <40 yr	Tends to be >40 yr (T2DM in youth becoming an epidemic)
Family History	Usually none	Often present
Treatment	Requires exogenous insulin for survival	Requires diet modification and exercise, oral hypoglycemic agents, and possibly insulin

2. **Secondary DM:** accounts for <10% of all DM; causes include monogenic forms (MODY genes, e.g. HNFα), endocrinopathies (e.g. Cushing's disease, acromegaly, pheochromocytoma), destruction of pancreas, drugs (e.g. commonly prednisone)
3. **Gestational DM:** mainly caused by increased human placental lactogen (hPL) in the 3rd trimester in susceptible individuals (with underlying insulin resistance, which may resolve)

Focused History

- Document details of diagnosis (age, time, presenting signs, symptoms), family and past medical history (including other autoimmune disorders)
- Ask questions related to risk factors for diabetes: family history, ethnicity, central obesity, lifestyle (exercise, dietary patterns)
- Ask questions related to blood sugar control: diet, exercise, oral hyperglycemic agents, drugs, home blood glucose monitoring, hypoglycemia, diabetes education, symptoms and severity of complications

Common Chief Complaints

- T1DM: hyperglycemic symptoms (e.g. polyuria, polydipsia, nocturia, hyperphagia, weight loss, blurred vision, fatigue)
- T2DM: same, but often asymptomatic and identified on blood glucose screening[1]

Acute Complications

- Hyperglycemic conditions include diabetic ketoacidosis (DKA) and hyperglycemic hyperosmolar syndrome (HHS; formerly HONKS). Ask:
  - Polyuria, polydipsia, weight loss, extracellular fluid volume contraction
  - Neurologic symptoms with rapid progression: lethargy, coma

Chronic Complications

- Ask questions related to microvascular complications of DM:
  - Retinopathy: change in vision, last ophthalmologist visit
  - Nephropathy: urinary albumin excretion, HTN
  - Neuropathy
    - Autonomic: postural hypotension, gastroparesis, urinary retention, erectile dysfunction
    - Peripheral: numbness, tingling or decreased sensation in hands and/or feet, foot ulcers
- Ask questions related to macrovascular complications of DM:
  - Presence of chest pain, shortness of breath, claudication, symptoms of TIA/stroke
  - Risk Factors: smoking, HTN, dyslipidemia, family history of premature CAD (e.g. angina, MI, stroke, TIA, peripheral vascular disease [PVD], gangrene, infection)
- Other Complications: immune suppression: recommend Pneumovax®

Focused Physical Exam

- **General:** height, weight, waist circumference (central obesity), BMI, BP (supine and standing), pulse
- **H&N:** eyes (fundoscopy), thyroid
- **CVS:** signs of CHF, peripheral pulses and bruits
- **GI:** hepatomegaly from fatty liver
- **MSK:** foot inspection, limited joint mobility, arthropathy, color/temperature of limbs
- **Neuro:** screen for peripheral neuropathy using vibration tuning fork or monofilament
- **Derm:** inspection for cutaneous infections, problems with injection sites

Diagnostic Criteria

- Random plasma glucose (PG) ≥11.1 mM with symptoms (polyuria, polydipsia, unexplained weight loss) **OR**
- Fasting PG ≥7.0 mM seen on 2 occasions **OR**
- 2 h post 75 g oral glucose tolerance test (OGTT) ≥11.1 mM **OR**
- HbA1c ≥ 6.5%[2]

Screening for hyperglycemia should begin at age 40

Important Laboratory Markers

- Blood: HbA1c, glucose, lipids, creatinine, electrolytes, AST
- Urine: albumin/creatinine ratio

1.2 Hypoglycemia

Classification

- **Fasting:** resulting from an imbalance of hepatic glucose production (too little) and peripheral glucose utilization (too much)
  - Most commonly due to insulin or insulin secretagogues (iatrogenic)
  - Insulinoma
  - Non-β cell tumor: overproduction of insulin-like growth factor 2 (IGF-2)
  - Adrenal insufficiency, renal or liver failure
- **Postprandial** (within 4 h of food consumption): glucose levels fall more rapidly than insulin levels
  - Alimentary hypoglycemia post gastric surgery
  - Early T2DM
  - Idiopathic

Focused History

- Ask questions relating to common hypoglycemic symptoms:
  - Neurogenic: sweating, pallor, tachycardia, palpitations, tremor, anxiety, tingling and paresthesias of mouth and fingers, hunger, N/V
  - Neuroglycopenic: weakness, headache, fainting, dizziness, blurred vision, mental dullness/confusion, abnormal behavior, amnesia, seizures

Focused Physical Exam

- ↑HR, ↑BP, confusion which may escalate to seizures and coma
- Cold, diaphoretic skin

Diagnostic Test

- Plasma or capillary glucose <4.0 mM
- If suspect insulinoma: 72 h fast for levels of plasma glucose, insulin, C-peptide, proinsulin, plasma sulfonylurea

2. PITUITARY DISORDERS

- Disorders of the pituitary can present with one or more of the following: hyperfunction, hypofunction, or mass effect
- The pituitary hormones are:
  - Anterior pituitary: adrenocorticotropic hormone (ACTH), growth hormone (GH), prolactin (PRL), thyroid-stimulating hormone (TSH), follicle-stimuating hormone (FSH), luteinizing hormone (LH)
  - Posterior pituitary: antidiuretic hormone (ADH), oxytocin
- Mass Effect: any tumor can cause normal pituitary to underproduce hormones (by stalk compression); other mass effects include pressure on the optic nerve (CN II, leading to bitemporal hemianopsia), headache, effects on the cranial nerves of the cavernous sinus (e.g. CN III, IV, V1, V2, VI)
  - Classified as either micro (<1 cm) or macro (>1 cm)

2.1 Hyperfunction

Etiology

- Increased hormone secretion usually resulting from benign adenomas of the pituitary that overproduce PRL (prolactinoma) or GH (acromegaly) or ACTH (Cushing's syndrome), rarely TSH (see **Table 2** and **Table 3**)

Table 2. Focused History and Physical Exam for Pituitary Hyperfunction

Hormones	Focused History and Physical Exam	Diagnostic Criteria
PRL (30% of all pituitary adenomas)	Symptoms of galactorrhea, amenorrhea, infertility, erectile dysfunction, poor libido	↑ prolactin, rule out other causes
GH	HTN, "acral" enlargement: hands, fingers, and heel pad thickening, prominent eyebrows and jaw, misaligned teeth, macroglossia, frontal bossing, sleep apnea, osteoarthritis, carpal tunnel syndrome, colonic polyps, cardiomegaly, multinodular goiter, DM, small testes, reduced male pattern hair	↑ IGF-1 GH not fully suppressed with oral glucose test
ACTH	Central obesity, round facies, dorsal and supraclavicular fat pads, HTN, proximal weakness, osteoporosis, psychosis, purple striae, thin bruised skin, hirsutism, DM	see **Table 3**

Clinical Pearl: Prolactin Overproduction

Overproduction of PRL can be caused by pregnancy/breastfeeding/nipple stimulation, pituitary tumor (prolactinoma or nonsecretory with stalk effect), decreased clearance as in liver and renal failure, drugs (psychiatric, GI), and/or primary hypothyroidism (via thyrotropin releasing hormone [TRH]).

Table 3. Summary of Laboratory Findings in Various Forms of Cushing's Syndrome

Type of Cushing's	Plasma ACTH	24 h Urine Cortisol	Low Dose DXM Test	High Dose DXM Test
Adrenal Cushing's				
Adenoma, carcinoma, bilateral nodular adrenal hyperplasia	↓ ACTH	↑ cortisol	Cortisol *not* suppressed	Cortisol *not* suppressed
Pituitary Cushing's				
Pituitary ACTH-producing adenoma stimulating adrenal cortisol overproduction	↑ ACTH	↑ cortisol	Cortisol *not* suppressed	Cortisol suppressed
Ectopic ACTH-Secreting Tumor				
Small cell lung cancer, bronchial carcinoma	↑↑ ACTH	↑ cortisol	Cortisol *not* suppressed	Cortisol *not* suppressed

DXM = dexamethasone

Goljan EF. Endocrine disorders. *Rapid Review: Pathology*, 3rd ed. Philadelphia: Mosby; 2010.

> **Clinical Pearl: Cushing's Syndrome**
> The commonest cause of Cushing's syndrome is iatrogenic use of glucocorticoid therapy.

2.2 Hypofunction

Etiology

- Hypopituitarism can occur by the following mechanism:
  - Compression of pituitary stalk/normal cells by pituitary adenomas
  - Loss of hypothalamic function
  - Pituitary infarction (e.g. Sheehan's syndrome) or hemorrhage (apoplexy)
  - Pituitary surgery or radiation
  - Other rare causes such as cell infiltration, inflammation
- For each individual pituitary hormone, there exists a factor that stimulates its release arising from the hypothalamus; e.g. for the **anterior pituitary** (stimulator → hormone): corticotropin releasing hormone (CRH) → ACTH, GH releasing hormone (GHRH) → GH, thyrotropin releasing hormone (TRH) → PRL/TSH, gonadotropin releasing hormone (GnRH) → FSH/LH
- Hypothalamic lesions (tumors, aneurysms, genetic syndromes) can cause pituitary hormone deficiencies, which are referred to as "tertiary" deficiencies

> **Clinical Pearl: Pituitary Hypofunction**
> *Go Look For The Adenoma Please* is a mnemonic for the order of hormone loss in pituitary hypofunction (GH, LH/FSH, TSH, ACTH, PRL).

Focused History and Physical Exam

Table 4. Focused History and Physical Exam for Pituitary Hypofunction

Hormones	Focused History and Physical Exam	Diagnostic Criteria
Anterior Pituitary		
ACTH	Signs and symptoms of adrenal insufficiency (see **Adrenal Disorders**, p.446)	↓ 8 AM cortisol
GH	Low energy, osteoporosis, dyslipidemia Short stature (in children)	↓ IGF-1
PRL	Inability to lactate	↓ prolactin
TSH	Signs and symptoms of hypothyroidism (see **Thyroid Disorders**, p.448)	↓ TSH and ↓ free T_4
FSH/LH	Women: amenorrhea, infertility Men: erectile dysfunction, loss of libido ↓ secondary sexual characteristics (body hair growth, breast development)	↓ LH ↓ FSH ↓ estradiol ↓ bioavailable testosterone
Posterior Pituitary		
ADH	Symptoms of diabetes insipidus: polyuria, polydipsia Confusion and coma from hypernatremia	May have hypernatremia

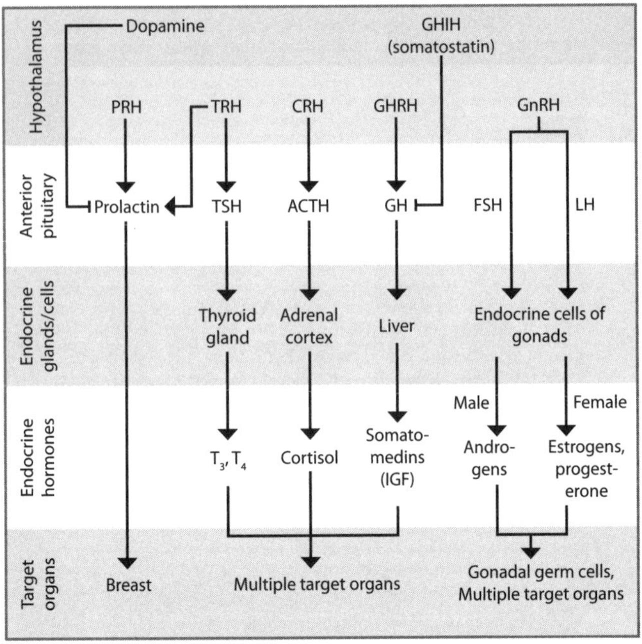

Figure 1. Hypothalamic-Pituitary Hormonal Axes
CRH = corticotropin-releasing hormone, GnRH = gonadotropin-releasing hormone, GHIH = growth hormone-inhibiting hormone, GHRH = growth hormone-releasing hormone, PRH = prolactin-releasing hormone, TRH = thyrotropin-releasing hormone

3. ADRENAL DISORDERS

- Disorders of the adrenal gland that cause problems related to endocrine functions leading to overproduction or underproduction of adrenal hormones
- The adrenal gland cortex makes 3 classes of steroid hormones:
  - **Glucocorticoids** (regulate blood sugar, metabolism, and immunity)
  - **Mineralocorticoids** (regulate Na^+ and K^+, blood volume, and BP)
  - **Androgens** (affect 2° sex characteristics: axillary/pubic hair, libido)
- The adrenal medulla produces catecholamines (epinephrine and norepinephrine)

3.1 Hyperfunction

Cushing's Syndrome

- See **Table 2** (ACTH) and **Table 3** (Adrenal Cushing's)

Conn's Syndrome

- Overproduction of aldosterone secondary to adrenal adenoma, hyperplasia or rarely carcinoma

Focused History and Physical Exam

- Severe or resistant HTN, often with hypokalemia

Diagnostic Criteria

- ↑aldosterone and ↑aldosterone/renin ratio
- Aldosterone does not suppress with salt load

Pheochromocytoma
- Overproduction of catecholamines and metanephrines by adrenal glands or extra-adrenal sympathetic nervous tissue

Focused History and Physical Exam
- Spells with headache, palpitations, and perspiration
- HTN

Diagnostic Criteria
- Elevated catecholamines and/or metanephrines in 24 h urine collection

3.2 Hypofunction

Etiology
- Can be caused by underproduction of adrenal gland hormones, as a result of destruction/dysfunction of the adrenal gland itself, or inadequate ACTH formation or release
  - Includes Addison's disease or adrenal insufficiency

Causes of Adrenal Insufficiency
- **Primary** (adrenal gland hypofunction, high ACTH):
  - Autoimmune destruction (may be associated with type 1 or 2 autoimmune polyglandular syndrome); infectious (TB, systemic fungal infection, opportunistic infection, e.g. in HIV); tumor (metastatic carcinoma, especially of breast, lung, kidney, or bilateral lymphoma); other (hemorrhage [e.g. Waterhouse-Friderichsen syndrome], necrosis, thrombosis, congenital)
- **Secondary** (pituitary hypofunction, low ACTH):
  - Tumor (pituitary, craniopharyngioma); pituitary surgery or radiation, necrosis (e.g. Sheehan's syndrome); hemorrhage (pituitary apoplexy), trauma; infection (e.g. histiocytosis X); other (lymphocytic hypophysitis, sarcoidosis, empty sella syndrome)
- **Tertiary** (low CRH secretion, low ACTH):
  - Hypothalamic tumors; long-term glucocorticoid therapy

Focused History
- **Common Chief Complaints:**
  - Fatigue, weakness, loss of appetite, weight loss
- **Other Complaints:**
  - Hyperpigmentation of skin (seen in 1° adrenal insufficiency), N/V or abdominal pain (signs of adrenal crisis), hypotension, muscle and joint pain, salt craving
- **Associated Symptoms:**
  - Fatigue that worsens on exertion and improves with rest, weakness; anorexia, weight loss; salt craving; N/V, abdominal pain; amenorrhea; more severe cases present with postural lightheadedness and frank hypotension
- Ask questions related to **cause of adrenal disease:**
  - Consider secondary adrenal insufficiency: pituitary tumor symptoms (headache, loss of peripheral vision, symptoms of low levels of other pituitary hormones)
- Ask questions related to **consequences and complications:**
  - Adrenal crisis (shock = hypotension with loss of consciousness; preceded by fever, N/V, and abdominal pain, weakness and fatigue, and confusion) can occur in primary adrenal insufficiency often due to infection, trauma or other stress; symptoms of hypoglycemia are more common in secondary/tertiary adrenal insufficiency because they are accompanied by GH deficiency

Focused Physical Exam

- **H&N:** assess pituitary findings (headache [on history], visual symptoms), articular calcification
- **CVS:** postural hypotension
- **GI:** tenderness on palpation
- **MSK:** diffuse, nonspecific weakness
- **Derm:** vitiligo, hyperpigmentation (primary adrenal insufficiency) especially in areas exposed to light (e.g. face, neck, backs of hands) and to chronic mild trauma (e.g. elbows, knees, spine, knuckles, waist, shoulders, buccal mucosa along dental occlusion and inner surface of lips)

Diagnostic Criteria

- Low plasma cortisol (classically less than 100 nM at 8 AM), especially if still less than 500 nM after Cortrosyn® (cosyntropin) stimulation testing (ACTH)

4. THYROID DISORDERS

- Disorders of the thyroid gland that cause problems related to endocrine function or mass effect leading to overproduction or underproduction of thyroid hormones
- The thyroid gland makes two main forms of thyroid hormone: main circulating hormone T_4 and small amounts of the active hormone T_3
- T_4 enters cells and is converted to T_3; T_3 has nuclear receptors that have different effects depending on the organ; in general, T_3 increases metabolic rate, heart rate, and energy levels, and regulates bone health

> **Clinical Pearl: Thyrotoxicosis vs. Hyperthyroidism**
> Thyrotoxicosis is any condition that results in elevated levels of thyroid hormone, including hyperthyroidism. Hyperthyroidism is the excess production of thyroid hormone by the thyroid gland itself.

4.1 Thyrotoxicosis

- **Excess Production** (Hyperthyroidism):
  - **Primary** (↓TSH, ↑T_4/T_3): Graves' disease (most common cause), toxic multinodular goiter, toxic adenoma, hyperemesis gravidarum, trophoblastic tumors, struma ovarii, drugs (e.g. amiodarone)[3]
  - **Secondary** (↑TSH, ↑T_4/T_3): TSH-secreting anterior pituitary adenoma; pituitary resistance to T_4/T_3[3]
- **Excess Hormone Release** (Thyroiditis, ↓TSH, ↑T_4/T_3): thyroid gland inflammation and release of stored hormone; can be subacute, postpartum, drug-induced (e.g. amiodarone), or radiation-induced
- **Exogenous Thyroid Hormone** (↓TSH, ↑T_4/T_3): thyroid medications (excess dosage or surreptitious use); hamburger thyrotoxicosis

Focused History

- **Common Chief Complaints:**
  - "Anxiety", weight loss with increased appetite, fatigue and weakness, frequent bowel movements, heat intolerance/sweating, palpitations, chest pain, shortness of breath, insomnia
- Ask questions related to the **cause of thyroid disease:**
  - Personal or family history of autoimmune, thyroid or endocrine disorders (e.g. DM, gonadal dysfunction), past management (drugs, surgery, head/neck irradiation), medication use (e.g. amiodarone, Li), pregnancy, goitrogen ingestion (e.g. seaweed, kelp, iodine)
- Ask questions related to **symptoms associated with enlarged thyroid:**
  - Enlarged thyroid/nodule, "mass effects": dysphagia, dyspnea, dysphonia (pressure on laryngeal nerve)

- Ask questions related to **symptoms associated with high thyroid hormone** (see **Table 5**); eye symptoms (e.g. Graves' exophthalmos, eye grittiness, discomfort, excess tearing)
- Ask questions related to **symptoms of complications of elevated thyroid hormone**: e.g. thyrotoxicosis can cause decompensation in heart disease leading to chest pain and osteoporosis leading to bone fractures
  - Thyroid storm is a rare, life-threatening condition characterized by an exaggeration of the usual symptoms of thyrotoxicosis; it may develop in cases of untreated thyrotoxicosis or may be precipitated by stress such as surgery, trauma or infection

Focused Physical Exam

Table 5. Physical Signs and Symptoms of Thyrotoxicosis

System	Symptoms	Signs
General	Weight loss with good appetite, heat intolerance	Fever, decreased LOC in thyroid storm
H&N	Anxious, irritability	Eyes: exophthalmos, stare, lid lag
CVS	Palpitations	Tachycardia, wide pulse pressure, bounding pulse, aortic systolic murmur, atrial fibrillation, systolic HTN
GI	Increased bowel movements	None
GU	Women: menstrual irregularities	None
Neuro	Feeling shaky	Fine tremor, proximal muscle weakness, hyperreflexia
Derm	Warm, smooth and silky skin, increased perspiration, hair thinning	Diaphoresis, pretibial myxedema (Graves')

Reid JR, Wheeler SF. 2005. *Am Fam Physician* 72(4):623-630.

4.2 Hypothyroidism

- **Primary** (↑TSH, ↓T_4/T_3):
  - Iatrogenic: post-thyroid surgery or radioactive iodine ablation (e.g. in treatment of thyroid cancer or Graves' disease)
  - Autoimmune: Hashimoto's thyroiditis, recurrent thyroiditis
  - Drug-induced: goitrogens (iodine), thionamides (propylthiouracil, methimazole), Li, amiodarone
  - Infiltrative disease: progressive systemic sclerosis, amyloid
  - Other: iodine deficiency, congenital, subacute granulomatous thyroiditis (De Quervain's), subacute lymphocytic thyroiditis
- **Secondary** (↓TSH, ↓T_4/T_3):
  - Insufficiency of pituitary TSH
  - Bexarotene treatment
  - Hypopituitarism: tumors, surgery, trauma, infiltrative disorders
- **Tertiary:** hypothalamic disease leading to TRH release

Focused History

- **Common Chief Complaints:**
  - Weight gain, fatigue, constipation, cold intolerance
- Ask questions related to **cause of thyroid disease, and to symptoms associated with enlarged thyroid**

- Ask questions related to **symptoms associated with low thyroid hormone** (see **Table 6**)
- Ask questions related to **symptoms of complications of low thyroid hormone:**
  - Myxedema coma is a severe disease where the body cannot adapt to the hypothyroidic changes causing organ failure and is usually precipitated by another illness (leading to coma, hypothermia, hypotension, bradycardia and respiratory failure)

Focused Physical Exam

Table 6. Physical Signs and Symptoms of Hypothyroidism

System	Symptoms	Signs
General	Weight gain, cold intolerance, fatigue, depression	Increased weight, hypothermia
H&N	Periorbital edema, hoarseness	Queen Anne's sign: loss of lateral third of eyebrow, signs of goiter
CVS	Dizziness	Diastolic HTN, bradycardia, hyperlipidemia
GI	Constipation	None
GU	Women: menorrhagia	None
Neuro	Difficulty concentrating; tingling, pain or weakness in hands	Delirium, coma, proximal muscle weakness, carpal tunnel syndrome, delayed relaxation of reflexes
Derm	Dry skin, hair loss	Dry skin, brittle hair and nails, yellow skin from beta-carotene, skin may be pale from associated anemia

ENDOCRINOLOGY

5. POLYCYSTIC OVARIAN SYNDROME (PCOS)

- PCOS is a metabolic syndrome characterized by oligomenorrhea, hirsutism, obesity, and polycystic appearing ovaries
- **Prevalence:** 5-10% of reproductive age women, leading cause of infertility, may be underdiagnosed because condition is masked by oral contraceptive pills[4]. Age of onset is often around menarche, adolescence or in young adults
- **Etiology:** causes are not well understood, both genetic and environmental influences

Diagnostic Criteria

- 2003 Rotterdam European Society of Human Reproduction and Embryology (ESHRE)/American Society for Reproductive Medicine (ASRM) criteria require 2 of the following 3[5,6]:
  1. Oligoovulation and/or anovulation
  2. Clinical and/or biochemical signs of hyperandrogenism
  3. Polycystic ovaries on transvaginal ultrasound (ovary size >10 mL and/or >12 follicles 2-9 mm)
- PCOS is a diagnosis of exclusion
- Rule out androgen excess disorders, such as congenital adrenal hyperplasia (21-hydroxylase deficiency) (see **Table 7**)

Focused History

- Ask questions related to **presenting symptoms:** menstrual history, hair growth on face, back, chest, and abdomen
- Ask questions related to **associated symptoms:** irregular vaginal bleeding, recent weight gain, infertility, sleep apnea

- Ask questions related to **family history** of infertility, insulin resistance, DM, and androgen excess
- Ask questions related to **complications of PCOS:** past medical history of T2DM, HTN, cardiovascular disease, miscarriage, endometrial hyperplasia/cancer

Focused Physical Exam

- **General:** height, weight, BMI, waist circumference (>80 cm in women and >88 cm in men)
- **H&N:** thyroid exam, androgenic alopecia (male pattern baldness)
- **CVS:** blood pressure
- **GU:** adnexal size and masses
- **Derm:** acanthosis nigricans (hyperpigmented skin, usually in the posterior folds of the neck, axilla, groin, and umbilicus), hirsutism, acne, frontal balding

Table 7. Conditions for Exclusion for the Diagnosis of PCOS

Differential Diagnosis	Clinical Features	Laboratory Features
Androgen-Secreting Tumor	Virilization (clitoromegaly, extreme hirsutism, increased muscle bulk, frontal balding)	↑↑↑ DHEAS and/or ↑↑↑ testosterone
Amenorrhea: Primary (or Secondary)	May be related to other autoimmune disorders	↑, normal or ↓ FSH + LH; ↓ estradiol
Acromegaly	see **Table 2**	↑ IGF-1
Congenital Adrenal Hyperplasia	Family history of infertility and hirsutism	↑ 17-hydroxypro-gesterone
Cushing's Syndrome	Obesity, hirsutism, moon facies, HTN, striae	↑ 24 h urinary cortisol
Hyperprolactinemia	Galactorrhea, amenorrhea	↑ prolactin
Thyroid Dysfunction	Goiter, signs of hypothyroidism (see **Table 6**)	↑ TSH and ↓ T_4
HAIR-AN Syndrome	Hyperandrogenism, insulin resistance, acanthosis nigricans	↑↑↑ insulin following oral glucose challenge
Idiopathic Hirsutism	No menstrual irregularities	Normal serum androgen
Exogenous Androgen Administration	History of androgen therapy or Danazol use	

6. PARATHYROID GLAND DISORDERS

- Parathyroid hormone (PTH) function[7]:
  - On kidney:
    - Stimulates reabsorption of calcium in the distal convoluted tubule
    - Inhibits phosphate reabsorption
    - Stimulates production of 1,25-$(OH)_2$D (calcitriol)
  - On bone:
    - Stimulates resorption of calcium and phosphate
    - PTH is stimulated by hypocalcemia and hyperphosphatemia
    - PTH is suppressed by hypercalcemia and hypophosphatemia

ENDOCRINOLOGY

6.1 Hyperfunction (Hyperparathyroidism [HPT])

Primary Hyperparathyroidism (↑serum calcium, ↑PTH)[7]:

- Elevated secretion of PTH, leading to hypercalcemia and hypophosphatemia
- Etiology: parathyroid adenoma (most common), primary hyperplasia of parathyroid glands, carcinoma
- Familial forms are associated with multiple endocrine neoplasia (MEN) I, and MEN IIa syndromes (autosomal dominant inheritance)
- MEN I is associated with parathyroid tumors, pituitary tumors, pancreatic endocrine tumors
- MEN IIa is associated with parathyroid tumors, medullary thyroid carcinoma, pheochromocytoma

Focused History

- **Common Chief Complaints:**
  - Usually asymptomatic; otherwise, fatigue, pain from kidney stones (if severe: constipation, polyurea, decreased level of consciousness, abdominal pain)
- Ask questions related to **symptoms of hypercalcemia:**
  - History of renal stones, bone pain, myalgias, arthralgias ("stones, bones, moans, and groans")
- Ask questions related to **family history** of primary HPT, MEN I or MEN IIa disorders (parathyroid, pituitary, thyroid or pancreatic tumors)

Focused Physical Exam

Table 8. Physical Signs and Symptoms of Hyperparathyroidism

System	Symptoms	Signs
General	Depression	Diastolic HTN
H&N	Jaw pain/mass (osteitis fibrosa cystica: bone lesions due to increased osteoclastic activity)	Eyes: band keratopathy (deposition of calcium in the limbis of the eye) Neck mass
GI	Constipation, abdominal pain	None
GU	Flank pain, dysuria	Renal stones
MSK/Neuro	Muscle cramps, myalgias	Paresthesias, bone pain, clinical evidence of osteoporosis/ osteopenia

Palazzo F. Epocrates Online Diseases. San Mateo: Epocrates, Inc. 2012. *Primary Hyperparathyroidism*. Available from: http://www.epocrates.com.
Stack, BC Jr, Chou FF, Schneider V. Epocrates Online Diseases. San Mateo: Epocrates, Inc. 2012. *Secondary Hyperparathyroidism*. Available from: http://www.epocrates.com.

Secondary Hyperparathyroidism (↓serum calcium, ↑PTH)[8]:

- Any disorder that results in hypocalcemia and subsequently causes compensatory elevation of PTH levels
- Most common causes: hypovitaminosis D due to chronic kidney disease, malabsorption syndromes, and inadequate sunlight exposure

Common Chief Complaints/Focused History

- Ask questions regarding history of malabsorption syndromes (Crohn's disease, celiac disease, Whipple's disease, history of bariatric surgery), inadequate intake of vitamin D (poor intake, decreased sun exposure), and chronic kidney disease

- In patients with malabsorption syndromes, ask questions regarding bowel habits, current management of disease
- In patients with chronic kidney disease, ask about fatigue, nausea, pruritus, anorexia, arthralgias

Focused Physical Exam

- **MSK:** muscle cramps, bone pain, Chvostek and Trousseau signs (demonstrates neuromuscular excitability due to hypocalcemia)
- In patients with chronic renal failure look for: discolored skin, periorbital/ peripheral edema, ecchymoses, elevated BP

6.2 Hypofunction (Hypoparathyroidism)

Causes of Hypoparathyroidism (↓serum calcium,↓PTH):

- Most common cause is iatrogenic: following thyroid/parathyroid surgery
- Other causes: autoimmune (e.g. DiGeorge syndrome), impaired PTH secretion (hypomagnesemia, alcohol ingestion), HIV/AIDs

Focused History

- **Common Chief Complaints:** muscle twitches or spasms; tingling around lips, fingers or toes
- Ask questions regarding history of thyroid or parathyroid surgery, congenital disorder
- Ask questions regarding malabsorption syndromes, malnutrition, recent alcohol use, HIV infection
- Ask questions regarding history of autoimmune diseases (hypoparathyroidism may be associated with Addison's disease and autoimmune polyglandular syndrome type I)

Focused Physical Exam

- **H&N:** cataracts (chronic hypocalcemia)
- **MSK:** muscle twitches/spasms, Chvostek sign (tapping of facial nerve will cause twitching of facial muscles), Trousseau sign (inflating blood pressure cuff over brachial artery can cause flexion of the wrist and extension of the interphalangeal joints)
- **Neuro:** confusion, disorientation, numbness/paresthesias (perioral and in fingers/toes)
- **Derm:** dry skin/hair, brittle nails

ENDOCRINOLOGY

7. PHARMACOLOGICAL THERAPIES

Table 9. Pharmacological Therapy for Common Clinical Scenarios in Endocrinology

Common Clinical Scenario	Pharmacological Therapy
T1DM	• Insulin: rapid (aspart, lispro, glulisine), short (regular insulin), intermediate (NPH), long (glargine, detemir)
T2DM	• Sulfonylureas: glyburide, gliclazide, glimepiride • Biguanides: metformin • Glucosidase inhibitor: acarbose • Thiazolidinediones: pioglitazone • Meglitinides: nateglinide, repaglinide • Insulin • DPP-IV inhibitors: sitagliptin, saxagliptin • GLP-1 analog: liraglutide

Table 9. Pharmacological Therapy for Common Clinical Scenarios in Endocrinology (continued)

Common Clinical Scenario	Pharmacological Therapy
Hyperthyroidism	• Methimazole, propylthiouracil (PTU), radioactive iodine therapy to ablate thyroid tissue, β-blocker to alleviate symptoms
Hypothyroidism	• Levothyroxine (Synthroid®, Eltroxin™)
Addison's Disease	• Hydrocortisone and fludrocortisone; patients are instructed to increase dose of glucocorticoids during surgery and during any stressful conditions/infection
Hypercalcemia	• Start with fluid resuscitation with normal saline ± furosemide to prevent volume overload • Bisphosphonates to inhibit osteoclast activity • Calcitonin in patients with serum calcium >3.5 mM • Glucocorticoid therapy (for hypercalcemia due to lymphoma, or granulomatous disease) • Dialysis for severe hypercalcemia
PCOS	• Weight reduction if obese • Low-dose oral contraceptives/spironolactone if unable to tolerate oral contraceptives • ± metformin
Hyperparathyroidism	• Surgery, bisphosphonates, calcimimetics
Hypoparathyroidism	• Calcium, vitamin D supplements

ENDOCRINOLOGY

REFERENCES

1. Laffel L, Svoren B. *Epidemiology, Presentation, and Diagnosis of Type 2 Diabetes Mellitus in Children and Adolescents*. Waltham: Wolters Kluwer Health. 2012. Available from: http://www.uptodate.com/contents/epidemiology-presentation-and-diagnosis-of-type-2-diabetes-mellitus-in-children-and-adolescents.
2. Canadian Diabetes Association Clinical Practice Guidelines Expert Committee. 2013. Canadian Diabetes Association 2013 Clinical Practice Guidelines for the Prevention and Management of Diabetes in Canada. *Canadian Journal of Diabetes* 37(SI 1):S1-S212.
3. Reid JR, Wheeler SF. 2005. Hyperthyroidism: Diagnosis and treatment. *Am Fam Physician* 72(4):623-630.
4. Ehrmann DA. 2005. Polycystic ovary syndrome. *N Engl J Med* 352(12):1223-1236.
5. Franks S. 2006. Controversy in clinical endocrinology: Diagnosis of polycystic ovarian syndrome: In defense of the Rotterdam criteria. *J Clin Endocrinol Metab* 91(3):786-789.
6. Rotterdam ESHRE/ASRM-Sponsored PCOS consensus workshop group. 2004. Revised 2003 consensus on diagnostic criteria and long-term health risks related to polycystic ovary syndrome (PCOS). *Hum Reprod* 19(1):41-47.
7. Palazzo F. Epocrates Online Diseases. San Mateo: Epocrates, Inc. 2012. *Primary Hyperparathyroidism*. Available from: http://www.epocrates.com.
8. Stack, BC Jr, Chou FF, Schneider V. Epocrates Online Diseases. San Mateo: Epocrates, Inc. 2012. *Secondary Hyperparathyroidism*. Available from: http://www.epocrates.com.
9. Fauci AS, Braunwald E, Kasper D, Hauser S, Longo D, Jameson J, et al (Editors). *Disorders of the Anterior Pituitary and Hypothalamus*. In: *Harrison's Principles of Internal Medicine*, 17th ed. New York: McGraw-Hill; 2008.

The Essentials of Fluids, Electrolytes, and Acid/Base Disturbances

Editors:
Anandita Gokhale
Emily Trenker
Brad Wiggers

Faculty Reviewers:
Martin Schreiber, MD, MEd, FRCS(C)
Jeffrey Zaltzman, MD, FCFP(C)

TABLE OF CONTENTS

1. VOLUME STATUS

1.1 Clinical Features of Volume Overload

- Symptoms
  - Swelling of ankles, especially at the end of the day
  - Generalized swelling, including hands (rings feel tight) and around the eyes
  - Shortness of breath on exertion, paroxysmal nocturnal dyspnea, orthopnea
  - Recent weight gain

- Signs
  - Peripheral edema (ankle edema in patients who are ambulatory; sacral edema in patients who are mainly in bed)
  - Evidence of ascites and/or pleural effusion
  - Bibasilar crackles on lung auscultation (i.e. indicating pulmonary edema)
  - Elevated JVP, positive abdominojugular reflux
  - BP may be elevated

1.2 Clinical Features of Volume Depletion

- History
  - Excessive fluid loss
  - GI: vomiting, diarrhea
  - Renal: diuretics, polyuria
  - Skin: excessive sweating (fever, exercise, hyperthermia), burns
  - Hematologic: blood loss
  - Neurologic: altered mental status leading to reduced intake
- Symptoms
  - Recent weight loss
  - Excessive thirst
  - Postural dizziness
  - Fatigue
  - Weakness
  - Cramps
- Signs
  - Dry mucous membranes
  - Dry axilla
  - Oliguria or anuria
  - Hemodynamic changes
    - Resting supine tachycardia and hypotension
    - Orthostatic tachycardia (rise in HR >30 from supine to standing)
    - Orthostatic hypotension (fall in systolic BP >20 on standing, any fall in dystolic BP)
    - Low JVP
  - Soft fontanelles, reduced skin turgor, dry cry, dry diaper (in newborns)

EBM: Hypovolemia

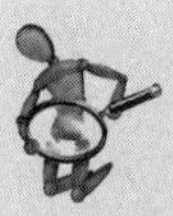

The finding of dry axilla has a LR+ of 2.8 and a LR- of 0.6 while the finding of orthostatic tachycardia has a LR+ of 1.7 and a LR- of 0.8.

Simel DL. Update: Hypovolemia, Adult. In Simel DL, Rennie D (Editors). *The Rational Clinical Examination: Evidence-Based Clinical Diagnosis*. New York: McGraw-Hill Medical; 2009.

2. DISORDERS OF SODIUM CONCENTRATION

2.1 Hyponatremia

- Serum sodium <135 mM

Clinical Features

- Symptoms: vary depending on severity and speed of onset
  - Slow onset, mild hyponatremia:
    - Often asymptomatic (due to compensation)
    - Nausea, anorexia, malaise
  - Rapid onset, severe hyponatremia:
    - Headache, lethargy, decreased LOC
    - Seizures and death may occur

Classification and Causes

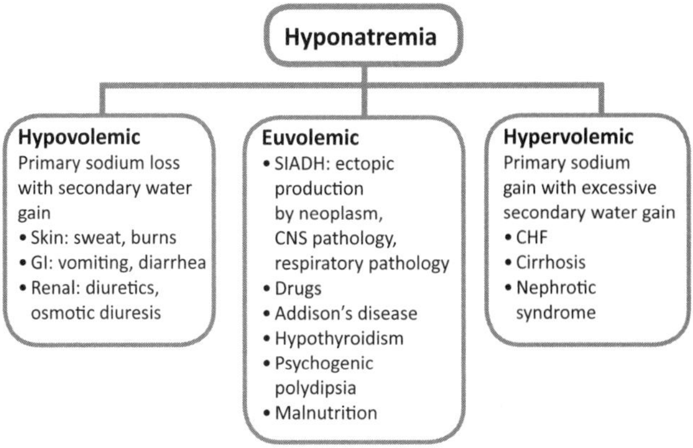

Hyponatremia
Hypovolemic
Primary sodium loss with secondary water gain
• Skin: sweat, burns
• GI: vomiting, diarrhea
• Renal: diuretics, osmotic diuresis
Euvolemic
• SIADH: ectopic production by neoplasm, CNS pathology, respiratory pathology
• Drugs
• Addison's disease
• Hypothyroidism
• Psychogenic polydipsia
• Malnutrition
Hypervolemic
Primary sodium gain with excessive secondary water gain
• CHF
• Cirrhosis
• Nephrotic syndrome

Figure 1. Classification and Causes of Hyponatremia
SIADH = syndrome of inappropriate antidiuretic hormone secretion

Other

- Pseudohyponatremia
  - Normal osmolality
    - Hyperlipidemia
    - Hyperproteinemia
  - Increased plasma osmolality
    - Hyperglycemia
    - Hypermannitolemia

> **Clinical Pearl: Adjusting for Hyperglycemia**
> The plasma sodium concentration should be corrected for hyperglycemia by adding 1.6 mM to the reported sodium level for every 5.6 mM increase in glucose above 5.6 mM.

Investigations

- Assess volume status (HR, BP, signs of edema or volume depletion)
- Measure serum sodium, osmolality
- Measure urine sodium, osmolality

Management

- Treat underlying cause
- Water restrict
- Monitor serum sodium and urine osmolality to ensure that chronic hyponatremia is not corrected too rapidly (serum [Na^+] should never increase more than 8 mM/d in patients with chronic hyponatremia)
- For acute, symptomatic hyponatremia (seizures) treat with intravenous 3% NaCl (1-2 mL/kg/h) until symptoms stop. Aim to correct [Na^+] by 3-5%
- For chronic, symptomatic hyponatremia, aim to correct [Na^+] by 4-6 mM in first several h and not more than 8 mM in the first 24 h

2.2 Hypernatremia

- Serum sodium >145 mM

Clinical Features

- Symptoms: mild unless thirst mechanism is defective or water access is restricted
- Weakness, lethargy, irritability, confusion
- Intracerebral hemorrhage, seizures, coma, and death if severe

Classification and Causes

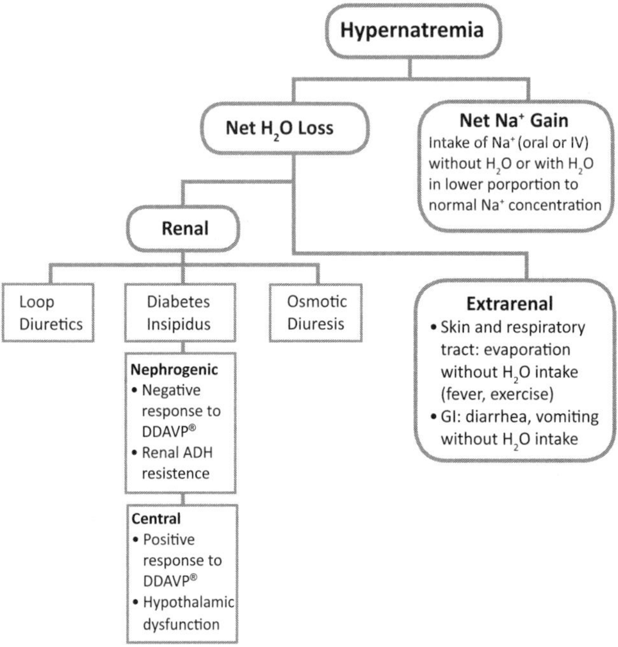

Figure 2. Classification and Causes of Hypernatremia
ADH = antidiuretic hormone, DDAVP = desmopressin

Investigations

- Assess extracellular fluid (ECF) volume status
- Serum electrolytes, creatinine, urea, glucose
- If hypovolemic:
  - Check urine osmolality (UOsm) and sodium (UNa)
    - Renal loss: UOsm 300-600 and UNa >20
    - Nonrenal loss: UOsm >600 and UNa <20
- If euvolemic:
  - Check UOsm
    - UOsm <300 suggests diabetes insipidus

Management

- **Hypovolemic Hypernatremia**
  - If evidence of hemodynamic instability, correct with bolus of NS:
    - Calculate free water deficit and replace with water PO/NG or IV hypotonic infusates (maximum 12 mM decrease of [Na^+] over 24 h)
    - Free H_2O deficit = Total body water (TBW) x (serum [Na^+] -140) / 140

- **Hypervolemic Hypernatremia**
  - Loop diuretic (or dialysis if renal failure):
    - Replace water deficit with 5% dextrose in water (D5W)

> **Clinical Pearl: Overcorrection of Serum Sodium**
> Correcting chronic hyponatremia and hypernatremia too quickly can lead to neurological damage (demyelination and brain swelling, respectively).

3. DISORDERS OF POTASSIUM CONCENTRATION

3.1 Hypokalemia
- Serum potassium <3.5 mM

Clinical Features
- Symptoms
  - Skeletal muscle: fatigue, myalgia, cramps, weakness
- Signs
  - Metabolic alkalosis
  - Heart: arrhythmia (ventricular premature beats [VPBs], ventricular tachycardia)
  - ECG changes: flattened T waves, premature ventricular beats, prolonged QT interval, U waves

Classification and Causes

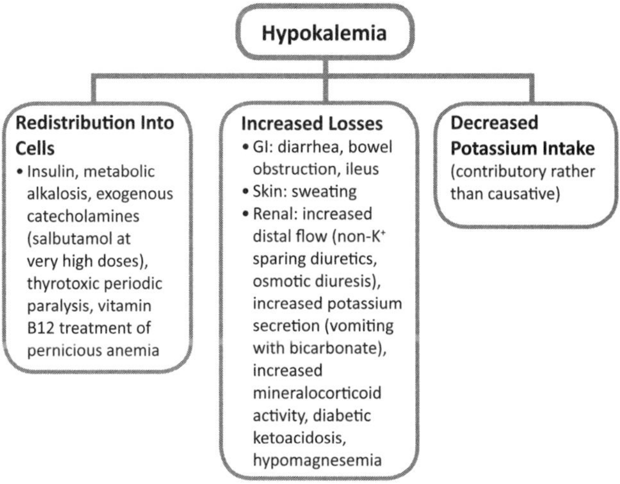

Figure 3. Classification and Causes of Hypokalemia

Investigations
- Rule out shift into cells
- 24 h urine K^+ excretion (UK)
  - UK <20 mEq/d suggests extrarenal loss
  - UK >40 mEq/d suggests renal loss
- Transtubular potassium gradient (TTKG) = (UK/PK) / (Uosm/Posm)
  - UK = urine [K^+], PK = plasma [K^+], Uosm = urine osmolality, Posm = plasma osmolality
  - TTKG >4 suggests renal loss due to increased distal K^+ secretion
- If renal loss, check BP and acid-base status
- Assess serum renin, aldosterone, and [Mg^{2+}]

Management

- ECG if potassium level <3.0 mM
- Treat underlying cause (if fluid repletion needed, avoid dextrose-containing solutions since dextrose → ↑ insulin → intracellular potassium shift)
- Potassium repletion: difficult to quantitate precisely
- 100-200 mEq of K^+ raises serum [K^+] by ~1 mEq/L
- Mild-moderate hypokalemia:
  - KCl (40 mEq) PO BID
- Severe hypokalemia or patient not able to take oral therapy:
  - Maximum IV [KCl] is 40 mEq/L in peripheral veins or 60 mEq/L in central lines

3.2 Hyperkalemia

- Serum potassium >5.0 mM
- Note serum potassium >7.0 mM is life-threatening

Clinical Features

- Symptoms: none if mild
  - Skeletal muscle: weakness, stiffness
- Signs
  - Heart: arrhythmia (sinus bradycardia, heart block, asystole, junctional rhythms, etc.)
  - ECG changes (if severe): peaked T waves, widened QRS, small/absent P waves, prolonged PR interval, "sine wave", asystole

Classification and Causes

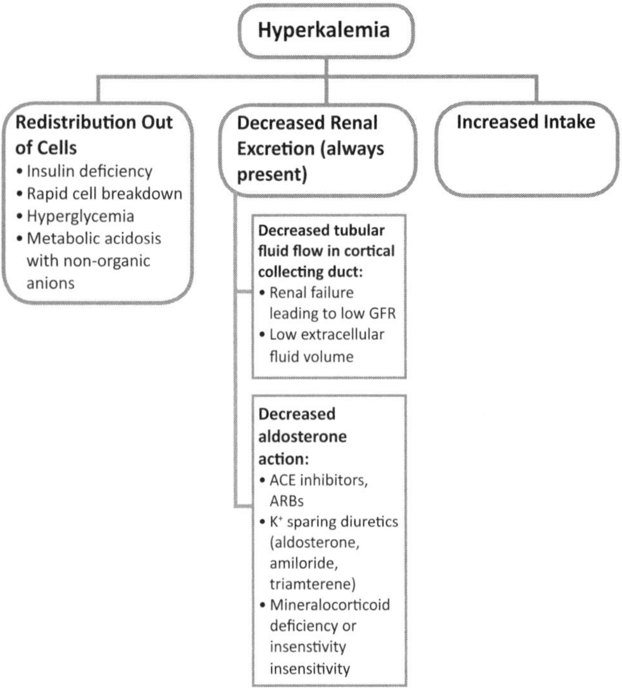

Figure 4. Classification and Causes of Hyperkalemia
ARBs = angiotensin receptor blockers, GFR = glomerular filtration rate

Specific Physical Findings Depending on Cause of Hyperkalemia

- If patient is hypovolemic or euvolemic consider these possibilities:
  - Decreased renal function and decreased potassium secretion
  - Decreased mineralocorticoid level
    - Bronzing of skin due to excess proopiomelanocortin (POMC) secretion from anterior pituitary
    - Mineralocorticoid resistance
    - Aldosterone blockers (spironolactone), blockage of Na^+ channel in cortical collecting duct (amiloride, trimethoprim, triamterene), other medications (ACE inhibitors, ARBs, direct renin inhibitor [DRI])
- If patient is hypervolemic, consider these possibilities:
  - Due to enhanced chloride absorption in cortical collecting duct (and therefore reduced intraluminal negative charge to attract potassium secretion)
  - Gordon's syndrome (rare)
  - Calcineurin toxicity (i.e. cyclosporine, tacrolimus)
  - Hyporeninemic hypoaldosteronism of diabetes

Investigations

- Rule out factitious hyperkalemia (e.g. hemolysis during venipuncture)
- Check to make sure that if receiving IVF, there is no KCl in fluid
  - Rule out shift of K^+ out of cells
  - Estimate glomerular filtration rate (GFR)
  - If normal GFR, calculate TTKG (see **Hypokalemia**, p.459)
  - TTKG <7 in patient with hyperkalemia → hypoaldosteronism
  - TTKG >7 in patient with hyperkalemia → normal aldosterone function

Management

- Emergent reaction if symptoms, ECG changes, or serum $[K^+]$ >6.5 mEq
- Tailor response to severity of increase in K^+ and ECG changes

Table 1. Treatment of Hyperkalemia

Intervention	Onset	Dose	Mechanism
Calcium Gluconate	min	1-2 amps (10 mL of 10% solution) IV	Protect heart
Insulin	15-30 min	1 amp D50W IV then 10-20 units insulin R IV	Shift K^+ into cells
Bicarbonate	15-30 min	1-3 amps IV	Shift K^+ into cells
β2-agonists	30-90 min	Salbutamol: 10 mg inhaled	Shift K^+ into cells
Diuretics	30 min	≥40 mg furosemide IV ± IV NS to prevent hypovolemia	Enhance K^+ removal via urine
Cation-Exchange Resins	1-2 h	Sodium polystyrene sulfonate 15-30 g; likely limited benefit; need to be given with laxative – avoid sorbitol due to risk of intestinal necrosis	Enhance K^+ removal via gut; not for acute hyperkalemia!
Dialysis			Enhance K^+ removal

4. DISORDERS OF CALCIUM CONCENTRATION

- Calcium (Ca^{2+}) Measurement
  - Total serum calcium includes calcium bound to albumin and free calcium (aka ionized calcium)
  - Ionized calcium is the most physiologically relevant, but measurement is difficult and can be compromised by exposure to air and the presence of anticoagulants in the tube
  - Adjusting the total serum Ca^{2+} for the albumin level is the intermediate choice
  - Adjusted Ca^{2+} (mM) = Total Ca^{2+} (mM) + 0.02 (40 - albumin [g/L])

> **Clinical Pearl: Correcting Calcium**[1]
> Rule of thumb: add 0.2 mM Ca^{2+} for every 10 g/L albumin drop.

4.1 Hypocalcemia

- Total serum Ca^{2+} <2.2 mM

Clinical Features

- Symptoms
  - Acute, mild hypocalcemia: paresthesia, hyperreflexia
  - Acute, severe hypocalcemia: tetany, confusion, seizures, laryngospasm, bronchospasm
  - Chronic hypocalcemia: parkinsonism, dementia, cataracts, abnormal dentition, dry skin
- Signs
  - Chvostek's sign
    - Facial spasm when facial nerve or branch is tapped
  - Trousseau's sign
    - Carpal spasm induced with arterial occlusion using a BP cuff (1-3 min above systolic on the forearm)
  - Papilledema
  - ECG: prolonged QT interval

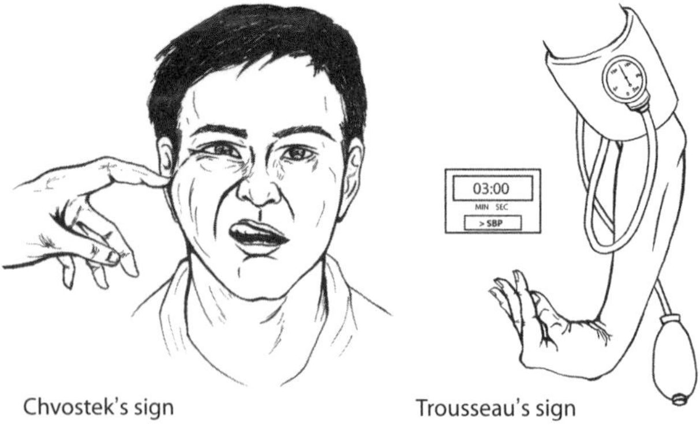

Wendy Gu

Figure 5. Chvostek's and Trousseau's Signs

Classification and Causes

Associated with Low PTH Levels (Hypoparathyroidism)

- Genetic disorders
- Surgical removal of parathyroid glands
- Autoimmune hypoparathyroidism
- Hypomagnesemia

Associated with Elevated PTH Levels (Secondary Hyperparathyroidism)

- Deficiency of vitamin D
- Renal failure (low calcitriol levels)
- Malabsorption syndromes
- Drugs: phosphate, calcitonin, aminoglycosides
- Shift out of circulation: sepsis, osteoblastic metastases, pancreatitis, post-parathyroidectomy (hungry bone syndrome)
- Respiratory alkalosis (total calcium level is normal, but a greater fraction is bound to albumin, so ionized fraction falls)
- Hyperphosphatemia
- Hypoalbuminemia (ionized calcium will be normal)

Investigations

- Measure serum ionized calcium, phosphate, magnesium, creatinine, and PTH
- Serum phosphorus usually elevated except in hypocalcemia from vitamin D deficiency
- Serum PTH usually elevated except in hypoparathyroidism and magnesium deficiency

Management

- Treat underlying cause
- Do not treat hypocalcemia if suspected to be transient response
- Mild/asymptomatic
  - Oral Ca^{2+} 1000-2000 mg/d (of elemental Ca^{2+})
- Acute/symptomatic
  - Calcium gluconate: 1 g IV over 10 min ± slow infusion (10 g in 1000 mL D5W over 10 h)
  - Check serum Ca^{2+} q4-6h
  - If hypomagnesemia present, must be treated to correct hypocalcemia
- If parathyroid hormone (PTH) recovery not expected (e.g. hypoparathyroidism), treat with vitamin D and calcium long-term (use calcitriol for vitamin D replacement if patients have hypoparathyroidism or renal failure)

4.2 Hypercalcemia

- Total serum Ca^{2+} >2.6 mM

Clinical Features

- Symptoms
  - "Bones, stones, abdominal groans with mental overtones"
    - Skeleton "bones": bone pain
    - Renal "stones": renal colic, polyuria, polydipsia
    - "Abdominal groans": N/V, anorexia, constipation, pancreatitis, peptic ulcer disease
    - "Mental overtones": cognitive changes, decreased level of consciousness
- Signs
  - Hypotonia, HTN
  - Evidence of dehydration, may lead to acute kidney injury (AKI)
  - ECG: shortened QT interval

Clinical Pearl: Causes of Hypercalcemia[2]
90% of cases of hypercalcemia are caused by primary hyperparathyroidism or malignancy.

Classification and Causes
- Parathyroid hormone
  - Primary hyperparathyroidism
  - Tertiary hyperparathyroidism of renal failure
- Malignancy
  - Humoral hypercalcemia of malignancy (paraneoplastic parathyroid hormone related peptide [PTHrP])
- Squamous cell carcinoma (lung), renal carcinoma, bladder carcinoma, breast cancer, leukemia
- Solid tumors causing local bone resorption
- Hematologic malignancy (e.g. multiple myeloma)
- Vitamin D elevation (sarcoidosis, TB or exogenous)
- Drugs: thiazides, lithium, calcium carbonate (milk alkali syndrome)
- Familial hypocalciuric hypercalcemia, Addison's disease, hyperthyroidism

Investigations
- Intact PTH is first step in work-up
- Further investigations: phosphate, bicarbonate, PTHrP, albumin, globulin, ALP, serum free light chains, radiographic imaging

Management
- Treat underlying cause
- Normal saline to restore extracellular fluid volume
- Use furosemide if, and only if, extracellular fluid volume overload develops
- Bisphosphonates (e.g. pamidronate) for hypercalcemia of malignancy
- If emergency situation, can use calcitonin subcutaneously
- In primary hyperparathyroidism, symptomatic patients and some asymptomatic ones should be referred for parathyroidectomy or Cincalcet® management (if not surgical candidates)

5. DISORDERS OF PHOSPHATE CONCENTRATION

5.1 Hypophosphatemia
- Serum phosphate <0.84 mM

Clinical Features
- Symptoms
  - Generally absent
  - Proximal muscle weakness, paresthesia, seizures, delirium, coma
- Signs
  - Hemolytic anemia
  - Muscle weakness, ventilatory failure, rhabdomyolysis
  - Heart failure
  - Delirium

Classification and Causes
- Decreased intestinal absorption
  - Poor intake
  - Aluminum- or magnesium-containing antacids
  - Fat malabsorption
  - Vitamin D deficit
- Excessive renal excretion of phosphate (tends to be chronic)
  - Hyperparathyroidism
  - Fanconi syndrome
- Rapid shift of phosphate from extracellular fluid to bone or soft tissue
  - Insulin (either exogenous [treatment of diabetic ketoacidosis] or endogenous [refeeding in patients with severe malnutrition])

- Acute respiratory alkalosis
- Hungry bone syndrome

Investigations
- Measure serum phosphate, PTH
- Measure urine phosphate

Management
- Treat underlying cause
- Chronic cases can be treated with oral phosphate supplementation
- Can treat acute or symptomatic hypophosphatemia with IV potassium phosphate or sodium phosphate

5.2 Hyperphosphatemia
- Serum phosphate >1.8 mM

Clinical Features
- Ectopic soft tissue calcification leading to hypocalcemia
- Clinical features of hypocalcemia (see p.462)

Classification and Causes
- Increased intake
  - Phosphate-containing laxatives
- Decreased output
  - Renal failure
  - Hypoparathyroidism
- Shift of phosphate out of cells
  - Massive cell death (rhabdomyolysis, tumor lysis, hemolysis)
  - Respiratory acidosis

Investigations
- Measure serum phosphate, PTH
- Measure urine phosphate

Management
- Treat underlying cause
- Oral phosphate binders in Stage 3-4 chronic kidney disease (CKD): calcium carbonate, calcium acetate, lanthanum, or sevelamer carbonate given with largest meal

6. DISORDERS OF MAGNESIUM CONCENTRATION

6.1 Hypomagnesemia
- Serum Mg^{2+} <0.7 mM

Clinical Features
- Symptoms
  - CNS: apathy, depression, delirium, seizures, paresthesias
  - Neuromuscular: muscle cramps
- Signs
  - Neuromuscular: increased deep tendon reflexes, tetany
  - Cardiac: arrhythmias (VPBs, ventricular tachycardia)
  - Metabolic: refractory hypokalemia and hypocalcemia

Classification and Causes
- Decreased intake
  - Malabsorption/malnutrition
- Increased losses

- Renal
  - Diuretics (thiazide, furosemide)
  - Alcohol
  - Nephrotoxic drugs (amphotericin, cisplatin, cyclosporine)
  - Rare inherited renal tubular disorders (Bartter syndrome, Gitelman syndrome)
  - Diarrhea

Investigations

- Measure 24 h urine Mg^{2+} excretion (>2 mEq/d indicates excessive renal loss)
- Normal serum Mg^{2+} does not exclude total body Mg^{2+} deficiency

Management

- Mild/chronic: oral magnesium oxide or magnesium lactate
- Severe symptomatic: 1-2 g magnesium sulphate IV over 15 min followed by infusion of 6 g in ≥1 L over 24 h, repeated over 7 d to replete Mg^{2+} stores

6.2 Hypermagnesemia

- Serum Mg^{2+} >1.2 mM

Clinical Features

- Symptoms
  - Mild hypermagnesemia: N/V, skin flushing, bradycardia
  - Moderate hypermagnesemia: weakness, somnolence
  - Severe hypermagnesemia: muscle paralysis, coma
- Signs
  - Mild hypermagnesemia: decreased deep tendon reflexes
  - Moderate hypermagnesemia: hyporeflexia, hypotension
  - Severe hypermagnesemia: refractory hypotension, bradycardia, respiratory failure, decreased LOC

Classification and Causes

- Increased intake
  - Iatrogenic (most commonly in setting of treatment of preeclampsia)
- Decreased output
  - Renal failure (most common cause)

Investigations

- Measure serum Mg^{2+}
- Assess kidney function (creatinine, urea)

Management

- Asymptomatic: stop magnesium-containing products
- Severe symptomatic: 1-2 g calcium gluconate IV over 10 min (plus dialysis in severe renal failure)

7. DISORDERS OF ACID-BASE BALANCE

Information required to evaluate the status of a patient with an acid-base disturbance:

- Arterial blood gases (for ABG see **Respiratory Exam,** p.355)
- Plasma anion gap (see below)
- Clinical evaluation of respiration

Table 2. Normal ABG Values

Normal ABG Values	
pH	7.35-7.45
pCO_2	35-45 mmHg
pO_2	80-100 mmHg
HCO_3^-	22-28 mM

7.1 Respiratory Acidosis

- Pathophysiology: hypoventilation leads to accumulation of CO_2 from metabolism, which lowers the pH of body fluids

Common Causes

- COPD or any severe lung disease associated with excessive work of breathing can eventually lead to respiratory muscle fatigue and hypoventilation
- Drugs (excess amounts of opioids, benzodiazepines, sedating antihistamines, tricyclic antidepressants, barbiturates, anesthetics) or other causes of decreased LOC, hypothyroidism
- Problem with respiratory muscles or chest wall (e.g. nerve problem such as Guillain-Barré syndrome; neuromuscular junction disorder such as myasthenia gravis; severe chest wall abnormality such as kyphoscoliosis)

Normal Compensation

- Increased levels of bicarbonate raises the pH and buffers against respiratory acidosis
- Acute: bicarbonate increases 1 mM for every 10 mmHg increase in pCO_2
- Chronic (after 2-3 d): the kidney increases rate of production of new bicarbonate, resulting in a rise of 3 mM for every 10 mmHg increase in pCO_2

7.2 Respiratory Alkalosis

- Pathophysiology: hyperventilation lowers pCO_2 and thereby raises pH of body fluids

Common Causes

- Any lung disease tends to cause hyperventilation and therefore respiratory alkalosis (provided work of breathing not so great that patient develops respiratory muscle fatigue) (e.g. pneumonia, pulmonary embolism, asthma, pulmonary fibrosis, pulmonary edema)
- Sepsis
- Pregnancy
- Liver failure
- ASA overdose

Normal Compensation

- Decreased levels of bicarbonate lowers the pH and buffers against respiratory alkalosis
- Acute: bicarbonate decreases 2 mM for every 10 mmHg decrease in pCO_2
- Chronic: the kidney reduces bicarbonate production, resulting in a drop of 5 mM for every 10 mmHg decrease in pCO_2

7.3 Metabolic Acidosis

- Pathophysiology: reduction in ECF bicarbonate concentration results in a lower pH
  - This can be caused directly by the addition of H^+ (which binds to bicarbonate to reduce the concentration), loss of bicarbonate from the body; or the failure of the kidneys to produce bicarbonate at the usual rate
  - Use plasma anion gap to help determine etiology

Plasma Anion Gap (PAG)

- PAG = $Na^+ - (HCO_3^- + Cl^-)$, normal value is 12 (range 10-14)
- Proportional to albumin concentration
- If the compound that caused the acidosis contributes an anion, this will be reflected in an increased PAG because the newly ingested substance dissolutes into H^+ and an anion in the body; this new H^+ is mopped up by HCO_3^- and is now reflected in the above formula as a lower amount of HCO_3^-, thus elevating the PAG
- In a pure increased anion gap acidosis, the drop in bicarbonate closely matches the increase in PAG
- If the drop in bicarbonate is significantly greater than the increase in PAG, then there is both an increased anion gap type of metabolic acidosis and also a normal anion gap type of acidosis
- If the drop in bicarbonate is significantly less than the increase in PAG, then there is both an increased anion gap type of metabolic acidosis and also a metabolic alkalosis

Common Causes of Increased PAG Metabolic Acidosis: MUDPILES

- **M**ethanol
- **U**remia
- **D**iabetic ketoacidosis
- **P**araldehyde or Propylene glycol (in car radiator fluid)
- **I**soniazid
- **L**actic acidosis
- **E**thylene glycol
- **S**alicylates

Common Causes of Non-Anion Gap Metabolic Acidosis

- Diarrhea
- Mild to moderate renal failure
- Renal tubular acidosis
- Mineralocorticoid deficiency

Normal Compensation

- Hyperventilation should decrease the pCO_2 (in mmHg) by the same amount as the decrease in bicarbonate (in mM)
- Kussmaul's breathing: respiratory compensation (i.e. hyperventilation) for metabolic acidosis may be clinically detectable in terms of deep and perhaps rapid breathing

7.4 Metabolic Alkalosis

- Pathophysiology: a rise in pH due to an increase in ECF bicarbonate secondary to:
  - Exogenous source
  - Stomach production from emesis
  - Renal production
- Under normal conditions, the kidneys excrete the extra bicarbonate, which corrects the elevated bicarbonate levels, thus preventing metabolic alkalosis
  - During volume and/or potassium depletion, the kidneys retain the extra bicarbonate and thus cause metabolic alkalosis

Common Causes

- Diuretics
- Vomiting
- Excess mineralocorticoid activity

Normal Compensation

- Hypoventilation with a variable increase in pCO_2 (range is 3-8 mmHg for each 10 mM rise in bicarbonate level)

> **Clinical Pearl: Acidosis vs. Acidemic** (Alkalosis vs. Alkalemic)
> AcidOSIS (alkalOSIS) is the final diagnOSIS. The terms acidEMIC or alkalEMIC are solely used to define the pH nature of the blood. Then other variables such as pCO_2 and HCO_3^- are taken into account to arrive at the final diagnOSIS.

Approach to Evaluating Acid-Base Disorders

1. Assess pH – is it acidemic or alkalemic?[10]
2. Determine primary acid-base disorder
   - If pH is acidemic, then there is either metabolic acidosis (reflected by low HCO_3^- level) or respiratory acidosis (reflected by high pCO_2)
   - If pH is alkalemic, then there is either metabolic alkalosis (reflected by high HCO_3^- level) or respiratory alkalosis (reflected by low pCO_2)
   - If pH is normal, then the patient either has no abnormalities, or has two abnormalities that happen to balance each other (e.g. metabolic acidosis and respiratory alkalosis)
3. Determine compensation
   - If primary disorder is metabolic acidosis, then for compensation expect to observe hyperventilation leading to a fall in pCO_2
   - If primary disorder is respiratory acidosis, then for compensation expect to observe increase in HCO_3^- level
   - If primary disorder is metabolic alkalosis, then for compensation expect to observe hypoventilation leading to rise in pCO_2
   - If primary disorder is respiratory alkalosis, then for compensation expect to observe decrease in HCO_3^- level
4. Always calculate PAG

Figure 6. Algorithm for Evaluation of Acid-Base Status

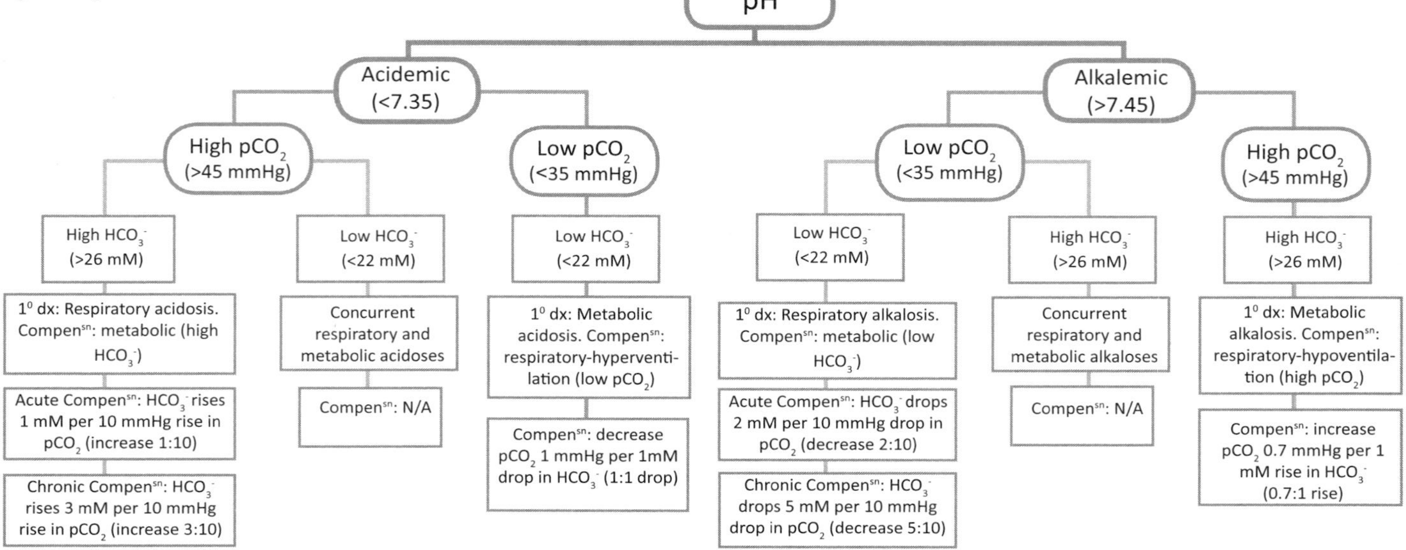

*Failure of normal compensation or overcompensation indicates the presence of a second acid-base disturbance. For example, a patient with a bicarbonate of 10 mM (i.e. a drop of 15) with a pCO_2 of 35 (i.e. a drop of only 5) would represent a combined metabolic and respiratory acidosis – manifested by a failure to reach normal compensation for the metabolic acidosis. When comparing changes in pCO_2 and HCO_3^- levels, use middle values of normal ranges: for pCO_2, 40 mmHg; for HCO_3^- level, 24 mM.

8. INTRAVENOUS FLUIDS

Table 4. Commonly Used IV Solutions (Crystalloids)

Fluid	Components	Tonicity	Indications
D5W (5% dextrose in water)	50 g/L Dextrose	Hypotonic (100% free water)	• Hypernatremia
0.9% NaCl (Normal Saline [NS])	154 mM Na 154 mM Cl	Isotonic	• Fluid resuscitation • Fluid maintenance • Large volumes can cause hyperchloremic non-anion gap metabolic acidosis
0.45% NaCl (½ NS)	77 mM Na 77 mM Cl	Hypotonic (50% free water)	
Ringer's Lactate	130 mM Na 109 mM Cl 4 mM K 3 mM Ca 28 mM Lactate	(nearly) Isotonic	• Avoid in hyperkalemia • Useful in large volume resuscitation (lactate metabolized by liver to bicarbonate)
2/3rds 1/3rd	33 g/L Dextrose 51 mM Na 51 mM Cl	Hypotonic (66% free water)	
3% NaCl	513 mM Na 513 mM Cl	Hypertonic	• Cerebral edema due to hyponatremia

Fluid Balance

- TBW = 60% total body weight = 2/3 ICF + 1/3 ECF (where ICF = intracellular fluid and ECF = 3/4 interstitial + 1/4 intravascular)

Maintenance Fluids

- To calculate maintenance fluids (4/2/1 Rule):
  - 4 mL/kg/h for 1st 10 kg of patient's body weight
  - 2 mL/kg/h for 2nd 10 kg
  - 1 mL/kg/h for the patient's remaining weight
- To calculate maintenance electrolytes:
  - Na^+: 3 mEq/kg/d
  - K^+: 1 mEq/kg/d

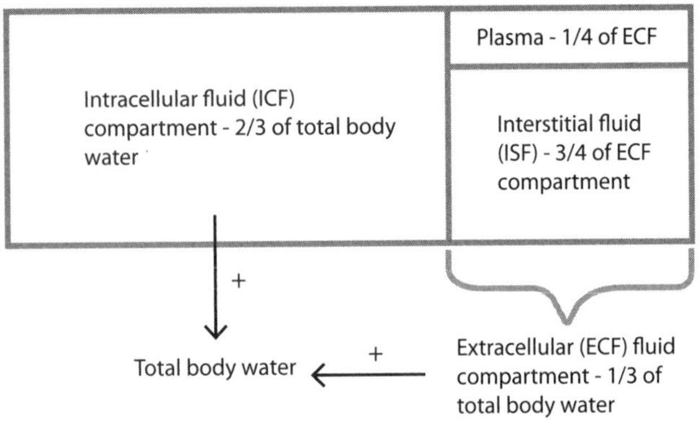

Plasma compartment changes manifest as changes in blood pressure and JVP. IV fluids are added to this compartment initially. The fluid will then equilibrate over the other body fluid compartments as per its tonicity.

For example, if isotonic saline is given it will equilibrate ¼ to plasma and ¾ to ISF. If hypotonic saline is given, the free water component will distribute 2/3 into ICF and 1/3 into ECF (of this amount, ¾ will go to ISF, and ¼ will stay in the plasma). If hypertonic saline is given, it will cause water to move out of the ICF and into the ECF (distributing in proportion), causing cells to shrink.

Increases in ISF will manifest as edematous states.

ICF changes will determine swelling or shrinkage of cells (i.e. especially affects brain cells and cognition).

Figure 7. Concept of Total Body Water
Dr. Martin Schreiber's 2nd year U of T Medicine Lecture on IV Fluids and Homeostasis, 2012.

REFERENCES

1. Baird GS. 2011. Ionized calcium. *Clinica Chimica Acta* 412:696-701.
2. Bilezikian JP, Khan AA, Potts JT. 2009. Guidelines for the management of asymptomatic primary hyperparathyroidism: Summary statement from the third international workshop. *J Clin Endocrinol Metab* 94:2335-2339.
3. Chiasson JL, Aris-Jilwan N, Bélanger R, Bertrand S, Beauregard H, Ekoé JM, et al. 2003. Diagnosis and treatment of diabetic ketoacidosis and the hyperglycemic hyperosmolar state. *CMAJ* 168(7):859-866.
4. McPhee SJ, Papadakis M. *Current Medical Diagnosis and Treatment 2010*. New York: Lange Medical Books/McGraw-Hill, Medical Publications Division; 2010.
5. Moe SM. 2008. Disorders involving calcium, phosphorous and magnesium. *Prim Care* 35(2):215-237, v-vi.
6. Simel DL, Rennie D (Editors). *The Rational Clinical Examination: Evidence-Based Clinical Diagnosis*. New York: McGraw-Hill Medical; 2009.
7. Tierney LM, McPhee SJ, Papadakis MA. *Current Medical Diagnosis and Treatment 2007*. McGraw-Hill Professional; 2006.
8. Cooper DH, Krainik AJ, Lubner SJ, Micek ST, Reno HEL. *The Washington Manual of Medical Therapeutics*. Philadelphia: Lippincott Williams & Wilkins; 2007.
9. Smetana GW, Macpherson DS. 2003. The case against routine preoperative laboratory testing. *Med Clin North Am* 87(1):7-40.
10. ED4Nurses. *6 Easy Steps to ABG Analysis*. 2012. Available from: www.ed4nurses.com.
11. Fauci AS. *Harrison's Principles of Internal Medicine*, 17th ed. New York: McGraw-Hill; 2008.

The Essentials of General Surgery

Editors:
Bailey Dyck
Esther Lau

Faculty Reviewer:
John Bohnen, MD, FACS, FRCS(C)

TABLE OF CONTENTS

1. SURGICAL HISTORY AND PHYSICAL EXAM

In addition to general history taking and physical exam, important aspects of assessing a surgical patient include:

- Cardiac, respiratory, and abdominal H&P (see **Table 1**)
- Assessing risk of cardiac complication in a noncardiac surgical setting using the Revised Cardiac Risk Index (see **Table 2**)
- Assessing risk of pulmonary complication using the Canet Risk Index (see **Table 3**)
- Assessing overall surgical risk using the American Society of Anesthesiologists Physical Status Classification (see **Table 4**)

Table 1. Cardiac, Pulmonary, and Abdominal Evaluation

	History	Physical Exam
CV	Symptoms: SOB, angina, syncope, palpitations Diagnoses: DM, MI, valvular heart disease, CHF Procedures: CABG, angioplasty, prosthetic heart valve	See **Cardiovascular Exam**, p.52
Resp	Habitus: smoking Hx, occupational exposure, obesity Symptoms: sputum production, exertional dyspnea, functional status (e.g. walk up a flight of stairs), wheezing Diagnoses: COPD, asthma	See **Respiratory Exam**, p.351

GENERAL SURGERY

Table 1. Cardiac, Pulmonary, and Abdominal Evaluation (continued)

	History	Physical Exam
Abdo	Symptoms: pain, changes in bowel habits, vomiting, bleeding (hematemesis, melena, hematochezia)	See **Abdominal Exam**, p.20

CABG = coronary artery bypass surgery, SOB = shortness of breath
Lee TH, et al. 1999. *Circulation* 100(10):1043-1049.

Table 2. Assessing Cardiac Risk: Revised Cardiac Risk Index

Factors	Points
History of CHF	1
History of Ischemic Heart Disease	1
History of Cerebrovascular Disease	1
Preoperative Treatment with Insulin	1
Preoperative Serum Creatinine Level >177 μM	1
High-Risk Surgical Procedure	1
Probability of Major Cardiac Complication: 0 points, 0.4 - 0.5%; 1 point, 0.9 - 1.3%; 2 points, 4.0 - 7.0%; 3+ points, 9.0 - 11.0%	

Canet J, et al. 2010. *Anesthesiology* 113(6):1338-1350.

Table 3. Assessing Pulmonary Risk: Canet Risk Index

Factors	Points
Age	
≤50 yr	0
51-80 yr	3
>80 yr	16
Preoperative O_2 Saturation	
≥96%	0
91-95%	8
≤90%	24
Respiratory Infection in the Last Month	17
Preoperative Anemia: Hemoglobin ≤100 g/L	11
Surgical Incision	
Upper abdominal	15
Intrathoracic	24
Duration of Surgery	
≤2 h	0
2-3 h	16
>3 h	23
Emergency Surgery	8
Probability of Pulmonary Complication: <26 points, low risk (1.6%); 26-44 points, intermediate risk (13.3%); ≥45 points, high risk (42.1%)	

Table 4. Assessing Surgical Risk: American Society of Anesthesiologists (ASA) Physical Status Classification

Class	Patient Status
I	Healthy patient
II	Patient with mild systemic disease
III	Patient with severe but not incapacitating systemic disease
IV	Patient with severe systemic disease that poses constant threat to life
V	Moribund patient who is not expected to survive without surgery
VI	Patient who has been declared brain-dead and whose organs are being removed for donor purposes

ASA classes I and II correspond to low risk; class III corresponds to moderate risk; and classes IV and V correspond to high risk.

Dripps RD, Lamont A, Eckenhoff JE. 1961. *JAMA* 178:261-266.

2. PREOPERATIVE MANAGEMENT

Preoperative Admission[1]

Investigations

- CXR: in patients with cardiopulmonary disease, or >50 yr undergoing major surgery
- ECG
- See **Table 5** for indications for other investigations

Laboratory Tests

- CBC, Hb, electrolytes, creatinine, sickle test in high risk groups[2]
- Type and Screen for ABO and Rh status: if expected blood loss, want minimum 2 units packed RBCs
- Coagulation: anticoagulants should be discontinued prior to surgery (ASA, 7-10 d prior; Plavix, 5 d prior; Warfarin, 3-5 d prior); check INR

Forms

- Informed consent
- Code status: discuss advance directives

Calls and Contacts

- Consult: appropriate services if required
- Book the operating room (OR): call Anesthesia, nurses

Table 5. Indications for Preoperative Laboratory Investigations

Investigations	Indications
Hb	Procedure associated with significant blood loss
WBC	Infection symptoms, myeloproliferative disease, myelotoxic medications
Platelets	Bleeding disorder, myeloproliferative disease, myelotoxic medications
PTT and INR	Bleeding disorder, chronic liver disease, malnutrition, long-term antibiotic or anticoagulant use
Electrolytes	Renal insufficiency, CHF, diuretic, digoxin, ACE inhibitors

Table 5. Indications for Preoperative Laboratory Investigations (continued)

Investigations	Indications
Creatinine and BUN	Age >50 yr, DM, HTN, cardiac disease, medications that influence renal function (ACE inhibitors, NSAIDs), major surgery
Glucose	Obesity, known DM or symptoms thereof, infection or suspected infection
Albumin	Liver disease, serious chronic illness, recent major illness, malnutrition
Urinalysis	No indication
Chest X-ray	Age >50 yr, known cardiopulmonary disease or symptoms thereof
ECG	Males >40 yr, females >50 yr, CAD, HTN, DM

Smetana GW, Macpherson DS. 2003. *Med Clin North Am* 87(1):7-40.

3. OPERATIVE MANAGEMENT

Operative Note

- Date and time of procedure
- Preoperative diagnosis
- Postoperative diagnosis
- Procedures
- Names of surgeons and assistants
- Operative findings
- Complications
- Anesthesia (e.g. general, regional, local)
- Estimated blood loss (EBL)
- Crystalloid replaced (type and volume)
- Blood products administered
- Tubes and drains (e.g. nasogastric [NG], Foley, Jackson-Pratt [JP])
- Urine output
- Specimens collected: cultures, blood, pathology
- Intraoperative X-rays
- Condition of patient on transfer to post-anesthesia care unit (PACU)
- Disposition after PACU

Sutures

- See **Figure 1**

Timing of Suture Removal[3]

- Face (including lips): 5-7 d
- Eyelids: 3-5 d
- Hands/feet: 10-14 d
- Trunk: 7-10 d
- Breast: 7-10 d

Note: if staples were used as opposed to sutures, remove as early as day 3 (regardless of site) and replace with Steri-strips

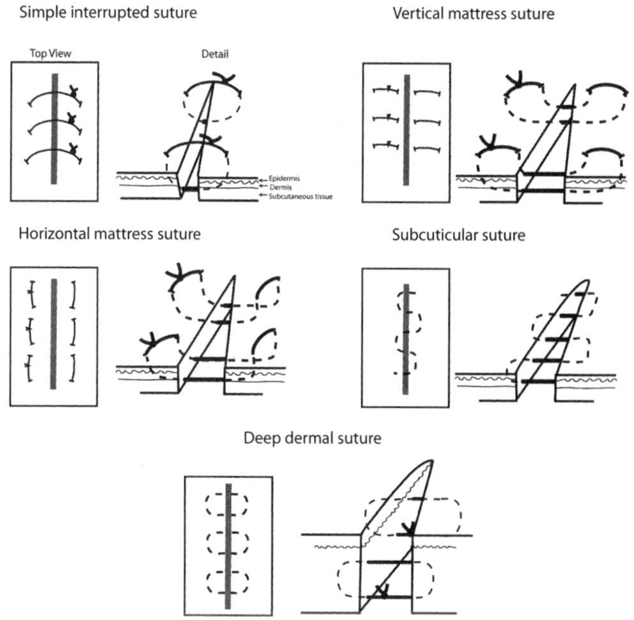

Prerna C. Patel and Miliana Vojvodic

Figure 1. Common Suturing Techniques

4. POSTOPERATIVE MANAGEMENT

4.1 Postoperative Orders: ADDAVID

Admit to ward/service (under the care of Dr.______)

Diagnosis Pre/Postoperatively

Diet

- Preoperative: NPO (*nil per os* = nothing by mouth) → must have IV, see below
- Postoperative: NPO → sips/clear fluids (CF) → diet as tolerated (DAT)
- Total parenteral nutrition nutrition (TPN); requires Interventional Radiology consult to insert peripherally inserted central catheter (PICC) line

Activity

- Activities as tolerated (AAT)
- Bed rest/elevate head of bed/other special positions

Vital Signs

- Vital signs routine (VSR, as per floor)
- Vitals q4h (vitals every 4 h)
- Notify MD if: systolic BP <90 mmHg, HR >120 bpm, temperature >38.5°C or O_2 saturation <92%

IV, Ins/Outs, Investigations

- IV
  - Normal saline (NS) at 125 cc/h (+10-20 mEq/L KCl, avoid K if oliguric)

- If dehydrated, bolus with NS or Ringer's lactate
  - If patient drinking well postoperatively
    - IV to keep vein open when drinking well (IV TKVO WDW; means IV running at 5 cc/h)
    - IV to SL (saline lock)
    - D/C (discontinue) IV
- Ins/Outs
  - NG tube (to suction/straight drain); especially upper GI obstruction; if excessive losses via NG, then replace losses 1:1 with NS + 20 mEq/L KCl
  - JP drains to bulb suction
  - Foley catheter to straight drain/urometer
  - Measure IV/PO in and all fluids out
  - Maintain O_2 saturation >92%
- Lab Investigations
  - Routine blood work (b/w): CBC, electrolytes, BUN, creatinine
  - Assess for coagulopathy: partial thromboplastin time (PTT), INR, platelet count (in CBC differential)
  - Imaging/tests (as indicated):
    - CXR, X-ray of extremity
    - ECG
  - Consults (as indicated)
    - Internal Medicine
    - Anesthesia, Acute Pain Service

Drugs (6 A's)
- **A**nalgesics
  - Morphine 5-10 mg SC q3h PRN for pain
  - Tylenol® #3 1-2 tabs PO q4h PRN for pain
    - ***Note:*** maximum acetaminophen from all sources is 4 g/24 h
  - NSAID often used to reduce opioid need: choice of ketorolac (Toradol) parenteral; indomethacin suppository; or oral ibuprofen. Keep course short to avoid risk of GI bleed, coagulopathy, other complications in elderly
    - ***Note:*** unless fresh GI anastomosis, may order stool softener with opioid pain medications (constipating)
- **A**ntiembolics: Heparin 5000 units SC q12h
- **A**ntecedents
  - While NPO, may need to withhold oral medications taken prior to admission (e.g. antihypertensives, thyroid, hormone replacement, etc.) or replace with IV medications
  - Note potential contribution of medications to coagulopathy (see **Essentials of Pharmacology and Toxicology**, p.389)
    - ASA (Aspirin®) = antiplatelet
    - Warfarin (Coumadin®) = anticoagulant
    - NSAIDs = reversible COX-1, 2 inhibitors
  - Postoperative: restart medications
- **A**ntibiotics
  - Base empiric treatment on likely causative organisms until culture results are available. Common organisms include: *E. coli* and *B. fragilis* in community-acquired abdominal infections; hospital organisms and fungi in hospital-acquired abdominal infections; Group A streptococcus, gram positive (GP) cocci, gram negatives (GNs) in cellulitis; GN rods in UTI; and GN rods and *S. aureus* in pneumonia (including anaerobes if aspiration)
  - Hospital resistance patterns should guide therapy once culture results obtained

- Refer to *The Sanford Guide to Antimicrobial Therapy* and/ or *Compendium of Pharmaceuticals and Specialties* (CPS) for comprehensive and updated information

- **A**ntiemetics
  - Dimenhydrinate (Gravol®) 25-50 mg IV/IM/PO q3-4h for nausea
- **A**nxiolytics
  - Benzodiazepines (e.g. diazepam, lorazepam)
- CAUTION: Do NOT order medications PO with concurrent NPO order

4.2 Progress Note: SOAP

- Date/Time, Service, POD (postoperative day) #, your name (legibly)

S̲ubjective

- Changes in symptoms, significant events, physical complaints in patient's own words, pain control

O̲bjective

- Vital signs
- Intake and output (urinary output [UO], NG, JP)
- Physical exam: check incision site (take off dressing from 48 h onward), lines, chest, neurovascular status
- Investigations: CBC, electrolytes, imaging, etc.

A̲ssessment and P̲lan

- Increase activity; plan discharge in advance
- For each identified problem, devise an appropriate therapeutic regimen

4.3 Postoperative Pain Management

- See **Figure 2**

4.4 Postoperative Complications

Table 6. Presentation and Management of Common Postoperative Complications

Complication	Presentation	Management
Fever	If caused by infection, tend to reach higher temperatures (>38.5°C) and associated with moderately elevated WBC on POD 3 or later	**Investigations:** WBC, respiratory exam (cough, sputum, respiratory effort), check lines, further work-up as indicated (CXR, sputum cultures, blood cultures, urinalysis, CT abdomen) **Treatment:** discontinue any unnecessary Tx, treat underlying cause; think **4 W**'s: **W**ind (atelectasis), **W**ater (UTI), **W**ound (SSI), **W**hat did we do (DVT/PE, hospital acquired infections, drug reaction)
Pneumonia	Fever, SOB, hypoxia, productive cough, and rales on lung auscultation	**Investigations:** CXR, sputum cultures **Treatment:** see **Postoperative Note** (Drugs – Antibiotics), p. 478

GENERAL SURGERY

Table 6. Presentation and Management of Common Postoperative Complications (continued)

Complication	Presentation	Management
Surgical Site Infection (SSI)	Pain, erythema, swelling at the surgical site; usually not before POD 5	**Investigations:** cultures of purulent material from SSI **Treatment:** open and drain the wound, allow to heal by secondary intention, antibiotics depending on presence of cellulitis and for remote endoprosthesis
Deep Vein Thrombosis (DVT)	Lower extremity pain or one leg is noticeably more swollen than the other; physical exam unreliable	**Investigations:** venous duplex U/S **Treatment:** heparin infusion, switch to warfarin when patient is stable
Pulmonary Embolism (PE)	Decreased O_2 saturation or SOB, chest pain, tachycardia, diaphoresis	**Investigations:** spiral CT ± venous duplex U/S **Treatment:** heparin infusion (may be appropriate to start before Dx is confirmed)

POD = postoperative day, SOB = shortness of breath
Ashley SW (Editor). *ACS Surgery: Principles and Practice*. Hamilton: BC Decker; 2012.

4.5 Discharge Note

- Date and time
- Diagnoses
- Therapy and operations during hospital stay
- Investigations: ECG, CXR, CT
- Discharge medications
- Follow-up arrangements

EBM: Prevention of Surgical Site Infections (SSI)

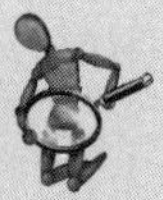

Timing of prophylactic antibiotics: Prophylactic antibiotics should be administered within 60 min of skin incision. In a study of 2847 surgical patients, compared to patients who received antibiotics within 2 h before the incision, those who received antibiotics earlier (2-24 h before incision), perioperatively (within 3 h after incision) or postoperatively (3-24 h after incision) had a higher chance of having SSI (relative risk = 6.7, 2.4, and 5.8, respectively).*

Maintenance of normothermia: Patient's core temperature should be maintained intraoperatively. In a study of 200 patients undergoing colorectal surgery, SSI were found in 19% of patients in the hypothermia group (34.7 ± 0.6°C), compared to 6% in the normothermia group (36.6 ± 0.5°C).†

Skin preparation: Chlorhexidine-alcohol should be used for preoperative cleansing of the patient's skin instead of povidone-iodine. In a study of 849 patients, the overall rate of SSI was significantly lower in the chlorhexidine-alcohol group than in the povidone-iodine group (9.5% vs. 16.1%).‡

*Classen DC, et al. 1992. *N Engl J Med* 326(5):281-286.
†Kurz A, Sessler DI, Lenhardt R. 1996. *N Engl J Med* 334(19):1209-1216.
‡Darouiche RO, et al. 2010. *N Engl J Med* 362(1):18-26.

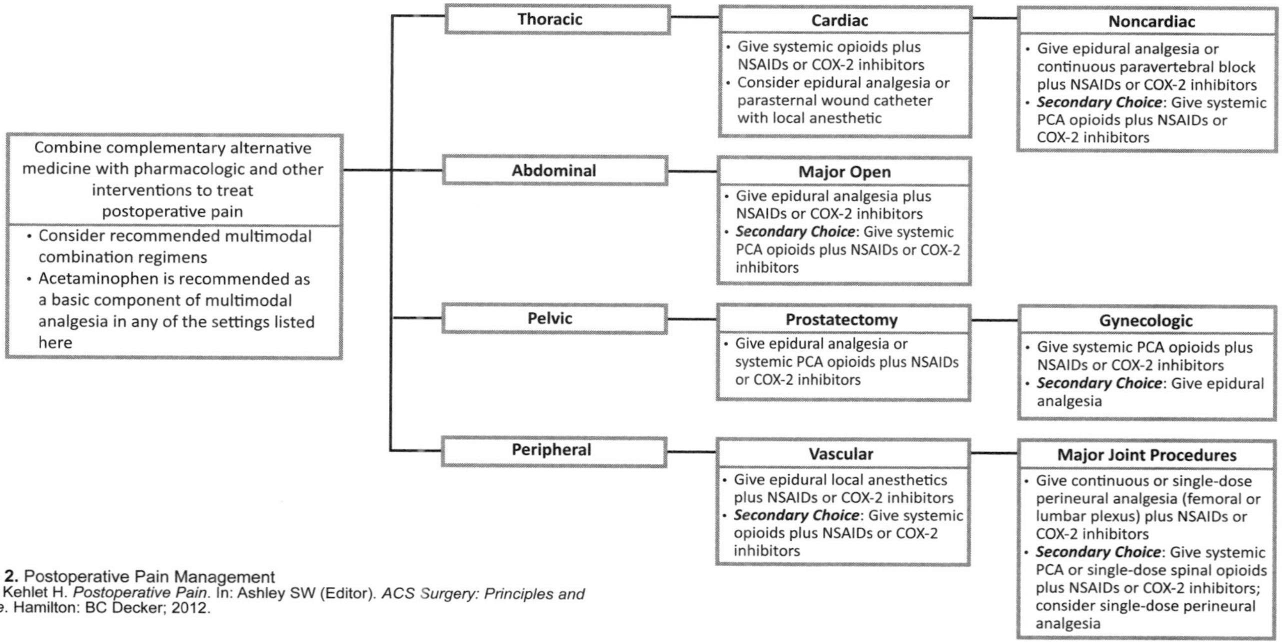

Figure 2. Postoperative Pain Management
Liu SS, Kehlet H. *Postoperative Pain*. In: Ashley SW (Editor). *ACS Surgery: Principles and Practice*. Hamilton: BC Decker; 2012.

5. SPECIAL CIRCUMSTANCES

Common Emergency Neonatal Surgical Problems[4]
- Congenital diaphragmatic hernia (CDH)
- Esophageal atresia
- Congenital lobar emphysema
- Intestinal obstruction
- Omphalocele, gastroschisis
- Exstrophy of the bladder
- Meningomyelocele

Common Surgical Problems in Infants and Children[4]
- Pyloric stenosis
- Gastroesophageal reflux
- Neck and soft tissue masses
- Inguinal hernia
- Undescended testes
- Acute appendicitis
- Intussusception
- Meckel diverticulum and lower GI hemorrhage

Approach to Acute Abdominal Pain in the Pregnant Patient[4]
- History, physical exam (3rd trimester: appendix is in right upper quadrant [RUQ])
- Place IV, start fluids as needed
- Insert NG tube if significant vomiting
- Perform routine labs
- Use fetal monitor after 24 wk
- Limit X-rays, avoid radionuclide scans, use abdominal and pelvic U/S

Table 7. General Surgical Approaches for the Elderly, Pregnant, and Pediatric Patient

Elderly Patient[4-6]	
Preoperative Assessment[7]	• Comprehensive geriatric assessment (CGA), including: functional status, comorbidities, nutrition, cognition, depression, social support, polypharmacy • DVT prophylaxis
Intraoperative Considerations	• Prolonged operative time
Postoperative Management	• Initiate respiratory therapy early • Encourage early ambulation • Pressure ulcer prevention (i.e. frequent turning, visual inspection) • Monitor for delirium
Pregnant Patient[4,8]	
Preoperative Assessment[9]	• Assess for Hx of DVT/PE, thrombocytopenia, bleeding disorders • Assess for Hx of CV disease, involve specialists as needed • If asthmatic: assess severity, watch Sx in context of histamine-releasing opioids (will worsen Sx) • Confirm antepartum HIV testing, on HAART if HIV+
Intraoperative Considerations	• Watch for severe preeclampsia, fetal bradycardia → emergent C-section

GENERAL SURGERY

Table 7. General Surgical Approaches for the Elderly, Pregnant, and Pediatric Patient (continued)

Pregnant Patient	
Postoperative Management[10]	• Slightly higher rates of complications due to cholecystectomy: VTE; infection; return to OR • 20% and 5% chance of fetal loss during surgery for perforated appendicitis and Sx of cholelithiasis, respectively
Pediatric Patient[4,11,12]	
Preoperative Assessment	• Assess for the following in the context of increasing postoperative risk of complications: not full term; ASA score >3; undergoing CV or neurological surgery; receiving intraoperative albumin transfusion • Assess for the following in the context of increasing intraoperative complications: not full term; ASA score >3; Hx of CV disease; undergoing CV, neurological, ortho surgery
Postoperative Management	• Infants in the first year experience highest rates of failure to rescue, infection, postoperative hemorrhage/hematoma, PE/DVT, and postoperative sepsis

CV = cardiovascular, HAART = Highly Active Anti-Retroviral Therapy, Sx = symptom, VTE = venous thromboembolism

6. COMMON CLINICAL SCENARIOS

6.1 Acute Appendicitis[4]

- **Signs and Symptoms:** acute abdominal pain (<48 h), pain periumbilical → right lower quadrant (RLQ), ± N/V, anorexia, diarrhea, constipation, fever
- **Physical Exam:** assess general appearance and positioning (i.e. pain), vitals; auscultate heart and lungs; perform abdominal exam, including DRE and groin inspection; perform pelvic exam
- **Investigations:** abdominal CT scan if diagnosis not obvious; ECG in elderly with heart Hx
- **Laboratory Tests:** CBC, hematocrit, serum electrolytes, BUN, serum creatinine, urinalysis
- **Treatment:** laparoscopy or laparotomy: immediately if spreading peritonitis, very sick or worsening clinically

6.2 Acute Cholecystitis[4]

- **Signs and Symptoms:** acute abdominal pain, localized to RUQ, ± referred pain (R subscapular area), ± N/V, anorexia, diarrhea, fever
- **Physical Exam:** assess general appearance and positioning (i.e. pain), vitals; auscultate heart and lungs; perform abdominal exam, including DRE and groin inspection; perform pelvic exam
- **Investigations:** abdominal U/S; ECG in elderly with heart Hx
- **Laboratory Tests:** CBC, hematocrit, serum electrolytes, LFTs (serum bilirubin, ALP, albumin, INR, PTT, ALT/AST), amylase, urinalysis
- **Treatment:** laparoscopic cholecystectomy (may require conversion to laparotomy)

6.3 Perforated Bowel[4]

- **History:** Hx of peptic ulcer disease? NSAID use?
- **Signs and Symptoms:** Phase 1 (<2 h): sudden onset severe abdominal pain, usually epigastric → generalized; tachycardia, weak pulse, low temperature; Phase 2 (2-12 h): lessened pain, abdominal rigidity, ± loss of liver dullness, tender on DRE; Phase 3 (>12 h): increasing abdominal distention, elevated temperature, hypovolemia, signs of peritonitis

- **Physical Exam:** assess general appearance and positioning (i.e. pain), vitals; auscultate heart and lungs; perform abdominal exam focusing on peritoneal signs, include DRE
- **Investigations:** CXR, abdominal X-ray
- **Laboratory Tests:** CBC, hematocrit, serum electrolytes, LFTs (serum bilirubin, ALP, albumin, INR, PTT, ALT/AST), amylase, urinalysis; rule out *C. difficile*, *Cytomegalovirus*, *E. coli*
- **Treatment:** urgent laparotomy or laparoscopy

6.4 Bowel Obstruction (BO)[4]

- **History:** previous episodes of BO? Previous abdominal/pelvic surgery? Hx of abdominal cancer? Hx of intra-abdominal inflammation, e.g. IBD, pelvic inflammatory disease (PID), pancreatitis, trauma? Recent change in bowel habits? Weight loss? Passage of flatus? Metabolic conditions? Radiation exposure? Current medications? (e.g. anticoagulants, anticholinergics)
- **Signs and Symptoms:** abdominal pain or distention, N/V, obstipation
- **Physical Exam:** assess general appearance, vitals, hydration status, cardiopulmonary system; perform abdominal exam – special considerations: auscultate 1 min, thoroughly search for hernias, perform DRE
- **Investigations:** determine if small BO (OR often unnecessary) or colonic BO (commonly cancer needing OR, cecum may burst if distended) with abdominal X-rays (supine, upright, lateral decubitus; usually CT and/or water-soluble contrast enema); alarm if cecum >10 cm; sometimes GI endoscopy
- **Laboratory Tests:** serum electrolytes, hematocrit, serum creatinine, coagulation profile
- **Treatment:** place NG tube, Foley catheter, IV; complete and/or colonic BO = immediate or urgent operation; partial and/or small BO = may try conservative management with NG suction, reassess hourly then q4h; repeat X-rays

REFERENCES

1. Blankstein U, Blankstein M. 2012. The 'perfect' pre-operative admission: A practical guide. *UTMJ* 89:170-171.
2. National Institute for Clinical Excellence. *Preoperative Tests: The Use of Routine Preoperative Tests for Elective Surgery*. Clinical Guideline 3. 2003. Available from: http://www.nice.org.uk/nicemedia/pdf/CG3NICEguideline.pdf.
3. Souba WW, Fink MP, Jurkovich GJ, Kaiser LR, Pearce WH, Pemberton JH, et al. *ACS Surgery: Principles and Practice*, 6th ed. Hamilton: BC Decker; 2007.
4. Ashley SW (Editor). *ACS Surgery: Principles and Practice*. Hamilton: BC Decker; 2012.
5. Kirshhtein B, Perry ZH, Mizrahi S, Lantsberg L. 2009. Value of laparoscopic appendectomy in the elderly patient. *World J Surg* 33(5):918-922.
6. Sprung J, Gajic O, Warner DO. 2006. Age related alterations in respiratory function – Anesthetic considerations. *Can J Anesth* 53(12):1244-1257.
7. Egol KA, Strauss EJ. 2009. Perioperative considerations in geriatric patients with hip fracture: What is the evidence? *J Orthop Trauma* 23(6):386-394.
8. Corneille MG, Gallup TM, Bening T, Wolf SE, Brougher C, Myers JG, et al. 2010. The use of laparoscopic surgery in pregnancy: Evaluation of safety and efficacy. *Am J Surg* 200(3):363-367.
9. Hinova A, Fernando R. 2010. The preoperative assessment of obstetric patients. *Best Pract Res Clin Obstet Gynaecol* 24(3):261-276.
10. Erekson EA, Brousseau EC, Dick-Biascoechea MA, Ciarleglio MM, Lockwood CJ, Pettker CM. 2012. Maternal postoperative complications after nonobstetric antenatal surgery. *J Matern Fetal Neonatal Med* 25(12):2639-2644.
11. Miller MR, Zhan C. 2004. Pediatric patient safety in hospitals: A national picture in 2000. *Pediatrics* 113(6):1741-1746.
12. Weinberg AC, Huang L, Jiang H, Tinloy B, Raskas MD, Penna FJ, et al. 2011. Perioperative risk factors for major complications in pediatric surgery: A study in surgical risk assessment for children. *J Am Coll Surg* 212(5):768-778.

The Essentials of Infectious Diseases

Editors:
Mackenzie Howatt
Jennifer M. Tran

Faculty Reviewers:
Wayne L. Gold, MD, FRCP(C)
Susan M. Poutanen, MD, MPH, FRCP(C)

TABLE OF CONTENTS

1. UPPER RESPIRATORY TRACT INFECTION

An infection of the upper respiratory tract that can range from self-limiting to lethal presentations depending on patient age, immune status, and infectious agent.

Etiology

- Mostly viral, but can be bacterial, mycobacterial or fungal in origin

Focused History

- Signs and Symptoms (see **Table 1**)

Focused Physical Exam

- See **Respiratory Exam**, p.351
- See **Head and Neck Exam**, p.108
- If specific localization of symptoms is observed – such as sinus, ears, pharynx, lower airway – then specific examination of those structures is required
- Ear and mastoid: pneumatic otoscopy, focused neurological exam of CN VIII (see **Neurological Exam**, p.180)
- Larynx: direct laryngoscopy

Table 1. Common Upper Respiratory Tract Infections

Diagnosis	Presenting Signs/ Symptoms	Investigations	Complications
Common Cold	Sneezing, nasal congestion and discharge (rhinorrhea), sore throat, cough, low grade fever, headache, and malaise	Clinical diagnosis; suspect alternative dx if >2 wk or high fever	Secondary bacterial rhinosinusitis, lower respiratory tract infections (LRTIs), otitis media
Acute Rhinosinusitis	Nasal congestion, obstruction, discharge, maxillary tooth pain, facial pain, fever, cough, headache	Clinical diagnosis; suspect bacterial etiology if >10 d without improvement; severe symptoms at the onset of illness; worsening symptoms after initial improvement	Bacterial sinusitis, meningitis, orbital cellulitis
Pharyngitis	Sore throat, tonsillar edema/exudate, tender anterior cervical lymph nodes, splenomegaly; cough and significant rhinorrhea are usually absent	Swab for culture, rapid streptococcal antigen testing (RSAT)	Peritonsillar/ retropharyngeal abscess, post-strep glomerulonephritis (GN), rheumatic fever

Note: Epiglottitis should always be considered on the differential diagnosis. May find drooling, respiratory distress, and dysphagia. This can lead to respiratory compromise and is a medical emergency[1].
Mandell GL, Bennett JE, Dolin R (Editors). *Mandell, Douglas, and Bennett's Principles and Practice of Infectious Diseases*, 7th ed. New York: Churchill Livingstone/Elsevier; 2010.

Investigations

- The common cold is generally self-resolving with nonspecific laboratory examinations, and thus should not be routinely investigated
- Pharynx and oral cavity: key investigation is to distinguish Group A streptococcal pharyngitis from viral pharyngitis
  - Throat swab culture (takes 24-48 h)
  - Rapid antigen detection testing for Group A β-hemolytic streptococci (GABHS) (less sensitive)
- Epiglottitis: Fiber optic laryngoscopy in the OR for visualization, or "thumb-printing" on lateral neck X-ray[2] (direct visualization in the examination room with tongue blade and laryngoscope NOT recommended)

Management

- Antibiotic therapy not indicated for uncomplicated common colds; symptomatic management includes decongestants, NSAIDs, dextromethorphan (for cough), lozenges, etc.
- Pharyngitis: see **EBM: Sore Throat Score** (p.487) for management criteria

EBM: Sore Throat Score

Symptom or Sign	Points
History of Fever or Temperature >38°C	1
Absence of Cough	1
Swollen, Tender, Anterior Cervical Adenopathy	1
Tonsillar Swelling or Exudate	1
Age 3-14 yr	1
Age ≥45 yr	–1

Total Points	Likelihood Ratio	Management
-1 or 0	0.05	No further testing or antibiotics required
1	0.52	
2	0.95	Culture ALL: antibiotics only for positive results
3	2.5	
4 or 5	4.9	Treat empirically with antibiotics

McIsaac WJ, et al. 2004. *JAMA* 291(13):1587-1595.

2. LOWER RESPIRATORY TRACT INFECTIONS

Acute Bronchitis

- Etiology: primarily viral
- Focused history: similar to URTI with cough ± sputum >5 d
- Focused physical exam (see **Respiratory Exam**, p.359)
- Investigations: no cultures recommended; CXR if pneumonia is suspected
- Management: no antibiotics indicated

Pneumonia

- Etiology: bacterial, viral, and less often fungal in origin
- Focused history: fever, productive cough, pleuritic chest pain, dyspnea
- Focused physical exam (see **Respiratory Exam**, p.360)
- Investigations: CXR, sputum and blood cultures; consider nasopharyngeal swab for influenza during influenza season
- Management: empiric antibiotic therapy; during influenza season, consider empiric antivirals for influenza while awaiting influenza test results; see **EBM: CURB-65 Criteria** below for admission criteria

EBM: CURB-65 Criteria

Score of 0 = low mortality rate, send home with oral antibiotics
Score of 1,2 = moderate severity, consider admission
Score of 3,4 = high severity, urgent admission, empiric antibiotics

Sign	Point
Confusion (urea >7 mM)	+1
Respiratory Rate >30	+1
BP Systolic <90 or Diastolic <60	+1
Age >65 yr	+1

Lim WS, et al. 2003. *Thorax* 58(5):377-382.

3. TUBERCULOSIS

- Caused by the *Mycobacterium tuberculosis* complex, manifesting as pulmonary and extrapulmonary disease (see **Table 2**)
- Transmission via airborne droplets produced by coughing from individuals with active pulmonary TB

Table 2. Extrapulmonary Tuberculosis

Location	History	Physical Findings
Lymph Nodes	Accompanying HIV infection, immunosuppression	Painless swelling of lymph nodes, most commonly at cervical and supraclavicular sites
Upper Airways	Hoarseness, chronic productive cough	Ulcerations
Pleura	Asymptomatic, fever, pleuritic chest pain, dyspnea	Pleural effusion, dullness to percussion, absence of breath sounds
Pericardial	Subacute or acute with fever, dull retrosternal pain	Friction rub, cardiac tamponade, constrictive pericarditis
Peritoneal	No specific history	Abdominal/pelvic masses
Genitourinary	Asymptomatic, urinary frequency, dysuria, hematuria, flank pain	**Females:** infertility, pelvic pain, menstrual abnormalities **Males:** epididymitis, prostatitis, orchiditis
Musculo-skeletal (spine)	Back pain, paraplegia, paraparesis	Kyphosis (gibbus deformity)
Sites Outside Spine	Monoarticular destructive arthritis	Hip, knee, ankle, or elbow pain
Miliary or Disseminated	Accompanying HIV infection, fever, night sweats, anorexia, weakness, weight loss	Hepatomegaly, splenomegaly, lymphadenopathy, choroidal tubercles in retina
CNS	Headache, mental lethargy, altered sensorium, neck rigidity	Obtundation, cranial nerve palsies

Long R, Ellis E (Editors). *Canadian Tuberculosis Standards*, 6th ed. Ottawa: Public Health Agency of Canada; 2007.
Heymann DL (Editor). *Control of Communicable Diseases Manual*, 19th ed. Washington: American Public Health Association; 2008.

INFECTIOUS DISEASES

3.1 Pulmonary Tuberculosis

Focused History

- Risk Factors
  - Endemic areas: Eastern Europe, Mediterranean, Russia, China, Southeast Asia, India, Pakistan, Africa, and South America (assume exposure regardless of whether the patient recognizes an exposure or not)
  - HIV/AIDS
  - First Nations peoples
  - Homelessness, individual with a history of imprisonment, lack of social support, joblessness, and poverty
  - Substance abuse
  - Family members with TB
  - Actual exposure to known TB cases

- Immunosuppression (organ transplant, long-term corticosteroids, DM, chronic kidney disease [CKD])
- Nonspecific Symptoms: fever that persists more than 2 wk, night sweats, weight loss, chills, general malaise, weakness
- Pulmonary Symptoms
  - Cough: may be initially nonproductive and subsequently purulent
  - Sputum ± hemoptysis
  - Pleuritic chest pain
  - Dyspnea or acute respiratory distress syndrome (ARDS)

Focused Physical Exam

- General inspection: age, degree of nutrition, emotional and anxiety states, cyanosis
- Fever
- Wasting
- Chest examination (see **Respiratory Exam**, p.351)
- Tachypnea
- Persistent rales in involved areas during inspiration, especially after coughing
- Rhonchi due to partial bronchial obstruction
- Whispered pectoriloquy may be helpful in finding small areas of local consolidation
- Amphoric breath sounds in areas with large cavities
- Percussion: fluid accumulation suggested by flat, wooden sounds
- Grocco's sign: presence of paravertebral area of dullness on the opposite side
- May have no detectable abnormalities

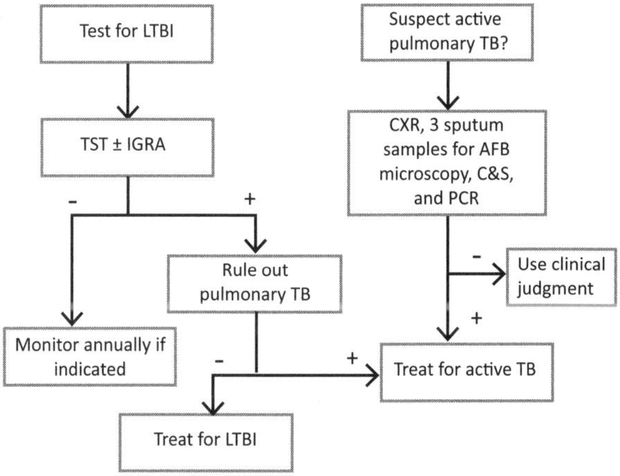

Figure 1. Flow Chart for TB Diagnosis
AFB = acid fast bacilli, IGRA = IFN-γ release assay, LTBI = latent TB infection, PCR = polymerase chain reaction, TST = tuberculin skin test

Investigation Notes

- Tuberculin skin test (TST) (used for latent infection, not for active TB infection; sensitivity = 90%, specificity >95% for 10 mm induration)[3,4]
  - False negatives common in immunosuppressed patients
  - False positives with nontuberculosis mycobacteria (NTM) and by BCG vaccination
  - Induration NOT erythema should be measured (see **Table 3**)
- Interferon gamma (IFN-γ) release assays
  - Can be used in conjunction with TSTs

- CXR
  - Usually shows upper lobe infiltrates with cavities but in immunosuppressed patients, atypical pattern of lower lobe infiltration without cavities seen
- 3 sputum specimens
  - Used to detect TB through microscopy for acid fast bacilli (AFB), C&S, and PCR (amplified mycobacterium tuberculosis direct test)
- CT and MRI can be used for imaging of extrapulmonary TB

Table 3. Tuberculin Skin Test Interpretation

Induration	Condition in which Size is Considered Positive
0-4 mm	HIV infection with immune suppression AND the expected likelihood of TB infection is high
5-9 mm	HIV infection, close contact of active contagious case, children suspected of having tuberculosis disease, abnormal chest X-ray with fibrotic disease, other immune suppression: TNF-α inhibitors
10-15 mm	Recent immigrants from endemic countries, IV drug users, people working in high-risk settings (e.g. mycobacteriology laboratory personnel), children <4 yr or children exposed to adults in high-risk categories, people with clinical conditions that place them at high risk
>15 mm	Any person, even if no known risk factors for TB

Long R, Ellis E (Editors). *Canadian Tuberculosis Standards*, 6th ed. Ottawa: Public Health Agency of Canada; 2007.
Jensen PA, Lambert LA, Iademarco MF, Ridzon R. 2005. *MMWR Recomm Rep* 54(RR17):1-141.

Simplified Management Plan

- See **Table 4**
- Referral to Public Health is mandatory
- Completion of treatment is defined by total doses taken and not duration of treatment
- Drug resistance and poor rates of adherence:
  - Direct observation of treatment (DOT), especially during the initial phase, can be used to ensure adherence
  - Concurrently with treatment, monthly sputum examination is conducted until AFB and cultures become negative

Table 4. Treatment for Pulmonary TB

TB Status	Drug Regimens
Latent	INH for 9 mo OR RMP for 4 mo*
Active	INH/RMP/PZA ± EMB for 2 mo, then INH/RMP for 4 mo OR INH/RMP for 9 mo
MDR-TB†	Individualized therapy based on susceptibility/clinical situation, DOT should be carried out

*This regimen should only be used if INH cannot be used
†If you suspect multidrug resistant TB, referral to a specialized center is recommended
EMB = ethambutol, INH = isoniazid, MDR-TB = multidrug resistant TB, PZA = pyrazinamide, RMP = rifampin
Long R, Ellis E (Editors). *Canadian Tuberculosis Standards*, 6th ed. Ottawa: Public Health Agency of Canada; 2007.

INFECTIOUS DISEASES

4. HIV/AIDS

- Infection with the human immunodeficiency virus (HIV) (subtypes 1 or 2) causing immunodeficiency through the progressive depletion of CD4+ lymphocyte populations
- Acquired Immunodeficiency Syndrome (AIDS) is characterized by CD4+ cell counts below 200/mL or diagnosis of an AIDS defining illness

Epidemiology

- Approximately 34 million people infected worldwide
- Risk Factors
  - Unprotected sexual activity, injection drug use
  - Men who have sex with men (MSM), sex workers, marginalized populations, immigrants from endemic countries

Table 5. Natural Progression of HIV/AIDS

Stage	Characteristics
Primary Infection/ Acute HIV Syndrome	• 50-70% experience this after primary infection • Unexplained fatigue, sore throat, myalgias, malaise, fevers/night sweats, diarrhea, rash, weight loss, aseptic meningitis, lymphadenopathy, resolves spontaneously
Asymptomatic Phase	• Clinical latency, average 10 yr for untreated patients • May note generalized lymphadenopathy with minor opportunistic infections (e.g. herpes zoster, oral candidiasis), chronic diarrhea • Progressive decline in CD4+ cells, but viral load can increase or remain stable
Progression to AIDS	• Persistent fever, fatigue, weight loss, diarrhea • CD4+ count <200/mL or AIDS defining illness (e.g. *Pneumocystis jiroveci* [previously known as *P. carinii*] pneumonia [PJP], TB – pulmonary or extrapulmonary, recurrent bacterial pneumonia, cryptococcal meningitis, CNS toxoplasmosis, CMV retinitis), or neoplasms (Kaposi's sarcoma [KS], lymphoma), clinical neurological disease – progressive multifocal leukoencephalopathy, HIV dementia

CMV = cytomegalovirus

Focused History

- Clinical presentation can vary widely depending on the stage of infection, underlying comorbid illness, and various aspects of patient history

History of Present Illness

- Pertinent medical assessments:
  - Date and place of HIV testing and confirmation of test results
  - Any history of prior testing (e.g. for insurance, giving blood, pregnancy, other)
  - CD4+ count and viral load
  - TB skin test results
  - Syphilis test results
  - Date and results of last Pap smear (women)
- Occurrence of opportunistic infections, malignancies, STIs, intravenous drug use (IVDU) associated conditions
  - STIs: hepatitis B and C, syphilis, genital warts, herpes simplex, gonorrhea, chlamydia
  - Other infections or malignancies (bacterial infections, fungal infections, parasitic infections, mycobacterial infections)

- Travel history, illness while away and use of preventative vaccines
- Medication history (certain clinical manifestations are due to side effects of medication and antiretrovirals)
  - Antiretroviral (ARV) history (include response, CD4+, viral load), adherence, toxicity, any resistance testing and results
  - Participation in clinical trials
  - Toxicity of ARV

Social History

- Sexual history: use of barrier protection
- Pregnancy: dates, mode of delivery, testing of offspring
- Significant relationships and support systems
- Disclosure
- Physical or emotional violence
- Work
- Housing
- Drug plan, % coverage, and financial resources
- Depression, previous suicidal attempts or ideations
- Alcohol, tobacco, recreational drug use

Review of Systems

- For history taking on HIV/AIDS patients, it is very important to do a thorough review of systems (see **General History and Physical Exam**, p.15)

Focused Physical Exam

- **General**
  - Vitals (including temperature)
  - Lipodystrophy and metabolic syndrome: central obesity and wasting of extremities and face
- **Head and Neck**
  - Fundoscopy (e.g. HIV retinopathy [cotton wool spots], cytomegalovirus [CMV] retinitis)
  - Examine oral cavity
    - Candidiasis (thrush)
    - Kaposi's sarcoma (KS) lesions
    - Hairy leukoplakia on lateral tongue
    - Gingivitis
    - Bruises or bleeding from gums
    - Ulcers
  - Lymphadenopathy
- **Cardiovascular**
  - Signs of heart failure (edema, dyspnea)
  - HTN
- **Respiratory**
  - Focal chest findings associated with bacterial pneumonia
  - Chest findings may also be associated with TB
  - Absent chest findings compatible with *Pneumocystis jiroveci* pneumonia (PJP)
- **Abdominal**
  - Liver (hepatitis B and C, drug toxicity): stigmata of chronic liver disease, ascites, jaundice, hepatomegaly
  - Spleen: splenomegaly
  - Masses (lymphoma)
- **GU**
  - Ulcers or warts
  - Pelvic exam/Pap smear: cervical carcinoma
  - Rectal exam: anal/rectal carcinoma

- **Neurological**
  - Mental status: depression, memory loss, dementia, and psychosis
  - Sensory and motor exams
    - Focal neurological findings (e.g. weakness, photophobia) suggest CNS infection or tumor
    - Unsteady gait, poor balance, tremor
    - Loss of bladder or bowel control with myelopathy
    - Increased tone and deep tendon reflexes
    - Peripheral neuropathies
  - Meningeal irritation (see **Meningitis**, p.500)
- **MSK**
  - Arthritis in large joints: suggests HIV/AIDS-associated arthropathy
- **Dermatological**
  - Macular rash (seen with acute seroconversion syndrome)
  - Dermatitis, folliculitis, seborrhea
  - Herpes zoster
  - KS

Investigations

- HIV antibody test (ELISA: >99% sensitivity, Western blot: >99% specificity)[5,6]
- CD4+ T cell count
- HIV RNA level
- HIV genotyping (i.e. HLA-B*5701 allele testing prior to prescription of abacavir)
- Routine blood work (CBC, electrolytes, Cr, LFTs, blood glucose, lipids)
- STI testing
- TB skin test
- Pap smear

Management

- Education and counseling
- Prophylaxis of opportunistic infection
- Highly Active Anti-Retroviral Therapy (HAART)
- Immunizations (Pneumovax®, hepatitis A and B, influenza)

5. SEXUALLY TRANSMITTED INFECTIONS

Bacterial, viral or parasitic organisms transmitted by any mode of sexual activity (oral, vaginal, anal).

Focused History

- Predisposing Factors
  - History of previous STI
  - New sexual partner in past 3 mo
  - Multiple partners
  - Not using barrier precautions
  - Oral contraceptive pill usage
  - Contact with infected person
  - Injection drug use leading to risky behaviors
- Signs and symptoms: see **Table 6**
- Children
  - Infections typically acquired during childbirth include conjunctivitis, lower respiratory infection, pharyngitis
  - Suspect abuse if vaginal infection is found in prepubertal female prior to sexual activity
- Women and MSM
  - Rectal infections are possible: perianal discomfort, rectal discharge, mucopus coating on stools
  - Oral-genital contact can cause pharyngitis: usually asymptomatic, but can have sore throat, pain/discomfort on swallowing

- Both men and women can develop a reactive arthritis syndrome following *C. trachomatis* infection: conjunctivitis, urethritis or cervicitis, arthritis, and mucocutaneous lesions

Focused Physical Exam

- **General Inspection**
  - Vitals (including temperature)
  - Examine conjunctiva, inspect mouth and tonsils, look for skin lesions
- **Adnexal Masses**
  - Tenderness and guarding in lower quadrants
  - Inspect perianal area and stool for mucopus
- **GU**
  - In men: inspect and palpate penis (especially meatus) and scrotum (espically epididymis), inspect for secretions
  - In women: inspection of vaginal orifice and Bartholin's gland for erythema and exudate, pelvic exam including inspection of cervix for redness, friability, discharge
  - Lymphadenopathy
- **MSK**
  - Arthritis
  - Polyarthralgias (especially wrists, knees, fingers, ankles)
  - Myalgias

Investigations

- See **Table 6**
- Direct microscopic examination of tissue scrapings
  - Gram stain of urethral discharge in men and women; cultures of pharynx, rectum
- Chlamydia cell culture of isolated organisms
  - Low and variable sensitivity (60-80%)[5], high cost, technically difficult
  - Only available in major medical settings
- Antigen and nucleic acid detection by immunologic and hybridization methods for both *N. gonorrhoeae* and *C. trachomatis*
  - Low and variable sensitivity (60-80%)[5]
  - High specificity (97-99%)[5]

Table 6. Signs/Symptoms and Diagnosis of Common STIs

Signs/Symptoms	Diagnosis	Treatment
Chlamydia (*Chlamydia trachomatis*) Asymptomatic (most); mucopurulent cervical discharge; erythematous cervix, often with infected erosion urethral syndrome (dysuria, increased frequency, urgency, pyuria with no bacteria)	PCR	Azithromycin
Gonorrhea (*Neisseria gonorrhoeae*) Similar to chlamydia; offensive yellow-white discharge; tends to be thicker, more copious and painful than chlamydia	PCR (urine); Gram stain; culture of urethral or cervical discharge	Dual therapy with ceftriaxone/cefixime plus azithromycin or doxycycline (for MSM, ceftriaxone is recommended)

Table 6. Signs/Symptoms and Diagnosis of Common STIs (continued)

Signs/Symptoms	Diagnosis	Treatment
Trichomoniasis (*Trichomonas vaginalis*) Asymptomatic (up to 50%); profuse thin, frothy gray/yellow-green discharge, often foul-smelling; occasionally irritated, tender vulva; dysuria; petechiae on vagina and cervix (10%)	Saline wet mount	Metronidazole
Condylomata Acuminata/Genital Warts (HPV) • Latent: no visible lesions, asymptomatic • Subclinical: visible after acetic acid use • Clinical: visible, wart-like hyperkeratotic, verrucous or flat, macular lesions; vulvar edema • Lesions usually enlarge in pregnancy	Cytology (Pap); colposcopic biopsy HPV DNA (nucleic acid probes – not routine)	Podophyllotoxin, imiquimod; trichloroacetic acid; excisional surgery or laser ablation
Herpes Simplex (HSV) • May be asymptomatic • Prodromal: tingling, burning, pruritus • Multiple painful shallow ulcerations with small vesicles – may coalesce • First infection: inguinal lymphadenopathy, malaise, fever • If affect urethral mucosa: dysuria, urinary retention • Recurrent: decreased duration, frequency, severity	Viral culture; cytologic smear; electron microscope	Antiviral therapy acyclovir, famciclovir, or valacyclovir
Syphilis (*Treponema pallidum*) • 1°: usually single, painless penile/vulval/vaginal/cervical chancre, inguinal lymphadenopathy 3 d to 4 wk after infection • 2°: (up to 3 mo later): • malaise, anorexia, headache, adenopathy; fever • generalized maculopapular rash; condylomata lata • 3°: CNS/ascending aorta • progressively destroyed; may involve other organs • Congenital: possible fetal anomalies/stillbirth/neonatal death • Latent: asymptomatic	Serology	Benzathine penicillin G dosed according to stage

PCR = polymerase chain reaction

Canadian Guidelines on Sexually Transmitted Infections. Ottawa: Public Health Agency of Canada; 2010.

6. URINARY TRACT INFECTIONS

- See **Urological Exam**, p.376

7. INFECTIOUS DIARRHEA

- Liquid or unformed stool passed at a higher frequency than usual >200 g/d
- 3 categories: acute (<2 wk), persistent (2-4 wk), chronic (>4 wk)

Etiology
- Infectious (90% of cases), see **Table 7**

Table 7. Common Signs, Symptoms, and Epidemiology of Infectious Diarrhea

	Signs and Symptoms	Epidemiology
Parasitic		
Giardia, Cryptosporidia, Cyclospora, Isospora	Persistent diarrhea (never blood), bloating, cramps, no fever; may have malabsorption	
Amoebiasis (*E. histolytica*)	Colitis with blood and mucus; absence of stool leukocytes	Rare, but serious
Bacterial		
Campylobacter, Salmonella, Shigella	Watery diarrhea progressing to bloody diarrhea; severe lower abdominal cramps, vomiting, fever	Increasing incidence of *Campylobacter* in travelers; *Shigella* more common in children, MSM
Listeria	Diarrhea followed by muscle aches, fever, and nausea	Often foodborne (cold cuts, cheeses)
ETEC	Watery diarrhea, mild cramps, no fever	Traveler's diarrhea
EHEC (*E. coli* 0157:H7)	Bloody diarrhea; may cause hemolytic uremic syndrome (HUS)	Often foodborne
Clostridium difficile	Diarrhea with mucus ± blood	Associated with antibiotic use, often in long-term care homes and hospitals, but increasing community-acquired cases
Viral		
Hepatitis A	Light-colored diarrhea	Often foodborne (raw seafood)
Rotavirus, Norwalk-like Virus (Norovirus)	Vomiting and diarrhea	Rotaviruses: children <2 yr Noroviruses: adults and children

EHEC = enterohemorrhagic *E. coli*, ETEC = enterotoxigenic *E. coli*

Focused History
- Travel history
- Recent stay in daycare center, hospital, ICU, recent antibiotic exposure
- Features of diarrhea: frequency, duration
- Appearance of stool: blood, mucus
- Associated signs and symptoms
  - Fever
  - Abdominal pain
  - Tenesmus
  - Vomiting

Focused Physical Exam

- Assess for intravascular volume depletion
  - Vitals
  - Postural lightheadedness and a reflex tachycardia >30 min indicates moderate to severe intravascular volume depletion
  - Urine output
  - Skin turgor
  - Axillary moistness
  - Mental status changes

Investigations

- Fecal WBC count
- Stool microbiology
  - Gram stain
  - Culture
  - PCR (e.g. for noroviruses)
  - Electron microscopy (e.g. for noroviruses, rotaviruses)

Differential Diagnosis

- Pseudo-diarrhea (frequent passage of stool but total <200 g/d)
- Fecal incontinence
- Overflow diarrhea due to fecal impaction
- Postinfectious IBD
- Secondary lactose intolerance

Management

- Fluid and electrolyte replacement
- In mild cases, observe
- In nonfebrile moderate cases without bloody stool or elevated WBC, antidiarrheal agents
- In febrile moderate to severe cases (significant volume depletion), consider empiric treatment with quinolone
- ***Note:*** antibiotic treatment of *E. coli* O157:H7 is contraindicated due to increased risk of progression to HUS and thrombotic thrombocytopenic purpura (TTP)[7,8]

8. VIRAL HEPATITIS

- 5 classes: hepatitis A-E (HAV, HBV, HCV, HDV, and HEV)
- Can be classified into two categories: fecal-oral (HAV, HEV) vs. parenteral/sexual (HBV, HCV, HDV)
- Of the 5 classes, HBV and HCV can cause chronic disease
- All RNA viruses except for HBV
- Wide range of symptoms from mild to severe

Etiology

- HAV
  - Incubation period: ~4 wk
  - From raw seafood or food prepared by an individual with active HAV
  - Usually self-limiting, but occasionally fulminant, life-threatening disease
- HBV
  - Incubation period: 8-12 wk
  - Parenteral and sexual exposure
  - Two peaks of exposure: infancy and adolescence
  - Exposure in infancy usually leads to chronic infection, while exposure in adolescence can lead to acute infections that may become chronic
  - Severe chronic and fulminant hepatitis can lead to cirrhosis and hepatocellular carcinoma

- HCV
  - Incubation period: ~7 wk
  - Parenteral exposure (some sexual transmission)
  - At risk groups: injection drug users, tattoo recipients, prison inmates, HIV patients, healthcare workers
  - At least six different genotypes with different patterns of worldwide distribution
  - Due to diversity, patients exposed to HCV will not have immunity against subsequent HCV infections
  - Associated with cutaneous disorders such as porphyria cutanea tarda and lichen planus
- HDV
  - Incubation period: ~8-12 wk
  - Absolute co-infection or superinfection with HBV (i.e. never alone)
  - Cause of fulminant hepatic deterioration in individuals with active HBV
- HEV
  - Incubation period: ~5-6 wk
  - Enteric virus predominantly in India, Asia, Africa, and Central America
  - Animal reservoir in pigs and other animals

Focused History

- Associated Signs and Symptoms
  - Constitutional symptoms: N/V, anorexia, fatigue, malaise, arthralgia, myalgia, headaches, photophobia, pharyngitis, cough, coryza
  - Fever: low grade (38-39°C) for HAV and HEV, others may have higher temperatures
  - Dark urine and clay-colored stool
  - Jaundice
- Predisposing Factors
  - IV drug user
  - Prison inmate
  - Healthcare worker
- Exposure History
  - Diet
  - Travel
  - Drugs/medications
  - Alcohol usage

Focused Physical Exam

- Focused abdominal exam
  - Palpation of enlarged masses (see **Abdominal Exam**, p.24)
  - Surface examination for signs of liver disease

Investigations

- Most common investigation for patients suspected of viral hepatitis is a panel of serological tests: HBV surface antigen (HBsAg), HBV surface antibody (HBsAb), IgM anti-HBc, IgM anti-HAV, and anti-HCV, plus viral load testing in patients with active HBV and HCV (see **Table 8** for diagnostic approach)
- Liver enzymes (AST, ALT)
- Liver function tests (albumin, INR, bilirubin, platelets)

Table 8. Simplified Approach to Diagnosis of Suspected Viral Hepatitis

HBsAg	IgM Anti-HAV	IgM Anti-HBc	Anti-HCV	Interpretation
--	+	--	--	Acute hepatitis A
+	--	+	--	Acute hepatitis B
+	--	--	--	Chronic hepatitis B
--	--	+	--	Acute hepatitis B (HBsAg below detection threshold)
--	--	--	+	Acute hepatitis C

Fauci AS. *Harrison's Principles of Internal Medicine*, 17th ed. New York: McGraw-Hill; 2008.

Differential Diagnosis

- **Vascular**
  - Right ventricular failure with passive hepatic congestion
  - Hypoperfusion syndromes (e.g. left ventricular failure or shock)
- **Infectious/Inflammatory/Autoimmune**
  - Infectious mononucleosis (especially CMV, herpes simplex, acute HIV infection)
  - Toxoplasmosis
  - Other causes of liver injury by microbial pathogens
  - Acute cholecystitis
  - Ascending cholangitis
  - Common duct stone
  - Autoimmune hepatitis
  - Primary sclerosing cholangitis
  - Primary biliary cirrhosis
- **Neoplastic**
  - Metastatic malignancy to the liver
  - Hepatoma
- **Drug-Induced Congenital/Developmental/Inherited**
  - α-1-antitrypsin deficiency
  - Hemochromatosis
  - Wilson's disease
  - Porphyria
- **Other**
  - Complications of pregnancy: acute fatty liver of pregnancy, cholestasis of pregnancy, eclampsia, HELLP (hemolysis, elevated liver enzymes, low platelet count) syndrome
  - Primary parenchymal liver disease
  - Alcoholic liver disease
  - Nonalcoholic steatohepatitis (NASH)

Management

- HBV/HDV
  - No intervention needed unless disease is chronic/persistent (HBeAg+) (adefovir or lamivudine)
- HCV
  - Long-acting pegylated interferon plus ribavirin, most successful in genotype 2/3 disease
- In general, specific treatment not necessary
  - If pruritus present, give bile salt-sequestering resin cholestyramine

9. MENINGITIS

Inflammation of the meninges which can be infectious or noninfectious in origin.

Epidemiology

- Viral and bacterial meningitis are most common (fungal/parasitic causes less common)
- Pneumococcal and meningococcal infections are the most common causes of bacterial meningitis in adults
- Predisposing factors for meningitis:
  - Infectious contacts
  - Travel to endemic regions
  - STIs (HSV, syphilis, HIV)
  - Infection with *Mycobacterium tuberculosis*
  - Parameningeal infections (e.g. otitis media, sinusitis)
  - Compromised immunity
  - Head trauma
  - Persistent CSF leaks
  - Anatomical defects (including dermal sinuses)
  - Previous neurosurgical procedures

Focused History

- Altered LOC: irritability/confusion/drowsiness/stupor/coma
- Seizures
- Neonates: signs of sepsis (fever, respiratory distress, apnea, jaundice)
- Infants: fever, vomiting, irritability, convulsions, high-pitch cry, poor feeding, lethargy
- Older children and adults:
  - Fever
  - Headache
  - Neck stiffness
  - Photophobia

Focused Physical Exam

- Vitals (fever, tachycardia/bradycardia, irregular respiration)
- Neonates and infants: inspect anterior fontanelle for bulging or tightness
- Nuchal rigidity (stiff neck)
  - **Brudzinski's Sign:** abrupt neck flexion with patient in supine position – involuntary flexion of hips and knees is positive sign
  - **Kernig's Sign:** strong passive resistance to attempts to extend knee from flexed thigh position
- Jolt accentuation
- Assess lethargy, level of consciousness (MMSE, Glasgow coma scale [GCS])
- Cranial nerves: typically IV, VI, VII affected by raised ICP or basilar inflammation
- Petechial or purpuric rash (typically in extremities)

Investigations

- CBC and differential, electrolytes
- Blood cultures
- CT to exclude elevated ICP and mass lesion
- Lumbar puncture
- Opening pressure
  - Protein, glucose, cell count and differential, Gram stain

Differential Diagnosis of Acute Bacterial Meningitis

- Bacterial endocarditis
- Early tuberculous meningitis
- Amoebic meningoencephalitis
- Lyme disease
- Herpes simplex encephalitis
- Cerebral toxoplasmosis
- Cerebral malaria
- Chemical or drug-induced meningitis
- Carcinomatous meningitis
- Sarcoid meningitis
- Parameningeal foci secondary to other lesions

Management Principles

- Do not delay IV antibiotics
- The chosen antimicrobial agent should be bactericidal and penetrate the CSF
- Examples of empiric antibiotic treatment of bacterial meningitis include:
    - Ceftriaxone 2g IV q12h
    - Vancomycin 1.5g IV q12h
    - Ampicillin 2g IV q4h for individuals >50 yr or immunocompromised to cover *L. monocytogenes*
- Adjuvant dexamethasone treatment in adults with acute pneumococcal meningitis lowers mortality/risk of unfavorable outcome

EBM: Adult Meningitis

History alone is not useful in establishing a diagnosis of meningitis. Physical exam is useful in ruling out meningitis, and in determining which patients should proceed to more definitive testing (lumbar puncture).

Physical Exam Finding	Sensitivity (%)
Fever	77
Neck Stiffness	83
Altered Mental Status (GCS <15)	69

The absence of all three signs of the classic triad of fever, neck stiffness, and altered mental status virtually eliminates a diagnosis of meningitis (sensitivity of >1 sign present = 99%). 95% of patients will have at least 2/4 of headache, fever, neck stiffness, and altered mental status.

Note: The applicability of these results is severely limited by the fact that most of the studies included in the analysis described were retrospective chart reviews, which lacked control populations. Only sensitivities could therefore be determined, and these are likely to overestimate the true sensitivities because the clinical examinations would have been performed with knowledge of the LP results.

Van de Beek D, et al. 2004. *N Engl J Med* 351(18):1849-1859.

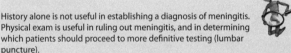

10. SEPSIS

- **Systemic Inflammatory Response Syndrome (SIRS)**
  - 2 or more of:
    - Temp <36°C or >38°C
    - HR >90 bpm
    - RR >20 breaths/min
    - WBC <4,000 or >12,000 cells/mm^3
- **Sepsis**
  - Clinical evidence of infection and SIRS
- **Severe Sepsis**
  - Sepsis associated with organ dysfunction due to hypoperfusion or hypotension, manifested by:
    - Oliguria
    - Lactic acidosis
    - Acute alteration in mental status
- **Septic Shock**
  - Severe sepsis (as above) with refractory hypotension: from patient's baseline
  - This clinical presentation persists despite fluid resuscitation of at least 500 mL saline solution

Epidemiology/Etiology

- Approximately 2/3 of new cases are due to nosocomial infection
- See **Table 9** for common microorganisms that may generate sepsis response

Table 9. Common Microorganisms Generating Sepsis Response

Microorganism	Common Examples
Gram-Negative Bacteria	Enterobacteriaceae, *P. aeruginosa*
Gram-Positive Bacteria	*S. aureus*, enterococci, *S. pneumoniae*, other streptococci
Classic Pathogens	*N. meningitidis, S. pneumoniae, H. influenzae, S. pyogenes*

Focused History

- Signs and Symptoms
  - Related to the site of origin of infection (skin and soft tissue, abdomen, genitourinary tract, lungs, CNS)
- Exposure history (diet, travel, infectious contacts)
- Predisposing Factors
  - **Previous medical or surgical interventions**
    - e.g. chemotherapy, surgery, transplantation
  - **Use of immunosuppressive agents or history of immunosuppression**
    - e.g. HIV/AIDS, chemotherapy, splenectomy, organ transplant, corticosteroid therapy, immunomodulatory biologic therapy (anti-TNF therapy), hypogammaglobulinemia
- **Previous infections and antimicrobial treatments** including medications and drug reactions (microbiological data from studies and investigations performed in the few weeks prior to presentation can be quite useful)
- Underlying chronic diseases affecting prognosis include:
  - DM
  - Alcoholism and/or cirrhosis
  - Renal failure
  - Respiratory diseases
  - Hematological malignancies and solid tumors

- Invasive procedures or indwelling devices, vascular catheterization
- Structural abnormalities in urogenital tract

Focused Physical Exam

- **Vitals** (including temperature, RR, HR, BP)
- **Respiratory**
  - Cyanosis
  - Pulmonary infiltrates
- **CVS**
  - Signs of hypovolemia
- **Abdominal**
  - Jaundice
  - Hepatosplenomegaly
- **Dermatological**
  - Exanthems, i.e. ecthyma gangrenosum in *P. aeruginosa*
  - Contusions
  - Purpuric rash
- **Neurological**
  - Altered mental status

Investigations

- Culture and sensitivity of microorganisms:
  - Local site
  - Blood samples (2 x 10 mL samples from different venipuncture sites)
  - Midstream urine/catheter specimen if needed
- CBC with differential, comprehensive metabolic panel
- Chest X-ray

Differential Diagnosis

- **Infectious** (with or without a source)
  - Bacterial (bacteremia, endocarditis)
  - Viral (e.g. viral hepatitis, dengue)
  - Parasitic (e.g. malaria)
- **Noninfectious**
  - Acute pancreatitis
  - Anaphylaxis
  - Drug intoxication/withdrawal
  - Heat stroke
  - Massive tissue injury (e.g. infarction, rhabdomyolysis)
  - Vasculitis

Management

- IV antibiotics (following sample collection)
- Source management (e.g. abscess drainage)
- Oxygen saturation and fluid management
- Respiratory support

11. OSTEOMYELITIS

An infection of bone, characterized by progressive inflammatory destruction of bone, bone necrosis, and new bone formation.

Epidemiology/Etiology

- Often community-acquired
- Commonly caused by staphlococci, streptococci, may be caused by *P. aeruginosa* and other gram negative rods (GNRs), anaerobic bacteria, and mycobacteria
- Microorganisms enter bone from a penetrating wound, or by spreading from a contiguous infectious focus or via hematogenous dissemination

Focused History

- HPI
  - Pain history (onset, duration, severity, localized skeletal pain, similar pain previously)
  - Trauma history
  - Constitutional symptoms (fever, malaise, night sweats)
- PMHx (predisposing factors)
  - Sickle cell anemia
  - Immunodeficiency
  - IV drug abuse
  - Prosthetic joints
  - DM
  - Vascular insufficiency
  - Endocarditis
  - Chronic skin ulcers

Focused Physical Exam

- Vitals
- Inspection:
  - Evidence of injury/trauma
  - Local source of infection (ingrown toenail, wound infection)
  - Cellulitis
- Peripheral vascular exam
- Probe-to-bone test

Investigations

- CBC, ESR, CRP
- Blood cultures
- Bone biopsy: culture/sensitivity and histology
- X-ray, MRI

Differential Diagnosis

- **MSK**
  - Traumatic or stress fractures
  - Altered biomechanics
- **Vascular**
  - Bone infarcts/avascular necrosis
- **Inflammatory**
  - Inflammatory arthritis
  - Psoriatic arthritis
  - Reactive arthritis
  - Gout
- **Neoplastic**
  - Sarcoid
  - Lymphoma
  - Metastases

Management

- **Medical**
  - Acute infection: IV antibiotics x 4-6 wk, can step-down to PO in selected cases
  - Chronic infection: as for acute followed by additional antibiotics using ESR/CRP, clinical signs and symptoms, and follow-up imaging as aids to determine antibiotic stop date
- **Surgical**
  - Acute infection: debridement of dead tissue
  - Chronic infection: debridement of all devitalized bone and soft tissue and removal of foreign bodies

12. SKIN, MUSCLE, AND SOFT TISSUE INFECTIONS

Tissue infection that involves the skin, subcutaneous fat, the fascia and/or muscle.

Epidemiology/Etiology

- Nosocomial vs. community-acquired
- Disruption of the epidermal layer by burns or bites, abrasions, foreign bodies, primary dermatologic disorders, surgery, or vascular/pressure ulcers allows penetration of bacteria to the deeper structures
- Hair follicles are a route of infection either for normal flora (e.g. staphylococci) or for extrinsic bacteria (e.g. *P. aeruginosa*)

Focused History

- HPI
  - Fever, chills, sweats
  - Pruritus
  - History of insect, tick, or animal/human bites
  - Travel history
  - Skin lesions
  - Erythema, warmth, edema
  - Pain, tenderness, myalgia
- PMHx
  - IV drug use
  - History of past disease (e.g. varicella zoster virus, herpes simplex virus)
  - Immune status
  - DM

Focused Physical Exam

- **Lesion(s)**
  - Type of lesion (see **Essentials of Dermatology**, p.398 and **Table 10**)
  - Exudates, hemorrhage
  - Arrangement (e.g. linear, clustered, annular, arciform, dermatomal)
  - Distribution and location (e.g. exposed surfaces, extremities, along skin folds)
  - Color (e.g. erythema in cellulitis)
  - Pain, tenderness, crepitus
  - Associated lymphangitis and regional lymph node involvement
  - Generalized lymph node enlargement
- **Fever**

Table 10. Common Skin Lesions and Conditions

Lesion	Associated Conditions
Vesicles	Smallpox, chickenpox (primary varicella zoster virus infection), shingles (herpes zoster virus), "cold sores" (herpes simplex virus), genital ulcers (herpes simplex virus), hand, foot and mouth disease (coxsackievirus)
Bullae	Necrotizing fasciitis (group A streptococci, mixed Gram-negative, anaerobic infections, community-acquired methicillin-resistant *Staphylococcus aureus* [CA-MRSA]), staphylococcal scalded skin syndrome, gas gangrene (clostridial myonecrosis)
Crusted Lesions	Impetigo (streptococcal, staphylococcal), ringworm (dermatophytes), histoplasmosis, blastomycosis, sporotrichosis, cutaneous leishmaniasis
Papules and Nodules	Onchocerciasis nodule (Calabar swelling), lepromatous leprosy, secondary syphilis

Table 10. Common Skin Lesions and Conditions (continued)

Lesion	Associated Conditions
Ulcers	Anthrax, leprosy, chancroid, primary syphilis (chancre)
Necrotizing Fasciitis	Staphylococcal necrotizing fasciitis (CA-MRSA), streptococcal gangrene (*S. pyogenes*), mixed aerobic and anaerobic bacteria, including Fournier's gangrene
Myositis and Myonecrosis	Pyomyositis (*S. aureus*), streptococcal necrotizing myositis (*S. pyogenes*), nonclostridial (crepitant) myositis (mixed infection), synergistic nonclostridial anaerobic myonecrosis (mixed infection), gas gangrene (*Clostridium* spp.)

Table 11. Common Soft Tissue Infections

Epidemiology/ Risk Factors	Location	Appearance of Lesions	Degree of Pain
Impetigo Common in children	Face, often perioral	Nonbullous honey-crust lesions, bullous-thin crust	Mild
Erysipelas Any age; may be spontaneous or post-traumatic; may complicate lymphedema	Face or extremities; involving the epidermis and dermis	Abrupt onset of fiery red swelling, well-defined indurated margins	Intense
Cellulitis As above	Epidermis, dermis, and subcutaneous fat	Swelling, erythema, warmth	Localized
Necrotizing Fasciitis Any age	Subcutaneous fascia	Swelling, edema, hemorrhagic bullae, cutaneous necrosis, patchy cutaneous anesthesia	Early reported pain may be out of proportion to the extent of skin findings

Investigations

- Aspiration or punch biopsy
- CT or MRI

Differential Diagnosis

- **Infectious**
  - Localized to the skin or soft tissues versus systemic viral and bacterial infections (e.g. measles, bacterial meningitis, infective endocarditis)
- **Noninfectious**
  - Drug reaction (e.g. Stevens-Johnson syndrome)
  - Inflammatory dermatologic conditions (e.g. psoriasis)
  - Vasculitis

Management

- Appropriate empirical antibiotic treatment (dependent on site, route of infection, exposure history)
- Early/aggressive surgical management if necrotizing fasciitis, myositis or gangrene is suspected:
  - Visualization of deep structures
  - Removal of necrotic tissue
  - Reduction of compartment pressure
  - Obtain samples for Gram stain and culture

13. TRAVEL-RELATED ILLNESSES

- Fever from the tropics is:
  - A medical emergency and assumed to be malaria until proven otherwise (i.e. it is imperative to rule out malaria in any febrile traveler returning from the tropics or subtropics)
  - However, travel-related illnesses are often not tropical diseases

Epidemiology

- The risk of acquiring tropical diseases is dependent on the travel environment, location, and duration
- Disease distribution varies with seasons (e.g. rainy seasons)
- For up-to-date information, it is best to visit a comprehensive website such as the Centers for Disease Control and Prevention (CDC)

Focused History

- Pre-Travel Preparation
  - Immunizations (e.g. hepatitis, meningitis, rabies, typhoid, yellow fever, etc.)
  - Malaria chemoprophylaxis (drug dose, adherence, duration)
  - Medications
- Travel Itinerary
  - Countries visited, dates and duration
  - Accommodations (urban and/or rural, living conditions)
  - Purpose of travel
- Exposure history
- Ingestion of:
  - Raw, undercooked or "exotic" foods
  - Contaminated mild or unpasteurized dairy products
  - Contaminated water
- Fresh water exposure
- Walking barefoot
- Sexual contact with local residents or fellow travelers
- Transfusions, injections, receiving tattoos or body piercings
- Insect bites (time of day, urban or rural)
- Exposure to or bites from animals
- Sick contacts
- Accommodation (e.g. mud/thatched huts)
- Fever Hx (see **Table 13**)
- Onset, duration, peak temperature, pattern
- Signs and symptoms (see **Table 14**)

Table 12. Incubation Periods for Selected Tropical Diseases

Incubation Period	Infection
Short (<10 d)	• Enteric bacterial infections • Arboviral infections (dengue fever) • Marburg viral disease
Intermediate (10-21 d)	• American trypanosomiasis (can include enteric fever) • Leptospirosis • Malaria (except *P. malariae*) • Rickettsial infections (Rocky Mountain spotted fever, scrub typhus, Q fever, tick-bite fever, enteric fever)
Long (>21 d)	• Malaria (*P. malariae*) • Schistosomiasis • Tuberculosis • Viral • Hepatitis B virus • Visceral leishmaniasis • Filariasis (*W. bancrofti*)

Table 13. Fever Pattern for Selected Tropical Diseases

Pattern	Infection
Continuous	Enteric (typhoid or paratyphoid) fever, Lassa fever
Remittent	Tuberculosis
Intermittent	Malaria, tuberculosis
Relapsing	Relapsing fever, dengue fever, *P. malariae*

Focused Physical Exam

- **General**
  - Hydration, level of consciousness, malnourishment
  - Inspect the skin and sclera for jaundice, dermatological findings
- **Head and Neck**
  - Inspect the conjunctiva for infection
  - Assess for lymphadenopathy (see **Table 15**)
- **Respiratory**
  - Signs of pneumonia
- **GU**
  - Hepatosplenomegaly, diarrhea
- **MSK**
  - Myalgia

Table 14. Basic Epidemiology and Symptoms of Major Tropical Diseases

Illness	Vector or Exposure	Distribution	Symptoms
African Sleeping Sickness (African Trypanosomiasis)	Tsetse flies	Africa	Skin sore at the bite site, muscle and joint pain, swollen lymph nodes, fever
Chagas Disease (American Trypanosomiasis)	Night-biting reduviid bugs; mud, thatch or adobe houses	South and Central America	Pain and swelling in the area of an infected bug bite followed by a systemic illness including fever

Table 14. Basic Epidemiology and Symptoms of Major Tropical Diseases (continued)

Illness	Vector or Exposure	Distribution	Symptoms
Dengue Fever	Mosquitoes	Tropical regions of Africa, South and Central America, Caribbean, Asia, and Oceania	Fever, bone and joint pain, headache, swollen glands, hepatomegaly, fatigue, eschar, rash (hemorrhagic dengue fever)
Filariasis	Mosquitoes	South and Central America, Africa, Asia, India, Caribbean	Most asymptomatic or lymphedema of leg, scrotum, penis, arm, or breast
Leishmaniasis	Night-biting sandflies	Widespread	1) Cutaneous: slow healing skin sores 2) Visceral: fever, weight loss, hepatosplenomegaly and anemia; months to years after exposure
Malaria	Mosquitoes	Widespread	Fever, chills, headache, myalgia, malaise, hepatosplenomegaly, jaundice
Onchocerciasis (River Blindness)	Day-biting black flies	Africa and South America	Dermatitis, subcutaneous nodules, lymphadenitis, ocular lesions (can lead to blindness); may occur months to years after exposure
Schistosomiasis (Bilharziasis)	Wading, swimming or bathing in fresh water	Sub-Saharan Africa, southern China, the Philippines, and Brazil	Most acute infections asymptomatic; acute syndrome: Katayama fever – fever, anorexia, weight loss, abdominal pain, hematuria, weakness, headaches, joint and muscle pain, diarrhea, nausea, and cough
Yellow Fever	Mosquitoes	Sub-Saharan Africa, Panama, Trinidad, South America	Sudden onset of fever, backache, headache, N/V, bradycardia, bleeding, jaundice

Diagnostic Investigations

- Blood films (thick and thin) × 3 (malaria) or rapid diagnostic test
- CBC, LFTs
- Blood, urine, stool cultures
- Serology (e.g. for dengue fever, schistosomiasis)
- Chest X-ray

14. IMMUNOCOMPROMISED POPULATION

Table 15. Important Opportunistic Infections and Common Associated Symptoms in HIV-Infected Individuals

Infections	Common Signs and Symptoms
Hepatitis C	Jaundice, splenomegaly, stigmata of chronic liver disease
Pneumocystis jiroveci Pneumonia (previously *P. carinii*)	Fever, progressive dyspnea, nonproductive cough, fatigue; O/E: tachypnea, fever, inspiratory rales
Tuberculosis (pulmonary)	Fever, cough, sputum production, night sweats, weight loss, anorexia
Mycobacterium avium **Complex in HIV-Infected Individuals**	Nonspecific symptoms: high fever, night sweats, weight loss, anorexia, fatigue; hepatosplenomegaly, lymphadenopathy, diarrhea
Cytomegalovirus	Retinitis: floaters, visual field defects, scotoma; O/E: creamy white retinal exudates with hemorrhage, lesions obscure visualization of underlying vessels and other retinal structures; colitis: fever, diarrhea, weight loss, colon ulceration (± bleeding); esophagitis: fever, odynophagia, retrosternal pain
Candida **Species**	Thrush: white patches in oral cavity, scrape off with tongue depressor; esophagitis: fever, anorexia, dysphagia, retrosternal pain
Toxoplasmic Encephalitis/ Cryptococcal Meningitis	Insidious onset; fever, headache, mental status changes; focal neurologic signs, seizures

REFERENCES

1. Mandell GL, Bennett JE, Dolin R (Editors). *Mandell, Douglas, and Bennett's Principles and Practice of Infectious Diseases*, 7th ed. New York: Churchill Livingstone/Elsevier; 2010.
2. Glynn F, Fenton JE. 2008. Diagnosis and management of supraglottitis (epiglottitis). *Curr Infect Dis Rep* 10(3):200-204.
3. Long R, Ellis E (Editors). *Canadian Tuberculosis Standards*, 6th ed. Ottawa: Public Health Agency of Canada; 2007.
4. Heymann DL (Editor). *Control of Communicable Diseases Manual*, 19th ed. Washington: American Public Health Association; 2008.
5. Porter RS (Editor). *The Merck Manual of Diagnosis and Therapy*, 19th ed. Whitehouse Station: Merck Research Laboratories; 2011.
6. McPhee SJ, Papadakis M. *Current Medical Diagnosis and Treatment 2012*. New York: McGraw-Hill Medical; 2012.
7. Wong CS, Jelacic S, Habeeb RL, Watkins SL, Tarr PI. 2000. The risk of the hemolytic-uremic syndrome after antibiotic treatment of Escherichia coli O157:H7 infections. *N Engl J Med* 342(26):1930-1936.
8. Safdar N, Said A, Gangnon RE, Maki DG. 2002. Risk of hemolytic uremic syndrome after antibiotic treatment of Escherichia coli O157:H7 enteritis: A meta-analysis. *JAMA* 288(8):996-1001.
9. Attia J, Hatala R, Cook DJ, Wong JG. 1999. The rational clinical examination. Does this patient have acute meningitis? *JAMA* 282(2):175-181.
10. Fauci AS. *Harrison's Principles of Internal Medicine*, 17th ed. New York: McGraw-Hill; 2008.

The Essentials of Medical Imaging

Editors:
Michal Bohdanowicz
Ashley Leckie
Ryan Lo

Faculty Reviewer:
Nasir Jaffer, MD, FRCP(C)

TABLE OF CONTENTS

1. ESSENTIALS OF IMAGING

X-ray (Radiography)
- Denser structures are more opaque (metal > bone > fat > water > air)
- Poor delineation of soft tissues

Computed Tomography Scan
- Multiplanar imaging using X-rays
- Delineates surrounding soft tissue better than a plain film

Magnetic Resonance Imaging
- No ionizing radiation but magnetic field exposure
- T1- vs.T2-weighted scans accentuate different tissues
- T1-weighted: fat is bright, water and CSF are dark
- T2-weighted: fat is dark, water is bright
- Excellent delineation of soft tissues

Ultrasound
- Image produced from reflected acoustic waves
- No ionizing radiation but can heat tissue

Nuclear Imaging
- Radioactive nucleotides in patient show physiological functioning
- Location and amount of activity can be seen on scans

Clinical Pearl: Importance of Clinical Context
Medical images can be misleading if interpreted without clinical context or correlates.

2. APPROACH TO THE CHEST X-RAY

Types
- Posterior-Anterior (PA) and left lateral
- Portable: Anterior-Posterior (AP) – done supine or upright

> **Clinical Pearl: Optimal Patient Positioning**
> PA upright chest films are preferred because AP supine films obfuscate air-fluid levels and magnify mediastinal structures.

Interpretation
Identifying Data
- Exam date, name, sex, age, history number, position (supine, decubitus, upright), view (e.g. AP, PA), markers (R and L)

Quality of Radiograph: RIP
- **R**otation
  - Medial ends of the clavicle should be equidistant from the spinous process
  - Left and right ribcages, if not superimposed, should be within ~1-2 cm of each other on the lateral film (ideally <0.5 cm)
- **I**nspiration
  - Both the anterior segment of the 6th rib and the posterior segment of the 9th rib should be above the diaphragm (if inspiratory effort appropriate)
- **P**enetration
  - Vertebral bodies should be just visible through the cardiac shadow
  - Overexposed (vertebral bodies are very visible); underexposed (invisible)

Looking for Pathologies: ABCDS x2 and Mediastinum
- **A**irway
  - Follow trachea to carina and main bronchi (midline and patent)
- **A**orta
  - Follow arch to descending aorta on both frontal and lateral views
- **B**reathing (Lungs and Pleura)
  - Lung fields: upper, middle, and lower
    - » Lung volumes, symmetry of markings (on frontal film)
    - » Air space pathologies, interstitial pathologies, lobar collapse, and nodules
    - » Lung periphery for pneumothorax and effusions
    - » Examples of lung findings:
      - Silhouette sign: loss of normally appearing interfaces implying opacification usually due to consolidation
      - Air bronchogram: bronchi become visualized because the lungs are opacified indicating air space disease, consolidation, etc.
      - Kerley B lines: thickened connective tissue planes that commonly occur in pulmonary edema
      - Net-like/reticular appearance: interstitial disease
      - "Batwing" or "butterfly" appearance: alveolar edema
  - Pleura: costophrenic angles, entire perimeter of lung fields, position of fissures
    - » Minor fissure from the right hilus to the 6th rib
    - » Major fissure laterally from T4-5 to the diaphragm
    - » Check for: blunting of costophrenic angles, focal or diffuse areas of pleural thickening, shifting of fissures, calcification, fluid collection
- **B**ones
  - Vertebrae, clavicles, ribs, sternum (best seen on lateral film)

  - Check for vertebrae and disc spaces, lytic or sclerotic lesions, rib fractures, osteoporosis (osteopenia, compression fracture, wedged)
- **C**irculation (including hila)
  - Central pulmonary arteries, veins, lymph nodes; mainstem and lobar bronchi
    - Deviation: left hilum should be 1-2 cm above the right (deviation may be due to lobar collapse or lobectomy)
    - Hilar enlargement
      - Smooth enlargement suggests arteries
      - Lobulated enlargement suggests lymphadenopathy
- **C**ardiac
  - Assess width of heart borders via the cardiothoracic ratio
    - Maximum heart width/greatest thoracic diameter should be <0.5
    - Right border = edge of right atrium
    - Left border = edge of left ventricle
  - Enlargement/distortion of cardiovascular shadow
    - Cardiomegaly, poor inspiration, supine position, obesity, pectus excavatum
    - Cardiomegaly suggests either myocardial hypertrophy, cardiac chamber dilatation or pericardial effusion
    - Cardiothoracic ratio <0.5 when cardiomegaly occurs alongside a hyperexpansive chest disorder (i.e. emphysema)
    - On expiration, heart size appears larger and mediastinum appears wider
- **D**iaphragm
  - Assess: position and costophrenic angles
    - Right hemidiaphragm may be up to 2 cm higher than the left
    - Check for: free air, calcifications, high or low diaphragm
      - Air underneath diaphragm: pneumoperitoneum (abnormal) or gastric bubble (normal)
      - Calcifications on diaphragm: asbestosis
      - Deviated diaphragm: either increased or decreased volume of peritoneal/thoracic structure
      - Elevated diaphragm: abdominal distention, lung collapse, pneumonectomy, pregnancy, pleural effusion
      - Depressed diaphragm: asthma, emphysema, pleural effusion, tumor
- **D**eformities
  - Assess: spine for deformity, asymmetry of pedicles/spinous processes
- **S**oft Tissues
  - Assess: neck, supraclavicular area, axillae, breast tissue, muscles
  - Check for: soft tissue masses, amount of soft tissue present
- **S**houlder
  - Look at bones and periphery
  - Continue in superior soft tissues/bones, up anterior chest wall, and down posterior ribs to the costophrenic angles
- **M**ediastinum
  - Mediastinal shift, abnormal widening and masses
  - Great vessels and mediastinal contours
  - Determine the mediastinal compartment where the abnormality is located (**Table 1**)

Table 1. Differential Diagnosis for a Mediastinal Mass

Anterior Mediastinal Mass	**4 T**'s (thyroid lesions, thymic lesions, teratoma, terrible lymphoma), parathyroid lesions
Middle Mediastinal Mass	Bronchial carcinoma, bronchogenic cysts
Posterior Mediastinal Mass	Neurogenic tumors, esophageal lesions, hiatus hernia
All Compartments	Lymphoma, hematoma, abscess, aortic aneurysm

3. CHEST PATHOLOGIES AND FINDINGS

3.1 Pneumothorax

- Air or gas in the pleural space

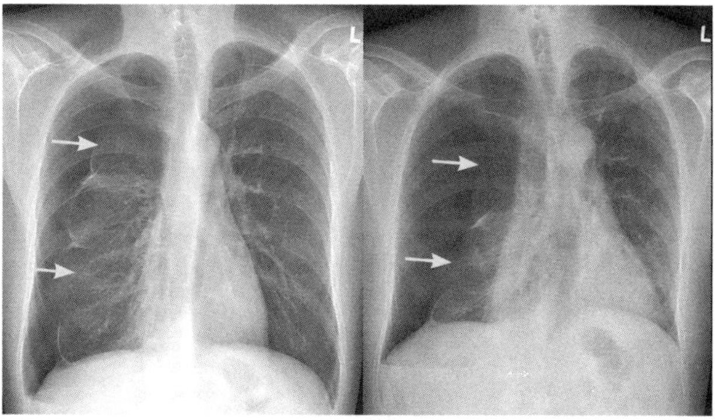

Figure 1. (A) CXR showing a right lung pneumothorax. With expiration, the tracheal and mediastinal shift becomes more pronounced.

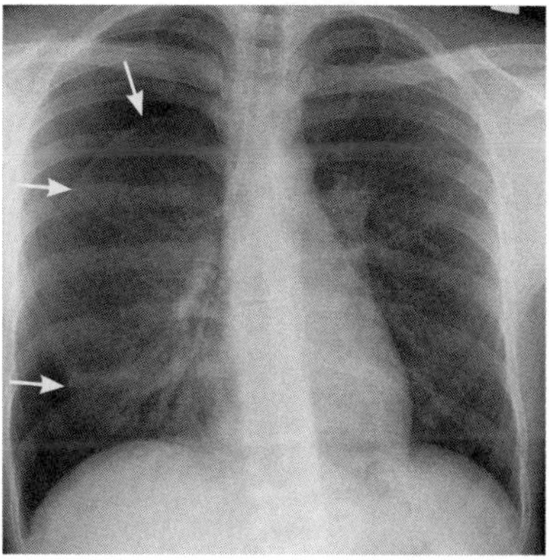

Figure 1. (B) CXR showing a right lung pneumothorax.

1st Modality	2nd Modality	3rd Modality
CXR: decreased lung markings, partial or complete collapse of ipsilateral lung, contralateral mediastinal shift. **Tension pneumothorax**: severe contralateral mediastinal shift, inversion of hemidiaphragm. Sensitivity: 52% Specificity: 100%	**CT**: the gold standard imaging investigation; lung markings will be absent in region of pneumothorax. **Perform when**: an underlying pathology is suspected, for example: apical pleural blebs or bullae; pulmonary interstitial disease (lymphangiomyomatosis). Look for thin-walled cysts.	**CXR**: if a chest tube is inserted to re-expand the lung, repeat study after placement of chest tube. Look for proper placement. Then repeat CXR post chest tube removal.

Ding W, et al. 2011. *Chest* 140(4):859-866.
Murphy FB, et al. 1990. *AJR Am J Roentgenol* 154(1):45-46.

3.2 Atelectasis (Loss of Volume)

- Collapse of a subsegment, segment, lobe or entire lung
- Atelectasis or loss of volume can be subsegmental, segmental, lobar, or involve the entire lung
- Atelectasis is often qualified by descriptors such as linear, discoid, or plate-like

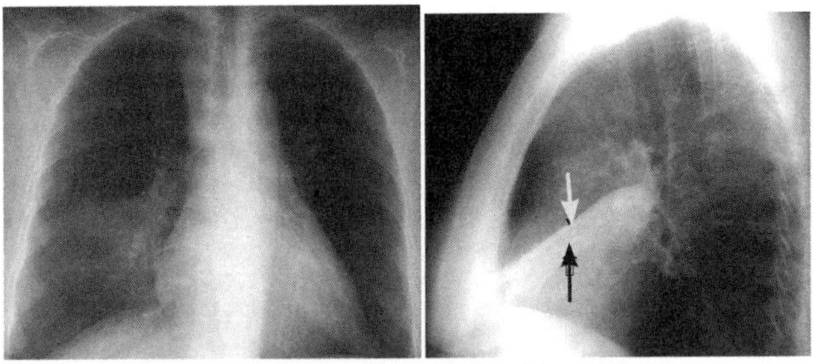

Figure 2. Complete right middle lobar atelectasis. Local increased density is seen in the region of the collapsed lung (see arrows).

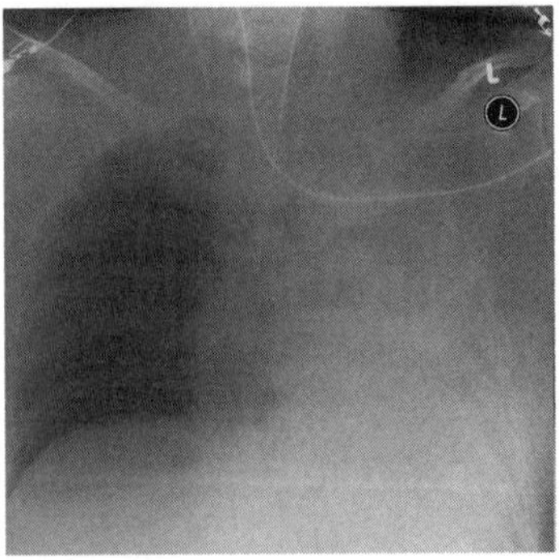

Figure 3. Complete atelectasis of left lung with air bronchogram and shift of the mediastinum to the left. The endotracheal tube is in the right lower bronchus resulting in the atelectasis.

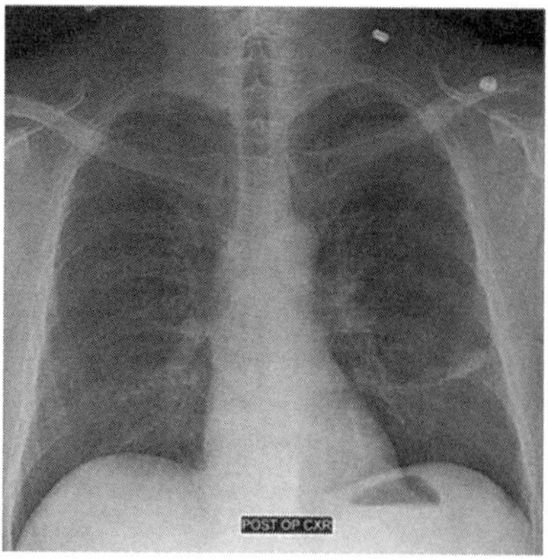

Figure 4. There is subsegmental atelectasis on the left lower lobe (postoperative).

1st Modality	2nd Modality
CXR: look for signs of loss of volume. Direct signs: Displacement of fissures Indirect signs: Local increased density, elevation of diaphragm, mediastinal displacement, compensatory hyperinflation, displacement of hila, absence of air bronchogram or increased opacity of the collapsed lung segment.	**CT**: look for reduced volume and decreased attenuation in the affected part of the lung. Atelectasis is often associated with abnormal displacement of fissures, bronchi, vessels, diaphragm, heart, or mediastinal structures. **Perform when**: only in cases where a malignant process is the suspected etiology, such as an endobronchial lesion (mucous plug, tumor or foreign body), intramural lesion (tumor or inflammatory lesion) or extrinsic lesions such as lymphadenopathy. CT is also used for staging the tumor.

3.3 Pneumonia

- Inflammation and possible consolidation of the respiratory units of the lung

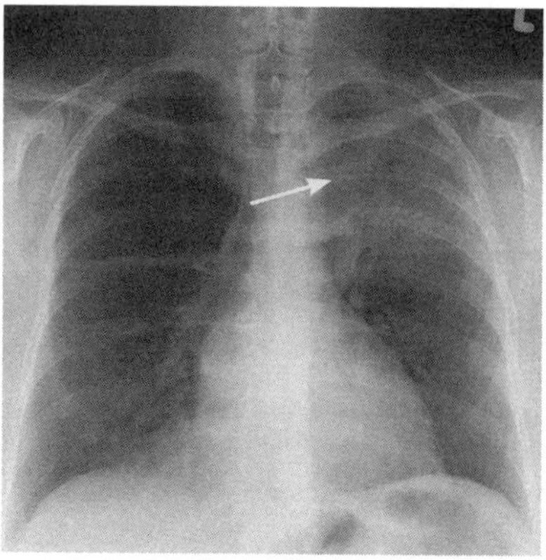

Figure 5. Left upper lobe pneumonia characterized by consolidation of the affected segment.

1st Modality	2nd Modality
CXR: look for increased opacity of affected segment (consolidation) with air bronchogram, the hallmark for pneumonia. Other signs include silhouette sign of mediastinal structures and the spine sign on lateral CXR with increased opacity of lower lobes posterior. Some pneumonias may cause slight loss of volume (atelectasis) or increased volume (such as *Klebseilla* and *Legionella* bacteria). Sensitivity: 67%[1] Specificity: 85%	**CT**: the gold standard imaging investigation. Consolidation appears as a homogeneous increase in pulmonary parenchymal attenuation that obscures the margins of vessels and airway walls. An air bronchogram may be present. The attenuation characteristics of consolidated lung rarely helpful in differential diagnosis (e.g. decreased attenuation in lipoid pneumonia and increased in amiodarone toxicity). **Perform when**: atypical pneumonia on CXR or not resolving post treatment.

3.4 Obstructed Upper Airway

- Physical blockage of the upper respiratory tract

1st Modality	2nd Modality
Depends on the patient's age group and the possible etiology and location of obstruction. **X-ray of the lateral soft tissue of the neck**: look for epiglottitis or foreign body. The classic radiographic findings of epiglottitis are a swollen epiglottis (i.e. a thumb sign; normal epiglottis is 3-5 mm thick), thickened aryepiglottic folds, and obliteration of the vallecula (vallecula sign).	**CXR**: look for air trapping on an exhalation phase film. Additionally, atelectasis may be present in the obstructed region. **Perform when**: to assess for other causes of patient's dyspnea; the obstructed airway could affect any segments of the tracheobronchial tree. Sensitivity: 66%[2]

3.5 Interstitial Lung Disease

- Disease of the nonconducting and nonrespiratory tissues of the lung

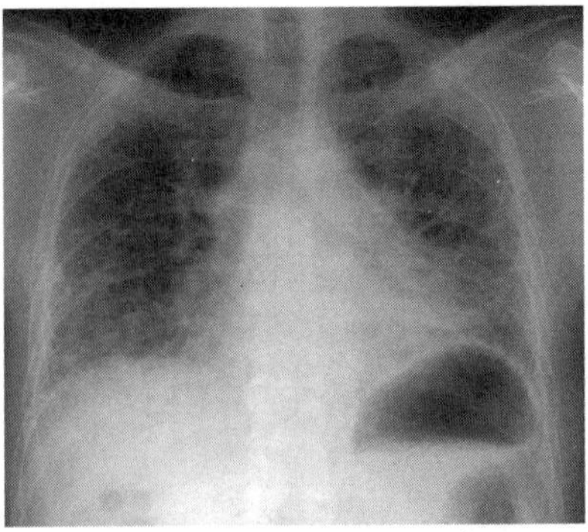

Figure 6. Interstitial lung disease characterized by a honeycomb appearance.

1st Modality	2nd Modality
CXR: interstitial lines fine, medium, and coarse (Kerley lines, septal) honeycomb with decreased or increased lung volume. Sensitivity: 59% Specificity: 40%[3]	**High Resolution CT (HRCT)**: the imaging modality of choice. Look for reticular opacities, honeycomb, ground glass opacities, and architectural distortion. **Perform when**: to distinguish the different types of interstitial disease including: interstitial pulmonary fibrosis, sarcoidosis, interstitial pneumonia, and hypersensitivity pneumonitis. Sensitivity: 77-79%[3] Specificity: 85-88%

Hunninghake GW, et al. 2001. *Am J Respir Crit Care Med* 164(2):193-196.

3.6 Acute Bronchitis

- Inflammation of conducting bronchi (a clinical diagnosis)

1st Modality
CXR: bronchial wall thickening in more severe cases.

3.7 COPD

- Irreversible obstruction of airways

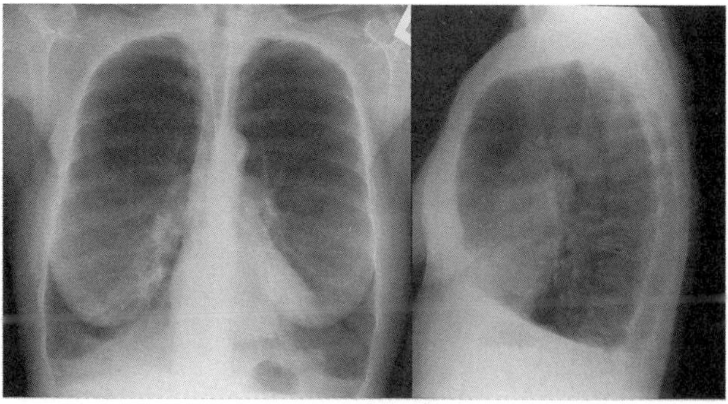

Figure 7. CXR showing hyperinflation and flattened diaphragms consistent with COPD.

1st Modality	2nd Modality
CXR: hyperinflation, decreased vascularity, flattened diaphragms, increased retrosternal air space. Basal emphysema suggestive of α-1-antitrypsin deficiency.	**CT**: imaging modality of choice. Similar findings as CXR but certain imaging findings suggestive of either panacinar or centrilobular emphysema. **Perform when**: as an adjunct to find out the morphologic type of emphysema. Sensitivity: 63%[4] Specificity: 88%

Mets OM, et al. 2011. *JAMA* 306(16):1775-1781.

3.8 Bronchiectasis

- Irreversible dilation of airways

1st Modality	2nd Modality
CXR: the findings depend on the severity and type of bronchiectasis: 1) bronchial wall thickening: tram tracks (parallel line shadows) and 2) cystic type: cystic spaces, honeycombing, ring opacities. Other findings: finger-in-glove opacities result from mucous plugs within dilated bronchi. Sensitivity: 87%[5] Specificity: 74%	**HRCT**: perform to distinguish types of bronchiectasis. Look for bronchial wall thickening and dilatation when bronchus is larger than the adjacent pulmonary artery (signet ring sign) or when bronchi are visible within 1 cm of the pleura; finger-in-glove mucous plugs in dilated bronchi. Three different forms of bronchiectasis will show different patterns: 1) cylindrical bronchiectasis, which shows smooth bronchial dilatation, 2) varicose bronchiectasis, which is characterized by beaded bronchial dilatation, and 3) cystic bronchiectasis, which is characterized by bronchial dilatation of greater 1 cm. **Perform when**: to distinguish between the 3 different types of bronciectasis. Sensitivity: 84-95%[6] Specificity: 93-100%

Naidich DP, et al. 1982. *J Comput Assist Tomogr* 6(3):437-444.
Hartman TE, et al. 1994. *Radiographics* 14(5):991-1003.

3.9 Pulmonary Embolism

- Embolus blocking the arterial vessels in the lung

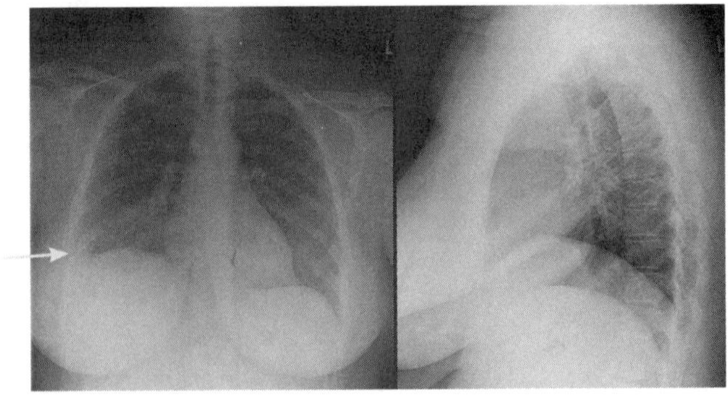

Figure 8. Hampton's hump at the right costophrenic sulcus shown in right lower lobe which is characteristic of a pulmonary embolism.

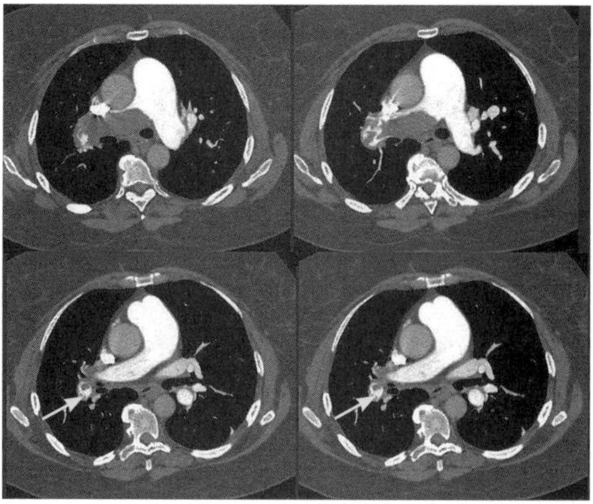

Figure 9. CT pulmonary angiogram showing a large embolus in the right main pulmonary trunk with smaller ones in left upper lobe pulmonary artery branch.

1st Modality	2nd Modality
CXR: most commonly normal (25%). Uncommon findings include: cardiomegaly (27%), pleural effusion (23%), elevated hemidiaphragm (20%), pulmonary artery enlargement (19%), atelectasis (18%), ill-defined opacity (17%), pulmonary edema (14%), oligemia (Westermark's sign) (8 %), overinflation (5%).[7] Sensitivity: 33%[8] Specificity: 59%	**CT Pulmonary Angiogram**: imaging of choice in moderate to high probability of pulmonary embolism. CT scan done with venous injection of contrast and imaging done at 20 s after. **Direct Findings**: railway track sign, rim sign, vessel cut-off, thrombus partially or completely occluding the artery with or without enlargement of artery. **Indirect Findings**: pulmonary hemorrhage or infarct, oligemia of affected segment, atelectasis, and small effusions. **Perform when**: moderate or high probability of pulmonary embolism based on the Wells score. Sensitivity: 80%[9] Specificity: 85.7%

Greenspan RH, et al. 1982. *Invest Radiol* 17(6):539-543.
Sood S, et al. 2006. *IJIR* 16(2):215-219.

3.10 Pulmonary Edema

- Fluid accumulating in lung parenchyma or air spaces

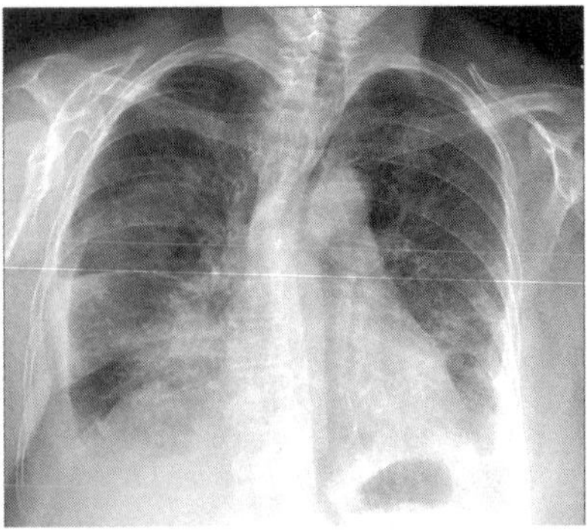

Figure 10. AP CXR showing a mixed interstitial and alveolar pulmonary edema with bilateral pleural effusions and cardiomegaly. Kerley B lines are seen at the bases.

1st Modality	2nd Modality
CXR: look for vascular redistribution, indistinct hilar vessels, interstitial edema (Kerley A and B lines), alveolar edema (consolidation), cardiomegaly, pleural effusions, and enlarged azygous vein. **Pulmonary Wedge Pressures (in mmHg)**: normal CXR (4.5-12), cephalization of pulmonary veins (12-17), Kerley lines (A, B, and C) (17-20), alveolar pulmonary edema (>25). Sensitivity: 57%[10] Specificity: 78%	**CT**: look for extensive vascular markings and possible underlying lung pathologies. **Perform when**: acute respiratory distress syndrome is present in order to detect underlying lung pathology and complications.

Fonseca C, et al. 2004. *Eur J Heart Fail* 6(6):807-812.

3.11 Lung Cancer

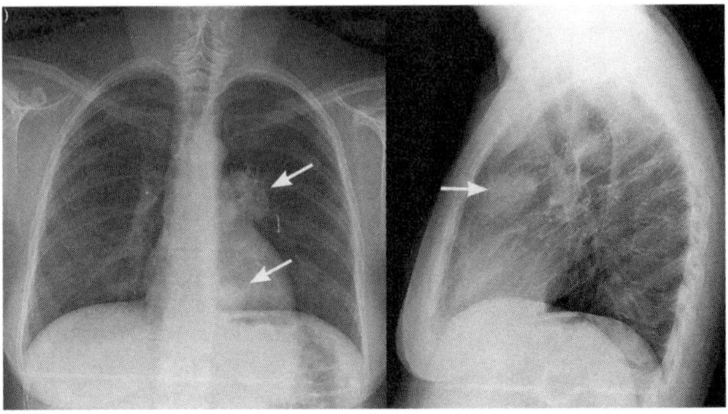

Figure 11. Left lung cancer demonstrated showing a 2.5 cm mass in the anterior segment of the left upper lobe. There is an additional lesion in the left lower lobe (behind the cardiac shadow).

1st Modality	2nd Modality
CXR: **Malignant Characteristics**: pulmonary nodule or mass that: 1) doubles in volume within 1 to 18 mo, 2) irregular, speculated or lobulated edges, 3) noncalcified or calcification pattern that is not central nidus, laminated, popcorn or diffuse, 4) larger than 3 cm in diameter. **Adenocarcinoma**: solitary pulmonary nodule or mass usually in the upper lobe. Margins can be well-circumscribed, irregular, lobulated, or speculated. Can have a chronic airspace disease pattern. **Squamous Cell Carcinoma**: postobstructive pneumonia, atelectasis, Golden S sign, apical mass with ill-defined borders and central lucency, asymmetrical pleural thickening. **Large Cell Carcinoma**: mass greater than 3 cm in diameter usually located in the lung periphery. **Small Cell Carcinoma**: hilar or perihilar mass, mediastinal widening, may be disseminated. **Nonbronchogenic Metastases**: multiple, noncalcified pulmonary nodules. Sensitivity: 78.3%[11] Specificity: 97%	**CT**: preferred imaging because of better soft tissue delineation. **Adenocarcinoma**: solitary pulmonary nodule or mass usually in the upper lobe. Often have air bronchograms. **Squamous Cell Carcinoma**: subpleural mass with cavitation. **Large Cell Carcinoma**: mass greater than 3 cm in diameter. **Small Cell Carcinoma**: extensive lymph node involvement and soft tissue infiltration of the mediastinum. **Nonbronchogenic Metastases**: multiple, noncalcified pulmonary nodules. **Perform when**: require better characterization of the primary tumor, visualization of metastases and cancer staging. Sensitivity: 88.9%[11] Specificity: 92.6%

3.12 Lung Abscess

- Necrosis of lung tissue and cavitation

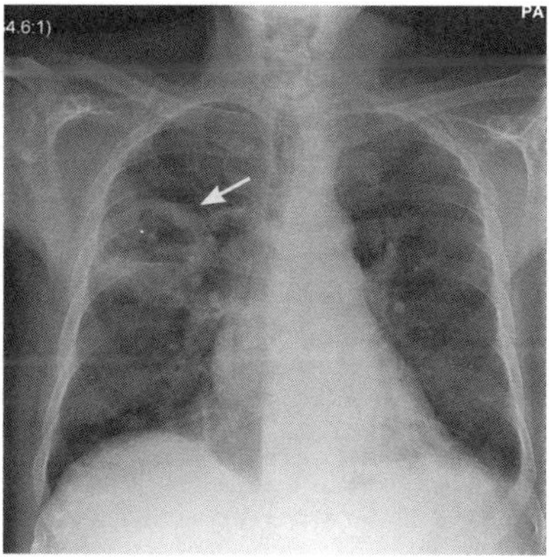

Figure 12. There is a large irregular cavitary lesion with air-fluid level in the right upper lobe.

1st Modality	2nd Modality
CXR: round, peripheral thoracic lesion. Has ill-defined margins (due to surrounding parenchymal inflammation) and may have cavitation with irregular margins and air-fluid levels. May be single or multiple (latter may be secondary to septicemia [e.g. from drug injection sites]).	**CT**: look for thick wall, nonuniform width, no pleural separation, no compression of uninvolved lung, acute chest wall angle, round shape, small size. **Perform when**: CXR is inconclusive or not definitive.

Stark DD, et al. 1983. *AJR Am J Roentgenol* 141(1):163-167.

3.13 Rib Fracture

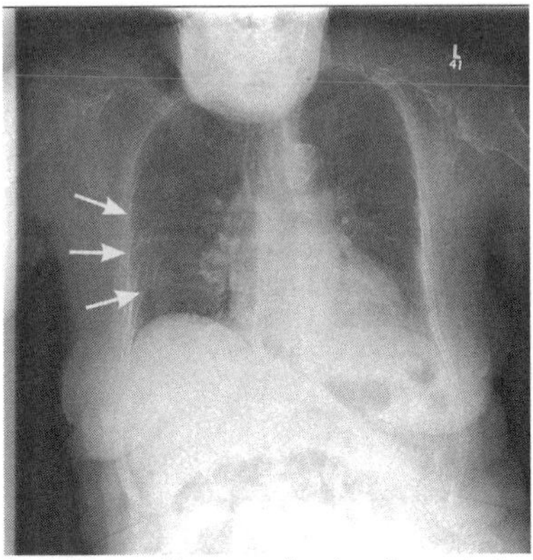

Figure 13. Right rib fracture. Since more than two ribs are broken in two places, a flail chest is seen.

1st Modality	2nd Modality
CXR: displaced or nondisplaced rib fracture, can be associated with pneumothorax or hemothorax. Sensitivity: 40%[12]	CXR usually sufficient. Perform **rib series** if high suspicion of traumatic rib fracture without evidence on plain CXR. Perform a **bone scan** in the case of stress fractures. **Perform when**: high suspicion of traumatic rib fracture without evidence on plain film or if suspecting stress fracture.

MEDICAL IMAGING

3.14 Mitral Valve Stenosis

- Narrowing of mitral valve opening

1st Modality	2nd Modality
CXR: signs of left atrial hypertension (enlargement of the left atrium, right ventricle, and pulmonary trunk). Cephalization of pulmonary vasculature, septal (Kerley B lines), rarely calcification of mitral valve.	**Transthoracic Echocardiogram and Doppler**: considered gold standard. Look for thickened mitral leaflets with reduced motion during diastole. Doming of the mitral valve. Enlarged left atrium and right ventricle with normal-sized left ventricle. **Perform when**: to allow visualization of abnormal leaflet motion and blood flow consistent with mitral valve stenosis.

Habib G. 2006. *Heart* 92(1):124-130.

3.15 Angina with Nondiagnostic ECG and Negative Serum Markers

1st Modality	2nd Modality
Stress Radionuclide Myocardial Perfusion Imaging: extensive reversible ischemia in multiple segments, left ventricular dilatation, increased lung uptake of radionuclide.	**CT Coronary Angiogram**: gold standard imaging technique. Look for reduced coronary artery cross-sectional diameter. **Perform when**: to determine the degree of arterial stenosis. Sensitivity: 99%[13] Specificity: 96%

3.16 Myocardial Infarction

1st Modality
CXR: may be normal or associated with nonspecific signs of CHF. Imaging is not usually recommended.

3.17 Aortic Dissection

- Separation of the walls of the aorta

1st Modality	2nd Modality
CXR: widening of the aorta (ascending and descending) especially when compared to previous CXR, displaced intimal calcification from outer surface of the aorta (>10 mm), left apical pleural soft tissue cap (dissected left subclavian artery or apical pleural hemorrhage), widened mediastinum, left pleural effusion (hemothorax: rare). Sensitivity: 67%[14] Specificity: 86%	**CT Angiogram**: look for dilated aorta, intimal flap with two distinct lumens (false lumen and true lumen), beak sign, cobweb sign, intraluminal thrombus, pericardial effusion. **Perform when**: to determine the type of aortic dissection in order to direct treatment. Sensitivity: 98% Specificity: 100%[15]

MEDICAL IMAGING

3.18 Esophageal Rupture

1st Modality	2nd Modality	3rd Modality
CXR: rupture common on left side of distal esophagus. Pneumomediastinum, air in the prevertebral space, widened lower thoracic mediastinum, left pleural effusion, subcutaneous emphysema. Pneumoperitoneum (if rupture extends toward gastric fundus).	**CT**: look for esophageal wall thickening and irregularity. Extra-esophageal air, mediastinal widening, air and fluid in left pleural space, abscess abutting the esophagus (in undiagnosed rupture). **Perform when**: to detect smaller esophageal ruptures.	**Contrast Esophagography**: look for extravasation of contrast material, extraluminal gas. **Perform when**: CXR and CT are inconclusive in making a diagnosis.
Sensitivity: 86%[16]	Sensitivity: 95%[16]	Sensitivity: 91%[16]

3.19 Pericarditis

- Inflammation of pericardium

1st Modality	2nd Modality
CXR: often normal. In severe cases, enlarged cardiac silhouette with clear lung fields, rapid cardiomegaly.	**CT**: look for pericardial fluid, pericardial thickening/enhancement, and pneumopericardium (rare). **Perform when**: for a definitive diagnosis.

3.20 Spontaneous Pneumomediastinum

- Air in the mediastinum

1st Modality	2nd Modality
CXR: mediastinal lucencies that outline the aorta and pulmonary artery and distend the mediastinal pleura laterally or into the neck. Continuous diaphragm sign. Spinnaker sign. V sign of Naclerio (for esophageal rupture). Ring around the artery sign. Subcutaneous emphysema.	**CT**: look for the same signs as on CXR. **Perform when**: to improve sensitivity and provide a more definitive diagnosis.

4. ABDOMINAL PATHOLOGIES AND FINDINGS

4.1 Peritoneal Hemorrhage

- Bleeding within the peritoneum[17-21]

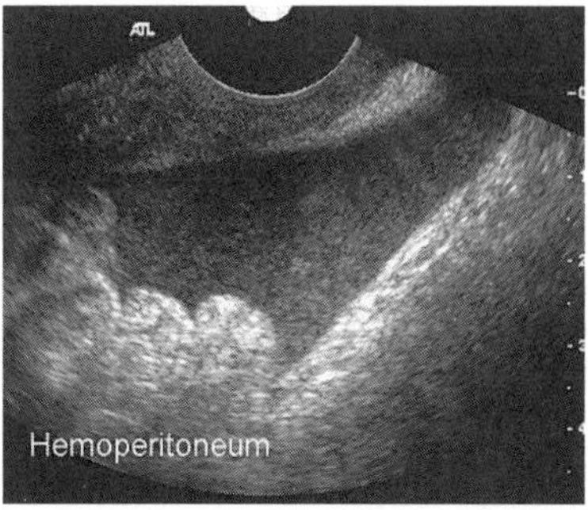

Figure 14. U/S of the pelvis showing hyperechoic fluid collection with small bowel (rounded structures) floating (not anechoic).

1st Modality	2nd Modality
U/S (FAST – Focused Assessment with Sonography in Trauma): a hyperechoic fluid collection in the most dependent spaces (Morison's pouch, pouch of Douglas, and paracolic gutters) of the peritoneum. Sensitivity: 85%[20] Specificity: 96%	**CT**: look for hyperdense fluid in the dependent spaces of the abdomen. Blood obscures, displaces or compresses the normal peritoneal structures. It can be distinguished from ascites since it has a higher attenuation than ascitic fluid. **Perform when**: to determine cause of hemorrhage, better visualize surrounding structures, and plan therapeutic intervention. Patients must be hemodynamically stable to undergo CT scan. Sensitivity: 97.2%[20] Specificity: 94.7%

4.2 Intussusception

- Invagination of a bowel loop with its mesenteric fold (intussusceptum) into the lumen of a contiguous portion of bowel (intussuscipiens) as a result of peristalsis[22-27]

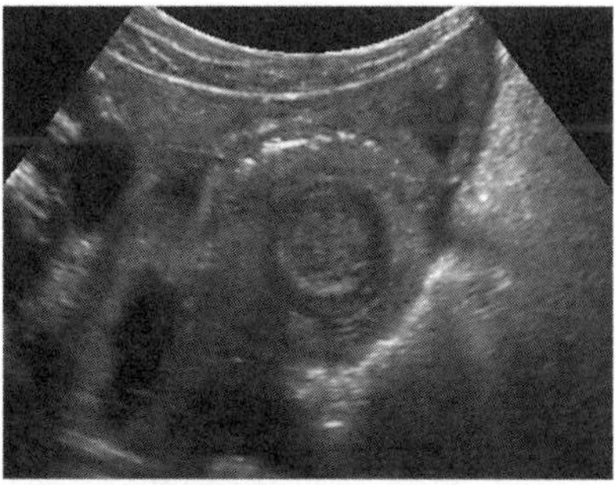

Figure 15. An U/S showing the target sign which is characteristic of intussusception. Intussusception of the jejunum is seen here.

1st Modality	2nd Modality	3rd Modality
Abdominal Plain Film: look for distended bowel with absence of colonic gas. Crescent sign of air outlining the intussusceptum within the intussuscipiens (target sign). Signs better seen in children. Sensitivity: 80% Specificity: 58%[22]	**U/S**: target sign or coiled spring lesion. Useful especially in pediatric age group. **Perform when**: if you require a more sensitive and specific test for intussusception. This aids in determining the severity and complications of the pathology. Sensitivity: 97.9%[26] Specificity: 97.8%	**CT Scan with Oral and IV Contrast**: useful in the adult population. Better visualization of surrounding structures allows for determination of cause of intussusception and assesses for complications such as bowel obstruction and strangulation. **Perform when**: to determine etiology of intussusception. Sensitivity: 71.4-87.5%[26] Specificity: 100%

4.3 Ascites

- Pathologic fluid collection within the abdominal cavity (typically diagnosed based on clinical history and physical exam, imaging useful when suspect small volumes of ascitic fluid)[28-32]

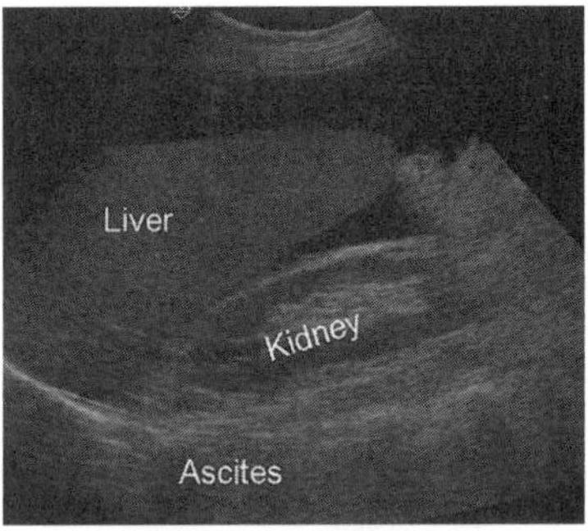

Figure 16. (A) Ascitic fluid collection seen as the hypoechoic density between the liver and kidney in Morison's pouch.

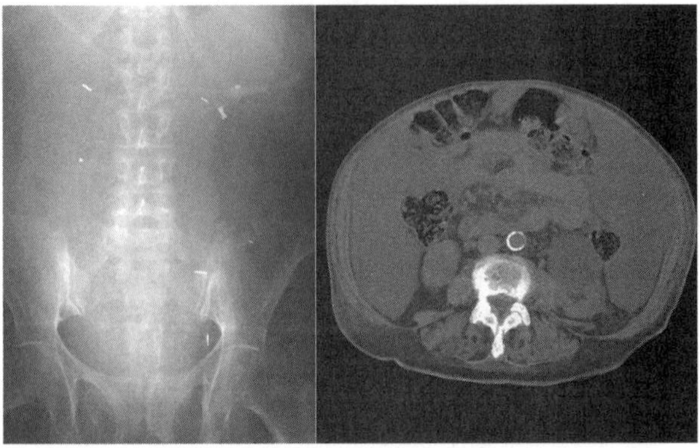

Figure 16. (B) The plain film of the abdomen (left image) shows a "ground glass appearance", and the corresponding axial CT image (right) shows large volume of clear fluid ascites.

1st Modality	2nd Modality
Abdominal Plain Film: look for loss of posterior liver edge (Morrison's pouch), Mickey Mouse ear sign in pelvis (fluid in supravesicular peritoneal space), displacement of bowel loops, and increased haziness (large volume ascites). **U/S**: ascitic fluid is free-flowing and is typically found in the subhepatic recess, paracolic gutters, and in-between organs. If the fluid is transudative, the fluid is typically hypoechoic; whereas exudative fluids typically have multiple echoic foci. Sensitivity: 98%[32] Specificity: 97%	**CT**: look for a hypodensity specifically in the perihepatic and subhepatic spaces. Can detect very small quantities of fluid. **Perform when**: to determine cause of ascites, such as liver disease or malignancy.

4.4 Small Bowel Obstruction

- Low grade or high grade blockage of the small intestine
- The small bowel is considered dilated when it exceeds 3 cm in diameter (3,6,9 rule)

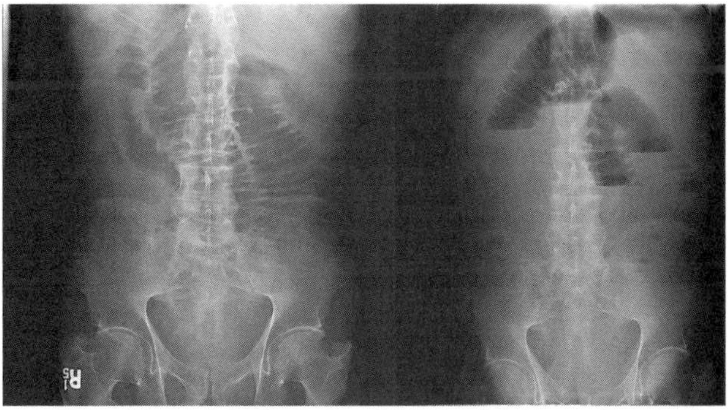

Figure 17. Small bowel obstruction is characterized by dilated loops of bowel and "string of pearls" appearance. Plicae circulares are seen which confirms small bowel dilation with multiple air-fluid levels and minimal gas in the colon.

1st Modality	2nd Modality
Abdominal Plain Film: look for distended loops with multiple differential air-fluid levels, step ladder fluid levels, string of pearls sign, and minimal or no gas beyond point of obstruction. Sensitivity: 69%[33] Specificity: 57%	**CT Scan with Oral and IV Contrast**: look for a transition point of where the bowel abruptly changes. Absence of air or fluid in areas distal to this point. Proximal loops are distended and filled with fluid and gas. **Perform when**: to determine etiology of bowel obstruction such as adhesions and strangulation. Sensitivity: 81-94%[33] Specificity: 96%

Frager D, et al. 1994. *AJR Am J Roentgenol* 162(1):37-41.
Burkill GJC, Bell JRG, Healy JC. 2001. *Clin Radiol* 56(5):350-359.

4.5 Large Bowel Obstruction

- Partial or complete blockage of the colon or rectum

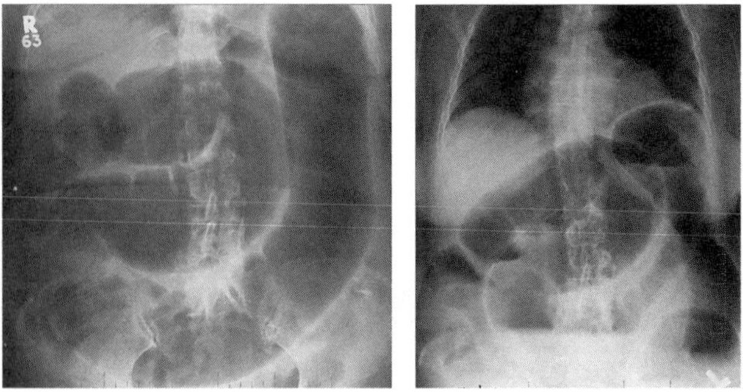

Figure 18. Large bowel obstruction characterized by dilated loops of bowel as defined by the 3, 6, 9 rule. Haustra are seen on the portions of dilated bowel which confirms that it is large bowel.

1st Modality	2nd Modality
Abdominal Plain Film: distended loops of bowel filled with gas and fluid proximal to point of obstruction. The colon is considered dilated when it exceeds 6 cm in diameter and the cecum is dilated when it exceeds 9 cm in diameter (3, 6, 9 rule). Sensitivity: 77%[34] Specificity: 50%	**CT Scan with IV, Oral, and Rectal Contrast**: look for dilated colon with an abrupt point of obstruction. Also can see associated complications such as ischemia and possible localized perforation (cecum). **Perform when**: to determine etiology (colon cancer, diverticulitis), severity and complications of obstruction. Sensitivity: 94%[34] Specificity: 96%

Megibow AJ, et al. 1991. *Radiology* 180(2):313-318.
Khurana B, et al. 2002. *AJR Am J Roentgenol* 178(5):1139-1944.

4.6 Perforated Bowel

- A hole penetrating through the wall of the intestines

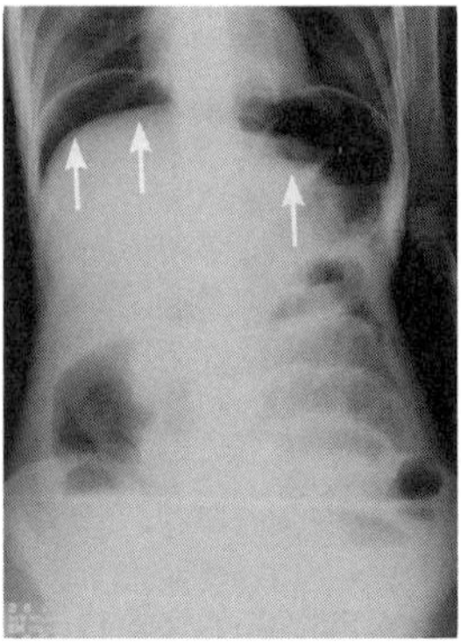

Figure 19. Free air (arrows) under the diaphragm is seen and is characteristic of a bowel perforation.

1st Modality	2nd Modality
Abdominal Plain Films (Supine and Upright): two types of free air – intraperitoneal and retroperitoneal air. **Intraperitoneal Air**: • **Upright Film**: air under the diaphragm. • **Supine Film**: signs include: outlining of the falciform ligament, and Rigler's sign (bowel wall outlined on luminal and peritoneal sides). **Retroperitoneal Air**: "streaky air" • Look for air/gas outlining retroperitoneal organs: kidney, ascending/descending colon, and duodenum.	**CT Scan with Oral and IV Contrast**: look for a collection of air or leakage of oral contrast locally around region of perforated bowel. There may be inflammatory changes shown in the pericolonic soft tissues and resultant focal abscess may be seen. **Perform when**: suspect a small perforation since there is better visualization of small quantities of air/gas. Sensitivity: 92%[35] Specificity: 94%

Sherck J, et al. 1994. *Am J Surg* 168(6):670-675.

4.7 Peptic Ulcer Disease

- Mucosal erosions forming ulcers in the stomach or duodenum

1st Modality	2nd Modality
Single-Contrast or Double-Contrast Barium Studies: poor mucosal coating of the barium and filling defects in the ulcerated regions are observed. Sensitivity: 80-90%[36]	**Esophagogastroduodenoscopy**: the imaging investigation of choice. Look for erosions and active bleeding sites in stomach lining. Additionally, can take a biopsy with this imaging method. **Perform when**: for confirmatory diagnosis and also to aid in determining cause of peptic ulcer disease. Sensitivity: >90% Specificity: >90%[36]

Ramakrishnan K, Salinas RC. 2007. *Am Fam Physician* 76(7):1005-1012.

4.8 Appendicitis

- Inflammation of the appendix

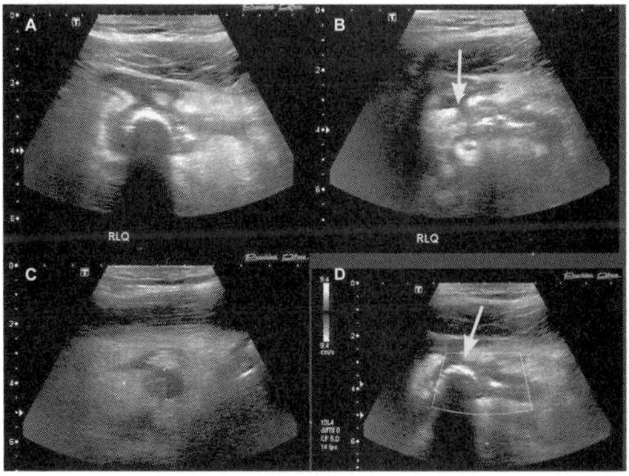

Figure 20. The healthy appendix is not normally seen on U/S. Here an inflamed appendix is seen surrounded by periappendiceal fluid. White semicircular area with shadowing in A and D display an appendicolith. Arrow points to a perforation in B.

1st Modality	2nd Modality
U/S: a healthy appendix is not normally seen on U/S. An inflamed appendix presents as a noncompressible structure >7 mm in diameter. The structure lacks peristalsis and typically has periappendiceal fluid surrounding it. Sensitivity: 66%[37] Specificity: 95%	**CT with IV Contrast Only**: look for an appendix with thickened walls which do not fill with contrast. May see appendicolith, mesoappendiceal inflammation, localized or diffuse perforation, and abscess. **Perform when**: U/S is inconclusive and there is a high degree of suspicion. Also, can aid in developing a treatment plan since gives good visualization of surrounding structures. Sensitivity: 98.5% Specificity: 98%[37]

Barloon TJ, et al. 1995. *Abdom Imaging* 20(2):149-151.

4.9 Diverticulitis

- Outpouching of the inner lining of the intestine which becomes infected or inflamed

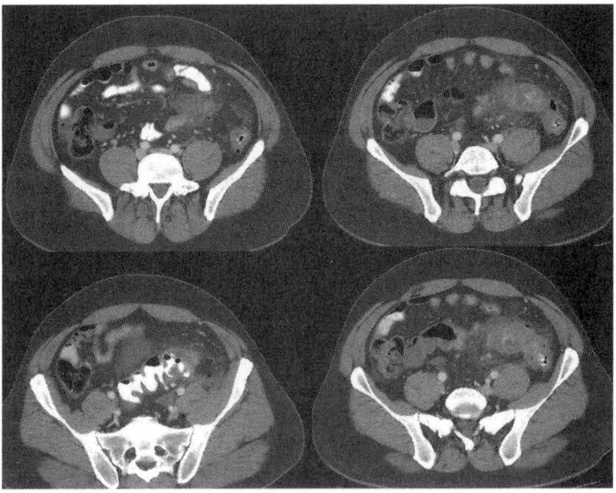

Figure 21. CT of pelvis with positive rectal contrast in sigmoid shows thickened sigmoid colon with few diverticula and inflamed mesentery.

1st Modality
CT with Oral, Rectal, and IV Contrast: the gold standard in the diagnosis of diverticulitis. Look for pericolic fat infiltration, colonic diverticula, bowel wall thickening, phlegmon, abscesses, and localized perforation. Sensitivity: 97%[38] Specificity: 97%

Miller FH, et al. *Reston: American College of Radiology*; 2011.

4.10 Cholecystitis

- Inflammation of the gallbladder

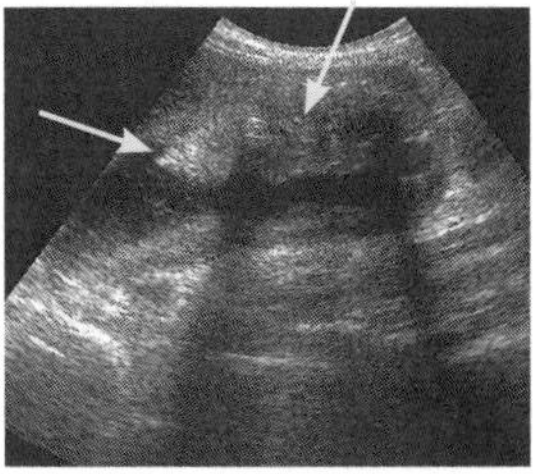

Figure 22. Thickened gallbladder walls visualized above are findings suggestive of cholecystitis.

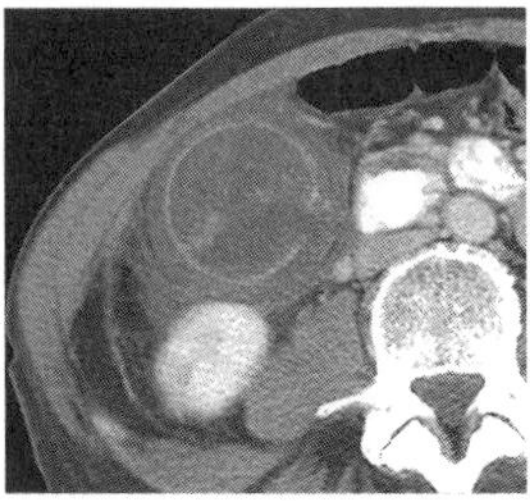

Figure 23. Pericholecystic fluid and thickened gallbladder wall are seen on the CT suggestive of cholecystitis.

1st Modality	2nd Modality
U/S: look for pericholecystic fluid, gallbladder wall thickening (>4 mm), and gallstones. Sensitivity: 90-95%[39] Specificity: 78-80%	**CT**: look for gallbladder wall thickening (>4 mm), pericholecystic fluid, edema without the presence of ascites, and intramural gas. **Perform when**: require better visualization of the surrounding structures, which can aid in developing a treatment plan. Sensitivity: 95%[40]

4.11 Pancreatitis

- Inflammation of the pancreas (typically a clinical diagnosis; however, imaging more useful to assess complications or pre-existing chronic pancreatitis)[41-45]

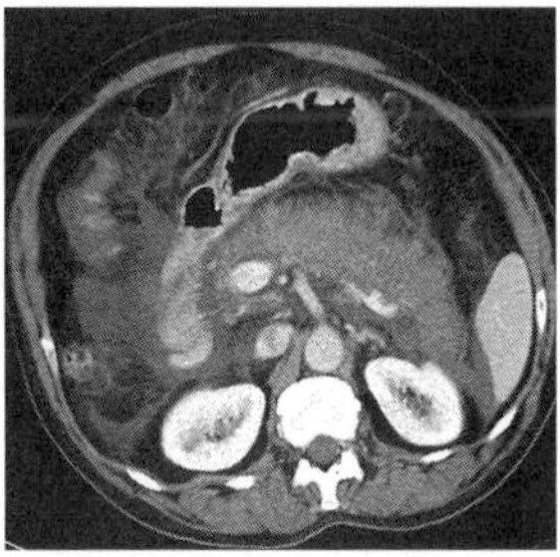

Figure 24. Diffuse enlargement of the pancreas and blurring of the peripancreatic fat planes is seen, which is consistent with pancreatitis.

1st Modality	2nd Modality
U/S: look for pancreatic enlargement, peripancreatic fluid, hypoechoic foci suggestive of necrosis, and pancreatic pseudocysts. Sensitivity: 60-70%[43] Specificity: 80-90%	**CT with IV Contrast**: look for pancreatic enlargement, heterogeneous enhancement of the gland, irregular contour, blurring of peripancreatic fat borders, pseudocysts, abscesses, and necrosis. **Perform when**: to visualize complications of pancreatitis. Sensitivity: 70-90%[45] Specificity: 85%

4.12 Peritonitis

- Inflammation of the peritoneum

1st Modality
CT: look for free intraperitoneal air, peritoneal thickening with enhancement, bowel wall and mesenteric thickening, and ascites. CT is only indicated if a clinical diagnosis of peritonitis is not definitive. ***Note:*** plain film not useful

Demirkazik FB, et al. 1996. *Acta Radiol* 37:517-520.

4.13 Renal Colic

- Acute abdominal pain due to kidney stones

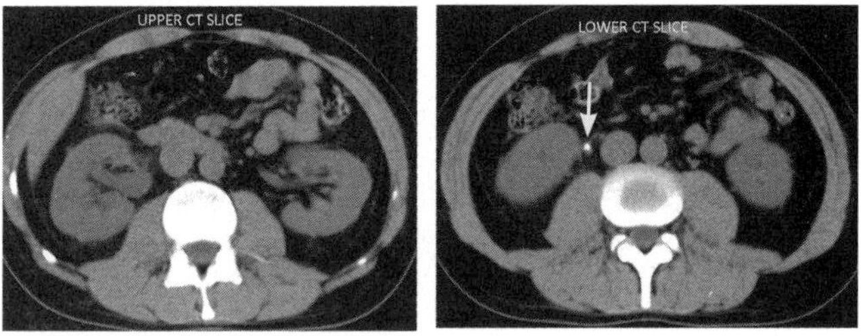

Figure 25. (A) A small, calcified kidney stone (see arrow), seen as hyperdensity, is visualized in right ureter.

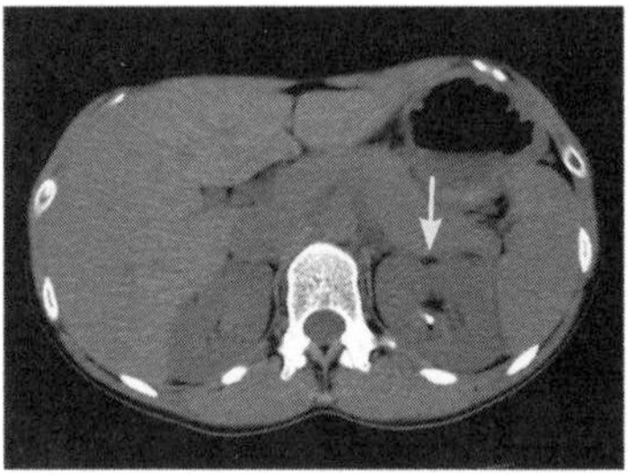

Figure 25. (B) A small, calcified kidney stone, seen as hyperdensity, is visualized in left pelvis.

1st Modality	2nd Modality
CT (No Contrast): often considered the gold standard. Look for renal pelvis and collecting system dilation, and obstructing kidney stones. Perinephric stranding or rarely urinoma may occur. **Perform when**: for treatment planning since can visualize surrounding structures and can better determine characteristics of obstructing stone. Sensitivity: 91%[46] Specificity: 91%	**Abdominal Plain Film**: used for pre-lithotripsy planning. Look for location, radiopacity of stone (calcium containing), and size of kidney stones. Sensitivity: 69%[46] Specificity: 82%

Jindal G, Ramchandani P. 2007. *Radiol Clin North Am* 45(3):395-410, vii.
Heneghan JP, et al. 2003. *Radiology* 229(2):575-580.

4.14 Small Bowel Mesenteric Ischemia

- Insufficient blood flow from the mesenteric circulation resulting in ischemia and eventually necrosis of the small bowel wall

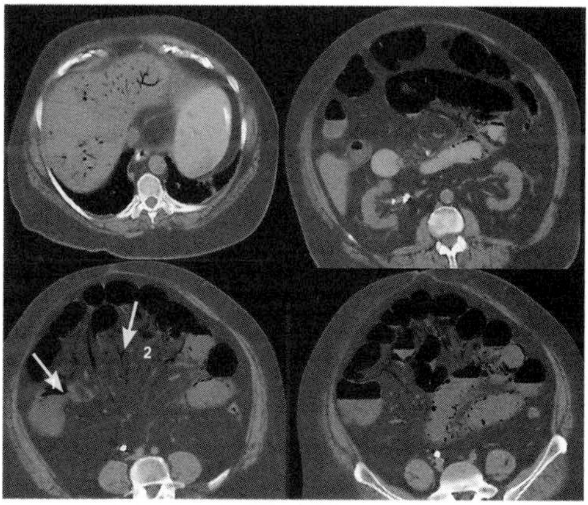

Figure 26. Small bowel ischemia visualized by bowel wall thickening and perienteric fat stranding (arrow 1). Additionally, portal venous gas and pneumatosis (arrow 2) are also shown.

1st Modality	2nd Modality
Abdominal Plain Film: sometimes done as first-line imaging as clinical diagnosis often not apparent. Common findings: normal bowel gas pattern. Uncommon findings: ileus, wall thickening ("pinky printing"), pneumatosis, portal venous gas at periphery of liver edge (distinguishing portal versus biliary air).	**CT Ischemic Protocol (Plain, Arterial, and Venous)**: look for bowel wall thickening, dilation, perienteric fat stranding, ascites, mesenteric arterial or venous thrombus, bowel infarction: pneumatosis and portal venous gas. **Perform when**: to better characterize complications and severity of ischemia. Sensitivity: 96-100%[47] Specificity: 89-94%

Kirkpatrick IDC, Kroeker MA, Greenberg HM. 2003. *Radiology* 229(1):91-98.

4.15 Ectopic Pregnancy

- Pregnancy that occurs outside the uterus

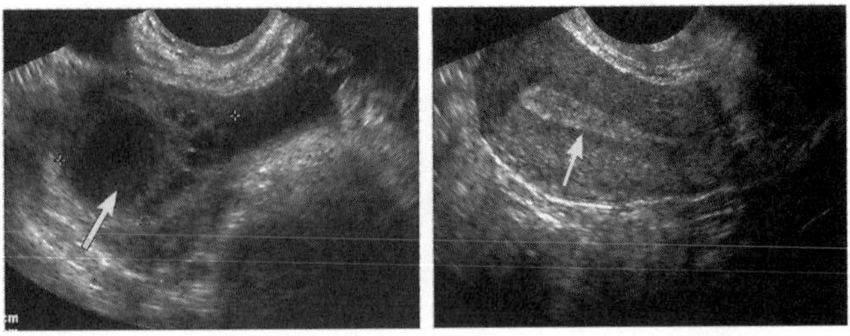

Figure 27. A gestational sac is seen outside the uterus and there is no embryo present within the uterus. The uterine cavity has decidual reaction but no fetus.

1st Modality

U/S: usually performed transvaginally. A bright echogenic, ring-like structure located outside the uterus that contains a gestational sac with a fetal pole, a yolk sac, or both is indicative of an ectopic pregnancy.
Additional findings may include: an adnexal mass and hyperechoic free fluid in cul-de-sac (hemorrhage).

Sensitivity: 87-99%[48]
Specificity: 94-99.9%

4.16 Gastritis

- Inflammation of the lining of the stomach

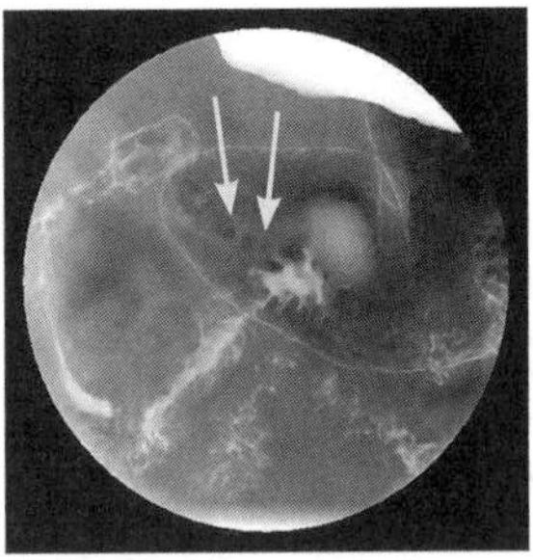

Figure 28. Gastric erosions and mucosal nodules seen, which is typical of gastritis.

1st Modality

Double-Contrast Upper GI Barium Studies: look for thick gastric folds, gastric mucosal nodules, and gastric erosions.

Sensitivity: 72%[49]
Specificity: 77%

Thoeni RF, et al. 1983. *Radiology* 148(3):621-626.

4.17 Pyelonephritis

- Infection of the kidney

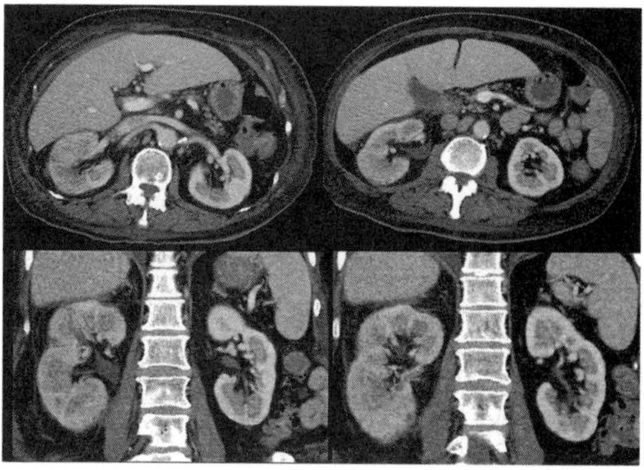

Figure 29. Pyelonephritis of the right kidney seen characterized by kidney enlargement and decreased enhancement.

1st Modality	2nd Modality
U/S: often done as first-line imaging due to vague flank symptoms. Look for renal enlargement, loss of cortical medullar differentiation, mild hydronephrosis, and possible renal abscess.	**CT**: the imaging investigation of choice. Contrast-enhancement typically indicated. Look for enlargement of kidney, dilation of the collecting system, multi-focal abscess regions, and linear parenchymal striations. **Perform when**: to better detect severity and complications of pyelonephritis. Sensitivity: 86.8%[50] Specificity: 87.5%

Majd M, et al. 2001. *Radiology* 218(1):101-108.

4.18 Ischemic Colitis

- Insufficient blood supply to the colon resulting in ischemia and eventually necrosis

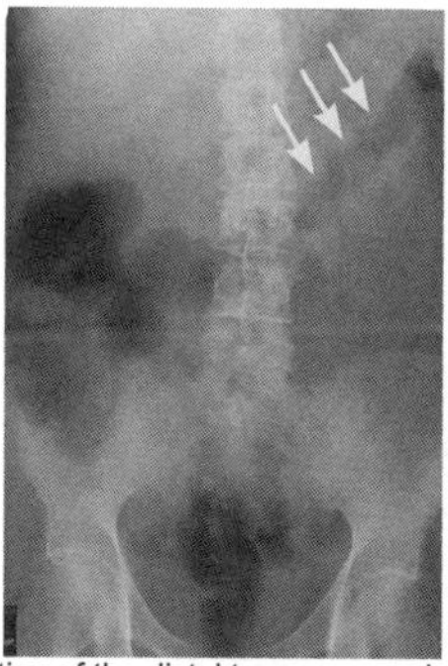

Figure 30. There is thumbprinting of the distal transverse colon (arrows) and narrowed descending colon: acute ischemic colitis in watershed area. The watershed area (branches from both the superior mesenteric artery [SMA] and inferior mesenteric artery [IMA]) is most vulerable to ischemia since the SMA and the IMA do not have as many collaterals.

1st Modality	2nd Modality
Abdominal Plain Film: common radiographic findings include: normal gas pattern or ileus. Uncommon findings include: dilatation of a section of the colon (watershed area), mucosal edema (thumbprinting), pneumatosis.	**CT Ischemic Protocol**: look for thromboembolism in the inferior mesenteric vessels, thickening of the bowel wall, absence of bowel wall enhancement with contrast-enhanced CT, narrowing of the bowel lumen due to mucosal edema, and bowel dilatation proximal to the ischemic segment of the bowel. **Perform when**: the patient has abdominal pain and/or rectal bleeding or bloody diarrhea. The presence of any of the following risk factors elevates the pretest probability: age >60 yr, hemodialysis, HTN, DM, hypoalbuminemia, and constipation-inducing medications. Sensitivity: 82%[51]

Balthazar EJ, Yen BC, Gordon RB. 1999. *Radiology* 211(2):381-388.
Wiesner W, et al. 2003. *Radiology* 226(3):635-650.

4.19 Large Bowel Volvulus

- Twisting of the sigmoid or cecum on its respective mesentery leading to obstruction and ultimately ischemia

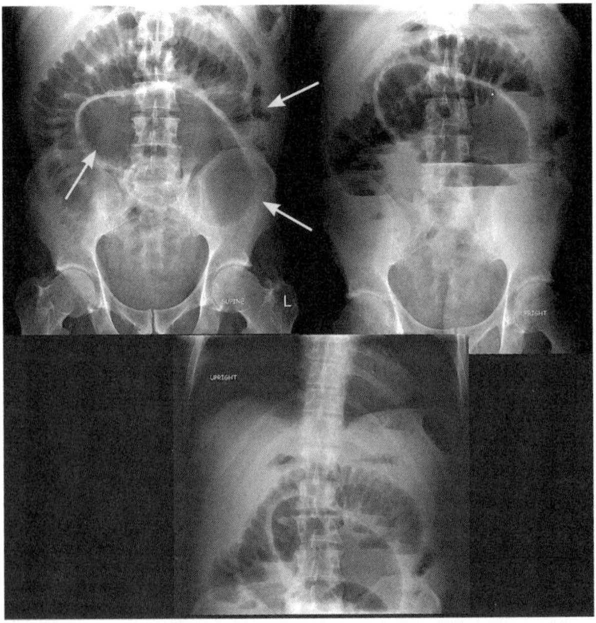

Figure 31. Abdominal plain films show dilated cecum in the midline with no air in the rest of the colon and dilated small bowel with air-fluid levels indicating a cecal volvulus.

1st Modality	2nd Modality
Abdominal Plain Film: **Cecal Volvulus**: look for dilated cecum in left upper quadrant, small bowel obstruction, and no gas in the rest of colon (from hepatic flexure to rectum). **Sigmoid Volvulus**: Look for dilated sigmoid colon extending from pelvis to epigastrium (coffee bean sign), and dilated and/or stool filled proximal colon.	**CT**: **Cecal Volvulus**: look for dilated edematous cecum, small bowl obstruction, whirl sign of twisted mesenteric and mesenteric vessel, ascites, rarely pneumatosis or free air. **Sigmoid Volvulus**: look for coffee bean sign of obstructed sigmoid and dilated colon proximally, whirl sign of twisted inferior mesenteric artery vessels and mesentery, and ascites.

Peterson CM, et al. 2009. *Radiographics* 29(5):1281-1293.

4.20 Small Bowel Volvulus

- Obstruction and ischemia of the small bowel as a result of a loop of small bowel twisting

1st Modality	2nd Modality
Abdominal Plain Film: look for bowel wall thickening and/or pneumatosis involving the affected segment of bowel. Poor sensitivity and specificity.	**CT Abdomen and Pelvis with Oral, IV, and Rectal Contrast**: the imaging modality of choice. Look for single loop of dilated small bowel with two points of narrowing close to each other (bird beak), edema, delayed mucosal enhancement, and whirl sign of twisted vessels, and ascites. **Perform when**: to allow for better visualization of surrounding structures, and for treatment planning. Sensitivity: 94%[52]

4.21 Ileus

- Bowel obstruction in the absence of mechanical obstruction

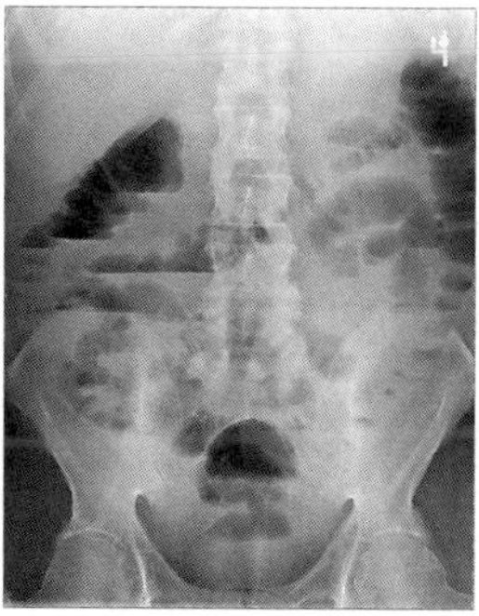

Figure 32. An upright view of the abdomen showing multiple air-fluid levels in nondilated small and large bowel including the rectum indicating ileus.

1st Modality	2nd Modality
Abdominal Plain Film: look for extensively gas-filled bowels without dilation. There are several types of ileus depending on the etiologies and possible outcomes: **Localized Ileus (Sentinel Loop Sign)**: secondary to underlying inflammatory process such as pancreatitis (C-Loop of duodenum); ileocecal ileus (appendicitis) or ileus affecting hepatic flexure (cholecystitis). **Diffuse Ileus**: usually either postoperative or infectious cause (*C. difficile* or garden variety gastroenteritis or electrolyte imbalance). **Ileus in ICU or Bedridden Orthopedic Patients**: colonic dilatation with competent ileocecal valve may lead to cecal dilatation and perforation – Ogilvey's syndrome.	**CT**: may be required if symptoms getting worse and/or colon dilating despite treatment to rule out early perforation. **Perform when**: helpful in determining etiology and allow for treatment planning.

Frager DH, et al. 1995. *AJR Am J Roentgenol* 164(4):891-894.

5. CENTRAL NERVOUS SYSTEM PATHOLOGIES AND FINDINGS

5.1 Epidural Hemorrhage

- Bleeding in between skull and dura mater from injury

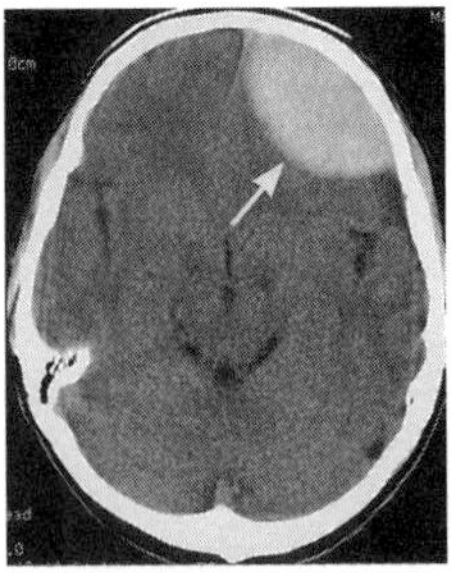

Figure 34. Epidural hematoma (see arrow) characterized by a biconvex hyperdensity between the skull and dura mater.

1st Modality
CT: biconvex high density lesion between dura and skull.

5.2 Subdural Hemorrhage

- Bleeding in between dura and arachnoid mater from ruptured veins

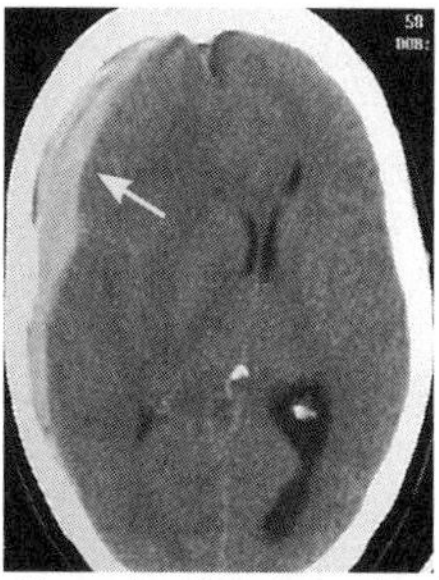

Figure 34. Crescent-shaped hyperdensity between the dura and arachnoid mater (see arrow) associated with the acute phase of a subdural hemorrhage.

1st Modality	2nd Modality
CT: **Acute Phase**: crescent-shaped area of high density between dura and arachnoid. **Chronic Phase**: crescent-shaped, low attenuation (fluid density). Sometimes there is an acute-on-chronic subdural bleed (fluid-fluid level).	**MRI**: Better visualization of small collections of fluid and isodense hematomas.[41] **Perform when**: in chronic presentations of subdural hemorrhage, since allows for better contrast.

Senturk S, et al. 2010. *Swiss Med Wkly* 140(23-24):335-340.

5.3 Subarachnoid Hemorrhage (SAH)

- Bleeding underneath arachnoid mater from ruptured cerebral aneurysm or trauma

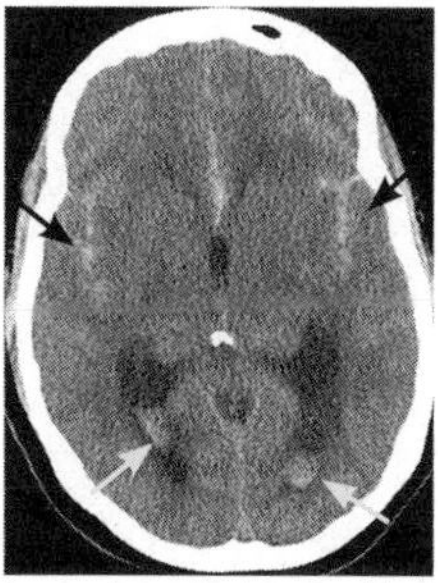

Figure 35. Interventricular hemorrhage is visualized by hyperdensities in the posterior horns of the lateral ventricles (white arrows). Subarachnoid hemorrhage is visualized by hyperdensity in the subarachnoid spaces (Sylvian fissure) (black arrows).

1st Modality	2nd Modality	3rd Modality	4th Modality
CT: high density blood in CSF spaces around brainstem, Sylvian fissure, and sometimes the ventricles.	**CT Angiogram**: useful to determine cause of SAH. Aneurysm can be visualized with remodelling techniques.	**Conventional Angiogram**: detection and coiling of aneurysm during interventional procedure.	**MRI**: may be used to detect an aneurysm.[53] Increased signal intensity on fluid attenuated inversion recovery (FLAIR).
	Perform when: to determine cause of SAH. Sensitivity: 99%[54] Specificity: 88%[54]	**Perform when**: to locate aneurysm and allow for targeted treatment.	**Perform when**: to determine cause of SAH if not well visualized on CT.

Eisenberg RL, Johnson NM. *Comprehensive Radiographic Pathology*, 4th ed. St. Louis: Mosby Elsevier; 2007.

5.4 Hydrocephalus

- Accumulation of CSF in ventricles from obstruction

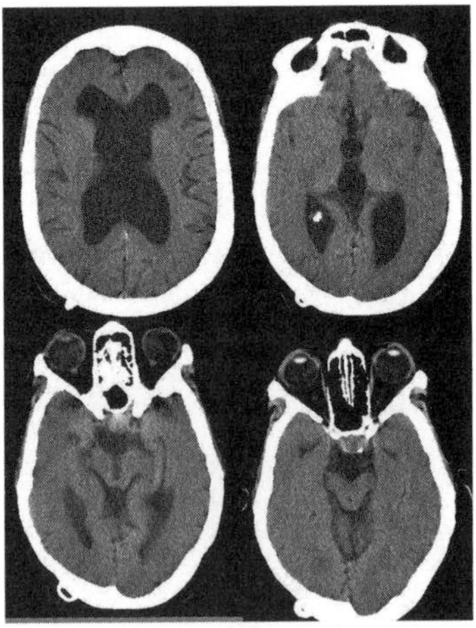

Figure 36. Markedly dilated ventricular system (lateral, third, and fourth ventricles) consistent with hydrocephalus.

1st Modality	2nd Modality
Contrast CT: enlargement of ventricles. Cause (e.g. colloid cyst) can be detected.	**MRI**: more specific findings to determine underlying cause (communicating vs. non-communicating). Useful to visualize hyperintense white matter surrounding hydrocephalus demonstrating extent of edema from condition. **Perform when**: the cause of hydrocephalus is unknown and needs to be determined for treatment. MRI has higher resolution images showing causes (e.g. blockages) better than CT.

Shprecher D, Schwalb J, Kurlan R. 2008. *Curr Neurol Neurosci Rep* 8(5):371-376.

5.5 Cerebral Abscess

- Accumulation of a pus-filled cavity due to an infectious process

1st Modality	2nd Modality
Contrast CT: ring enhancement with a hypodense, necrotic core with contrast.	**MRI**: T1-weighted image shows low intensity signal mass with isointense capsule. T2-weighted image demonstrates hyperintensity in mass and edema which frames abscess. **Perform when**: patient has more specific clinical and imaging findings of abscess. Findings on MRI are more specific for cerebral abscess and can help distinguish from other pathologies (e.g. ring-enhancing gliomas).

Eisenberg RL, Johnson NM. *Comprehensive Radiographic Pathology*, 4th ed. St. Louis: Mosby Elsevier; 2007.
Holmes TM, Petrella JR, Provenzale JM. 2004. *AJR Am J Roentgenol* 183(5):1247-1252.

5.6 Stroke (Ischemic Infarction)

- Loss of blood to brain region due to an emboli

Day 1

Day 2

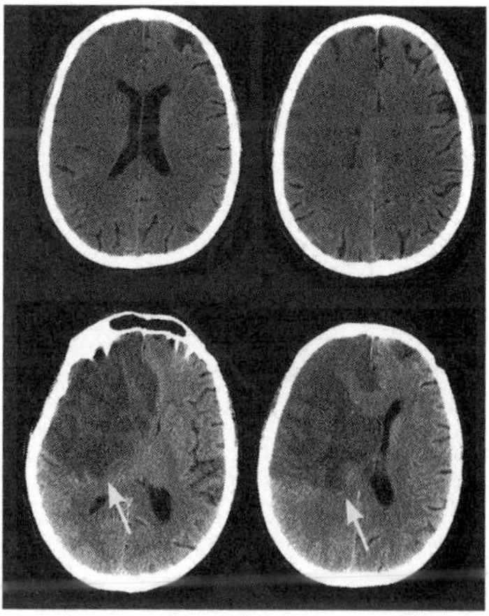

Figure 37. Day 1: Contrast CT shows mild decreased attenuation of right fronto-parietal lobe with effacement of sulci. Day 2: A significant change with further decreased attenuation and mass effect compressing the ventricles (see arrows) and displacing the midline structure to the left. Hypodense area corresponding to area of ischemic stroke.

1st Modality	2nd Modality
CT: low density, wedge-shaped area corresponding to vascular distribution with little or no mass effect. Sensitivity: 61%[55]	**MRI**: used for patients who present within a couple of hours of onset. T2-weighted image shows hyperintense white matter with low differentiation between white/gray matter. **Perform when**: completed for all patients within a couple hours of onset as the test has greater sensitivity. Sensitivity: 91%[55]

Srinivasan A, et al. 2006. *Radiographics* 26(Suppl 1):S75-95.

MEDICAL IMAGING

5.7 Multiple Sclerosis

- Demyelinating, autoimmune disease affecting the CNS

1st Modality
MRI: T2-weighted image shows round or ovoid white matter plaques often with periventricular or subcortical distribution. Plaques tend to be hyperintense, confluent and >6 mm in diameter. New lesions with active demyelination enhance with gadolinium while old lesions do not. Sensitivity: 57%[56] Specificity: 95%[56]

5.8 Cord Compression

- Decreased space in the spinal canal causing deficits which follow affected nerve distribution

1st Modality	2nd Modality
MRI: T1-weighted image shows narrowing of spinal cord in canal by disc herniation, fracture, tumors, etc. Sensitivity: 94%[57] Specificity: 98%[57]	**CT**: better visualization of vertebrae involved around cord compression. Impingement of spinal cord at site of injury. **Perform when**: to determine treatment plan, specifically surgical interventions, since able to visualize bony structures well.

Yadav RK, Agarwal S, Saini J. 2008. *J Indian Med Assoc* 106(2):79-82.

6. MUSCULOSKELETAL PATHOLOGIES AND FINDINGS

6.1 Colles Fracture

- Fracture of the distal radius from a force causing posterior displacement: “dinner fork” deformity

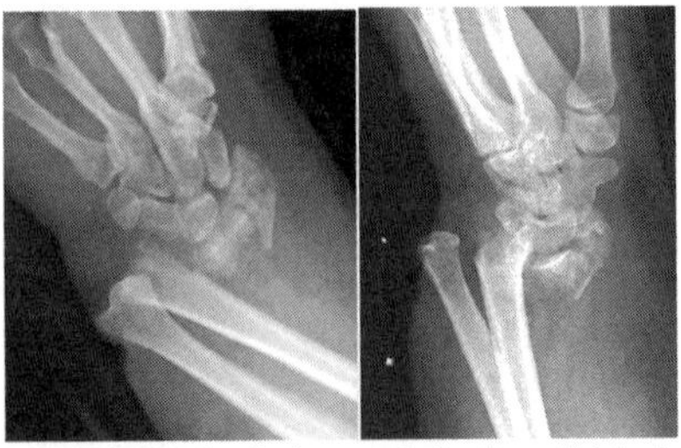

Figure 38. Fracture and posterior displacement of radius which is characteristic of a Colles fracture.

1st Modality
Plain Film (3 views): radial displacement with dorsal displacement of distal fragment.

6.2 Dislocated Shoulder (Anterior)

- Complete separation of humerus from glenoid fossa: commonly from "falling on outstretched arm or direct blow"

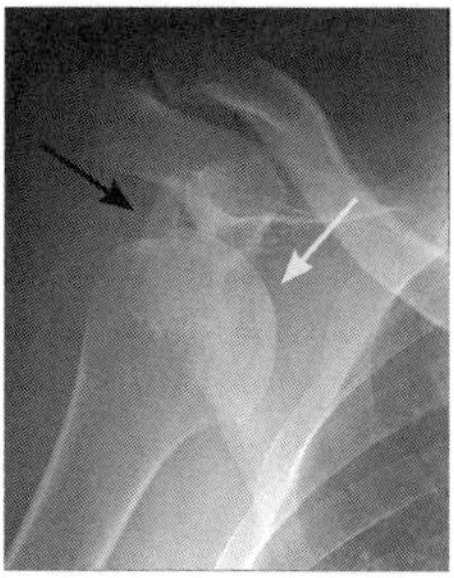

Figure 39. Dislocation of the shoulder characterized by displacement of humeral head (white arrow) from glenoid fossa (black arrow).

1st Modality
Plain Film (3 views): anterior displacement of humeral head on axillary view.

6.3 Hip Fracture (Subcapital)

- Fracture of the proximal femur: femoral neck

1st Modality
Plain Film (3 views): disruption of Shenton's line (line formed by top of obturator foramen and inner side of femur neck). Altered angle of neck shaft.

6.4 Dislocated Hip (Posterior)

- Complete separation of femoral head with acetabulum
- One leg will appear shorter in posterior dislocations

1st Modality	2nd Modality	3rd Modality	4th Modality
Plain Film (3 views): adducted and internally rotated femur with superolateral displacement of femoral head.	**MRI**: coronal T1-weighted image can detect early fractures if radiographs are inconclusive. **Perform when**: suspicion of early fractures and this is not conclusive on plain film.	**Bone Scan (Technetium 99m)**: useful in equivocal cases if suspicion of avascular necrosis. **Perform when:** suspicion of avascular necrosis.	**CT**: may be useful if more osseous details (e.g. degree of comminution and possible intra-articular bone fragments) are required. **Perform when**: to allow for better visualization of bony structures and help direct treatment planning.

Eisenberg RL, Johnson NM. *Comprehensive Radiographic Pathology*, 4th ed. St. Louis: Mosby Elsevier; 2007.
Alavi A, McCloskey JR, Steinberg ME. 1977. *Clin Orthop Relat Res* 127:137-141.

6.5 Torn Knee Ligaments

- Anterior cruciate ligament (ACL), posterior cruciate ligament (PCL), medial collateral ligament (MCL)

1st Modality
MRI: Poor visualization, an irregular contour or hyperintense signal in intrasubstance. Sensitivity (ACL): 76%[58] Specificity (ACL): 52%[58]

6.6 Osteomyelitis

- Inflammation in the bone due to an infectious process

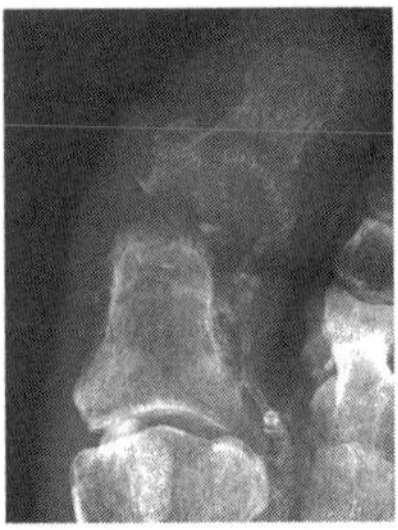

Figure 40. Lytic bone lesions and osteoporosis seen in the distal phalanx which is characteristic of osteomyelitis.

1st Modality	2nd Modality	3rd Modality	4th Modality
Plain Film (3 views): soft tissue swelling, focal osteoporosis, with lytic bone destruction and periosteal reaction. Sensitivity: 43-75%[59] Specificity: 75-83%[59]	**Bone Scan (Technetium 99m)**: active phase: increased uptake in affected area (bone and soft tissues). **Perform when:** to allow for early detection of osteomyelitis. Sensitivity: 65%[60]	**Gallium Scan**: demonstrates increased uptake in affected area. **Perform when**: higher sensitivity than Technetium 99m scan required; poorer visualization of bone/soft tissue. Sensitivity: 67-70%[59] Specificity: 92%[59]	**MRI**: active phase: marrow edema, appears hypointense on T1-weighted images and hyperintense on T2-weighted images. Periostitis, soft tissue inflammation, transphyseal disease. **Perform when**: extent of disease is required for treatment planning (surgery). Most sensitive and specific imaging, but ineffective at imaging osteomyelitis near metal joint implants due to artifact. Sensitivity: 72%[60]

Pineda C, Espinosa R, Pena A. 2009. *Semin Plast Surg* 23(2):80-89.

REFERENCES

1. Cortellaro F, Colombo S, Coen D, Duca PG. 2012. Lung ultrasound is an accurate diagnostic tool for the diagnosis of pneumonia in the emergency department. *Emerg Med J* 29(1):19-23.
2. Kwong JS, Adler BD, Padley SP, Müller NL. 1993. Diagnosis of diseases of the trachea and main bronchi: Chest radiography vs CT. *AJR Am J Roentgenol* 161(3):519-522.
3. Raghu G, Mageto YN, Lockhart D, Schmidt RA, Wood DE, Godwin JD. 1999. The accuracy of the clinical diagnosis of new-onset idiopathic pulmonary fibrosis and other interstitial lung disease: A prospective study. *Chest* 116(5):1168-1174.
4. Mets OM, Buckens CF, Zanen P, Isgum I, van Ginneken B, Prokop M, et al. 2011. Identification of chronic obstructive pulmonary disease in lung cancer screening computed tomographic scans. *JAMA* 306(16):1775-1781.
5. Van der Bruggen-Bogaarts BA, van der Bruggen HM, van Waes PF, Lammers JW. 1996. Screening for bronchiectasis. A comparative study between chest radiography and high-resolution CT. *Chest* 109(3):608-611.
6. Dodd JD, Souza CA, Müller NL. 2006. Conventional high-resolution CT versus helical high-resolution MDCT in the detection of bronchiectasis. *AMJ Am J Roentgenol* 187(2):414-420.
7. Hunninghake GW, Zimmerman MB, Schwartz DA, King TE Jr, Lynch J, Hegele R, et al. 2001. Utility of a lung biopsy for the diagnosis of idiopathic pulmonary fibrosis. *Am J Respir Crit Care Med* 164(2):193-196.
8. Elliott CG, Goldhaber SZ, Visani L, DeRosa M. 2000. Chest radiographs in acute pulmonary embolism. Results from the International Cooperative Pulmonary Embolism Registry. *Chest* 118(1):33-38.
9. Patel S, Kazerooni EA. 2005. Helical CT for the evaluation of acute pulmonary embolism. *AJR Am J Roentgenol* 185(1):135-149.
10. Gluecker T, Capasso P, Schnyder P, Gudinchet F, Schaller MD, Revelly JP, et al. 1999. Clinical and radiologic features of pulmonary edema. *Radiographics* 19(6):1507-1531.
11. Toyoda Y, Nakayama T, Kusunoki Y, Iso H, Suzuki T. 2008. Sensitivity and specificity of lung cancer screening using chest low-dose computed tomography. *Br J Cancer* 98(10):1602-1607.
12. Crandall J, Kent R, Patrie J, Fertile J, Martin P. 2000. Rib fracture patterns and radiologic detection – A restraint-based comparison. *Annu Proc Assoc Adv Automot Med* 44:235-259.
13. Pugliese F, Mollet NR, Runza G, van Mieghem C, Meijboom WB, Malagutti P, et al. 2006. Diagnostic accuracy of non-invasive 64-slice CT coronary angiography in patients with stable angina pectoris. *Eur Radiol* 16(3):575-582.
14. Nienaber CA, von Kodolitsch Y, Nicolas V, Siglow V, Piepho A, Brockhoff C, et al. 1993. The diagnosis of thoracic aortic dissection by noninvasive imaging procedures. *N Engl J Med* 328(1):1-9.
15. von Kodolitsch Y, Nienaber CA, Dieckmann C. 2004. Chest radiography for the diagnosis of acute aortic syndrome. *Am J Med* 116(2):73-77.
16. Hermansson M, Johansson J, Gudbjartsson T, Hambreus G, Jönsson P, Lillo-Gil R, et al. 2010. Esophageal perforation in South of Sweden: Results of surgical treatment in 125 consecutive patients. *BMC Surg* 10:31.
17. Alexander ES, Clark RA. 1982. Computed tomography in the diagnosis of abdominal hemorrhage. *JAMA* 248(9):1104-1107.
18. Sagel SS, Siegel MJ, Stanley RJ, Jost RG. 1977. Detection of retroperitoneal hemorrhage by computed tomography. *AJR Am J Roentgenol* 129(3):403-407.
19. Lee BC, Ormsby EL, McGahan JP, Melendres GM, Richards JR. 2007. The utility of sonography for the triage of blunt abdominal trauma patients to exploratory laparotomy. *AJR Am J Roentgenol* 188(2):415-421.
20. Liu M, Lee CH, P'eng FK. 1993. Prospective comparison of diagnostic peritoneal lavage, computed tomographic scanning, and ultrasonography for the diagnosis of blunt abdominal trauma. *J Trauma* 35(2):267-270.
21. Lubner M, Menias C, Rucker C, Bhalla S, Peterson CM, Wang L, et al. 2007. Blood in the belly: CT findings of hemoperitoneum. *Radiographics* 27(1):109-125.
22. Smith DS, Bonadio WA, Losek JD, Walsh-Kelly CM, Hennes HM, Glaeser PW, et al. 1992. The role of abdominal x-rays in the diagnosis and management of intussusception. *Pediatr Emerg Care* 8(6):325-327.
23. Gayer G, Apter S, Hofmann C, Nass S, Amitai M, Zissin R, et al. 1998. Intussusception in adults: CT diagnosis. *Clin Radiol* 53(1):53-57.
24. Zubaidi A, Al-Saif F, Silverman R. 2006. Adult intussusception: A retrospective review. *Dis Colon Rectum* 49(10):1546-1551.
25. Barbiera F, Cusma S, Di Giacomo D, Finazzo M, Lo Casto A, Pardo S. 2001. Adult intestinal intussusception: Comparison between CT features and surgical findings. *Radiol Med* 102(1-2):37-42.
26. Hryhorczuk AL, Strouse PJ. 2009. Validation of US as a first-line diagnostic test for assessment of pediatric ileocolic intussusception. *Pediatr Radiol* 39(10):1075-1079.
27. Kim YH, Blake MA, Harisinghani MG, Archer-Arroyo K, Hahn PF, Pitman MB, et al. 2006. Adult intestinal intussusception: CT appearances and identification of a causative lead point. *Radiographics* 26(3):733-744.
28. Testa AC, Ludovisi M, Mascilini F, Di Legge A, Malaggese M, Fagott A, et al. 2012. Ultrasound evaluation of intra-abdominal sites of disease to predict likelihood of suboptimal cytoreduction in advanced ovarian cancer: A prospective study. *Ultrasound Obstet Gynecol* 39(1):99-105.
29. Black M, Friedman AC. 1989. Ultrasound examination in the patient with ascites. *Ann Intern Med* 110(4):253-255.
30. Proto AV, Lane EJ, Marangola JP. 1976. A new concept of ascitic fluid distribution. *AJR Am J Roentgenol* 126(5):974-980.
31. Edell SL, Gefter WB. 1979. Ultrasonic differentiation of types of ascitic fluid. *AJR Am J Roentgenol* 133(1):111-114.

32. Gayer G, Hertz M, Manor H, Strauss S, Klinowski E, Zissin R. 2004. Dense ascites: CT manifestations and clinical implications. *Emerg Radiol* 10(5):262-267.
33. Maglinte DD, Reyes BL, Harmon BH, Kelvin FM, Turner WW Jr, Hage JE, et al. 1996. Reliability and role of plain film radiography and CT in the diagnosis of small-bowel obstruction. *AJR Am J Roentgenol* 167(6):1451-1455.
34. Suri S, Gupta S, Sudhakar PJ, Venkataramu NK, Sood B, Wig JD. 1999. Comparative evaluation of plain films, ultrasound and CT in the diagnosis of intestinal obstruction. *Acta Radiol* 40(4):422-428.
35. Kim SH, Shin SS, Jeong YY, Heo SH, Kim JW, Kang HK. 2009. Gastrointestinal tract perforation: MDCT findings according to the perforation sites. *Korean J Radiol* 10(1):63-70.
36. Levine MS. Peptic ulcers. In: Gore RM, Levine MS. *Textbook of Gastrointestinal Radiology*, 2nd ed. New York: Saunders Elsevier; 2000.
37. Doria AS, Moineddin R, Kellenberger CJ, Epelman M, Beyene J, Schuh S, et al. 2006. US or CT for diagnosis of appendicitis in children and adults? A meta-analysis. *Radiology* 241(1):83-94.
38. Sarma D, Longo WE. 2008. Diagnostic imaging for diverticulitis. *J Clin Gastroenterol* 42(10):1139-1141.
39. Håkansson K, Leander P, Ekberg O, Håkansson HO. 2000. MR imaging in clinically suspected acute cholecystitis. A comparison with ultrasonography. *Acta Radiol* 41(4):322-328.
40. Barakos JA, Ralls PW, Lapin SA, Johnson MD, Radin DR, Colletti PM, et al. 1987. Cholelithiasis: Evaluation with CT. *Radiology* 162(2):415-418.
41. Bastid C, Sahel J, Filho M, Sarles H. 1990. Diameter of the main pancreatic duct in chronic calcifying pancreatitis. Measurement by ultrasonography versus pancreatography. *Pancreas* 5(5):524-527.
42. Niederau C, Grendell JH. 1985. Diagnosis of chronic pancreatitis. *Gastroenterology* 88(6):1973-1995.
43. Badea R. 2005. Ultrasonography of acute pancreatitis – An essay in images. *Rom J Gastroenterol* 14(1):83-89.
44. Luetmer PH, Stephens DH, Ward EM. 1989. Chronic pancreatitis: Reassessment with current CT. *Radiology* 171(2):353-357.
45. Balthazar EJ, Robinson DL, Megibow AJ, Ranson JH. 1990. Acute pancreatitis: Value of CT in establishing prognosis. *Radiology* 174(2):331-336.
46. Eray O, Cubuk MS, Oktay C, Yilmaz S, Cete Y, Ersoy FF. 2003. The efficacy of urinalysis, plain films, and spiral CT in ED patients with suspected renal colic. *Am J Emerg Med* 21(2):152-154.
47. Wiesner W. 2003. Is multidetector computerized tomography currently the primary diagnostic method of choice in diagnostic imaging of acute intestinal ischemia? *Praxis* 92(31-32):1315-1317.
48. Kirk E. 2012. Ultrasound in the diagnosis of ectopic pregnancy. *Clin Obset Gynecol* 55(2):395-401.
49. Dheer S, Levine MS, Redfern RO, Metz DC, Rubesin SE, Laufer I. 2002. Radiographically diagnosed antral gastritis: Findings in patients with and without Helicobacter pylori infection. *Br J Radiol* 75(898):805-811.
50. Craig WD, Wagner BJ, Travis MD. 2008. Pyelonephritis: Radiologic-pathologic review. *Radiographics* 28(1):255-277.
51. Taourel P, Aufort S, Merigeaud S, Doyon FC, Hoquet MD, Delabrousse E. 2008. Imaging of ischemic colitis. *Radiol Clin North Am* 46(5):909-924, vi.
52. Sandhu PS, Joe BN, Coakley FV, Qayyum A, Webb EM, Yeh BM. 2007. Bowel transition points: Multiplicity and posterior location at CT are associated with small-bowel volvulus. *Radiology* 245(1):160-167.
53. Frager D, Medwid SW, Baer JW, Mollinelli B, Friedman M. 1994. CT of small-bowel obstruction: Value in establishing the diagnosis and determining the degree and cause. *AJR Am J Roentgenol* 162(1):37-41.
54. Teksam M, McKinney A, Casey S, Asis M, Kieffer S, Truwit CL. 2004. Multi-section CT angiography for detection of cerebral aneurysms. *AJNR Am J Neuroradiol* 25(9):1485-1492.
55. Fiebach JB. 2002. CT and diffusion-weighted MR imaging in randomized order: Diffusion-weighted imaging results in higher accuracy and lower interrater variability in the diagnosis of hyperacute ischemic stroke. *Stroke* 33(9):2206-2210.
56. Barkhof F, Filippi M, Miller DH, Scheltens P, Campi A, Polman CH, et al. 1997. Comparison of MRI criteria at first presentation to predict conversion to clinically definite multiple sclerosis. *Brain* 120(Pt 11):2059-2069.
57. Parmar H, Park P, Brahma B, Gandhi D. 2008. Imaging of idiopathic spinal cord herniation. *Radiographics* 28(2):511-518.
58. Rayan F, Bhonsle S, Shukla DD. 2009. Clinical, MRI, and arthroscopic correlation in meniscal and anterior cruciate ligament injuries. *Int Orthop* 33(1):129-132.
59. El-Maghraby TA, Moustafa HM, Pauwels EK. 2006. Nuclear medicine methods for evaluation of skeletal infection among other diagnostic modalities. *Q J Nucl Med Mol Imaging* 50(3):167-192.
60. Williamson MR, Quenzer RW, Rosenberg RD, Meholic AJ, Eisenberg B, Espinosa MC, et al. 1991. Osteomyelitis: Sensitivity of 0.064 T MRI, three-phase bone scanning and indium scanning with biopsy proof. *Magn Reson Imaging* 9(6):945-948.

ACKNOWLEDGEMENTS

We would like to thank Dr. Taebong Chung, Dr. Bob Bleakney, and Dr. Eugene Yu for their contribution of images for this chapter.

The Essentials of Oncology

Editors:
Yuliya Velykoredko
Shivangi Trivedi

Faculty Advisors:
Richard Tsang, MD, FRCP(C)
Raymond Jang, MD, FRCP(C)

TABLE OF CONTENTS

1. SCREENING GUIDELINES

Primary prevention is essential in the management of cancer. **Table 1** lists the rank estimates of cancer cases by incidence (excluding non-melanoma skin cancers) and mortality. **Table 2** lists the current Canadian Screening Guidelines for some common cancer types.

Table 1. Canadian Cancer Statistics, 2011 Estimates

Incidence		Mortality	
Male	**Female**	**Male**	**Female**
1. Prostate	1. Breast	1. Lung	1. Lung
2. Lung	2. Lung	2. Colorectal	2. Breast
3. Colorectal	3. Colorectal	3. Prostate	3. Colorectal

ONCOLOGY

Table 1. Canadian Cancer Statistics, 2011 Estimates (continued)

Incidence		Mortality	
4. Bladder	4. Uterus	4. Pancreas	4. Pancreas
5. Non-Hodgkin Lymphoma	5. Thyroid	5. Non-Hodgkin Lymphoma	5. Ovary
6. Melanoma	6. Non-Hodgkin Lymphoma	6. Leukemia	6. Non-Hodgkin Lymphoma
7. Kidney	7. Ovary	7. Esophagus	7. Leukemia

Canadian Cancer Society's Steering Committee on Cancer Statistics. *Canadian Cancer Statistics 2011*. Toronto: Canadian Cancer Society; 2011.

Table 2. Canadian Cancer Screening Guidelines

Cancer Type	Canadian Guidelines	
Breast Cancer[1,2]	Average risk	Age 40-49 yr: mammography not recommended[1] Age 50-74 yr: mammography every 2-3 yr[1]
	High risk (previous breast cancer, history of breast cancer in first degree relative, known BRCA1/BRCA2 mutation, received chest radiation, calculated as having >25% lifetime risk of breast cancer)	Age 30-69 yr: annual mammography + MRI[2]
Colon Cancer[4,5]	Average risk	Age 50-75 yr: • FOBT annually • Sigmoidoscopy every 10 yr • Colonoscopy every 10 yr (gold standard; recommended by major US societies, but not Canadian Association of Gastroenterology at the population level for asymptomatic patients)
	Higher risk (FAP, HNPCC, IBD, family history)	FAP: annual sigmoidoscopy starting at 10-12 yr HNPCC: colonoscopy at 20 yr or 10 yr before index case Previous colon cancer or polyps: colonoscopy every 3-5 yr IBD: colonoscopy 8-10 yr after diagnosis
Cervical Cancer[5,6]	Cytology (if HPV DNA test is not available/funded)	Age 21-70 yr: • Cytology testing for sexually active women every 3 yr • If not sexually active until 21 yr, then test when sexually active • Stop at age 70 yr if unremarkable Pap smear for 10 previous yr

Table 2. Canadian Cancer Screening Guidelines (continued)

Cancer Type	Canadian Guidelines	
Cervical Cancer[5,6]	HPV DNA test (preferred)	Age 30-65 yr: • HPV DNA testing every 3-5 yr (if positive, perform cytology testing) • Discontinue at age 65 yr if negative screening history in previous 10 yr and final negative HPV test at age 65 yr
Prostate Cancer[7,8]		Consider screening after discussion of risks/benefits: • DRE + PSA starting at age 50 yr (increases detection of early-stage cancers, but no evidence that screening decreases mortality) • High risk men can start screening at age 40 yr

FAP = familial adenomatous polyposis, FOBT = fecal occult blood test, HNPCC = hereditary nonpolyposis colorectal cancer
Canadian Task Force on Preventive Health Care, et al. 2011. *CMAJ* 183(17):1991-2001.

2. COLORECTAL CANCER

History

- Change in bowel habits: alternating constipation and diarrhea; decreased stool caliber (thinner)
- Hematochezia/melena
- Abdominal pain
- Intestinal obstruction
- Iron deficiency anemia
- Constitutional: anorexia, fatigue, weight loss
- Asymptomatic (detected by screening)

Risk Factors

- Age >50 yr
- Smoking, diet (low fiber)
- Family history
  - Familial adenomatous polyposis (FAP)
  - Hereditary nonpolyposis colorectal cancer (HNPCC)
  - Nonsyndromic familial colon cancer
- Personal history
  - Colon cancer
  - Adenomatous polyps (especially if villous, >1 cm or multiple)
  - IBD

Focused Physical Exam

- Often no findings on physical exam
- General appearance
  - Weight loss, cachexia
- DRE (see **Urological Exam**, p.368)
  - Mass may be palpable if rectal involvement (poor overall sensitivity)
  - Bright red blood per rectum may be evident
- Abdomen (see **Abdominal Exam**, p.21)
  - Palpable mass
- With advanced disease may see:
  - Liver mass
  - Distension/ascites

ONCOLOGY

Investigations

- Screening (see **Table 2**)
- Colonoscopy for lesion identification and biopsy
- CT chest/abdomen/pelvis
- CT head and bone scan (if symptoms)
- MRI pelvis or transrectal ultrasound (TRUS) if rectal involvement
- Blood work with carcinoembryonic antigen (CEA)

3. PROSTATE CANCER

History

- Frequently asymptomatic and detected by screening
- Lower urinary tract symptoms (LUTS) if locally advanced:
  - Voiding: hesitancy, double voiding, intermittent/slow stream
  - Storage: frequency, urgency, nocturia, dysuria
- If metastatic:
  - To bone: bone pain (frequently localized to back)
  - To pelvic nodes: lower extremity pain/edema (2° to lymphatic obstruction)
- Constitutional: anorexia, fatigue, weight loss

Risk Factors

- Race: African-American
- Family history
- High dietary fat
- Smoking

Focused Physical Exam

- General appearance: cachexia, weight loss, lower extremity edema
- DRE (see **Urological Exam**, p.368); can present as hard, irregular nodule in peripheral zone of prostate

Investigations

- Screening (see **Table 2**)
  - DRE, PSA, free/total PSA (<10% free PSA is suggestive of cancer)
  - Prediction algorithms can be of use in determining whether further testing is warranted. To calculate patient's prostate cancer risk, ProstateRisk.ca may be used as a tool
- TRUS of prostate and biopsy
- Metastatic work-up: bone scan, CT abdomen/pelvis

4. LUNG CANCER

History

- Chronic cough, dyspnea
- Hemoptysis
- Chest pain
- Persistent or recurrent pneumonia
- Pleuritic chest pain (with peripheral tumors)
- Constitutional: anorexia, fatigue, weight loss

Associated Presentations

- Due to locoregional spread:
  - Dysphagia (2° to esophageal compression)
  - Hoarseness (2° to recurrent laryngeal nerve paralysis)
  - Horner's syndrome (pancoast tumor)
  - Superior vena cava syndrome (see **Oncologic Emergencies**, p.557)

- Paraneoplastic syndromes:
  - Small cell carcinoma: syndrome of inappropirate antidiuretic hormone secretion (SIADH), Cushing's (2° to ACTH), Lambert-Eaton
  - Squamous cell carcinoma: hypercalcemia (2° to PTH)

ONCOLOGY

Risk Factors
- Smoking/second hand smoke
- Exposure to radon gas, asbestos
- Uranium mining

Focused Physical Exam
- General appearance: cachexia, weight loss, clubbing
- Respiratory exam
  - Variable findings: wheezing, atelectasis, pleural effusion
- Head and neck exam
  - Supraclavicular lymphadenopathy
  - Horner's syndrome (ptosis, miosis, anhydrosis)

Investigations
- Imaging: CXR, CT chest/abdomen/pelvis, CT or MRI brain
- Biopsy (bronchoscopy, percutaneous or endobronchial U/S)
- Patients deemed to be potentially curable: positron emission tomography (PET) scan and mediastinoscopy

5. BLADDER CANCER

History
- Painless gross hematuria
- LUTS: dysuria, frequency, urgency
- Voiding LUTS 2° to clot retention
  - Hesitancy, double voiding, intermittent/weak stream
- Ureter obstruction: uremia (N/V, diarrhea), flank pain
- Constitutional: anorexia, fatigue, weight loss

Risk Factors
- Smoking
- Environmental carcinogen exposure (e.g. aromatic amines in paints, pesticides, hair dyes) and chemical industries
- Drugs (cyclophosphamide, phenacetin)
- *Schistosoma haematobium* (trematode)
- Pelvic radiation
- Chronic bladder inflammation (stones, cystitis)

Focused Physical Exam
- Abdominal exam
  - Palpable midline pelvic mass (if invasion into bladder muscle): rarely present
- Inguinal lymphadenopathy

Investigations
- Urinalysis: chemical, C&S, and cytology
- Cystoscopy, bladder washings, and biopsy
- U/S to assess for hydronephrosis
- Metastatic work-up: CT chest/abdomen/pelvis

ONCOLOGY

6. PANCREATIC CANCER

History
- Usually asymptomatic until late stages (tumors of head of pancreas produce symptoms earlier)
- Jaundice, weight loss
- Abdominal pain (may radiate to back)
- N/V
- Sudden onset DM

Risk Factors
- Smoking
- High dietary fat and meat
- DM
- Chronic pancreatitis
- Obesity

Focused Physical Exam
- Painless jaundice
- Enlarged, palpable, but painless gallbladder in the presence of jaundice (Courvoisier's sign)

Investigations
- Imaging: abdominal U/S, CT chest/abdomen/pelvis
- Biopsy: endoscopic retrograde cholangiopancreatography (ERCP), endoscopic ultrasonography (EUS)
- Blood work including liver enzymes and CA19-9

7. BREAST CANCER
- See **Breast Exam**, p.39

8. SKIN CANCER
- See **Essentials of Dermatology**, p.413

9. LYMPHOMA
- See **Lymphatic System and Lymph Node Exam**, p.127

10. GYNECOLOGICAL CANCER
- See **Gynecological Exam**, p.93

11. GENERAL CANCER AND PALLIATIVE CARE HISTORY
- HPI
  - Symptoms: that led to investigations
  - Diagnostic results: imaging and pathology reports
  - Treatment received to date (surgery, chemotherapy, radiation, interventional procedures such as stents and drains)
  - Performance status: Eastern Cooperative Oncology Group (ECOG) scale
- PMHx
  - Medications, allergies
  - FHx of malignancies
  - SHx: occupation, living situation, family, support system, activities of daily living, smoking, EtOH
- Patient's understanding of disease and prognosis
- Other considerations for advanced disease:
  - Symptom burden assessment (e.g. the Edmonton Symptom Assessment Scale)

- End of life wishes (e.g. does the patient wish to die at home or hospital, Do Not Resuscitate [DNR] wishes)
- Power of Attorney, advance directives
- Spiritual or religious needs

12. FUNDAMENTALS OF CANCER THERAPY

Most cancers involve a multidisciplinary approach to treatment and management. A thorough discussion of each cancer-specific strategy is beyond the scope of this handbook. Below we discuss the role of biopsy, and outline the fields of surgical, medical, and radiation oncology.

12.1. Biopsies

All cancers are diagnosed through a biopsy that is ultimately read by a pathologist. Biopsies may be done with (e.g. CT or U/S) or without image guidance. Biopsies may also be done as part of endoscopic procedures (e.g. bronchoscopy, OGD) (see **Table 3**).

Table 3. Biopsy Types*

Biopsy Type	Description
Fine Needle Aspiration	Small needle, draw fluid out for cytology
Core Needle Biopsy	Large needle, preserves tissue architecture
Surgical (excisional)	Entire mass is removed

*As the molecular profiling of cancers becomes more prevalent, it may be more important to collect larger tissue samples.

12.2. Surgical Oncology

For most solid tumor malignancies, surgery offers the best chance for cure. Palliative surgery can sometimes be used to relieve symptoms in a noncurative setting.

12.3. Medical Oncology

Medical oncology is involved in the systemic treatment of cancer, especially in the presence of metastatic dissemination.

- Principles of Chemotherapy:
  - Adjuvant Chemotherapy: for patients with successful initial treatment (no evidence of residual disease), but high risk for relapse (e.g. post-surgery)
  - Neo-adjuvant Chemotherapy: for patients with bulky primary disease (not immediately amenable to initial therapy) with goal of reducing this bulk prior to initial treatment ("downstaging")
  - Palliative Chemotherapy: to prolong life and improve symptoms without the intention of cure; not the same as palliative care

12.4. Radiation Oncology

Radiation oncology is involved in locoregional eradication of cancer with preservation of the normal structure and function of surrounding tissues.

- Goals: treatment with curative vs. palliative intent
- Types of radiation therapy:
  - External beam radiation therapy
  - Brachytherapy
  - Unsealed radionuclide therapy (e.g. ^{131}Iodine, free or tagged to MAb)
- Contraindications to radiation therapy:
  - Previous radiation therapy to normal tissue tolerance
  - Pacemaker/defribillator within the direct radiation field

- Side effects of radiation therapy:
  - Early radiation-induced reactions: acute, local (e.g. local skin reactions, alopecia, nausea, mucositis, esophagitis) or constitutional (e.g. fatigue), and myelosuppression for large volume of bone marrow irradiation
  - Late radiation-induced reactions: dose-dependent (particularly sensitive to high dose per fraction), occurring months to years after treatment, progressive (e.g. lung fibrosis, bone necrosis, myelopathy)
  - Secondary malignancy: latency period generally >10 yr, risk is higher in conjunction with chemotherapy

13. ONCOLOGIC EMERGENCIES

13.1 Cancer-Associated Thrombosis

- Increased risk of both venous (DVT, PE), and to a lesser extent, arterial (stroke, MI) thromboembolic events
- Certain cancers (e.g. pancreas, stomach, lung, and lymphoma) are particularly associated with VTE
- Cancer chemotherapy further increases thrombosis risk
- Etiology: activate coagulation system resulting in a hypercoagulable state
- Signs and Symptoms:
  - DVT: calf pain, leg swelling/erythema
  - PE: dyspnea, cough, wheezing, chest pain, tachycardia, upper abdominal pain
- Investigations:
  - ECG/CXR, venous leg Doppler, CT angiography (if not, ventilation-perfusion [V/Q] scan)

13.2 Hypercalcemia

- See **Essentials of Fluids, Electrolytes, and Acid/Base Disturbances**, p.463
- Associated with the following cancers: breast, lung, thyroid, kidney, prostate, multiple myeloma
- Etiology: may be from bony metastasis or ectopic production
- Signs:
  - Volume depletion
- Symptoms:
  - Early: polyuria, polydipsia, nocturia, anorexia
  - Late: apathy, irritability, muscle weakness, N/V
- Investigations:
  - Blood work, including electrolytes, Ca^{2+}, Mg^{2+}, PO_4^{3-}, creatinine [Cr], and PTH
  - ECG

13.3 Tumor Lysis Syndrome

- Associated with acute leukemia, Burkitt's lymphoma, and other hematologic malignancies
- Occurs between hours and few days after treatment
- Etiology: massive release of potassium, phosphate, uric acid, and tumor breakdown products from successful chemotherapy
- Signs and Symptoms: lysis of tumors presents as electrolyte abnormalities (hypocalcemia, hyperphosphatemia, hyperkalemia, hyperuricemia) and possible renal failure (see **Essentials of Fluids, Electrolytes, and Acid/Base Disturbances**, p.460, 462, and 465)
- Investigations: Blood work, including electrolytes, Ca^{2+}, uric acid, K^+, PO_4^{3-}, and Cr

13.4 Febrile Neutropenia

- Definition: absolute neutrophil count <1.0 cell/mm^3 and temperature >38.0°C × 1 h or single temperature >38.3°C
- Investigations: blood work including CBC, blood cultures, urine culture, chest radiograph, and other investigations guided by symptoms
- Granulocytopenia carries risk of bacterial infection (usually patient's own endogenous flora), and fungal infection if prolonged

13.5 Superior Vena Cava Obstruction Syndrome

- Etiology: lung cancer (85%), advanced lymphoma (15%), metastatic disease
- Signs and Symptoms: tachypnea, neck vein swelling, facial plethora, upper extremity edema, vocal cord paralysis, Horner's syndrome (rare)
- Investigations: CXR, CT chest

13.6 Spinal Cord Compression

- Etiology: metastasis to the spine (thoracic spine is most common) involving the vertebral body, paravertebral tissue, or epidural space
- Signs and Symptoms: back pain, neurological deficits (muscle weakness, bladder and bowel dysfunction, and sensory deficit)
- Investigations: plain film, CT, MRI (whole spine)
- Note that residual neurological deficit is related to time from symptom onset to treatment; therefore spinal cord compression must be diagnosed and treated quickly!

14. APPROACH TO COMPLICATIONS IN ONCOLOGY

Table 4. DIMSH Approach to Complications in Oncology Patients

Type of Complication	Example
Drug (consider both oncology and non-oncology drugs)	• Febrile neutropenia • Chemotherapy-induced cardiomyopathy
Infectious	• Febrile neutropenia
Metabolic	• Electrolytes: hyponatremia, hypercalcemia, tumor lysis syndrome • Organ failure: renal, liver failure
Structural (Think anatomically)	• CNS: brain metastases, spinal cord compression • Organ obstruction: airway obstruction, biliary obstruction, bowel obstruction • Blood vessels: superior vena cava obstruction syndrome, pulmonary embolus • Excess fluid: pleural effusion, pericardial effusion, ascites
Hematologic	• Cytopenias: anemia, neutropenia, thrombocytopenia • Thrombosis • Disseminated intravascular coagulation (DIC)

ONCOLOGY

REFERENCES

1. Canadian Task Force on Preventive Health Care, Tonelli M, Connor Gorber S, Joffres M, Dickinson J, Singh H, et al. 2011. Recommendations on screening for breast cancer in average-risk women aged 40-74 years. *CMAJ* 183(17):1991-2001.
2. Cancer Care Ontario. *Ontario Breast Screening Program (OBSP): Women at High Risk for Breast Cancer.* Toronto: Cancer Care Ontario. 2011. Available from: https://www.cancercare.on.ca/common/pages/UserFile.aspx?fileId=99488.
3. Leddin D, Hunt R, Champion M, Cockeram A, Flook N, Gould M, et al. 2004. Canadian Association of Gastroenterology and the Canadian Digestive Health Foundation: Guidelines on colon cancer screening. *Can J Gastroenterol* 18(2):93-99.
4. Leddin DJ, Enns R, Hilsden R, Plourde V, Rabeneck L, Sadowski DC, et al. 2010. Canadian Association of Gastroenterology position statement on screening individuals at average risk for developing colorectal cancer: 2010. *Can J Gastroenterol* 24(12):705-714.
5. Cancer Care Ontario. *Updated Ontario Cervical Screening Cytology (Pap Test) Guidelines; 2012.* Toronto: Cancer Care Ontario. 2013. Available from: https://www.cancercare.on.ca/pcs/screening/cervscreening/.
6. Murphy J, Kennedy EB, Dunn S, McLachlin CM, Fung Kee Fung M, Gzik D, et al. 2012. Cervical screening: A guideline for clinical practice in Ontario. *J Obstet Gynaecol Can* 34(5):453-458.
7. Izawa JI, Klotz L, Siemens RD, Kassouf W, So A, Jordan J, et al. 2011. Prostate cancer screening: Canadian guidelines 2011. *Can Urol Assoc J* 5(4):235-240.
8. Greene KL, Albertson PC, Babaian RJ, Cater HB, Gann PH, Han M, et al. 2009. Prostate specific antigen best practice statement: 2009 update. *J Urol* 182(5):2232-2241.
9. Cavalli F, Hansen HH, Kaye SB (Editors). *Textbook of Medical Oncology*, 3rd ed. London: Informa Healthcare; 2009.
10. Chabner B, Lynch TJ, Longo DL. *Harrison's Manual of Oncology,* 1st ed. New York: McGraw-Hill Professional; 2007.
11. Feig BW, Ching CD, Fuhrman GM (Editors). *The M.D. Anderson Surgical Oncology Handbook*, 4th ed. Philadelphia: Wolters Kluwer/Lippincott Williams & Wilkins; 2012.
12. Govindan R (Editor). *Devita, Hellman, and Rosenberg's Cancer: Principles & Practice of Oncology*, 3rd ed. Philadelphia: Lippincott Williams & Wilkins; 2012.
13. Gunderson LL, Tepper JE. *Clinical Radiation Oncology*, 3rd ed. Philadelphia: Elsevier/Churchill Lingstone; 2012.
14. Yeung S-CJ, Escalante CP (Editors). *Holland-Frei Oncologic Emergencies*, 1st ed. Hamilton: BC Decker; 2002.

The Essentials of Pain Management and Pre-Operative Assessment

Editors:
Howard Meng
Marko Balan
Sharleen Gill

Faculty Reviewers:
Darryl Irwin, MD, FRCP(C)
Nick Lo, MD, FRCP(C)

PAIN MANAGEMENT

TABLE OF CONTENTS

1. PAIN BASICS

- Pain is an unpleasant sensory and emotional response associated with actual or potential tissue damage, or described in terms of such damage, subjectively modified by a patient's past experiences and expectations[1].

Common Pain Patterns and Symptoms

- **Acute Pain:** Lasts min to wk; concordant with degree of tissue damage and resolves spontaneously with tissue healing (e.g. dental extraction, surgery, renal calculi, trauma, acute illness)[2]
- **Chronic Pain:** Lasts >3-6 mo; can be associated with no underlying pathology identified to explain the pain, may be intermittent or persistent, may be associated with depression (e.g. chronic lower back pain, osteoarthritis, diabetic polyneuropathy, migraines, fibromyalgia)[2]
- **Localized Pain:** pain confined to site of tissue injury (e.g. cutaneous pain, some visceral pain, arthritis, tendonitis)
- **Referred Pain:** pain that is referred to a distant structure (e.g. pain produced by a MI may feel as if it is in the arm, diaphragmatic irritation causing shoulder tip pain)
- **Projected (transmitted) Pain:** pain transferred along the course of a nerve with a segmental distribution (e.g. herpes zoster) or a peripheral distribution (e.g. trigeminal neuralgia)
- **Dermatomal Pattern:** peripheral neuropathic pain
- **Nondermatomal Pattern:** central neuropathic pain, fibromyalgia
- **Hyperalgesia:** increased sensitivity to pain that is abnormally out of proportion to the painful stimuli; occurs from damage to nociceptors or peripheral nerves

- **Allodynia:** pain from a stimulus which does not normally cause pain; associated with neuropathic and chronic pain syndromes
- **Paresthesia:** a subjective skin sensation with no apparent physical cause that may be described as numbness, tingling, burning, prickling, pin pricks, pins and needles, etc.

2. FOCUSED PAIN HISTORY

- Pain history: full description of the pain
  - Characterize the features of the pain: OPQRST
  - Has the patient ever experienced this pain in the past? How is the pain affecting the patient's life and ability to perform daily activities?
- Progression of symptoms over time and response to treatment; can use validated tools to assess severity and change:
  - Visual Analog Scale: 100 mm line on which patient indicates his/her level of pain; a reduction of 30 mm or more is clinically significant
  - Numeric Rating Scale: patient rates pain on a scale of 0-10; a reduction of 3 digits or more is significant

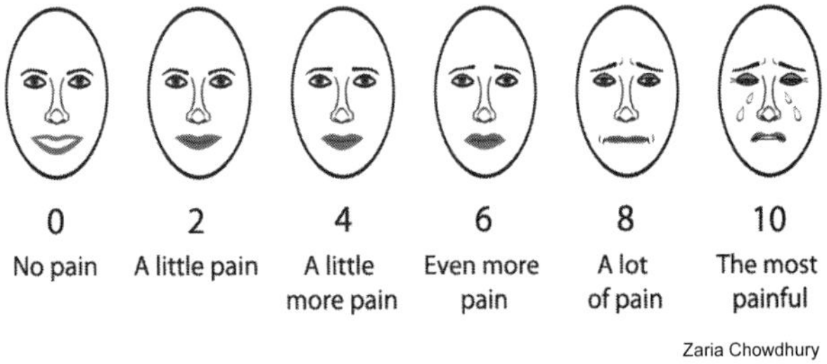

Figure 1. Numeric Rating Scale

- Pain medication history (prescription, nonprescription [i.e. OTC], naturopathic, recreational):
  - Previous experience with opioid therapy (including precise medication history: drug, dose, frequency, route)
  - Effectiveness on pain and function
  - Compliance
- Side effects of opioid therapy:
  - N/V, constipation, pruritus, sedation/respiratory depression, tolerance, addiction
  - Use of opioids for non-prescribed purposes (e.g. insomnia, stress, mood)
- FHx
  - Chronic pain
  - Substance abuse
- Psychiatric/psychosocial history
  - Recent life stressors, substance use (including alcohol and tobacco)
  - Patient expectations and goals of treatment (pain intensity, daily activities, quality of life)

3. FOCUSED PHYSICAL EXAM

- Consider performing MSK and neurological exams of the painful body locations (look for tenderness, trigger points)
- Look specifically for signs of neuropathic pain (hyperalgesia, allodynia, paresthesia)
- Look for secondary consequences of chronic pain (e.g. stiffness, disuse muscle atrophy, weakness)

- Document any physical stigmata of a substance use disorder (e.g. skin tracks, skin abscesses, stigmata of liver disease, edema, venous insufficiency, lymphadenopathy)
- Observe posture, gait, pain behaviors (e.g. favoring a limb or extremity, dyspnea/respiratory splinting)
- Assess the patient's pretreatment mental status and changes in mental status following treatment (e.g. Glasgow coma scale [GCS])

Table 1. Pain Classification

Classification	Description	Example
Nociceptive	Pain from normal activation of peripheral nociceptors by a noxious stimulant (e.g. heat, cold, pressure) Involves actual tissue damage Well-localized (can be diffuse if involve viscera or deep structures)	Soft tissue injuries (e.g. burn, laceration) Fracture Arthritis Abscess Ischemia
Neuropathic	Pain from direct injury to neural tissue Causes altered function of CNS or PNS Bypasses nociceptive pathways May or may not have tissue damage	**Peripheral Syndromes** Peripheral neuropathy Phantom limb **Central Syndromes** Post-stroke MS Spinal cord injury Trigeminal neuralgia
Cancer	Strong relationship between tissue pathology and level of pain, aggressive pain management permitted by limited time frame	**Primary** Inflammation from tumor **Metastatic** Back pain from bone metastasis
Chronic Non-Cancer	Weak relationship between tissue pathology and pain levels, prolonged potentially lifelong pain; can be associated with medicolegal, disability, and psychosocial issues	Fibromyalgia Headaches (tension, cluster, migraines) Complex regional pain syndromes

PAIN MANAGEMENT

4. GENERAL APPROACH TO PAIN MANAGEMENT

- Treat the underlying cause where possible (e.g. steroids for polymyalgia rheumatica, appendectomy for appendicitis)
- Use a multimodal approach where possible for additive effects of analgesics with fewer side effects
- Pain control should be continuous with regularly scheduled dosing and "PRN" dosing for intermittent breakthrough pain
- Manage pain preemptively (e.g. give pain control before painful procedures: i.e. before dressing changes, before physiotherapy)
- Multidisciplinary approach and nonpharmacological management also beneficial (see **Complementary and Alternative Therapies**, p.568)
- Ask the patient to rate the pain as mild, moderate or severe and treat according to the WHO approach to pain management (see **Figure 2**)
- Choice of analgesic and delivery method depend on:
  - Type of pain
  - Underlying medical condition
  - Patient restrictions: i.e. *nil per os* (NPO), swallowing problems, etc.
- ***Note:*** it may be necessary to switch therapies as clinical course changes

Table 2. Common Pain Management Medications

Class	Doses	Indications	Cautions	Side Effects	Comments
Acetaminophen	Acetaminophen 500 mg-1 g q6h PO	first-line for mild acute pain	Liver disease Elderly	Liver failure (rare)	Analgesia and antipyretic but no anti-inflammatory properties
NSAIDs	Naproxen 250-500 mg q12h PO Ibuprofen 200-400 mg q6h PO Celecoxib 50-200 mg q12h PO	Mild to moderate acute pain	Asthma Coagulopathy GI ulcers Renal disease CAD Do not take if have sulfa allergy	Bleeding, pruritus, rash, worsen pre-existing renal disease	Analgesia Anti-inflammatory therefore good for tissue damage and inflammation
Opioids	Codeine Tramadol Morphine Hydromorphone Oxycodone See dosing in **Opioids Management Principles**, p.563	Mild to moderate acute pain Moderate to severe pain Chronic pain refractory to other treatments	History of substance abuse Drug-seeking Liver disease Renal disease COPD Sleep apnea	Constipation or decreased gastrointestinal motility, nausea, sedation, pruritus, respiratory depression, delirium	Caution with concurrent sedating medications (e.g. benzodiazepines) Switch from intravenous to oral administration when able to tolerate and taper dose as acute pain resolves

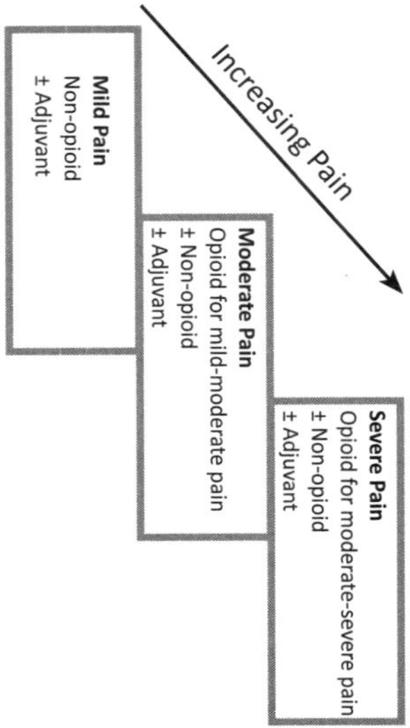

Figure 2. WHO Pain Ladder
http://www.who.int/cancer/palliative/painladder/en/

4.1 Medications

Opioids Management Principles

- Mild to moderate acute pain
  - Start with oral immediate release (IR)/short-acting (SA) opioids compounded with acetaminophen (e.g. Tylenol® #3 or Tramacet™) dosed 1-2 tablets, q4-6h PRN
    - Tylenol #3 = acetaminophen 300 mg + codeine 30 mg + caffeine 15 mg
    - Tramacet = acetaminophen 325 mg + tramadol 37.5 mg
  - If insufficient pain control and acetaminophen dose exceeds 3-4 g/d, switch to stronger compound (e.g. Percocet®) dosed 1-2 tablets, q4-6h PRN
    - Percocet = acetaminophen 325 mg + oxycodone 5 mg, no caffeine
  - Ensure acetaminophen dose from all sources does not exceed 4g/day
- Moderate to severe pain
  - Start with the maximum allowable dose of acetaminophen and add in an NSAID if appropriate. Consider an opioid for moderate to severe pain such as morphine, hydromorphone, or oxycodone either standing or as a PRN medication.
- Severe acute pain
  - Maximize acetaminophen and NSAID (if appropriate) and then titrate IV opioids to effect so pain becomes controlled. Switch as soon as appropriate to oral opioids as effect is longer lasting and easier to administer
  - ***Note:*** avoid IM opioid injections for acute, severe pain as absorption is slow and erratic
  - Taper dose as acute pain resolves
  - Pay attention to and treat side effects: constipation, sedation, nausea
  - Be wary of sedating medication: especially benzodiazepines for patients on opioids
  - Breakthrough doses of analgesia should be prescribed to manage sudden outbursts of pain. Two methods:
    1. Half the q4h standing dose of an opioid. For example, if someone is taking 10 mg of morphine PO every four hours and requires breakthrough pain medicine, a breakthrough dose of 2.5 mg IV morphine or 5 mg PO morphine every 2 h PRN is given
    2. 10% of the daily dose
- In palliative and end-of-life care: dose of morphine is titrated to patient's pain control requirements (no maximum dose)

Indications for/Contraindications to Opioids

- See **Table 2**
- In screening for opioid medication misuse or abuse, verified tools such as the Screener and Opioid Assessment for Patients with Pain (SOAPP) questionnaire (www.painedu.org/soapp.asp) can be used

> **Clinical Pearl: Opioid Therapy**
> For opioid therapy in older patients or those with severe renal/liver disease: Start LOW*, go SLOW.
> *Initial dose should be half the usual starting dose

Opioid Analgesic Equivalencies

- When converting from one opioid to another, use 50-75% of the equivalent dose to allow for incomplete cross-tolerance
- Rapid titration and PRN use may be required to ensure effective analgesia for the first 24 h
- Dose equivalencies provided in **Table 3** are approximate; individual patients vary

Table 3. Approximate Equivalent Doses

General Name	Oral (mg)	IV (mg)	Comments
Morphine	30	10	Parenteral 10 mg morphine is standard for comparison
Hydromorphone	6	2	
Oxycodone	20		Often formulated in combination with acetaminophen/Aspirin® (Percocet®/Percodan®) Use with caution if administering additional acetaminophen or Aspirin®
Codeine	200	120	Same as oxycodone
Fentanyl (transdermal)	60-134 mg morphine = 25 mcg/h transdermal fentanyl patch		Usually for stable chronic pain, especially in patients with GI dysfunction Refer to CPS for additional help Not used as first-line treatment for acute pain
Methadone	Equivalent dosing not reliably established	Equivalent dosing not reliably established	Long, variable half-life, which may complicate titration Variable conversion rates occur
Hydrocodone	20	Not available	Often combined with other analgesics Use with caution if administering additional acetaminophen or Aspirin®
Meperidine	300	75	Not a first-line opioid/rarely used; may cause seizures due to metabolite accumulation

*For all sustained release drugs: do not crush, break or chew oral controlled release medications

Opioid Overdose Management

- Opioid toxidrome classically presents with respiratory depression, pinpoint pupils as well as altered mental states, including unresponsiveness
- Opioid reversal: Naloxone (opioid antagonist)
  - Reverses effects of opioid overdose (hypoventilation, sedation) for 30-45 min
  - MUST BE diluted before use:
    - Initial concentration: 0.4 mg/mL
    - Dilution: 1 mL Naloxone + 9 mL saline = 0.04 mg/mL
  - Give 0.04 to 0.08 mg (1 to 2 mL) IV q3-5 min
  - If no change after 0.2 mg (5 mL), consider other causes
  - DDx: seizure, stroke, other medication effect, hyper/hypoglycemia, hyper/hyponatremia, hypoxia, HTN, MI, sepsis
- Relative overdose of naloxone may cause symptoms of opioid withdrawal: recurrence of pain, nausea, agitation, sweating, tachycardia, arrhythmias, HTN, seizures

Neuropathic Pain Management

- Neuropathic pain (e.g. postherpetic neuralgia, diabetic neuropathy) not usually relieved by typical analgesics (e.g. acetaminophen, NSAIDs)
- 4 main classes of treatment for neuropathic pain:
  - Anticonvulsants
    - Most common class of medication for treatment of neuropathic pain
    - e.g. gabapentin 300 mg TID PO
      - Titrate up starting from 100 mg TID PO to avoid excessive drowsiness
      - Usual effective dose: 300-1200 mg TID PO
      - Decrease dose in patients with impaired renal clearance
    - Others: pregabalin, carbamazepine
  - Tricyclic Antidepressants (TCAs)
    - e.g. amitriptyline
      - Starting dose: 10 mg qhs PO, then titrate up by 10 mg qwk
      - Max daily dose: 150 mg/d
    - Others: nortriptyline, desipramine
    - Contraindications: cardiac arrhythmias, recent MI, MAOI use, hyperthyroidism, narrow angle glaucoma
  - Opioid Analgesics
    - Can be effective, usually in conjunction with adjuvant medications
  - Topical Agents
    - e.g. lidocaine patch, capsaicin cream (substance P inhibitor)

> **Clinical Pearl: Analgesic Therapy**
> Use of multimodal anesthesia approach (various systemic medications ± regional anesthesia techniques) can improve pain management, reduce doses of individual medications, and thus reduce side effects.

4.2 Routes of Delivery

Local/Regional Anesthesia

- Definition: blockade of nerve fibers that transmit pain and sensation from the region of interest by local anesthetics; prevents conduction of electrical impulses by the nerve
- Uses:
  - Diagnostic procedures
  - Minor surgical procedures
  - Perioperative analgesia
  - Postoperative analgesia
  - Management of chronic pain
- Benefits:
  - Better pain control during the perioperative period
  - Avoids adverse effects of general anesthesia: myocardial and respiratory depression
- Side effects:
  - Block failure or excessive duration of anesthetic
  - Dizziness (rare) and hypotension
- Contraindications:
  - Infection at the block site/systemic infection
  - Allergy to anesthetics/analgesics
  - Anticoagulation
  - Patient refusal
  - Pre-existing nerve injury
  - Lack of skill
  - Lack of resuscitation equipment

- Complications:
  - Local Anesthetic Systemic Toxicity (LAST)
    - Low concentrations: drowsiness, lightheadedness, visual/auditory disturbances, restlessness, circumoral and tongue numbness, metallic taste
    - High concentrations: nystagmus, muscular twitching, tonic-clonic convulsions/seizures, arrhythmia
    - Treatment: Intralipid® 20%: 1.5 mL/kg bolus, followed by 0.25 mL/kg/min
  - Injury of targeted nerve or nerve plexus
  - Inadvertent injection of agent intravascularly or around nontargeted neurological tissues
  - Damage to other tissues around injection site (e.g. pneumothorax for blocks near thorax)
  - Infection
  - Perineural hematoma could result, especially in patients with an underlying bleeding disorder, or those on anticoagulation/antiplatelet therapy

Table 4. Regional Anesthesia Techniques

Regional Anesthesia Technique	Main Uses
Local Anesthesia	Small incisions, sutures, and excisions of small lesions
Infiltration Anesthesia	Small dermal surgeries/procedures
Bier Block (IV regional anesthesia)	Short procedures in the distal limbs (<60 min)
Tumescent Anesthesia	Liposuction procedures
Peripheral Nerve Blocks:	
Brachial Plexus Block	Shoulder and upper limb procedures
Paravertebral Sympathetic Ganglion Block	Treatment of reflex sympathetic dystrophy
Lumbar Plexus Block	Pelvic girdle, knee, and proximal tibia procedures
Femoral Nerve Block	Open knee procedures (total knee replacement)
Fascia Iliaca Block	Hip procedures (total hip replacement)
Sciatic Nerve Block	Foot and distal lower limb procedures
Neuroaxial Blocks:	
Spinal (subarachnoid anesthesia)	Procedures on anatomical structures below upper abdomen
Thoracic Epidural	Abdominal and chest wall procedures
Lumbar Epidural	Gynecological procedures, orthopedic surgery, general surgery, vascular surgery (for structures innervated by lumbar spine and below)

Systemic Analgesic Delivery

Patient-Controlled Analgesia (PCA)

- Use of computerized (usually parenteral) pumps that can deliver a predetermined dose of medication when requested by a patient, within set parameters, allowing patient to reach his/her own minimum effective analgesic concentration

- PCA parameters: bolus dose, lockout interval, continuous infusion (optional), maximum 4 h limit
- Most commonly used agents for PCA are morphine and hydromorphone
- Shown to lessen postoperative pain, decrease complications, lead to earlier discharge, and lessen the overall opiate level consumed[3]

5. COMPLEMENTARY AND ALTERNATIVE THERAPIES

Transcutaneous Electric Nerve Stimulation (TENS)
- Definition: application of electrical current through the skin for pain control
- Effects:
  - Activates opioid reception in CNS[4]
  - Reduces excitation of CNS nociceptive neurons
- Meta-analyses have shown effectiveness in treating chronic and acute pain[5,6]

Physiotherapy
- Effects[4]:
  - Inhibits pain perception by stimulation of sensory afferents (gate-control theory)
  - Avoids painful movements by improvement in the quality of movement (muscle strength and coordination)
- Indicated in all pain syndromes where motor dysfunction is involved and in chronic pain (to reduce depression)
- Active therapy should start early, discourage long-term immobilization
- Apply in combination with other treatments such as analgesic drugs

Acupuncture
- Definition: the technique of inserting and manipulating fine filiform needles into specific points on the body
- Effect: excites receptors and nerve fibers (mechanical activation of somatic afferents)[4]
- "Ashi points"
  - Near the source of pain (local points)
  - On the forearms and lower legs (distal points)
- Meta-analyses have yet to consistently show effectiveness for pain management[7]

Massage
- Synonyms: effleurage, petrissage, friction, tapotement, vibration
- Effects[8]:
  - Stimulates large diameter nerve fibers (gate-control theory)
  - Increases blood flow, temperature, and histamine release by dilatation of superficial blood vessels
  - Physical and mental relaxation
- Most consistently proven effect is decreased anxiety and perception of tension
- Contraindications: any area of acute inflammation, skin infection, nonconsolidated fracture, DVT, burns, active cancer tumors, advanced osteoporosis

Table 5. Examples of Complementary and Alternative Therapies

Mindful	Spiritual	Stimulation-Based	Movement-Based
Hypnosis Imagery Meditation Relaxation Biofeedback	Prayer Spiritual healing Psychic healing Yoga	TENS Acupuncture Massage Aromatherapy Therapeutic touch	Exercise Tai Chi Yoga
Mechanical	**Nutriceutical**	**Psychotherapy**	
Chiropractic Osteopathy Massage	Vitamins Diet Herbal medicine Homeopathy Aromatherapy	Counseling Relaxation Biofeedback Behavioral modification Hypnosis Cognitive behavioral therapy (CBT)	

Belgrade MJ, Schamber CD. Evaluation of Complementary and Alternative Therapies. In: Wilson PR, Jensen TS, Watson PJ, Haythornthwaite JA (Editors). *Clinical Pain Management: Chronic Pain*, 2nd ed. Oxford: Oxford University Press; 2008.

6. PREOPERATIVE ANESTHESIA ASSESSMENT

- History:
  - Identifying data (age, sex), proposed surgery and diagnosis
  - Previous anesthetics and adverse outcomes, previous postoperative N/V, history of difficult intubation, family history of anesthetic problems (e.g. malignant hyperthermia)
  - Drug allergies
  - Current medications (including dose and frequency)
  - PMHx/Review of systems (cardiovascular, respiratory, renal, neurology, MSK, GI, hematology, endocrinology)
- Physical Exam:
  - Vitals (HR, RR, BP, temperature, O_2 saturation)
  - Airway
    - Neck range of motion: flexion and extension (sniffing position)
    - 3-2-1 rule (3 fingers between thyroid cartilage and mandible, 2 fingers between upper and lower teeth with mouth open, 1 finger behind condylar process of mandible during anterior subluxation)
    - Dental anatomy (dentures/cap/crown, chipped/cracked/loose teeth)
    - Mallampati score (see **Figure 3**)
  - Cardiovascular exam
  - Respiratory exam
  - Other exams pertinent to surgery or medical conditions
- Investigations:
  - Consider investigations relevant to the surgical procedure and medical history of the patient (e.g. CBC, electrolytes, coagulation profile, blood group and screen or cross-match, ECG, CXR, etc.)
  - Review medical records: i.e. anesthesia records (adverse events, ease of intubation), previous testing (echocardiogram, pulmonary function testing, etc.)
- Preparation for Anesthesia and Surgery:
  - NPO Guidelines (Canadian Anesthesiologists' Society)
    - ≥2 h clear fluids
    - ≥4 h breast milk
    - ≥6 h light meal (i.e. toast and clear fluids)

        - ≥8 h regular meal
        - Medications should generally still be taken, with sips of water
    - Medications
        - Anticoagulants may need to be discontinued several days prior, depending on surgery and patient risk
        - Ensure patient takes usual pain medication (± NSAIDs) day of surgery
        - Many essential medications should be continued the day of surgery:
            - Blood pressure medication
            - Respiratory medications (i.e. puffers)
            - Reflux/heartburn medications
        - Diabetic medications are often held the day of surgery because patient is NPO
            - Glucose should be measured by patient in morning and on arrival to hospital
    - Optimization
        - Does the patient require further consultations, investigations, treatments prior to surgery?
    - Types of Anesthesia
        - Local anesthesia only
        - Local + light sedation (neurolept)
        - General anesthesia
        - Regional anesthesia
        - General anesthesia + regional anesthesia (for postoperative pain control)
    - Disposition
        - Does the patient require special care/monitoring in the postoperative phase (i.e. intensive care unit)?
- ASA score (see **Essentials of General Surgery**, **Table 4**, p.475)

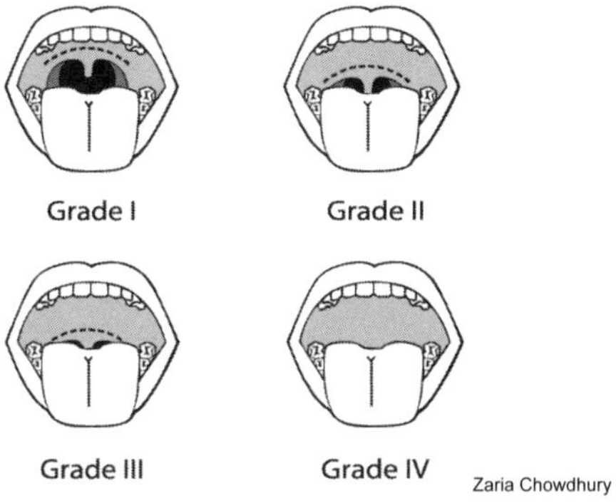

Figure 3. Mallampati Score

General Anesthesia

- Definition: a reversible state of amnesia, analgesia, loss of consciousness, immobility, and inhibition of sensory and autonomic reflexes
- Typical approach: induced with IV anesthetic agents and maintained with inhalational and/or IV anesthetics; may be used in combination with muscle relaxants

REFERENCES

1. Schmidt RF, Willis WD (Editors). *Encyclopedia of Pain*. Berlin: Springer-Verlag; 2007.
2. Barash PG, Cullen BF, Stoelting RK, Cahalan MK, Stock MC. *Clinical Anesthesia*, 6th ed. New York: Lippincott Williams & Wilkins; 2009.
3. Ballantyne JC, Carr DB, Chalmers TC, Dear KB, Angelillo IF, Mosteller, F. 1993. Postoperative patient-controlled analgesia: Meta-analyses of initial randomized control trials. *J Clin Anesth* 5(3):182-193.
4. Belgrade MJ, Schamber CD. Evaluation of Complementary and Alternative Therapies. In: Wilson PR, Jensen TS, Watson PJ, Haythornthwaite JA (Editors). *Clinical Pain Management: Chronic Pain*, 2nd ed. Oxford: Oxford University Press; 2008.
5. Johnson M, Martinson M. 2007. Efficacy of electrical nerve stimulation for chronic musculoskeletal pain: A meta-analysis of randomized controlled trials. *Pain* 130(2):157-165.
6. DeSantana J, Walsh DM, Vance C, Rakel BA, Sluka KA. 2008. Effectiveness of transcutaneous electrical nerve stimulation for treatment of hyperalgesia and pain. *Curr Rheumatol Rep* 10(6):492-499.
7. Hopton A, MacPherson H. 2010. Acupuncture for chronic pain: Is acupuncture more than an effective placebo? A systematic review of pooled data from meta-analyses. *Pain Pract* 10(2):94-102.
8. Paley CA, Johnson MI, Tashani QA, Bagnall AM. 2011. Acupuncture for cancer pain in adults. *Cochrane Database of Syst Rev* 1; CD 007753.
9. Swartz MH. *Textbook of Physical Diagnosis: History and Examination*, 6th ed. Philadelphia: Saunders Elsevier; 2010.
10. Wilson PR, Jensen TS, Watson PJ, Haythornthwaite JA (Editors). *Clinical Pain Management: Chronic Pain*, 2nd ed. Oxford: Oxford University Press; 2008.

Appendix 1: Concepts in Evidence-Informed Medical Practice

Editors:
Jonathan Fuller
Ashwin Sankar

Faculty Reviewer:
Ross Upshur, MD, MSc, FRCP(C)

APPENDIX: EBM

TABLE OF CONTENTS

1. WHAT IS EVIDENCE-INFORMED MEDICAL PRACTICE?

Evidence-informed practice is the dynamic process of distilling emerging evidence from the medical literature, integrating evidence with clinical experience, and applying evidence in conjunction with patient values and preferences to maximize clinical outcomes. It involves personalizing medical care based on evidence while preserving the centrality of patient goals and desires.[1]

2. THE EVIDENCE-BASED MEDICINE APPROACH

Evidence-based medicine (EBM) is a model for critically appraising medical literature and finding the best evidence for clinical decision-making. Study design criteria are used to determine the best clinical evidence for answering questions concerning therapeutic benefit, therapeutic harm, diagnosis, or prognosis (see **Figure 1**).[2,3]

3. SOURCES OF CLINICAL RESEARCH EVIDENCE

- **Synopsis:** summary of other pre-appraised evidence, sometimes including background information or recommendations
- **Clinical Practice Guideline:** produced by a consensus panel comprised of experts who summarize evidence and make recommendations to guide clinical decision-making
- **Systematic Review:** synthesis of a particular, well-defined body of evidence; includes both narrative review (narrated summary) and meta-analysis (pooling of quantitative data from multiple studies)
- **Primary Article:** report of the results of a single study

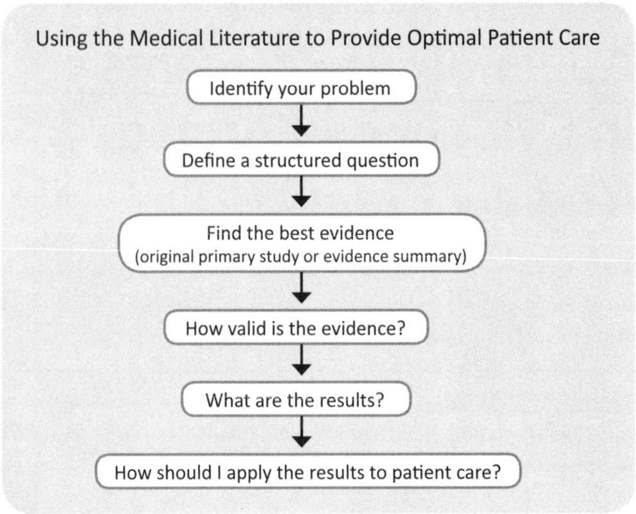

Figure 1. The EBM Approach to the Medical Literature
Guyatt G, Rennie D, Meade MO, Cook DJ. *Users' Guides to the Medical Literature: Essentials of Evidence-Based Clinical Practice*, 2nd ed. New York: McGraw-Hill Medical; 2008.

Common Synopses and Databases for Literature-Searching

- **UpToDate** (www.uptodate.com) is an online resource offering articles that are authored and edited by expert clinicians; they are the result of structured questioning, identification of evidence, and appraisal of the quality of evidence to provide recommendations and guidelines for practicing clinicians
- **ACP Journal Club** (www.acpjc.org) is a distillation of core healthcare and specialty journals that primarily targets internal medicine and its subspecialities; articles from journals are reviewed and those of highest clinical relevance are summarized as structured abstracts
- **Cochrane Database of Systematic Reviews** (www.cochrane.org/cochrane-reviews) is part of the Cochrane Library and includes rigorous reviews on therapeutic and preventive healthcare interventions
- **US National Guidelines Clearinghouse** (www.guideline.gov) is a web-based interface that allows comparison of different clinical practice guidelines that cover a broad range of topics
- **PubMed** (www.ncbi.nlm.nih.gov/pubmed) is a free service that indexes citations from MEDLINE, life science journals, and online books to allow the user to limit searches to studies of certain designs (such as systematic reviews) or to studies of particular clinical relevance (using **PubMed Clinical Queries**)

4. STUDY DESIGN CONSIDERATIONS

Table 1. Studies of Therapy and Harm

Type	Design Characteristics	Strengths and Weaknesses	Assessing Study Quality
Randomized Controlled Trial (RCT)	• Experimental • **Parallel-arm, placebo-controlled:** individuals randomized to receive either a placebo or a treatment • **Design variations: cluster:** groups of individuals randomized; **comparative effectiveness:** two or more treatments are compared; **crossover:** one study arm receives control then treatment, the other group receives these in reverse sequence; **pragmatic:** study is done under routine practice conditions	• **Strengths:** avoids selection bias; considered "gold standard" for establishing cause-effect relationships • **Weaknesses:** often expensive; strict inclusion and exclusion criteria means sample often is not representative of target population	• Was randomization done using accepted method? • Were subjects and assessors blinded? • Was follow-up complete? • Were patients analyzed in the groups they were randomized? • How large and precise was the treatment effect?
Cohort Study	• Observational, longitudinal • Two groups: exposed vs. not exposed to factor of interest; groups studied through multiple time-points • **Prospective** (groups followed into future until outcome) OR **Retrospective** (exposure and outcome have already occurred)	• **Strengths:** ethically permissible when exposure is harmful; sample may be representative of target population; can establish temporality of events (especially if prospective) • **Weaknesses:** exposure may be linked to a confounder; prone to selection bias; prone to recall bias (if retrospective)	• Were exposed and nonexposed groups similar in terms of known prognostic factors? • Were methods for detecting outcome similar? • Was follow-up complete? • How strong is the association between exposure and outcome? • How precise is the effect estimate?

Table 1. Studies of Therapy and Harm (continued)

Type	Design Characteristics	Strengths and Weaknesses	Assessing Study Quality
Case-Control Study	• Observational • Two groups: cases (with outcome) vs. controls (without outcome) • Groups assessed retrospectively for exposure to harmful agent	• **Strengths:** allows study of rare and long-term outcomes; ethically permissible when exposure is harmful • **Weaknesses:** prone to recall and selection bias; confounders may account for association; selection of control group is difficult	• Were cases and controls similar in terms of known prognostic factors? • Were methods for detecting exposure similar? • How strong is the association between exposure and outcome? • How precise is the effect estimate?
Cross-Sectional Study	• Observational • Two groups: exposed vs. not exposed to factor of interest • Exposure and outcome are measured at the same time-point	• **Strengths:** inexpensive, quick to conduct; useful in generating hypotheses • **Weaknesses:** direction of association difficult to determine; recall bias susceptibility; unequal distribution of confounders; unequal group sizes	• Were baseline and prognostic characteristics of exposed and non-exposed groups similar? • Was either group over or under-represented? • How strong is the association between exposure and outcome? • How precise is effect estimate?
Case Report and Series	• Observational • One (report) or multiple (series) cases with observed association between exposure and outcome	• **Strengths:** inexpensive; useful in generating hypotheses • **Weaknesses:** no comparison group	• Are patients being treated similar to reported case(s)? • Is it plausible that the exposure caused the outcome? • Were the findings dramatic enough to necessitate precautionary action?

Guyatt G, Rennie D, Meade MO, Cook DJ. *Users' Guides to the Medical Literature: Essentials of Evidence-Based Clinical Practice*, 2nd ed. New York: McGraw-Hill Medical; 2008.

Table 2. Studies of Diagnosis and Prognosis

Type	Design Characteristics	Assessing Study Quality
Differential Diagnosis	• Prospective cohort or case-control or cross-sectional study examining frequencies of different diagnoses among individuals with an initial clinical presentation	• Was the sample representative of the target population? • Were diagnostic evaluations complete for all causes in all cases? • What were the relative disease frequencies? How precise were the probability estimates? • Will the results apply in the present clinical setting?
Diagnostic Tests	• Prospective cohort, case-control or cross-sectional study with comparison of diagnostic test to reference "gold standard"	• Were a range of patient presentations observed? • Was the reference "gold standard" appropriate? • Were those interpreting the test blind to the other results? • Was the reference "gold standard" performed for all subjects? • What were the test sensitivity and specificity? What were the test's positive and negative likelihood ratios?
Prognosis	• Cohort or case-control studies assessing determinants of outcomes • Long-term follow-up of RCT participants	• Was the sample representative of the population? • Was follow-up sufficient? • Were outcomes measured objectively? • How likely are outcomes over time? • How precise is the likelihood estimate?

RCT = randomized controlled trial
Guyatt G, Rennie D, Meade MO, Cook DJ. *Users' Guides to the Medical Literature: Essentials of Evidence-Based Clinical Practice*, 2nd ed. New York: McGraw-Hill Medical; 2008.

Table 3. Common Qualitative Study Designs

Type	Design Characteristics	Advantages and Disadvantages
Interviews	• **Structured:** set, rigid interview questions/prompts • **Semi-Structured:** interview questions/prompts can be personalized • **Unstructured:** conversational • Question guide may or may not be adjusted in between interviews	• **Advantages:** allow for full exploration of each patient's experience and perspective; study questions can evolve between interviews; permit discussion of sensitive topics • **Disadvantages:** time-consuming; interviewer-patient relationship can affect responses to questions; current views may impact interpretations of past events
Focus Groups	• **Structured; semi-structured; unstructured** • Question guide may or may not be adjusted in between focus groups	• **Advantages:** allow pilot-testing of novel study questions; participants can benefit from/build on the responses of others; efficient use of time in obtaining multiple perspectives • **Disadvantages:** interviewer-group relationship can affect responses; responses can be affected by the group dynamic and contrived setting

APPENDIX: EBM

5. APPRAISING CLINICAL RESEARCH EVIDENCE

The GRADE Approach to Rating Quality of Quantitative Research Evidence

- The Grades of Recommendation, Assessment, Development, and Evaluation (GRADE) system rates the quality of a body of evidence relevant to a particular question, usually concerning therapy
- The quality of evidence reflects our confidence in the effect estimate
- In the GRADE approach to grading evidence in clinical practice guidelines, initial quality ratings are first assigned to the evidence; these ratings can then be upgraded or downgraded based on a number of criteria:
  - **Inconsistency:** widely varying differences in estimates among studies
  - **Indirectness:** study population or intervention differs in relevant ways from patients, the intervention in practice, surrogate outcomes measured or interventions not compared head-to-head
  - **Imprecision:** wide confidence intervals around the effect estimate or small sample population studied
  - **Publication Bias:** not all relevant studies were considered
  - **Bias:** systematic error in study design or execution

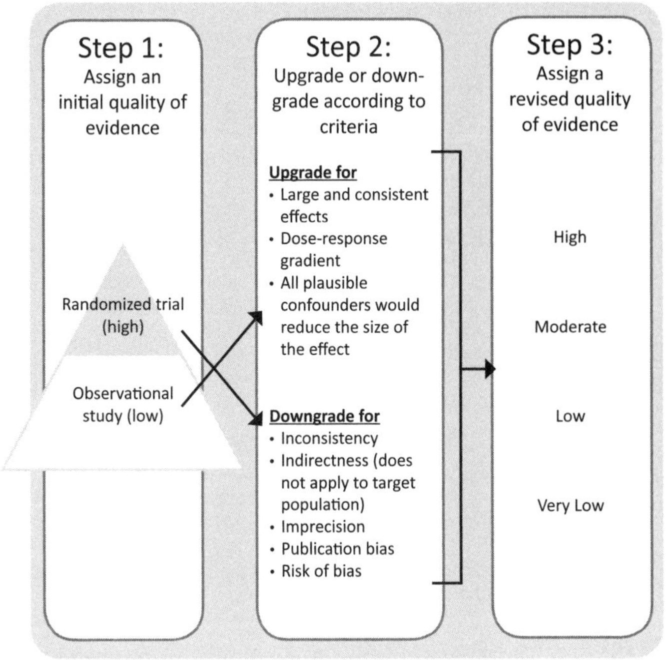

Figure 2. The GRADE Approach to Rating Quality of Evidence
Howick J. *The Philosophy of Evidence-Based Medicine*. Oxford: Wiley-Blackwell; 2011.

Critically Appraising Qualitative Research Evidence

- Critically appraising a qualitative study means evaluating its quality and its applicability in clinical practice
  - Quality reflects the appropriateness of choices made by the researchers and the transparency of the study
  - Applicability is concerned with the similarity between the study context and the context of clinical practice, or alternatively, the extent to which the study results inform clinically-applicable theory
- Six questions to consider when appraising a qualitative research study:[4]
  1. *Was the sample used in the study appropriate to the research question?* Did the sample have appropriate breadth and depth, and was the sociocultural context acknowledged?
  2. *Was the data collected appropriately?* Were methods chosen that were appropriate to the research question?
  3. *Was the data analyzed appropriately?* Is the study explicit about what was done, how, and by whom? Was the analysis conducted in a way that is congruent with the study's theoretical framework?
  4. *Does the study adequately address potential ethical issues?* Does the study address reflexivity or the researcher's influence on the research process?
  5. *Can I transfer the results of this study to my own setting?* Does the study advance our understanding of a particular situation? Careful attention should be paid to the influence of context on the applicability of the results for practice
  6. *In conclusion: is what the researchers did clear?*

6. APPLYING EVIDENCE IN PRACTICE

APPENDIX: EBM

Diagnosis

- Evidence of disease prevalence (reported for a general population, or from prognostic studies) can be used to foreground more probable diagnoses
- Evidence of sensitivity and specificity also assists in the interpretation of a diagnostic test result
  - If a test has high **Sen**sitivity, most **N**egative results are 'true negatives'. Thus, a negative result can be used to provisionally rule **out** a diagnosis (mnemonic: **SnNout**)
  - If a test has a high **Sp**ecificity, most **P**ositive results are 'true positives'. Thus, a positive result can be used to provisionally rule **in** a diagnosis (mnemonic: **SpPin**)
- It is important to assess the quality of the evidence and consider whether the research evidence is applicable to an individual patient, given his/her clinical presentation, compared to patients enrolled in the diagnostic study
- Clinical experience or intuition helps assess the 'fit' between a diagnosis and the particular clinical presentation
- An understanding of normal or abnormal structure and function can help to rule out implausible diagnoses or account for observed clinical features
- Qualitative evidence can help the clinician anticipate, understand, and empathically respond to a range of possible illness experiences

Prognosis or Risk

- Risk assessment tools determine the statistical risk of an adverse outcome given certain prognostic factors
- Confidence in the calculated risk will be higher if multiple assessment tools agree in their estimate
- To determine the applicability of a prediction tool to a particular case, it is important to ask whether the tool was validated in patients similar to this one (it is also important to consider other prognostic factors that are not accounted for by the risk assessment tool)
- Qualitative evidence can help the clinician anticipate how a patient might experience or prefer to receive certain difficult news

Therapy

- **Figure 3** represents a general approach to incorporating evidence in therapeutic decision-making. Note that evidence of comparative efficacy and harm among multiple treatments is not included here, but should be considered. The first step is to determine what positive and negative outcomes matter to the particular patient
- For initial therapy for symptomatic relief (e.g. pain relief) or cure (e.g. antibiotic treatment), the best evidence of benefit and harm comes from trial in the presenting patient, especially a trial in which the effects have been systematically observed
- Where evidence of effectiveness or harm in the presenting patient is unavailable or infeasible (e.g. risk reduction), an estimate of therapeutic efficacy can also be provided by clinical research evidence, especially experimental studies, but also observational studies (e.g. when the intervention demonstrates a dramatic treatment effect). Evidence of therapeutic harm can be provided by experimental or observational studies
- Studies report the average effect of the treatment, along with the precision of the estimate. The absolute risk reduction (ARR) and number needed to treat (NNT) are common, preferred measures of average

treatment effect, while the 95% confidence interval is the preferred measure of precision
- Based on the quality of the clinical research evidence, it is important to ask whether our confidence in the reported treatment effect is high enough to risk harm to the patient
- Is there other evidence that might modify our effect estimate? This might include other clinical research evidence, knowledge from the basic medical sciences, and evidence regarding the likelihood that this patient will adhere to the therapy
- Qualitative evidence can inform the clinician and patient as to how particular therapeutic options affect quality of life. It also brings to light the values and preferences that were important to patients in similar decision-making contexts, which may be relevant to clinicians, patients, or substitute decision makers
- Communicating effect estimates and the associated uncertainty to the patient allows for the reaching of a shared decision that incorporates the relative importance that the patient attaches to certain outcomes over others

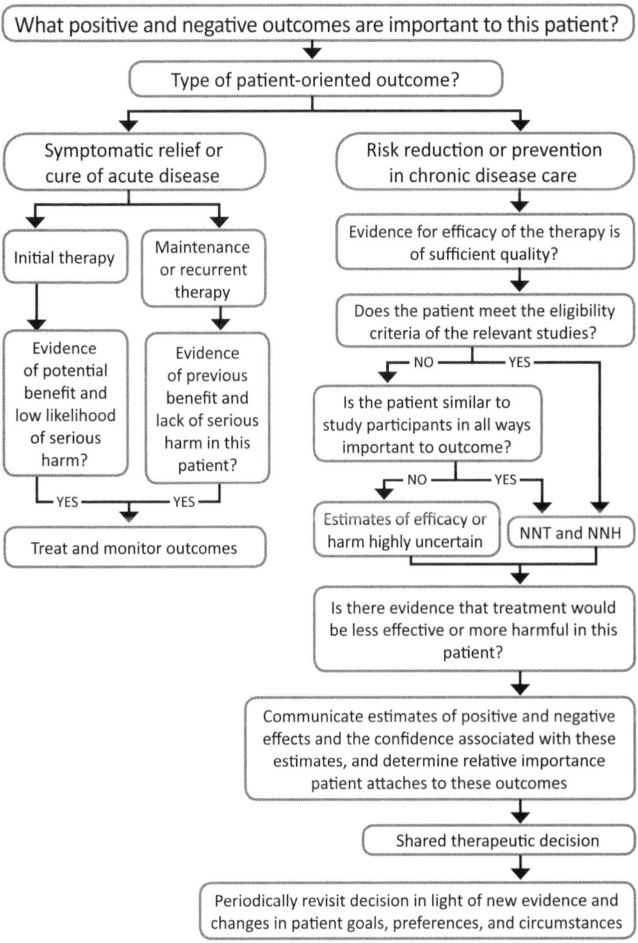

Figure 3. Using Evidence of Efficacy and Harm in Therapeutic Decision-Making

7. KEY CONCEPTS

- **Incidence:** the rate of occurrence of an event in a defined population in a defined period of time; this is also the probability (or risk) of an event occurring in the defined population
- **Prevalence:** the proportion of individuals in a defined population with a particular disorder in a defined period of time; this is also the pretest probability of anyone in the defined population having a particular disorder
- **Bias:** a methodological source of systematic deviation from true or reliable study results
- **Selection Biases** result when the groups being compared differ in baseline prognostic factors relevant to the outcome; common types of selection bias include:
  - **Volunteer Bias:** individuals who volunteer to participate in the study are different from non-volunteers
  - **Non-Respondent Bias:** responders and non-responders differ
- **Measurement Biases** result when systematic errors occur during the collection of data. Several types of measurement biases exist, including:
  - **Instrument Bias:** calibration errors lead to inaccurate measurements
  - **Insensitive Measure Bias:** lack of tool sensitivity precludes measurement of differences in variables of interest
  - **Expectation Bias:** prior expectations of those assessing the results influences their judgment
  - **Recall Bias:** individuals' responses to questions are dependent on memory
  - **Spectrum Bias:** differing case-mixes in various clinical settings affects the performance of diagnostic and screening tests
- **Intervention Biases** commonly affect research studies that compare groups, and include:
  - **Contamination Bias:** members of one group receive the intervention of the other group, therefore minimizing the difference between groups
  - **Compliance Bias:** subject adherence to interventions affects study outcomes
  - **Withdrawal Bias:** subjects who drop out of the study differ from those who remain
- **Confounder:** an extraneous variable (separate from the independent variable) that is related to the outcome of interest, potentially confusing the results
- **Internal Validity:** the extent to which the design and conduct of the study precludes systematic bias
- **External Validity:** the extent to which the results of a study can be generalized to the target population

Test Characteristics

- **Sensitivity:** a measure of how well a test detects a disorder when it is present (i.e. will test positively for a disorder when there is a disorder)
- **Specificity:** a measure of how well a test does not detect a disorder when it is not present (i.e. will test negatively for a disorder when there is not a disorder)
- **Positive Predictive Value (PPV):** the post-test probability of having a particular disorder when test results are positive (i.e. the proportion of people with a positive test that have the disorder) PPV = TP / (TP + FP)
- **Negative Predictive Value (NPV):** the post-test probability of not having a particular disorder when test results are negative (i.e. the proportion of people with a negative test who do not have the disorder) NPV = TN / (TN + FN)

- Predictive values vary with changes in the prevalence of a particular disorder, while sensitivity and specificity do not

Likelihood Ratio

- **Likelihood Ratio (LR):** the odds that a specific test result will be obtained in a patient with the condition compared to a person without the condition
  - If the LR is greater than 1, the finding is more likely among patients with the condition than patients without the condition
  - If the LR is less than 1, the finding is less likely among patients with the condition than patients without the condition
- A **nomogram** uses the pretest probability of a diagnosis, and the LR (obtained from test sensitivity and specificity; positive LR used if the test result is positive, while negative LR used if the test result is negative) to yield the post-test probability of the diagnosis

Effect Measures and Characteristics

- **Odds Ratio (OR):** ratio of the odds of event A among the exposed population compared to the odds of event A among the unexposed population
  - For rare diseases, the odds ratio is an estimate of the relative risk, but as the prevalence of the outcome increases, the odds ratio becomes a poor approximation of the relative risk
- **Absolute Risk (AR):** the proportion of individuals in a particular population who experience event A
- **Relative Risk (RR):** the absolute risk of event A in a population exposed to X, divided by the absolute risk of event A in a population not exposed to X. One needs to have sampled the population prior to exposure. Thus, the relative risk can be calculated from cohort studies, randomized trials, and controlled clinical trials, but cannot be calculated from case control studies or cross-sectional studies
- **Absolute Risk Reduction (ARR):** the absolute risk of adverse event A in a population exposed to the protective effects of X, compared to the absolute risk of adverse event A in a population not exposed to X
- **Absolute Risk Increase (ARI):** the absolute risk of adverse event A in a population exposed to the deleterious effects of X, compared to the absolute risk of adverse event A in a population not exposed to X
- **Relative Risk Reduction (RRR):** the reduction in rate of harmful outcomes in the exposed group compared to the nonexposed group, expressed as a proportion of the nonexposed group rate
- **Relative Risk Increase (RRI):** the increase in rate of harmful outcomes in the exposed group compared to the nonexposed group, expressed as a proportion of the nonexposed group rate
- **Number Needed to Treat (NNT):** the number of patients that would have to be treated with X in order for one patient to benefit by avoiding one harmful outcome
- **Number Needed to Harm (NNH):** the number of patients that would have to be treated with X in order for one patient to experience one harmful outcome
- **P-value:** the calculated probability of obtaining a test statistic as extreme as the observed result when the null hypothesis (often 'no difference between groups') is true
- **Statistical Significance:** the probability that a result occurred by chance.This concept is used to demonstrate whether a calculated or measured value represents a true effect and is not just the product of random error. By convention, this predetermined cut-off probability is less than 5%. In other words, the result would be observed once every 20 measurements if it is determined by chance alone

- **Clinical Significance:** the importance of the measured effect. Clinically significant effects are those that directly matter to patients and that are of a relevant magnitude
- **Confidence Interval:** the range of values in which one can be confident a measured or calculated value will reside, if the measurement or calculation is repeated. A confidence interval provides a summary of the precision of an estimate, that is, how much variability exists around a given estimate (e.g. for a 95% confidence interval, 19 of every 20 repeated measurements or calculations would produce a value that lies within this interval)

8. SUMMARY OF KEY FORMULAE

Table 4. Key Formulae in Evidence-Informed Medical Practice

Concept	Formula
Sensitivity	$\text{Sensitivity} = \frac{TP}{TP + FN}$
Specificity	$\text{Specificity} = \frac{TN}{TN + FP}$
Positive Predictive Value (PPV)	$PPV = \frac{TP}{TP + FP}$
Negative Predictive Value (NPV)	$NPV = \frac{TN}{TN + FN}$
Likelihood Ratio for a negative result (LR–)	$LR- = \frac{1 - \text{sensitivity}}{\text{specificity}}$
Likelihood Ratio for a positive result (LR+)	$LR+ = \frac{\text{sensitivity}}{1 - \text{specificity}}$
Absolute Risk (AR)	$AR = \frac{\text{Number of those with outcome in group}}{\text{Population of group}}$
Relative Risk (RR)	$RR = AR_{exposed} / AR_{unexposed}$
Absolute Risk Reduction (ARR)	$ARR = AR_{unexposed} - AR_{exposed}$
Absolute Risk Increase (ARI)	$ARI = AR_{exposed} - AR_{unexposed}$
Relative Risk Reduction (RRR)	$RRR = ARR / AR_{unexposed}$
Relative Risk Increase (RRI)	$RRI = ARI / AR_{unexposed}$
Number Needed to Treat (NNT)	$NNT = \frac{1}{ARR}$
Number Needed to Harm (NNH)	$NNH = \frac{1}{ARI}$

FN = false negatives, FP = false positives, TN = true negatives, TP = true positives

REFERENCES

1. Miles A, Loughlin M. 2011. Models in the balance: Evidence-based medicine versus evidence-informed individualized care. *J Eval Clin Pract* 17(4):531-536.
2. Guyatt G, Rennie D, Meade MO, Cook DJ. *Users' Guides to the Medical Literature: Essentials of Evidence-Based Clinical Practice*, 2nd ed. New York: McGraw-Hill Medical; 2008.
3. Straus SE, Glasziou P, Richardson WS, Haynes RB. *Evidence-Based Medicine: How to Practice and Teach it*, 4th ed. New York: Churchill-Livingstone; 2011.
4. Kuper A, Lingard L, Levinson W. 2008. Critically appraising qualitative research. *BMJ*, 337, a1035.
5. Balshem H, Helfand M, Schünemann HJ, Oxman AD, Kunz R, Brozek J, et al. 2011. GRADE guidelines: 3. Rating the quality of evidence. *J Clin Epidemiol*, 64(4):401-406.
6. Howick J. *The Philosophy of Evidence-Based Medicine*. Oxford: Wiley-Blackwell; 2011.

Appendix 2: Commonly Used Drugs

Editor:
Ayan K. Dey

Faculty Reviewers:
Cindy Woodland, PhD
Prateek Lala, MD, MSc
Marisa Battistella, BSc Phm, Pharm D, ACPR

APPENDIX: DRUGS

TABLE OF CONTENTS

1. COMMONLY USED PHARMACOLOGICAL AGENTS BY SUBCATEGORY/CLINICAL SCENARIO

Subcategory/ Clinical Scenario	Examples
Analgesia	
NSAIDs	Acetylsalicylic acid (Aspirin®) Diclofenac (Voltaren®, Pennsaid Solution®) Ibuprofen (Motrin®, Advil®) Indomethacin Ketorolac (Toradol®) Meloxicam (Mobicox®) Naproxen (Naprosyn®)
NSAIDs-COX-2 Selective Inhibitors	Celecoxib (Celebrex®)

Subcategory/ Clinical Scenario	Examples
Analgesia	
Opioid Analgesics (narcotics)	Codeine Fentanyl Hydromorphone (Dilaudid®) Hydrocodone (Hycodan®) Methadone (Metadol®) Morphine (Statex®)
Opioid Antagonists	Naloxone (Naloxone HCl Injection®) Naltrexone (ReVia®)
Other Analgesics	Acetaminophen (Tylenol®) Acetaminophen with codeine (Tylenol #2®, Tylenol #3®)
Anesthesia/Sedation	
General Anesthetics: IV	Propofol (Diprivan®) Ketamine injection (Ketalar®) Thiopental
General Anesthetics: Inhaled	Isoflurane Desflurane (Suprane®) Nitrous oxide Sevoflurane (Sevorane AF®)
Muscle Relaxants	Atracurium besylate Neostigmine (Prostigmin®) Rocuronium (Zemuron®) Succinylcholine (Anectine®)
Sedatives: Benzodiazepines	Diazepam (Diastat®, Valium®) Lorazepam (Ativan®) Midazolam (Midazolam Injection®)* Oxazepam (Serax®) Temazepam (Restoril®; primarily for insomnia) Triazolam (Halcion®; primarily for insomnia) *most common adjunct for anesthesia
Sedatives: Other	Chloral hydrate (Chloral Hydrate Odan®) Zopiclone (Imovane®)
Cardiology	
ACE Inhibitors	Captopril (Capoten®) Enalapril (Vasotec®) Fosinopril (Monopril®) Lisinopril (Zestril®) Perindopril (Aceon®) Ramipril (Altace®)
Angiotensin II Receptor Blockers (ARBs)	Candesartan cilexetil (Atacand®) Irbesartan (Avalide®, Avapro®) Losartan (Cozaar®) Telmisartan (Micardis®) Valsartan (Diovan®)
Antiadrenergics (central acting)	Clonidine (Catapres®; both central/peripheral) Methyldopa (Aldomet®, Supres®) Prazosin (both central/peripheral)
Antiadrenergic (peripheral acting)	Reserpine

Subcategory/ Clinical Scenario	Examples
Cardiology	
Anticoagulant	**Vitamin K Antagonist:** Warfarin (Coumadin®) **Low Molecular Weight Heparins (LMWH):** Dalteparin (Fragmin®) Enoxaparin (Lovenox®) Tinzaparin (Innohep®) **Direct Thrombin Inhibitors:** Bivalirudin (Angiomax®) Dabigatran (Pradax®)
Antiplatelet Agents	Acetylsalicylic acid (Aspirin®) Dipyridamole (Persantine®) Dipyridamole/ASA (Aggrenox®) **Adenosine Diphosphate Receptor Inhibitors:** Clopidogrel (Plavix®) Prasugrel (Effient®) Ticagrelor (Brilinta®) Ticlopidine (Ticlid®) **GP IIb/IIIa Inhibitors:** Abciximab (ReoPro®) Tirofiban (Aggrastat®)
β-Blockers	Atenolol (Tenormin®; β1 selective) Acebutolol HCl (Monitan®; β1 selective) Metoprolol (Lopressor®; β1 selective) Nadolol (nonselective) Propranolol (Inderal-LA®; nonselective) Timolol (Azarga®, Blocadren®; nonselective)
Calcium Channel Blockers	**Nondihydropyridine:** Diltiazem (Cardizem®) Verapamil (Chronovera®) **Dihydropyridine:** Amlodipine besylate (Norvasc®) Nifedipine (Adalat®)
Inotropes (increase contractility)	**Cardiac Glycosides:** Digoxin (Lanoxin®) **Phosphodiesterase Inhibitors:** Milrinone lactate (Primacor®) **Sympathomimetic Amines:** Dopamine (Intropin®) Dobutamine HCl Epinephrine (Alveda®) Norepinephrine bitartrate (Levophed®)
Nitrates	Isosorbide dinitrate (Isordil®) Isosorbide mononitrate Nitroglycerin (Minitran®)
Thrombolytics (lytics)	Alteplase (Activase®; tPA) Reteplase (Retavase®) Streptokinase (Streptase®) Tenecteplase (TNkase®)
Agents for Dyslipidemia	
Bile Acid Sequestrants	Cholestyramine (Olestyr®) Colestipol (Colestid®) Colesevelam (Lodalis®)

APPENDIX: DRUGS

Subcategory/ Clinical Scenario	Examples
Agents for Dyslipidemia	
HMG-CoA Reductase Inhibitors (statins)	Atorvastatin (Lipitor®) Fluvastatin (Lescol®) Lovastatin (Advicor®, Mevacor®) Pravastatin (Pravachol®) Rosuvastatin (Crestor®) Simvastatin (Zocor®)
Cholesterol Absorption Inhibitor	Ezetimibe (Ezetrol®)
Fibrates	Fenofibrate (Fenomax®) Gemfibrozil (Lopid®)
Nicotinic Acid	Niacin
Diuretics	
Carbonic Anhydrase Inhibitor	Acetazolamide (Diamox Sequels®)
Loop Diuretics	Bumetanide (Burinex®) Ethacrynic acid (Edecrin®) Furosemide (Lasix®)
Osmotic Diuretics	Mannitol (Osmitrol®) Glycerol Urea (Hydrophil®, Uremol®)
K^+ Sparing Diuretics	Amiloride (Midamor®) Spironolactone (Aldactone®)
Thiazide and Related Diuretics	Hydrochlorothiazide (Accuretic®, Altace HCT®) Chlorthalidone
Other Clinical Scenarios	
Acute MI	ACE inhibitors Acetylsalicylic acid (Aspirin®) β-blockers Clopidogrel Heparin Morphine Nitroglycerin Thrombolytics
Angina Pectoris	Acetylsalicylic acid (Aspirin®) β-blockers Calcium channel blockers Nitrates
CHF	ACE inhibitors Angiotensin receptor antagonists β-blockers Digoxin Diuretics
HTN	ACE inhibitors Angiotensin receptor antagonists β-blockers Calcium channel blockers Diuretics

Subcategory/ Clinical Scenario	Examples
Endocrinology (Agents for Clinical Scenarios)	
Addison's Disease	Fludrocortisone (Florinef®) Hydrocortisone
DM Type 1	**Intermediate-Acting Insulin:** NPH **Long-Acting Insulin:** Glargine **Rapid-Acting Insulin:** Aspart Lispro **Short-Acting Insulin:** Insulin
DM Type 2	**α-Glucosidase Inhibitor:** Acarbose (Glucobay®) **Biguanides:** Metformin (Sandoz®) **Gliptins (DPP-IV Inhibitors):** Sitagliptin (Januvia®) Sitagliptin + Metformin (Janumet®) **Insulin:** Rapid, short, intermediate, long **Meglitinides:** Nateglinide (Starlix®) Repaglinide (GlucoNorm®) **Sulfonylureas:** Chlorpropamide Glyburide (DiaBeta®) Gliclazide (Diamicron®) Glimepiride (Amaryl®) **Thiazolidinediones:** Pioglitazone (Actos®) Rosiglitazone (Avandia®)* *Rosiglitazone is not approved for use alone (i.e. as a "monotherapy"), unless metformin (another diabetes drug) treatment is inappropriate. Rosiglitazone is not recommended for use as part of a "triple therapy" (i.e. in combination with the diabetes drugs metformin and sulfonylurea). Rosiglitazone is not to be used (i.e. it is contraindicated) in patients with any stage of heart failure.
Hypercalcemia	**Bisphosphonate:** Pamidronate disodium (Aredia®) **Bone Reabsorption Inhibitor:** Calcitonin (Calcimar®, Miacalcin®) **Calcimimetic Agent:** Cinacalcet (Sensipar®) **Precipitating Agent:** Potassium phosphate* *poses significant risks

APPENDIX: DRUGS

Subcategory/ Clinical Scenario	Examples
Endocrinology (Agents for Clinical Scenarios)	
Hyperkalemia	**β-Agonist:** Salbutamol (Ventolin®) **Electrolyte Supplements:** Calcium chloride Calcium gluconate Furosemide (Lasix®) Insulin with Dextrose **Potassium Binding Resins:** Sodium polystyrene sulfonate (Kayexalate®) Sodium bicarbonate
Hyperthyroidism	β-blocker (alleviates symptoms) Iodine-131 Methimazole (Tapazole®) Propylthiouracil
Hypothyroidism	Levothyroxine (Levotec®, Eltroxin®; T4) Liothyronine (Cytomel®; T3)* *can be used in conjunction with levothyroxine
Gastroenterology	
Antacids	Aluminum hydroxide (Amphojel®) Calcium carbonate (Caltrate®) Magnesium hydroxide/carbonate **OTC Preparations:** Alka-Seltzer® Gaviscon® Maalox® Rolaids®
Antiemetics	**Anticholinergic Agent:** Scopolamine (Buscopan®) **Antihistamine:** Dimenhydrinate (Gravol®) **Dopamine Receptor Antagonists:** Metoclopramide (Maxeran®) Prochlorperazine **Serotonin Receptor Antagonists:** Dolasetron mesylate (Anzemet®) Ondansetron (Zofran ODT®) Granisetron (Kytril®)
H2-Receptor Antagonists	Cimetidine (Tagamet®) Famotidine (Pepcid®) Nizatidine (Axid®) Ranitidine (Zantac®)
Proton Pump Inhibitors (PPIs)	Esomeprazole (Nexium®) Lansoprazole (Prevacid®) Omeprazole (Losec®) Pantoprazole (Pantoloc®) Rabeprazole (Pariet®)

Subcategory/ Clinical Scenario	Examples
Gastroenterology	
Agents for Constipation	**Bulk-Forming Laxative:** Psyllium (Metamucil®) **Decompaction:** Mineral oil **Osmotic Agents:** Magnesium hydroxide Lactulose Magnesium citrate Magnesium Polyethylene glycol **Stimulant Laxatives:** Bisacodyl (Bi-PegLyte®, Correctol®) Senna (Senokot S®) **Surfactant:** Docusate (Colace®)
Agents for Diarrhea	Attapulgite (Kaopectate®) Bismuth subsalicylate (Pepto-Bismol®) Diphenoxylate (Lomotil®) Loperamide (Imodium®, Loperacap®) Oral rehydration therapy
Agents for GI Bleed	Pantoprazole (Pantoloc®) Octreotide
Agents for Irritable Bowel Syndrome	**Antidepressant:** TCA (for pain) **Bile Acid Sequestrant:** Cholestyramine (Questran®) **Bulk-Forming Laxative:** Psyllium (Metamucil®) **Opioid:** Loperamide (Imodium®, Loperacap®)
Agents for Inflammatory Bowel Disease	**Steroids:** Budesonide Hydrocortisone Prednisone **Other:** 5-Aminosalicylic acid (Salofalk®, Pentasa®) Azathioprine (Imuran®) Cyclosporine (Restasis®, Sandimmune®) Infliximab (Remicade®) Mercaptopurine (Purinethol®) Methotrexate Sulfasalazine (Salazopyrin®)
Head and Neck (Agents for Clinical Scenarios)	
Bell's Palsy	Artificial tears Corticosteroids Ocular ointment **Oral Antivirals:** Acyclovir Prednisolone
Acute Otitis Externa	Analgesics **Otic Drops:** Betamethasone + Gentamicin (Garasone®) Ciprofloxacin (Cipro®) Ofloxacin (Floxin®, Ocuflox®) Moxifloxacin (Vigamox®)

Subcategory/ Clinical Scenario	Examples
Head and Neck (Agents for Clinical Scenarios)	
Sudden Sensorineural Hearing Loss	Corticosteroids
Otitis Media	**First-Line Antibiotics:** Amoxicillin Sulphamethoxazole-Trimethoprim (Septra®) Macrolides **Second-Line Antibiotics (When Amoxicillin Fails):** Amoxicillin/Clavulanic acid (Clavulin®) Cephalosporins **For Symptoms:** Analgesics Antipyretics
Vertigo	**Anticholinergic Agent:** Transdermal scopolamine **Antihistamine:** Diphenhydramine (Benadryl®) **Benzodiazepine:** Diazepam (Valium®) **Ménière's Disease:** Betahistine (Serc®) **Phenothiazine Antiemetics:** Prochlorperazine maleate (Nu-Prochlor®)
Rhinorrhea	**Antihistamines:** Desloratadine (Aerius®) Diphenhydramine (Benadryl®) Fexofenadine (Allegra®) Loratadine (Claritin®) **Topical/Systemic Decongestants:** Phenylephrine (Neo-Synephrine®) Pseudoephedrine (Promatussin®) **Topical Glucocorticoids:** Budesonide (Rhinocort®) Fluticasone proprionate (Advair®)
Anterior Epistaxis	**Topical Vasoconstrictors:** Cocaine Oxymetazoline (Dristan®, Vicks Sinex®)
Infectious Diseases: Antibacterial	
Cell Wall Synthesis Inhibitors	Cephalosporins Carbapenems Glycopeptides (Vancomycin) Penicillin
DNA Complex Agent	Metronidazole (Flagyl®)* *The major mechanism of action involves cross-linking with, and inactivation of, cysteine-containing bacterial and protozoal enzymes
DNA-Directed RNA Polymerase Inhibitor	Rifampin (Rifadin®)
DNA Gyrase Inhibitor	Fluoroquinolones
Folic Acid Metabolism Inhibitors	Sulfamethoxazole (Bactrim®) Trimethoprim (Polytrim®)

Subcategory/ Clinical Scenario	Examples
Infectious Diseases: Antibacterial	
Protein Synthesis Inhibitors (50S ribosomes)	Clindamycin (Dalacin®) Macrolides
Protein Synthesis Inhibitors (30S ribosomes)	**Aminoglycosides:** Gentamicin Tobramycin Tetracyclines
Clinical Scenarios	
Community-Acquired Pneumonia	Amoxicillin/Clavulanic acid Cephalosporins Doxycycline (Doxycin®) Macrolides **Quinolones:** Gatifloxacin (Zymar®) Levofloxacin (Levaquin®) Moxifloxacin (Avelox®)
Otitis Media	Amoxicillin Amoxicillin/Clavulanic acid Cefixime (Suprax®) Cefuroxime axetil (Ceftin®) Sulfamethoxazole/Trimethoprim (Septra®)
TB	**1st Line:** Ethambutol (Etibi®) Isoniazid (INH) Vitamin B6 Pyrazinamide Rifampin (Rifadin®) Streptomycin (SteriMax®) **2nd Line:** Fluoroquinolones (Levofloxacin)
UTI	Amoxicillin Amoxicillin/Clavulanic acid Cephalexin (Keflex®) Nitrofurantoin **Quinolones:** Ciprofloxacin (Cipro®) Norfloxacin (Noroxin®) Trimethoprim/Sulfamethoxazole (Septra®)
Infectious Diseases: Antifungal	
Echinocandin	Capsofungin (Cancidas®; intravenous)
Polyenes	Amphotericin B (Fungizone®; systemic) Nystatin (Nyaderm®; topical)
Imidazoles	Clotrimazole (Lotriderm®) Ketoconazole (Ketoderm®) Miconazole (Desenex®)
Triazoles	Fluconazole (Diflucan®) Itraconazole (Sporanox®) Voriconazole (Vfend®)

Subcategory/ Clinical Scenario	Examples
Infectious Diseases: Antiviral	
HIV	Fusion inhibitors Protease inhibitors NNRTIs (non-nucleoside reverse transcriptase inhibitors) NRTIs (nucleoside reverse transcriptase inhibitors)
Nucleoside Reverse Transcriptase Inhibitors (NRTIs)	Abacavir sulfate (Ziagen®) Lamivudine (Epivir®) Stavudine (Zerit®) Zidovudine (Retrovir®)
Non-Nucleoside Reverse Transcriptase Inhibitors (NNRTIs)	Delavirdine mesylate (Rescriptor®) Efavirenz (Sustiva®; also known as EFV) Nevirapine (Viramune®)
Protease Inhibitors	Amprenavir Atazanavir Indinavir Lopinavir Nelfinavir Ritonavir Saquinavir
Integrase Inhibitor	Raltegravir potassium (Isentress®)
Combination Antiretrovirals	Abacavir + Zidovudine + Lamivudine (Trizivir®) Zidovudine + Lamivudine (Combivir®)
Fusion Inhibitors	Enfuvirtide (Fuzeon®) Maraviroc (Celsentri®)
Other Antivirals	Oseltamivir (Tamiflu®; against influenza virus) Ribavirin (Virazole®; inhibits wide range of viruses)
Nucleoside Polymerase Inhibitors	Acyclovir (Zovirax®) Ganciclovir (Cytovene®)
Musculoskeletal (Agents for Clinical Scenarios)	
Osteoarthritis	Acetaminophen (Tylenol®) Capsaicin topical (Rub A535®) Intra-articular glucocorticoid injection Intra-articular hyaluronan injection NSAIDs Opioids Selective COX-2 inhibitors
Osteoporosis	Alendronate (Fosamax®) Etidronate (Didrocal®) Risedronate (Actonel®) Calcium and Vitamin D supplementation Calcitonin (Calcimar®, Caltine®) Estrogen (Premplus®, Premarin®) Parathyroid hormone Raloxifene (Evista®)

Subcategory/ Clinical Scenario	Examples
Musculoskeletal (Agents for Clinical Scenarios)	
Rheumatoid Arthritis	**Disease Modifying Therapy (DMARDs):** Hydroxychloroquine sulfate (Plaquenil®) Sulfasalazine (Salazopyrin®) Methotrexate **Immunosuppressive Therapy:** Azathioprine (Imuran®) Cyclosporine (Restasis®) Cyclophosphamide (Procytox®) Leflunomide (Arava®) **NSAIDs**
Neurology (Agents for Clinical Scenarios)	
Alzheimer's Disease	**Cholinesterase Inhibitors:** Donepezil (Aricept®) Galantamine (Reminyl ER®) Rivastigmine (Exelon®) Memantine (Ebixa®)
CVA/TIA	Alteplase (Activase®; tPA) Acetylsalicylic acid (Aspirin®) Clopidogrel (Plavix®) Dipyridamole + Aspirin® (Aggrenox®) Warfarin (Coumadin®)
Epilepsy	**Atypical Absence/Myoclonic/Atonic:** Lamotrigine (Lamictal®) Topiramate (Topamax®) **Focal:** Carbamazepine (Tegretol®) Phenytoin (Dilantin®) **Generalized-Onset Tonic Clonic:** Lamotrigine (Lamictal®) Topiramate (Topamax®, Topiragen®) Valproic acid (Depakene®) **Partial Seizures (Narrow-Spectrum AEDs):** Gabapentin (Neurontin®) Vigabatrin (Sabril®) **Typical Absence:** Ethosuximide (Zarontin®) Valproic acid (Depakene®) **Other (Acute Therapy):** Diazepam (Valium®) Lorazepam (Ativan®)
MS	Glatiramer acetate (Copaxone®) Glucocorticoids Interferon-β1a (Avonex®) or 1b (Betaseron®)
Parkinson's Disease	**Dopamine Agonists:** Pramipexole (Mirapex®) Ropinirole (ReQuip®) Levodopa/Carbidopa (Sinemet®) **Other:** Anticholinergics (Benztropine) COMT inhibitors (Entacepone) MAO-B inhibitors (Selegiline) NMDA antagonists

Subcategory/ Clinical Scenario	Examples
Obstetrics and Gynecology (Agents for Clinical Scenarios)	
Nutritional Supplementation	Folic acid Multivitamins (Materna®, Pregvit®)
Antinausea	Benzamides (serotonin antagonists) Dimenhydrinate (Gravol®) Doxylamine + Pyridoxine (Diclectin®)
HTN	**Severe HTN (>160mmHg systolic or >90mmHg diastolic):** Hydralazine Labetalol (Trandate®) Nifedipine (Adalat®) **Non-Severe HTN:** Methyldopa (Aldomet®) Labetalol (Trandate®) Other β-blockers
Inducing Agents	Oxytocin Prostaglandin E2
Medical Abortion	Methotrexate + Misoprostol
Rh- Mother and Rh+ or Unknown Fetus	RHO immune globulin (RhoGAM®)
Psychiatry	
Antidepressants	
Selective Serotonin Reuptake Inhibitors	**SSRIs:** Citalopram (Celexa®) Escitalopram (Cipralex®) Fluoxetine (Prozac®) Paroxetine (Paxil®) Sertraline (Zoloft®)
Tricyclic Antidepressants	**TCAs:** Amitriptyline (Elavil®) Clomipramine (Anafranil®) Doxepin (Sinequan®) Imipramine (Tofranil®) Nortriptyline (Aventyl®)
Serotonin-Norepinephrine Reuptake Inhibitors	**SNRIs:** Duloxetine (Cymbalta®) Venlafaxine (Effexor®)
Monoamine Oxidase Inhibitors (MAOIs)	Phenelzine sulfate (Nardil®) Tranylcypromine sulfate (Parnate®)
Other	Bupropion (Wellbutrin®) Mirtazapine (Remeron®) Tryptophan (Tryptan®)
Antipsychotics	
Typical	Chlorpromazine (Largactil®) Flupenthixol (Fluanxol®) Haloperidol (Haldol®) Perphenazine (Trilafon®)

Subcategory/ Clinical Scenario	Examples
Psychiatry: *Antipsychotics*	
Atypical	Clozapine (Clozaril®) Olanzapine (Zyprexa®) Quetiapine (Seroquel®) Risperidone (Risperdal®) Ziprasidone (Zeldox®)
Other	
Antianxiety Agents	SSRIs TCAs MAOIs **Benzodiazepines:** Alprazolam (Xanax®) Clonazepam (Rivotril®) Lorazepam (Ativan®) Oxazepam (Serax®) Temazepam (Restoril®) Diazepam (Valium®) **β-Blockers:** Atenolol (Tenormin®) Oxprenolol (Trasicor®; non-selective) Pindolol (Visken®) Propranolol **Other:** Buspirone (BuSpar®) Hydroxyzine (Atarax®) Pregabalin (Lyrica®) Venlafaxine (Effexor®)
Mood Stabilizers (for bipolar disorder)	**Anticonvulsants:** Carbamazepine (Tegretol®) Lamotrigine (Lamictal®) Lithium (Lithane®, Carbolith®) Valproic Acid (Depakene®)
Opioid Agonists	Buprenorphine + Naloxone (Suboxone®; for opioid addiction) Methadone (Metadol®)

Notes for Psychiatry

- Cognitive behavioral therapy is an effective first-line treatment for mild to moderate depression and anxiety disorders
- Electroconvulsive therapy is indicated and effective for severe and medically refractory depression

Respirology (Agents for Clinical Scenarios)	
Asthma (relief medication)	**Anticholinergic:** Ipratropium bromide (Atrovent®) **β-Agonists:** Epinephrine Isoprenaline Salbutamol Terbutaline **Methylxanthine:** Theophylline (Uniphyl®)

Subcategory/ Clinical Scenario	Examples
Respirology (Agents for Clinical Scenarios)	
Asthma (long-term control medication)	**Inhaled Glucocorticoids:** Beclomethasone (Qvar®) Budesonide (Pulmicort®) Fluticasone (Flovent®) **Leukotriene Inhibitor:** Montelukast (Singulair®) **Mast Cell-Stabilizing Agents:** Cromolyn (Nascrom®) Nedocromil (Alocril®)
COPD	**Anticholinergics:** Ipratropium bromide (Atrovent®) Tiotropium (Spiriva®) **β-Agonists:** Salmeterol (can also be used for asthma) Salbutamol **Inhaled Glucocorticoids:** Beclomethasone (Qvar®) Budesonide (Pulmicort®) Fluticasone (Flovent®) **Methylxanthine:** Theophylline (Uniphyl®)
Urology (Agents for Clinical Scenarios)	
Benign Prostatic Hyperplasia	**5α-Reductase Inhibitor:** Finasteride (Proscar®) **α-Adrenergic Blockers:** Terazosin (Hytrin®) Doxazosin (Cardura®) Tamsulosin (Flomax®)
Chronic Renal Failure	ACE inhibitors Angiotensin receptor blockers Protein restriction
Erectile Dysfunction	Sildenafil (Viagra®) Tadalafil (Cialis®) Vardenafil (Levitra®)
Agents for Urinary Incontinence (hyperactive bladder)	**Anticholinergic Drugs:** Propantheline bromide *Antispasmodics*: Oxybutynin (Ditropan®) Tolterodine (Detrol®) Trospium (Trosec®) **TCAs**
Agents for Urinary Incontinence (stress incontinence)	Estrogen Pseudoephedrine hydrochloride **TCAs:** Imipramine Desipramine Amitriptyline

Subcategory/ Clinical Scenario	Examples
Vascular (Agents for Clinical Scenarios)	
DVT/PE	Heparin Warfarin (Coumadin®) **LMWH:** Dalteparin (Fragmin®) Enoxaparin (Lovenox®) Tinzaparin (Innohep®)
Temporal Arteritis (GCA)	Prednisone (high dose, starting at 60 mg/d PO for approximately 1 month)

2. DRUG CATEGORY NAMING SHORTCUTS

Although there are several exceptions, drugs in the same therapeutic/mechanistic category often have similar endings/beginnings. It is also worth noting that there may be other drugs that also belong to the classes described below that have different endings.

Endings/ Beginnings	Therapeutic Class	Examples
-afil	PDE-5 inhibitors	sildenafil, tadalafil, vardenafil
-ane	Inhaled general anesthetics	halothane, enflurane, isoflurane
-ase	Thrombolytics	streptokinase, alteplase, tenecteplase
-azine	Phenothiazine antipsychotics and Antihistamines	chlorpromazine, fluphenazine, perphenazine, promethazine
-azole	Antifungals	ketoconazole, itraconazole, fluconazole
-barbital	Barbiturates	phenobarbital, pentobarbital, secobarbital
Ceph-/Cef-	Cephalosporins	ceftriaxone, cefuroxime, cefazolin, cephalexin, cefprozil
-cillin	Penicillin antibiotics	penicillin, amoxicillin, cloxacillin
-curonium	Non-depolarizing neuromuscular blockers	pancuronium, rocuronium, vecuronium
-cycline	Tetracycline antibiotics	tetracycline, doxycycline, minocycline
-dipine	Dihydropyridine calcium channel blockers	nifedipine, felodipine, amlodipine
-dronate	Bisphosphonates	alendronate, etidronate, risedronate
-floxacin	Fluoroquinolones	moxifloxacin, levofloxacin, ciprofloxacin
Gli-/Gly-	Second generation sulfonylureas	gliclazide, glimepiride, glibenclamide/glyburide
-ipramine	Tricyclic antidepressants	clomipramine, imipramine, desipramine
-lol	β-blockers	propranolol, metoprolol, labetalol

APPENDIX: DRUGS

Endings/ Beginnings	Therapeutic Class	Examples
-mab	Monoclonal antibodies	rituximab, trastuzumab, bevacizumab
-micin/ -mycin	Aminoglycoside antibiotics	gentamicin, neomycin, tobramycin
-navir	Antiretroviral protease inhibitors	ritonavir, indinavir, saquinavir
-(pa)rin	Anticoagulants	heparin, warfarin, enoxaparin
-penem	Carbapenems	ertapenem, meropenem, imipenem
-platin	Platinating antineoplastics	cisplatin, carboplatin, oxaliplatin
-prazole	Proton pump inhibitors	omeprazole, pantoprazole, lansoprazole
-pressin	Antidiuretic hormones	desmopressin, vasopressin
-pril	ACE inhibitors	captopril, enalapril, lisinopril
-rubicin	Anthracycline antineoplastics	doxorubicin, daunorubicin, epirubicin
-sartan	Angiotensin II receptor blockers	losartan, irbesartan, valsartan
-(s)one	Corticosteroids	cortisone, prednisone, prednisolone
-statin	HMG-CoA reductase inhibitors	atorvastatin, lovastatin, pravastatin
-terol	β2-agonist bronchodilators	salmeterol, formoterol, albuterol
-thromycin	Macrolide antibiotics	erythromycin, clarithromycin, azithromycin
-tidine	H2-receptor antagonists	cimetidine, ranitidine, famotidine
-tilide	Class III antiarrhythymics	dofetilide, ibutilide
-triptan	Serotonin (5-HT) agonists	sumatriptan
-zepam/ -zolam	Benzodiazepines	midazolam, diazepam, lorazepam
-zosin	α-adrenergic blockers	prazosin, terazosin, doxazosin

Browne A, et al. *Pharmacology You See: A High-Yield Pharmacology Review for Health Professionals*, 1st ed. Toronto: McGraw-Hill; 2011.

REFERENCES

1. Browne A, Dugani S, Hutson J, McSheffrey G, Stefater M. *Pharmacology You See: A High-Yield Pharmacology Review for Health Professionals*, 1st ed. Toronto: McGraw-Hill; 2011.
2. Compendium of Pharmaceuticals and Specialties. Ottawa: Canadian Pharmacists Association. 2012. Available from http://www.e-therapeutics.ca.
3. Harvey R, Clark M, Finkel R, Rey J. *Lippincott's Illustrated Reviews: Pharmacology*, 5th ed. Baltimore: Lippincott Williams & Wilkins; 2011.
4. Micromedex Online. Greenwood Village: Thomson Reuters (Healthcare) Inc.; 2013.
5. Wells PS. Venous Thromboembolism. In Repchinsky C (Editor). *Therapeutic Choices*, 6th ed. Ottawa: Canadian Pharmacists Association; 2011.

Appendix 3: Common Laboratory Values

Editor:
Bhupinder Sahota

Faculty Reviewers:
Andrew Morris, MD, SM, FRCP(C)
Atul Prabhu, MD, FRCA

TABLE OF CONTENTS

1. HEMATOLOGY

Test	Conventional Units	SI Units/Notes
Complete Blood Count (CBC)		
Hemoglobin (Hb)	M: 13.3-16.2 g/dL F: 12.0-15.8 g/dL	M: 133-162 g/L F: 120-158 g/L
Hematocrit (Hct)	M: 38.8-46.4% F: 35.4-44.4%	M: 0.388-0.464 F: 0.354-0.444
Erythrocyte Count (RBC)	M: 4.3-5.6 x 10^6/mm^3 F: 4.0-5.2 x 10^6/mm^3	M: 4.3-5.6 x10^{12}/L F: 4.0-5.2 x10^{12}/L
Mean Corpuscular Volume (MCV=Hct/Hb)	79.0-93.3 fL/cell	79.0-93.3 μm^3
Mean Corpuscular Hb (MCH=Hb/RBC)	26.7-31.9 pg/cell	26.7-31.9 pg/cell
MCH Concentration (MCHC=MCH/MCV)	32.3-35.9 g/dL	323-359 g/L
Leukocyte Count (WBC)	4.5-11.0 x 10^3/mm^3	4.5-11.0 x 10^9/L
Differential Count	Percent (%)	Cells x 10^9/L
Neutrophils	40-70	1.42-6.34
Bands	0-5	0-0.45
Lymphocytes	20-50	0.71-4.53
Monocytes	4-8	0.14-0.72
Eosinophils	0-6	0-0.54
Basophils	0-2	0-0.18
Platelet Count	1.65-4.15 x 10^5/mm^3	1.65-4.15 x 10^{11}/L

Hematology (continued)

Test	Conventional Units	SI Units/Notes
Miscellaneous Hematology Values		
Erythrocyte Sedimentation Rate (ESR)	M: 0-15 mm/h F: 0-20 mm/h	M: 0-15 mm/h F: 0-20 mm/h
Reticulocyte Count	M: 0.8-2.3% of RBCs F: 0.8-2.0% of RBCs	M: 0.008-0.023 F: 0.008-0.020

2. COAGULATION

Test	Conventional Units	SI Units/Notes
International Normalized Ratio (INR)	0.8-1.1	0.8-1.1
Prothrombin Time (PT)	12.7-15.4 s	12.7-15.4 s
Partial Thromboplastin Time	60-70 s	1.5-2.5x greater with anticoagulants
Activated Partial Thromboplastin Time (aPTT)	25-35 s	
Bleeding Time	<7.1 min	<7.1 min
D-dimer	220-740 ng/mL FEU	Low: not thrombosis
Fibrinogen	233-496 mg/dL	Low: clotting

3. SERUM CHEMISTRY

Test	Conventional Units	SI Units/Notes
Electrolytes		
Sodium	136-146 mEq/L	Critical: <120, >160
Potassium	3.5-5.0 mEq/L	Critical: <2.5, >6.5
Chloride	102-109 mEq/L	Critical: <80, >115
Bicarbonate (HCO_3^-)	22-30 mEq/L	Critical: <15, >40
Anion Gap [$Na^+ - (Cl^- + HCO_3^-)$]	7-16 mEq/L	12-20 mEq/L with K^+
Calcium Total Ionized	 8.7-10.2 mg/dL 4.5-5.3 mg/dL	 2.2-2.6 mM 1.12-1.32 mM
Magnesium	1.5-2.3 mg/dL	Critical: <0.5, >3
Phosphorus	2.5-4.3 mg/dL	0.81-1.4 mM
Lactate	Arterial: 4.5-14.4 mg/dL	Venous: 4.5-19.8 mg/dL
Nonelectrolytes		
Blood Urea Nitrogen (BUN)	7-18 mg/dL	2.5-6.4 mM
Creatinine	M: 0.6-1.2 mg/dL F: 0.5-0.9 mg/dL	M: 53-106 μM F: 44-80 μM
Uric Acid	M: 3.1-7.0 mg/dL F: 2.5-5.6 mg/dL	M: 180-410 μM F: 150-330 μM
Glucose (fasting)	75-100 mg/dL	4.2-5.6 mM

Serum Chemistry (continued)

Test	Conventional Units	SI Units/Notes
Nonelectrolytes		
Osmolality	280-325 mOsm	Critical: <265, >320
Osmolal Gap	<10 mOsm/kg	<10 mOsm/kg
Liver/Pancreas Tests		
Alanine Aminotransferase (ALT)	8-20 U/L	Viral hepatitis: ALT/AST >1
Aspartate Aminotransferase (AST)	12-38 U/L	Liver disease: ALT/AST <1
γ-Glutamyltransferase (GGT)	M: 9-50 U/L F: 8-40 U/L	Marker of hepatobiliary disease and chronic alcohol use
Alkaline Phosphatase (ALP)	30-120 U/L	Liver disease if elevated with 5′-nucleotidase, otherwise bone
5′-Nucleotidase	0-11 U/L	
Bilurubin		
Total	0.3-1.3 mg/dL	5.1-22 μM
Conjugated (direct)	0.1-0.4 mg/dL	1.7-6.8 μM
Unconjugated (indirect)	0.2-0.9 mg/dL	3.4-15.2 μM
Amylase	20-96 U/L	Acute pancreatitis: rise in amylase paralleled with later rise in lipase
Lipase	3-43 U/L	
Albumin	4.0-5.9 g/dL	40-50 g/L
Lipids		
Total Cholesterol		
Recommended	<200 mg/dL	<5.2 mM
Moderate risk	200-239 mg/dL	5.2-6.2 mM
High risk	≥240 mg/dL	≥6.2 mM
HDL-Cholesterol	M: >29 mg/dL F: >35 mg/dL	M: >0.75 mM F: >0.91 mM
LDL-Cholesterol		
Recommended	<130 mg/dL	<3.37 mM
Moderate risk	130-159 mg/dL	3.37-4.12 mM
High risk	≥160 mg/dL	≥4.12 mM
Free Fatty Acids (FFAs)	8-25 mg/dL	0.28-0.89 mM
Triglycerides (TG)	M: 40-160 mg/dL F: 35-135 mg/dL	M: 0.45-1.81 mM F: 0.40-1.52 mM
Apolipoprotein A-1	119-240 mg/dL	Component: HDL
Apolipoprotein B	52-163 mg/dL	Component: LDL, VLDL
Serum Proteins		
Albumin	3.5-5.0 g/dL	High: dehydration; half-life of 12-18 d

Serum Chemistry (continued)

Test	Conventional Units	SI Units/Notes
Serum Proteins		
Immunoglobulins (Ig)	IgA: 70-350 mg/dL IgD: 0-14 mg/dL IgE: 0-212 mg/dL IgG: 700-1700 mg/dL IgM: 50-300 mg/dL	15% of Ig rarely detected allergic response 75% of Ig ABO blood types and rheumatoid factor (RF); does not cross placenta
Protein		
Total	6.7-8.6 g/dL	67-86 g/L
Electrophoresis of globulins	α_1: 0.2-0.4 g/dL α_2: 0.5-0.9 g/dL β: 0.6-1.1 g/dL γ: 0.7-1.7 g/dL	α_1: 2-4 g/L α_2: 5-9 g/L β: 6-11 g/L γ: 7-17 g/L
C-Reactive Protein (CRP)	<1.0 mg/dL	Cardiac risk indicator
Markers for Neoplasia		
α-Fetoprotein (αFP)	<8.5 ng/mL	Indicates fetal defects
Carcinoembryonic Antigen (CEA)	Non-smokers: <2.5 ng/mL	Smokers: <5.0 ng/mL
Prostate Specific Antigen (PSA)	<4.0 ng/mL	Cancerous: <10% free PSA
CA-125	0-35 U/mL	Indicates ovarian cancer
Markers for Cardiac/Skeletal Muscle Injury		
Lactate Dehydrogenase (LDH)	115–221 U/L	Peak: 2-3 d with MI
Isoenzymes	Fraction 1: 18-33% Fraction 2: 28-40% Fraction 3: 18-30% Fraction 4: 6-16% Fraction 5: 2-13%	Origin: heart, RBC Origin: heart, lung Origin: lung Origin: kidney, pancreas Origin: muscle, liver
Creatine Kinase	M: 0.87-5.0 µkat/L F: 0.66-4.0 µkat/L	M: 51-294 U/L F: 39-238 U/L
CK-MB Isoenzyme	0-5.5 ng/mL	Myocardial cell specific
Myoglobin	M: 20-71 µg/L F: 25-58 µg/L	Elevated within 3 h of MI
Cardiac Troponin I	0-0.04 ng/mL	Elevated until 7-10 d after MI
Cardiac Troponin T	0-0.1 ng/mL	Elevated until 10-14 d after MI
Nutrition		
Folate		
Serum	5.4-18 ng/mL	12.2-40.8 nM
Eyrthrocytes	150-450 ng/mL	340-1020 nM
Iron	41-141 µg/dL	7-25 µM
Ferritin	M: 15-200 ng/mL F: 12-150 ng/mL	M: 15-200 µg/L F: 12-150 µg/L

Serum Chemistry (continued)

Test	Conventional Units	SI Units/Notes
Nutrition		
Transferrin	200-400 mg/dL	Low: iron deficiency anemia
Total Iron Binding Capacity (TIBC)	300-360 µg/dL	Indirectly measures transferrin

4. SERUM ENDOCRINE TESTS

Tests	Conventional Units	SI Units/Notes
Adrenocorticotropic Hormone (ACTH)		
0800 h	10-60 pg/mL	2.2-13.3 pM
1600 h	<20 pg/mL	<4.5 pM
Aldosterone		
Supine	<16 ng/dL	<443 pM
Upright	4-31 ng/dL	111-858 pM
β-human Chorionic Gonadotropin (β-hCG)	<5.0 mIU/mL	<5.0 IU/L
Cortisol		
0800 h	8-20 µg/dL	251-552 nM
1700 h	3-13 µg/dL	83-359 nM
C-Peptide	0.8-3.5 ng/mL	0.27-1.19 nM
Dehydroepiandrosterone Sulfate (DHEAS)		
M:	10-619 µg/dL	0.9-17 µM
F: Premenopausal	12-535 µg/dL	0.9-9.9 µM
F: Postmenopausal	30-260 µg/dL	<4.8 µM
Estradiol		
M:	<20 pg/mL	<184 pM
F: Follicular phase	20-145 pg/mL	184-532 pM
F: Ovulatory peak	112-443 pg/mL	411-1626 pM
F: Luteal phase	20-241 pg/mL	184-885 pM
F: Postmenopausal	<59 pg/mL	<217 pM
Follicle-Stimulating Hormone (FSH)		
M:	1.0-12.0 mIU/mL	1.0-12.0 IU/L
F: Follicular phase	3.0-20.0 mIU/mL	3.0-20.0 IU/L
F: Ovulatory peak	9.0-26.0 mIU/mL	9.0-26.0 IU/L
F: Luteal phase	1.0-12.0 mIU/mL	1.0-12.0 IU/L
F: Postmenopausal	18.0-153.0 mIU/mL	18.0-153.0 IU/L
Growth Hormone (GH)	M: <5 ng/mL F: <10 ng/mL	M: <5 µg/L F: <10 µg/L
Hemoglobin A1c (HbA1c)	<6%	Poor diabetic control >9%
Luteinizing Hormone (LH)		
M:	2.0-12.0 mIU/mL	2.0-12.0 IU/L
F: Follicular phase	2.0-15.0 mIU/mL	2.0-15.0 IU/L
F: Ovulatory peak	22.0-105.0 mIU/mL	22.0-105.0 IU/L
F: Luteal phase	0.6-19.0 mIU/mL	0.6-19.0 IU/L
F: Postmenopausal	16.0-64.0 mIU/mL	16.0-64.0 IU/L

Serum Endocrine Tests (continued)

Tests	Conventional Units	SI Units/Notes
Progesterone		
M:	<1.0 ng/mL	<3.18 nM
F: Follicular phase	<1.0 ng/mL	<3.18 nM
F: Luteal phase	3-20 ng/mL	9.54-63.6 nM
Prolactin		
M:	2-18 ng/mL	2-18 µg/L
F: Non-pregnant	3-30 ng/mL	3-30 µg/L
F: Pregnant	10-209 ng/mL	10-209 µg/L
F: Postmenopausal	2-20 ng/mL	2-20 µg/L
Parathyroid Hormone (PTH)	8-51 pg/mL	Shows diurnal variation
Serotonin (5-HT)	50-200 ng/mL	0.28-1.14 µM
Testosterone		
Free	M: 90-300 pg/mL F: 3-19 pg/mL	M: 312-1041 pM F: 10.4-65.9 pM
Total	M: 270-1070 ng/dL F: 6-86 ng/dL	M: 9.36-37.10 nM F: 0.21-2.98 nM
Thyroid Stimulating Hormone (TSH)	0.5-5 µU/mL	Shows diurnal variation
Thyroxine (T_4)		
Free	0.7-1.24 ng/dL	9-16 pM
Total	5-12 µg/dL	65-155 nM
Triiodothyronine (T_3)		
Free	2.4-4.2 pg/mL	3.7-6.5 pM
Total	77-135 ng/dL	1.2-2.1 nM
Vasoactive Intestinal Polypeptide (VIP)	<60 pg/mL	<60 ng/L

5. URINE

Tests	Conventional Units	SI Units/Notes
Urinalysis		
pH	5.0-9.0	5.0-9.0
Specific Gravity	1.001-1.035	Easy to obtain
Osmolality	50-1200 mOsm/kg	More exact results
Creatinine	1.0-1.6 g/d	8.8-14 mmol/d
Creatinine Clearance	M: 82-125 mL/min F: 75-115 mL/min	M: 1.37-2.08 mL/s F: 1.25-1.92 mL/s
Urea Nitrogen	6-17 g/d	214-607 mmol/d
Sodium	100-260 mEq/d	100-260 mmol/d
Potassium	25-100 mEq/d	25-100 mmol/d
Calcium	<300 mg/d	>7.5 mmol/d
Phosphate	400-1300 mg/d	12.9-42.0 mmol/d

Urine (continued)

Tests	Conventional Units	SI Units/Notes
Urinalysis		
Uric Acid	250-800 mg/d	1.49-4.76 mmol/d
Glucose	50-300 mg/d	0.3-1.7 mmol/d
Albumin	10-100 mg/d	0.01-0.1 g/d
Protein	<150 mg/d	<0.15 g/d
Urine Sediment		
Leukocytes	0-2/high power field	0-2/high power field
Erythrocytes	0-2/high power field	0-2/high power field
Urinary Catecholamines	<100 µg/d	<5.91 nmol/d
Dopamine	60-440 µg/d	392-2876 nmol/d
Epinephrine	0-20 µg/d	0-109 nmol/d
Norepinephrine	15-80 µg/d	89-473 nmol/d

6. CEREBROSPINAL FLUID (CSF)

Tests	Conventional Units	SI Units/Notes
Cell Count	0-5 cells/mm^3	Presence of white blood cells is considered abnormal
Chloride	116-130 mEq/L	Decreased with meningeal infections, tubercular meningitis, and low blood chloride levels; increased levels correlated with blood levels
Glucose	40-70 mg/dL	2.2-3.9 mM; a level <60% of blood glucose level may indicate meningitis or neoplasm
Opening Pressure	50-180 mmH_2O	If blockage in CSF circulation is suspected in the subarachnoid space, perform a Queckenstedt-Stookey test
Protein		
Albumin	6.6-44.2 mg/dL	Increased levels indicate a breakdown in the blood-brain barrier
IgG	0.9-5.7 mg/dL	Increased levels may be suggestive of inflammatory and autoimmune diseases of the CNS (e.g. MS)
Lumbar	15-50 mg/dL	Most common method; needle placed in the subarachnoid space of the spinal column
Cisternal	15-25 mg/dL	Needle placed below the occipital bone; done with fluoroscopy
Ventricular	6-15 mg/dL	Rarely done; recommended in people with possible brain herniation

7. ARTERIAL BLOOD GASES

Test	Conventional Units	SI Units/Notes
pH	7.35-7.45	Critical: <7.25, >7.55
HCO_3^-	22–28 meq/L	Critical: <15, >40
pCO_2	35–45 mmHg	Critical: <20, >60
pO_2	80-100 mmHg	Critical: <40
SaO_2	95-100%	Critical: ≤75%

8. ASCITIC FLUID

Condition	Gross Appearance	Protein, g/L	Cell Count		Other Tests/Notes
			Red Blood Cells, 10,000/μL	White Blood Cells /μL	
Transudates	Serum albumin: ascites albumin difference >11 g/L				
Cirrhosis	Straw-colored or bile-stained	<25 (95%)	1%	<250 (90%); predominantly mesothelial	Hepatic sinusoids have been damaged
CHF	Straw-colored	Variable, 15-53	10%	<1000 (90%); usually mesothelial, mononuclear	Hepatic sinusoids are normal, which allows passage of protein into the ascitic fluid
Exudates	Serum albumin: ascites albumin difference <11 g/L				
Neoplasm	Straw-colored, hemorrhagic, mucinous, or chylous*	>25 (75%)	20%	>1000 (50%); variable cell types	Cytology, cell block, peritoneal biopsy
Tuberculous Peritonitis	Clear, turbid, hemorrhagic, chylous	>25 (50%)	7%	>1000 (70%); usually >70% lymphocytes	Peritoneal biopsy, stain and culture for acid fast bacilli
Pyogenic Peritonitis	Turbid or purulent	If purulent, >25	Unusual	Predominantly neutrophils	Positive Gram stain, culture
Nephrosis	Straw-colored or chylous	<25 (100%)	Unusual	<250; mesothelial, mononuclear	If chylous, ether extraction, Sudan staining
Pancreatic Ascites (pancreatitis, pseudocyst)	Turbid, hemorrhagic, or chylous	Variable, often >25	Variable, may be blood-stained	Variable	Increased amylase in ascitic fluid and serum

*chylous: milk-colored

9. PLEURAL FLUID

Condition	Gross Appearance	pH	Glucose mM	Amylase PF:Serum	Cell Count	
					Red Blood Cells ($1000/mm^3$)	White Blood Cells ($1000/mm^3$)
Transudates	Light's criteria: pleural fluid/serum protein <0.5 OR pleural fluid/serum LDH <0.6 OR pleural fluid LDH <2/3 upper normal serum limit					
CHF	Clear, straw-colored	>7.4	>3.3	≤1	0-1	<1 predominantly mononuclear
Cirrhosis	Clear, straw-colored	>7.4	>3.3	≤1	<1	<0.5 predominantly mononuclear
Pulmonary Embolus: Atelectasis	Clear, straw-colored	>7.3	>3.3	≤1	<5	5-15 predominantly mononuclear
Exudates	Light's criteria: pleural fluid/serum protein >0.5 OR pleural fluid/serum LDH >0.6 OR pleural fluid LDH >2/3 upper normal serum limit					
Pulmonary Embolus: Infarction	Turbid to hemorrhagic, small volume	>7.3	>3.3	≤1	Bloody in 1/3 to 2/3 of patients	5-15 predominantly neutrophils; may show many mesothelial cells
		≥7.3	>3.3	≤1	<5	5-40 predominantly neutrophils
Pneumonia	Turbid	5.50-7.29	<3.3	≤1	<5	25-100 predominantly neutrophils
Empyema	Turbid or purulent					
		<7.3 (20%)	1.7-3.3 (20%)	≤1	>10	5-10 predominantly mononuclear
TB	Straw-colored; serosanguinous in 15%	<7.3 (30%)	<3.3 (30%)	≤1	1 to >100	<10 predominantly neutrophils
Malignancy	Straw-colored to turbid to bloody	<7.3; usually ~7.0	<1.7 (95%)	≤1	<1	1-20 neutrophils in acute; mononuclear in chronic
RA Effusion	Turbid or green or yellow	<7.3 (30%)	<3.3 (30%)	>2		Neutrophils in acute; mononuclear in chronic
SLE	Straw-colored to turbid	6.0	N or D	Salivary type		Predominantly neutrophils
Rupture of Esophagus	Purulent	>7.3	>3.3	>2	1-10	5-20 predominantly neutrophils
Pancreatitis	Serous to turbid to serosanguinous					

REFERENCES

1. Longo DL, Fauci AS, Kasper DL, Hauser SL, Jameson JL, Loscalzo J (Editors). *Harrison's Online*, 18th ed. New York: McGraw-Hill; 2012.
2. Porter RS (Editor). *The Merck Manual of Diagnosis and Therapy*, 19th ed. Whitehouse Station: Merck Research Laboratories; 2011.
3. Pagana KD, Pagana TJ. *Mosby's Manual of Diagnostic and Laboratory* Tests, 4th ed. St. Louis: Mosby; 2010.

Index

Note: Page numbers followed by *f* and *t* indicate figures and tables, respectively. Boxed materials are indicated by *b*.

INDEX

B

INDEX

C

INDEX

D

INDEX

E

F

G

INDEX

H

INDEX

I

J

K

L

INDEX

M

N

INDEX

INDEX

INDEX

Q

R

S

INDEX

INDEX

T

INDEX

U

V

INDEX

W

X

Y